CLASSICS AND OTHER SELECTED READINGS IN MEDICAL LIBRARIANSHIP

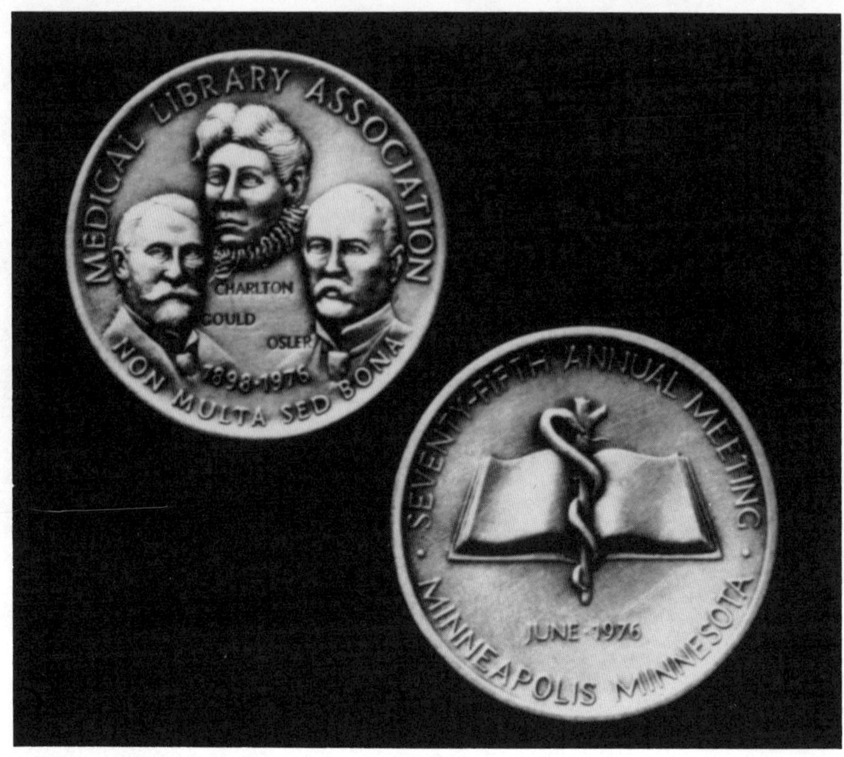

MEDICAL LIBRARY ASSOCIATION COMMEMORATIVE MEDAL, 1898-1976

Margaret Charlton, Dr. George Milbry Gould, and Sir William Osler were the creators of the Medical Library Association—an association dedicated to a cause—and were energetic contributors to growth and development of the medical librarian profession. The aphorism in Latin which reads *Non multa sed bona* translates to *Not many but good.*

One might enjoy "a quickening of the homiletic pulse" on reflecting on the history of the Medical Library Association and the appropriateness of this aphorism as a tribute to all who are or have been builders of a very special organization—relatively few in numbers, but excellent[1].

1. Key JD: The Medical Library Association Commemorative Medal, 1898-1976. Bull Med. Libr. Assoc. 64:45-47, 1976

CLASSICS AND OTHER SELECTED READINGS IN MEDICAL LIBRARIANSHIP

---

edited by

Jack D. Key, M.A., M.S.
Librarian, Mayo Clinic Library
and
Thomas E. Keys, M.A., Sc.D. (h.c.)
Librarian Emeritus,
Mayo Clinic Library

Robert E. Krieger Publishing Company
Huntington, New York • 1980

Original edition 1980

Printed and Published by
ROBERT E. KRIEGER PUBLISHING CO., INC.
P.O. Box 542
Huntington, NY 11743

Printed in the United States of America

Library of Congress Cataloging in Publication Data
Main entry under title:

Classics and other selected readings in medical librarianship.

Bibliography: p.
Includes index.
1. Medical libraries—Addresses, essays, lectures. I. Key, Jack D. II. Keys, Thomas Edward, 1908-
[DNLM: 1. Library science—Collected works. 2. Libraries, Medical—Collected works. Z657.M4 K42c]
Z657.M4S43 026'.61 78-9040
ISBN 0-88275-691-5

DEDICATION

All libraries should have friends. "Have friends," said Baltasar Gracian[1] in 1653. "It is a second life. Every friend is something good, and something wise to his friend: and between them everything comes off well. . . ."

With that quotation in mind, we dedicate this volume to Dr. Waltman Walters, Emeritus Surgeon of the Mayo Clinic, and to his charming wife, Phoebe Mayo Walters, as representative of the best of library friends.

Jack D. Key and Thomas E. Keys

1. Baltasar Gracian's A Truthtelling Manual and the Art of Worldly Wisdom. (Translated from a 1653 Spanish text by M Fischer) Second edition. Springfield, Illinois, Charles C Thomas, Publisher, 1945, p. 106

CONTENTS

"There is a marvelous piece where Galileo cries bitterly about how awful it is that there are no longer any 'classics'—you have to read books by people who are actually alive. We have been increasing the pace ever since, and it is this that gave birth to the scientific paper in the mid-17th century and to the abstract and bibliographic mechanism in the 18th century."[1]

We have, in this observation by Price, an historical perspective on the foundations of health sciences librarianship. It is based upon growth of the scientific endeavor and the provision of services, which in turn are affected by broader conditions of societal priorities, demographic changes, technological innovations, and economic conditions. As early as 1881, John Shaw Billings observed the steadily increasing production of medical books and warned of conditions to be expected a century hence[2]. The greatest rate of growth, however, occurred during a brief period after the Second World War (1953-1965), when federal support for science grew at a rate of nearly 20 percent each year.[3]

Health sciences librarianship is concerned with biomedical communication which encompasses the subsystems of generation, publication, correlation, retrieval, and dissemination of information. In *Classics and Other Selected Readings for Medical Librarians,* Jack Key and Thomas Keys have provided, through a choice of excellent papers, an overview of this specialty as it has responded to challenges in an era of great change. The papers, therefore, reflect a deep concern for the evolution of functions of the medical library and for the skills needed to support them. The new technology demanded specialized training, leading to a questioning of the identity of the health sciences librarian and to investigation of types of basic preparation and continuing education. The library was viewed as a complex organization, and norms were sought for resources, staffing, expenditures, and other relevant variables. In a world of shrinking resources and space, there was a concern for the ecology of health sciences libraries in the United States and for the development of various forms of networking and cooperation. It all added up to a different gestalt.

To cover developments from the use of handwritten cards in bibliographic control through direct, on-line access to computerized data bases is a formidable task. The editors have done a great service in bringing together those works which most effectively enlighten areas of a large landscape, so that we may stand back and see them more clearly over the perspective of time.

Susan Crawford, Ph.D.

REFERENCES

1. Price, D. "Invisible College Research: State of the Art" in Crawford, S., ed. Informal Communication Among Scientists: Proceedings of a Conference on Current Research. Chicago, American Medical Association, 1971. p. 27.
2. Rogers, F.B. Selected papers of John Shaw Billings, Chicago, Medical Library Association, 1965. p. 128.
3. Wolfle, D. The support of science in the United States. Sci. Am. 213:19, July 1965.

PREFACE

A book is the most varied product in the world. Its physical aspects are secondary to the range of thoughts and images it attempts to transfer to the mind of the reader. In this respect, a book is like a piece of rope; it takes on meaning only in connection with the things it holds together. What is carried by the book is nothing less than the life of the mind.[1]

The literature of medical librarianship today represents an accretive culmination of advances. This volume is intended to offer practicing medical librarians, library school students, and physicians interested in libraries a handy and concise anthology of some of the significant writings of the men and women who established the foundations for subsequent progress. Among the excellent papers, past and present, are several by physicians, like Osler and Billings, that relate to librarianship.

Representative writings of persons who have influenced medical librarianship are brought together to provide the reader ready access to these important works. Having them together in one volume for the first time should have appeal for both student and seasoned librarian. Brief biographies of the authors are included in the last chapter.

A close friend, Dr. James Eckman, retired Mayo Clinic medical editor and assistant professor of the history of medicine, authority on typography, insatiable traveler, and amused observer of his fellowman, wrote in the July 4, 1976, special issue of *The Mayo Alumnus:*

Mavericks are not evil gnomes. They simply arrive at objectives, usually desirable and sometimes even laudable, by inexplicable or mystic or tortuous means which their associates may erroneously regard as satanic or, at best, demented. A maverick of any standing knows instinctively that to achieve the shortest journey from Rochester to New York it makes sense to go by way of Bozeman, Montana, or Cape Girardeau, Missouri. To obtain orchids he plants peascods.

We hope that some of the flavor of the mavericks of our profession is reflected in what has been included.

Selections are based on work or personalities that appealed to us. Obviously, some may have more appeal to us than to others; also, we have probably omitted some that should have been included. In any case, we expect that every reader will find something satisfying and that collectively our book has value for the medical librarian.

1. Cousins N: Editor's odyssey: gleanings from articles and editorials by N.C. Saturday Review, vol. 5, no. 14, April 15, 1978, p. 11

ACKNOWLEDGMENTS

We are indebted to our Mayo Medical Library colleagues for their interest, support, and cooperation. We extend special thanks to Mary J. Knapp and Jean M. McDowall, our secretaries, for their patience; to Samuel Sohnen for his encouragement; to all the authors and publishers who allowed us to reprint from their publications; and to all others who have contributed to the literature of medical librarianship for making this endeavor such a pleasant experience.

All material from the *Bulletin of the Medical Library Association* is reprinted with the permission of the Medical Library Association.

Jack D. Key
Thomas E. Keys

I
JANET DOE LECTURES

Introduction

We are privileged to present in this chapter the *bibliotheca prima* of medical librarianship. The Janet Doe Lectureship, initiated in 1967, was named for a medical librarian who illustrated the best in professional medical librarianship and who also was a fine medical historian. Janet Doe, former librarian of the New York Academy of Medicine, is a past president of the Medical Library Association, editor of the first edition and coeditor of the second edition of the *Handbook of Medical Library Practice.* To be chosen a Janet Doe Lecturer is one of the highest honors that our profession bestows on one of its members.

Gertrude Annan, the first lecturer, reviews significant achievements and history of the Medical Library Association. Dr. F. B. Rogers considers medical subject cataloging and the importance of Medical Subject Headings (MeSH). Scott Adams celebrates the achievements of Dr. Rogers and the successful concept of the Medical Literature Analysis and Retrieval System (MEDLARS). Dr. Estelle Brodman defines and stresses pursuit of excellence and then considers applications of that concept to problems facing medical librarianship. Alfred Brandon reports on faculty status for librarians. Louise Darling examines the Medical Library Association's certification plan and its future implications. Jacqueline Felter stresses the importance of cooperation among libraries and worries about whether it will continue. Harold Bloomquist appraises the fads and fashions of management as they may relate to medical librarianship. David Bishop considers the use of diversity as a democratic approach to librarianship. Finally, Erich Meyerhoff examines the shift from historical inquiry to the scientific inquiry that in so many ways constitutes today's medical librarianship.

The Medical Library Association in Retrospect, 1937—1967*

By Gertrude L. Annan, *Librarian*

New York Academy of Medicine
New York, New York

ABSTRACT

The medical librarian of 1967 lives in a period of changing concepts, dramatic new methods, everwidening scientific horizons. In looking toward the immediate past he may think of the medical librarian of thirty years ago as a complacent follower of accepted procedures, not as a pioneer in a brave new world. Yet the corps of trained medical librarians today and the resources of our collections and their management are dependent upon the efforts of those who were then pioneers in medical librarianship. Training, standards, recruitment, literature control, international relations, all had continuing attention at a time when financial assistance through government funds, support by administrators, concern by scientists was almost nonexistent. In these years the day of the devoted amateur passed; the trained medical librarian came into being and matured.

This, the first Janet Doe Lecture, is named for one who illustrates the best in medical librarianship, serving with scholarly distinction. It is a brief survey pointing to some of the Association's significant achievements during the years of Miss Doe's greatest activity when she and her colleagues met their "Challenge of Change."

THE medical librarian of 1967 lives in a period of changing concepts, dramatic new methods, everwidening scientific horizons. To meet these challenges he must welcome the future with patient flexibility and ready enthusiasm. He is aware that no generation of librarians has seen such a swift transformation of techniques and that no generation has seen such a rapid expansion of scientific knowledge. In looking toward the immediate past he may think of the medical librarian of thirty years ago as a complacent follower of accepted procedures, not as a pioneer in a brave new world. Yet the corps of trained medical librarians today and the

*The first Janet Doe Lecture. Presented at the Sixty-sixth Annual Meeting of the Medical Library Association, Miami Beach, Florida, June 13, 1967.

Originally published in *Bulletin of the Medical Library Association,* Volume 55 (October, 1967), pp. 379-389. Reprinted by permission.

resources of our collections and their management are dependent upon the efforts of those who were then pioneers in medical librarianship. Training, standards, recruitment, literature control, international relations, all had continuing attention at a time when financial assistance through government funds, support by administrators, concern by scientists was almost nonexistent. Everyone using or administering medical libraries today is in their debt.

In 1937 the annual meeting was held in Richmond, Virginia, with Dr. William W. Francis of the Osler Library presiding. He was not the last on the list of physician presidents, but he served at a time when administration of the Association was becoming almost entirely in the hands of practicing librarians. Of the eighty-eight delegates representing seventy-two libraries at Richmond, only four were physicians and two dentists. Of the four physicians, one was President, one Vice President. Dr. Francis' presidential address was entitled, "At Osler's Shrine," and the formal program reflected the preoccupation with history which would continue to be evident for some years to come. The business of the Association, however, touched upon subjects and problems familiar to us today, and this small group attacked matters of significance.

As in 1967, so thirty years ago medical librarians looked to Washington, looked to an institution that had recently celebrated its centenary, the Army Medical Library. Appeals for funds were made by the Association, but these appeals were not for assisting libraries throughout the country; rather, they were for the support and maintenance of that great library itself. A depression coming in a period between two wars meant little interest in a military facility, and funds were cut drastically in 1933. Fluctuations of foreign currency further reduced the buying power to serious inadequacy. The Executive Committee of the Association reported in 1937 that, in response to action taken at a previous meeting, resolutions[1] were distributed "recommending the appropriation of adequate funds for the maintenance and growth of the Army Medical Library's Book Collection and Index Catalogue" and "requesting . . . appropriations sufficient to construct a building adequate for the purpose and . . . funds for its maintenance." These were sent to the President of the United States and to the Secretary of War and brought replies which were read at the meeting. The Secretary's report adds that "The matter was also brought before our own members, with the request that each one urge his organization to adopt similar resolutions to be sent to their local congressmen, asking their support of this measure. The same action was sought from national and state medical societies, and a further appeal was made to the medical profession in general to urge congressional support. . . . Altogether over 500 individuals, organizations and publications were approached." The report points out that, "Even if we do not accomplish our immediate purpose, we have done something toward awakening a consciousness of the great worth of the Army Medical Library and its *Index-Catalogue*." It is signed by the Association's Secretary, Janet Doe.

Response to appeals for sustaining the library was generous. The following year Colonel Jones as Librarian could announce in his Annual Report for 1937/8[2].

> The past year was noteworthy in the history of the Army Medical Library in that the Congress authorized the construction of a new Library and Museum Building, the legislation being approved by the President June 15, 1938. The whole-hearted support of the medical public and of numerous individuals, bodies, and institutions of learning...was a splendid tribute to the good service the Library and Museum have rendered through so many years. There were 4,104 bound volumes added . . . of which 2,292 were purchased. . . . The Library was fortunate in having the liberal appropriation of $24,500 for the purchase of books, journals, and equipment. . . . The Library receives more than 1,800 periodicals. . . . The Library loaned 14,102 items . . . more than 8 per cent over 2 years ago.

In the same report Colonel Jones told of a new service: "The Library is now prepared to assist in furnishing microfilms through the American Documentation Institute, in any quantity desired....A modern camera has been installed." These were heartening words, but several years followed with little progress noted. The Report of 1941[3] announces that the site for the new building has been selected and approved by the National Parks Planning Commission. "Nothing remains but to supply some of the funds. It is a race against time."

Although the new building was still years away, 1942 may be considered as the date of the beginning of a National Library of Medicine. In that year for the first time a trained librarian was appointed to the staff. Happily, the librarian was one of force as well as capability, for Helen Norris (later Mrs. Lucké) was not one to accept conditions as they were. She writes[4],

> I was the only library-trained person on the staff when I went there on the first of October in 1942—the first one the Library had ever had, I believe. What an appalling place it was. I asked for and received permission from Col. Jones to visit other libraries in Washington and vicinity. In New York, Dr. [Archibald] Malloch was most cordial; while I was in his office he telephoned Dr. [Alan] Gregg and announced that at last there was someone at the AML who was interested in doing something constructive. . . . On my return to Washington, I proposed to Colonel Jones that a survey of the AML be made by professional librarians, and that it be financed by the Rockefeller or Carnegie Foundation. Just the idea he had been looking for, so he said. Whereupon steps were taken to get the survey under way.

The stage was set. Colonel Jones on March 4, 1943, wrote the Executive Secretary of the American Library Association stating the approval of the War Department for a survey of the Library. Funds were made available by the Rockefeller Foundation, and a panel of distinguished librarians appointed—Keyes D. Metcalf, then Director of the Harvard University Library; L. Quincy Mumford, now Librarian of Congress; Andrew Osborn, at that time Assistant Librarian at Harvard; and three medical librarians, Janet Doe, Thomas P. Fleming, and Mary Louise Marshall. A report, but not the detailed findings, was published in 1944[5]. Those of you who know the National Library of Medicine only in its handsome building with a highly trained staff, electronic equipment, and expanding activities in scientific communication, can hardly conceive of the Army Medical Library so short a time ago. The conditions in the old building and its inadequacies have been described with appropriate humor, and need not be repeated. A few statements from the survey comparing that Library with the New York Academy of Medicine Library illuminate the situation. The Army Medical Library had twice the number of volumes, but maintained only four-fifths as many current subscriptions with a book budget 95 percent of the Academy's. There was one-tenth the number of readers, the same outside circulation, but, even then, considerably more activity in photoduplication. Of its reference services the report comments,

> In the matter of answering inquiries . . . all that can be said is that the Army Medical Library's reputation, among other libraries and those individuals whose opinions were asked, has not been good in this respect. So little satisfaction has been obtained that most inquirers turned elsewhere for help. This condition is rapidly changing, however, with the advent of trained library assistants in the Army Medical Library.

An analysis of the collection itself showed that "the situation with regard to periodical holdings is all too often deplorable;" that the acquisition of monographic material was by no means comprehensive; of international congresses and government documents, incomplete and by no means outstanding; and of publications relating to allied medical sciences, particularly weak. The detailed findings and recommendations may be found in transcripts of the report. A brief summary of essential needs are cited in the letter of transmittal, as follows: The constant improvement of the quality of the staff; the establishment of an emergency shelflist; a vigorous acquisitions program; the development of a classification scheme; adoption of a standard list of subject headings; a new card catalog; a ten-year rebinding program; and modification of the building plans. Janet Doe has summarized the findings and recommendations in her article, "The Survey and After." This and Mary Louise Marshall's "Reminiscences" are in the BULLETIN's special number, an anniversary issue[6], celebrating 125 years of the Library. This, then was the start of a new era for the old Library which soon would be transformed. Medical librarians would once more turn to Washington for assistance. In 1937, though, the idea of the Army Medical Library as a training ground for medical librarians would have been considered ludicrous; its present role in that respect was undreamed of. The training of medical librarians was such a novelty in 1937 that Isabelle T. Anderson reported on a new venture in Minnesota, commenting that

> There has never been a course in Hospital Librarianship or Medical Librarianship anywhere in the world. That statement may be challenged, but we haven't heard of any.... This last year Mr. Walter, the Librarian of the University of Minnesota, and Miss Perrie Jones, who was formerly Institution Librarian of the Minnesota Board of Control ... organized a course in Hospital Librarianship in connection with the University of Minnesota Library School. ... It is mainly a lecture course, although a six weeks' internship in an approved hospital has been arranged for. The lectures include selection of books for patients, and medical reference, as well as hospital and medical library administration....There have been eleven girls registered this year...[7].

Miss Anderson writes[8] that Miss Jones urged Mr. Walter that a course for potential hospital librarians should be part of the library school curriculum. "As a result, a one-quarter course was offered, which included lectures on medical library practices, given by several librarians and doctors from the Twin City area. As I remember, there were lectures on medical reference books, on book selection, and ordering, on medical history, on medical periodicals. ... Helen Norris and later Frida Pliefke participated." A young man named Thomas P. Fleming gave lectures on acquisitions and tells us, "with the exception of Norris and some of Anderson, the whole program was pointed toward the operation of a patients' library....Of course, the lectures by physicians on medical terminology and history of medicine were valuable in theory..."[9]. This pioneering venture was considered successful enough in its aim to provide graduates "doing excellent work in hospital, medical, institutional, and public libraries engaged in hospital library work."[10]. Mr. Fleming, then a member of the faculty of the University of Minnesota Library School, was soon to accept the position of Medical Librarian of Columbia University, New York, where he would carry to maturity those early efforts for training medical librarians in Minnesota. He wasted little time, and an announcement appeared in the BULLETIN that he would give a course on "Bibliographic and Reference Service in the Medical Sciences," in the 1939 Summer Session of the School of Library Service at Columbia. In 1948 the course was given at the same school by Estelle Brodman and was designed for the first time to cover all phases of medical library work. In 1951 a second approved course was taught by Mildred Jordan at Emory University.

These lecture courses were not supplemented by internships as were those in Minnesota. Mr. Walter had shown enthusiasm for this type of training and wrote: "One of the most practical features of the entire course is the six-weeks internship which follows the close of the classwork in June. Each student is assigned to one or more hospitals where she devotes her entire time to library work under the direction of the hospital librarian"[11]. A more extensive experiment, a year long "residency in medical library work," was inaugurated in October 1940 by Mary Louise Marshall in the libraries of the Orleans Parish Medical Society and Tulane School of Medicine. "The period of training was set at twelve months, with a two weeks' vacation, corresponding to that of a medical internship. . . . A stipend to cover board and room only has been paid. . . . The interns have worked as members of the staff under close personal direction, and have had a part in all phases of the libraries' work. Every effort has been made to explain not only methods used in our libraries, but in comparison with those used in other medical libraries"[12]. In this, her presidential address in 1946, she also cited a Program of Instruction in Library Schools, 1943[13], which advocated a year of internship after library school. She added that this would be "particularly advantageous in training for the special field of medicine in library work, since it furnishes opportunity for the student to learn the subject field, the nomenclature, the bibliography and the varying values of the different phases of medical library work. . . ."

Miss Marshall's address is a landmark in the history of medical librarianship. It was made at a time when the Association was ready and eager for action. It provoked at once animated and thoughtful discussion of varying efforts in library training and the urgent need of defining standards. William D. Postell moved that a committee be appointed to recommend the adoption of standards and a training program for medical librarianship. It was passed unanimously. There were, however, stormy years ahead. The most controversial was the program of certification. It was adopted, not without heated disagreement, at the Annual Meeting in April 1949 at Galveston, Texas. The presidential address by Janet Doe again was devoted to education. She commented, "Education for medical librarianship is at present in a healthy state of flux. A candidate taking the full library schedule of three semesters at the Columbia school, with the medical course included, will receive an M.S. degree. When there are enough applicants to justify additional facilities we hope that one or two other library schools in different sections of the country will inaugurate a medical course"[14]. It is interesting to note that since that time courses have now been given throughout the country, at Catholic University, Washington, D.C., Drexel in Philadelphia, Emory at Atlanta, at the Universities of California, Illinois, Maryland, Michigan, North Carolina, Pittsburgh, Southern California, Toronto, and Western Reserve.

The story is quickly told, but in its telling there is no way of indicating the enormous contributions of many members of this Association. Each of the courses requires monitoring, and this must be repeated every fifth year to make sure the quality and content are maintained so that Association approval can be granted. Committees on Standards, Curriculum, and Certification have been actively concerned. The Booklet of Information on Certification gives a brief history of its development and cites the code in detail. Under the separate items, number five should be read with care. Here are stipulated the types of certification, Grades 1, 2, and 3. Changes have been made over the years to meet new requirements, and each change has meant as much deliberation, discussion, soul searching, and argument as the first induced.

New trends in education have been watched and evaluated. In 1958 at the meeting in Rochester, Minnesota, the President, Thomas E. Keys, instituted a day of refresher courses on practical library procedures. The twelve brief lectures[15] were each given twice, enabling those so wishing to enroll for four. A total of 290 registered. Each year since that time, except for that of the International Congress, a day of the Annual Meeting has been reserved for this program, carried out since 1963 under the auspices of the Committee on Continuing Education. Here, again, responsive to changing needs, small, informal beginnings have developed into a "curriculum planned for cyclic presentation with advanced courses building on the foundations laid by previous ones"[16]. A recent offshoot of this national program has made the series of courses available regionally so that those unable to attend the Annual Meeting would have the opportunity of participation. Some have been coordinated with the national program, and all have been sponsored by regional groups of the Association.

The formation of regional groups was stimulated by the need of medical librarians to hold meetings during the war years when national meetings were omitted. In 1947 at the Annual Meeting in Cleveland, a preconvention session tackled the problem of "Regional Meetings for the Medical Library Association." Mildred Jordan reported that "letters requesting a reaction to this controversial subject were sent to administrative heads of 253 member libraries"[17]. Of those who replied 86 were for establishing groups, 22 against, and 49 uncommitted. Two years later Janet Doe wrote an editorial for the BULLETIN, "The New Venture: Regional Meetings"[18], telling that "the inclusion in the revised by-laws of the Medical Library Association of a section authorizing regional meetings marks the end of an old era. . . ." By that time local meetings had been held in New York, Chicago, and California. The vigorous growth of our regional groups, their effectiveness in bringing medical librarians from one locality together for educational, intellectual, and social purposes has not prevented the attendance of ever larger numbers of librarians at our annual meetings, as was feared in 1947; and some regional meetings today have a greater attendance than the 1947 meeting at which the subject was introduced.

The few librarians coming together in 1937, however, were not handicapped by the small size of the meeting, for they looked to wide horizons and were undaunted by the magnitude of problems needing solution. A Committee on Indexing Current Medical Literature, chaired by Eleanor Fair, reported on the results of a notice in the BULLETIN in 1936: "Wanted: a Clinical Abstract Journal"[19]. The Committee had made a study of the New York Academy of Medicine's journals to examine those carrying abstracts in English of articles appearing in foreign journals. There was not only the expected duplication in the 146 journals covered, but abstracts were so scattered that their usefulness was largely wasted. Responses to the notice varied; thirteen approvals, eight disapprovals. Questions were raised of cost and the desirability of first making sure that the duplication of abstracts would cease if a clinical abstract journal were published.

In the following year Eileen Cunningham came to the fore with a major contribution, "Problem of Abstract Publications in Medical and Allied Sciences"[20]. She began, "It has been evident for some time that there has been no effort to coordinate the abstracting services in clinical medicine and the clinical specialties. . . . At present, although a tremendous amount of money and time, as well as much sincere effort, often representing personal sacrifice on the part of editors and scientists, is being expended in the publication of abstracts of medical literature, the results fall far short of the reasonable goals that should be attained as to scope, cost, economic organization, promptness of issue, and elimination of duplication." A table listed thirty-one abstract journals with their 1936 prices. "The total cost," she said, "is the very considerable sum of $1,156.00," and she pointed out that only large and well-endowed libraries could afford some of the more expensive ones, which was "especially unfortunate because the value of an abstract journal is presumably greater in a small library, where large numbers of journals containing the original material are not available." The librarian of 1967 will be glad to learn that in 1936 *Biological Abstracts* was priced at $15 and *Chemcial Abstracts* at $12. Five of the German titles cost more than $100.

The chief difficulties were listed as expense, promptness, and elimination of duplication. The first recommendation was for a centralized bureau:

A rational, business-like approach to the problem would call for the establishment of an abstracting bureau which would be national, and perhaps international, in scope. This bureau might publish two major comprehensive abstractive journals, one in the biological sciences, which would include the so-called pre-clinical sciences, and one in the clinical sciences, including all specialties. It would be desirable to issue these publications with two sets of page numbering, those for complete volume numbering, and those for sections, and that subscriptions be made available to individuals for complete volumes and for sections and combinations of sections. . . . If it were found possible to make it international in scope, a French as well as English edition could be published.

Authors' abstracts were advocated, and editors should require them routinely. Overlapping of subjects might be avoided by publication of an abstract in full in but one journal or section, with cross references wherever needed. To finance this ambitious project a committee of librarians and scientists should work out a practical plan and submit it to foundations to try to get it funded for a five-year period when, presumably, it might become self-supporting. If this were impractical, a preliminary coordinating survey of all existing abstracting services would determine the exact amount of overlapping and the needs for further coverage made apparent.

Mrs. Cunningham, in November 1937, wrote to the editors of *Biological Abstracts* expressing dismay at the proposed schedule of service charges[21] and advising that the Committee on Periodical and Serial Publications regarded it as a dangerous and unfortunate move and proposed instead a flat subscription rate of $25 to $30 for libraries. Later it was reported that beginning with vol. 13, 1939, the subscription price for the complete volume with indexes was fixed at $25.

These were the early efforts in a long struggle. They deserve a separate paper, and the reader interested in a subject still of relevance in 1967 has only to look in the cumulated index of the first forty volumes of the BULLETIN. The entries indicate the story—Committee on Abstracting and Indexing; Committee on Coordinated Abstracting Service for Clinical Medicine; Joint Committee on Indexing and Abstracting Services; UNESCO Conference on Co-ordination of Medical Abstracting Services; UNESCO Conferences on Scientific Abstracting. These and other reports give convincing evidence of long, hard work and distinguished contributions. Perhaps the climax came at the annual meeting in Philadelphia in 1948 under New Business:

Resolved: that the Medical Library Association express to the directors of *Excerpta Medica* thanks and appreciation for their generous and genuine cooperation in endeavoring to meet the desires of medical librarians by providing a comprehensive abstract journal for medicine at reduced cost. We realize the great difficulties with which you have had to contend, and we do not mean to seem impatient. You have done remarkably well to have accomplished so much in so short a time. We look forward to the increased usefulness of *Excerpta Medica* through further lowered costs and expanded coverage as time and additional recognition and support makes these possible[22].

A report made at the same meeting by Mrs. Cunningham summarized progress and announced that "the steps taken by *Excerpta Medica* to become a non-profit organization under Dutch law were . . . practically complete. . . . The granting of a special discount price of $250.00 from the usual list price of $342.50 to libraries in the United States subscribing to all the sections was announced. This offer is particularly generous because the full quota of 200 subscriptions originally required to obtain this discount was not reached." Expanded coverage we have today in its twenty-five sections and two more promised; but lowered costs are an idle dream. In 1967 as we meekly accept spiraling prices, often with a burdensome higher pricing for libraries. Mrs. Cunningham's persistence seems tilting at windmills. Before the war she had been active and effective in fighting the high cost of German periodicals. After the war she continued and, with Wesley Draper, prepared a study whose findings compared subscription rates of 1939 with those of 1946. She was interested in all aspects of the literature, and a brief paper of 1936 can be read today with profit, "Looking Forward: Possible Developments in the Publication of Medical Literature." Among her conclusions are that a reduction in the total number of medical journals is desirable; the elimination of serials containing reprinted material would be advisable; as well as an awareness of new developments in photographic reproduction of literature. She ended, "No one can foresee the nature of the mature development of this literature and its publication. . . . The problem is a very serious one; it challenges the best mental efforts that those concerned have to offer; its solution will require the utmost of intellectual co-operation and endeavor"[23].

At the Association's meeting in Boston in 1938 a Symposium on Medical Literature[24] was conducted by Herman H. Henkle, then Director of the School of Library Science at Simmons College. He mentioned the need for a guide to medical literature and cited Mrs. Cunningham's paper on "Reference Works in Medicine" included in the symposium. It stressed the importance of having a comprehensive outline of medical reference works and listed about 200 reference books and review journals, and was surely the forerunner of her chapter and bibliography in the first edition of the *Handbook* in 1943. In the same symposium Mr. Henkle provided a thoughtful analysis of the periodical literature of biochemistry. He wrote, "The evaluation of printed materials is a matter of primary importance to librarians. . . This is especially true in respect to the periodical literature in the sciences. Attempts have been made with moderate success to apply objective methods of evaluation. In 1927 Gross and Gross set a pattern for the evaluation of chemical periodicals. . . ."

He concludes,

> The results of . . . such studies seem to make a definite contribution to the problem of selecting periodicals for the library; but also implicit in them is information of value in library administration. The objective data concerning the degrees of concentration and dispersion of the literature of particular subjects and the reflection in scientific literature of the interdependence of the sciences may prove especially useful in the determination of policies for the organization of subject departments and departmental libraries or for bringing together those already established.

Soon came the war years, and concern for the literature was limited chiefly to efforts to assist devastated libraries abroad and to acquire foreign publications for libraries here. With the war's end, attention once again turned to the problems of bibliographical control. In 1947 a Symposium on Medical Subject Headings was held at the Army Medical Library. Dr. Sanford Larkey said, "The bibliographical control of published materials has always been one of the major problems of librarians, and it is particularly vital and difficult in the scientific field. The difficulty was early realized by John Shaw Billings. . . .The increasing complexity of scientific literature has required elaborate and often very expensive means for dealing with it"[25]. Dr. Larkey stressed the serious problems consequent to expanded war research programs and predicted that the future peacetime programs would present similar questions, with the government's increased financial support for medical research. Well worth repeating today are some of his statements of 1949 in his announcement of The Army Medical Library Research Project at the Welch Medical Library:

> This problem of bibliographical control of the results of research is as serious in medicine as it is in the other fields of science. It is becoming increasingly difficult for our indexes and abstract journals to keep up with the growing number of medical publications and with articles of medical importance in other scientific journals. These difficulties will become greater in the future as more and more money is spent on research, and particularly if there is not commensurate support for our bibliographical facilities and for our scientific libraries. It is not necessary to convince this group, the Honorary Consultants to the Army Medical Library, of the importance of medical libraries and of our bibliographical research tools. But there does not seem to be enough general recognition of the vital significance to research of libraries and bibliographical facilities. One is dismayed to see that there is little if any provision made for them in the Report of the President's Scientific Research Board or in the plans for a National Science Foundation. . . .

Dr. Larkey reported that the Army Medical Library had asked the Welch Library to consider setting up a research project under contract with the

Army. Three aspects were determined upon: evaluation and study of the current indexes; a detailed study of subject headings; and a study of the possibility of using machine methods. He said, "The use of machine methods may appear somewhat Utopian, but one must look to the possibilities of the future. At present the machines are in a sense ahead of our ideas as to how they can be used and we must determine what we want them to do. Machines can probably be designed to do what we desire but it must be determined how well they do it and if it is worth doing, in terms of cost, in terms of the needs of medical research. . ."[26]

In 1951 a terminal report of the Research Project was prepared, and a new contract announced for continuing the study. Final reports in mimeographed form were ready in 1955. Those participating under Dr. Larkey's direction were a medical research bibliographer, Dr. Williamina A. Himwich, two medical librarians, Helen G. Field and John M. Whittock, and Eugene Garfield, whose later work in the field is widely known. One of the final reports related to subject headings and subject indexing; the other to machine methods for information searching. Advocating a large-scale machine information searching system, the report concluded: "We believe that, for any of these purposes, there are very definite possibilities in the machine methods developed by the Project, and by others, particularly with the expected future improvements in these machines or by the applications of the principles of these methods to other machines. Machine methods might have other applications in the field of medicine, such as the compilation of bibliographies on special subjects, the correlation and organization of basic factual information from many sources and for analyses of various forms of medical records." In a recent letter, Dr. Garfield makes the following evaluation:

> In my opinion, the work done at the Welch Medical Library Project is the foundation for most of the important work that has been done subsequently, particularly at the National Library of Medicine, and certainly a great deal of what has been done at the Institute for Scientific Information. Additionally, it had significant effects on other institutions, including *Chemical Abstracts* and *Biological Abstracts*.
>
> The most obvious and direct relationship that I can point to is the work of the Welch Medical Library Project and the existing MEDLARS system. Not only did we do the hard work on the MESH, which is still readily visible, including the system for categorization, but we also laid the foundation for the transition to the mechanized system and, of course, as you know, I, myself, was retained as a consultant in the second stage of the mechanization of the *Index Medicus*.
>
> It was at the Welch Medical Library that I first got the idea for citation indexing and if there were time and space, I could indicate any number of other benefits that derive from this project.

Estelle Brodman has called it "the first large-scale attempt to use the methods of experimental science in bibliographic problems; as such it can obviously be incomplete and inconclusive and still be the most important modern development in medical bibliography"[27].

This project had been initiated in 1948, just ten years after Colonel Jones announced that a microfilm camera was installed in the Army Medical Library. Our use of photocopy today is so essential a part of library practice that its comparatively recent advent is hard to realize. The BULLETIN in the forties reflected the interest in this new service. Mildred Walter, in "Practical Points on Microfilms," advocated its use for interlibrary loans. Thomas Keys in an editorial, January 1944, urged free microfilm copying in furtherance of research. The most prophetic words came from two librarians of the staff of Columbia University Library, Mary A. Bennett and D. H. Litchfield, who read a paper at the 1939 Annual Meeting in Newark, New Jersey, on "Problems of Microphotography"[28]. In response to a student request that the Photographic Department supply microfilms of manuscripts in a Spanish library, the authors wrote, "Perhaps this is not as ludicrous as it seems at first. Who knows but what some microphotographer will evolve a method of compensating for the curve in the earth's surface, so that a librarian in Spain will hold an open book at a west window while his colleague in New York will catch its image by means of a supertelescopic lens?"

We have not yet achieved such immediate communication with our colleagues abroad, but the Association's activities in the postwar period showed increasing awareness of the needs of foreign libraries. In 1947 a Committee on International and National Cooperation was proposed, stimulated by Mrs. Cunningham. One of its suggested purposes was to "assist in helping to bring medical librarians from other countries for study and work"[29]. Action was prompt. The Committee wrote to over sixty individuals connected with medical institutions abroad. "Twenty possible and eager applicants were discovered in this way. They represented ten countries: Bulgaria, Chile, China, Cuba, Hungary, India, Mexico, Sweden, Turkey, and Uruguay"[30]. Funds were made available by the Rockefeller Foundation. The Committee was chaired by Janet Doe, with Scott Adams, Eileen Cunningham, Sanford Larkey, and Mary Louise Marshall as members. Their work involved sending 270 member libraries questionnaires to determine what facilities could be offered for training and advanced study. Of these, fifty-one were willing to accept interns, and eleven would take them conditionally. The first successful candidate was Lydia Pazos, Assistant to the Librarian of the Medical School at the University of Havana. Twelve other applicants were under consideration.

The Committee modestly reported, "This is a time-consuming process, particularly for beginners like ourselves." In 1949 the Committee reported that two other scholarships were awarded and that the Rockefeller Foundation had renewed and increased their grant. The continuing success of this important project was due entirely to untiring efforts on the part of many librarians from coast to coast, whose functions as hosts went far beyond the training programs offered. The recent announcement of Mrs. Cunningham's generous bequest to the Association for training foreign medical librarians gives a touching reminder of her efforts in the past.

An evaluation of the first three years was included in her Committee report at the meeting in Denver, 1951[31]. A new program was also described. Funded, too, by the Rockefeller Foundation, it was a joint project with the U. S. Book Exchange for filling requests for foreign libraries. The material sent was either left over from Exchange lists or not wanted by member libraries. A total of 22,331 items were sent. The Association, with members in many countries, has ever been concerned with international activities relating to libraries and has participated in UNESCO and FID and IFLA. The high point came, of course, at the Second International Congress on Medical Librarianship in Washington in 1963, with Dr. Frank B. Rogers presiding, and with the new building he had done so much to attain available for inspection. Colonel Jones's race against time had taken twenty-one years.

These are some of the activities in which the Association has shown leadership. Some of its publications also led the way. The first edition of the *Handbook of Medical Library Practice*, with Janet Doe as editor, was surely a pioneering venture. It evolved from a primer prepared by Irene Jones from a card file compiled for her own use during her first years as a medical librarian. "Reference tools, various subject heading lists, catalogs, historical background texts, etc., in the medical and science subjects were an unknown field. Therefore, when or wherever I found something helpful in an article or book, or learned from someone, I made little file cards for future reference....I decided in 1936 to put it into written form with the idea it might possibly be of some help to others"[32]. This was generously turned over to a committee of the Association as a basis for a more comprehensive text that might "reflect the conclusions of many librarians instead of a single one." In 1939 the prospective *Handbook* was announced: "New libraries are constantly being organized; public librarians going into medical work wish to prepare themselves for their new field; library schools feel the want of a manual on this form of specialized library work; even seasoned medical librarians could benefit by a reliable guide in their professional problems. And yet no printed source for such information exists"[33]. A special committee was appointed to serve as authors covering the subjects: the medical library and librarian; book selection and ordering; cataloging; subject headings; classification; pamphlets and miscellaneous material; reference; rare books and the history of medicine. Miss Doe wrote in the introduction to the first edition, 1943, that half of the existing medical libraries had originated since 1910.

> To staff these libraries, workers have been enticed or commandeered from general and special libraries, from library schools, from the clerical staff of hospitals... from doctors' offices. Seldom, indeed, has it happened that a medical library could secure a librarian with both professional library training and education or experience in the medical sciences....An exceptionally definite need exists, therefore, for a means of liaison between the medical library and the sources from which it must draw its librarian. This *Handbook* attempts to fill that want.

The response was so favorable that by 1952 a fourth printing of about 1,000 copies was nearly exhausted, and plans for a revised edition were in progress, with Janet Doe and Mary Louise Marshall as editors. On its appearance in 1956, it was described in a review as "one of the most generally useful books on librarianship since the original publication of the old standby texts of Randall & Goodrich, Wilson & Tauber, Akers, Mann, and others of their kind"[34].

Another pioneering project was the inauguration of *Vital Notes on Medical Periodicals* in 1952. Mrs. Elizabeth F. Bready, then head of the Periodicals Department of the College of Physicians of Philadelphia, discussed with colleagues the time-consuming problems of establishing facts concerning the births and deaths and title changes of ever increasing numbers of journals. She suggested a continuing project and, together with Chizuru N. Boyea, of the New York Academy of Medicine Library staff, developed plans for cooperating medical librarians to pool all information of the kind. The chairman of the Association's Serials Committee, Harold Oatfield, and the President, William Postell, strongly backed the program, which was put into action by Lora Frances Davis. This important service has been well maintained by William Beatty and an alert Committee.

In 1954 a new series was inaugurated. Publication no. 1 was Estelle Brodman's contribution, *The Development of Medical Bibliography*. Slow to follow, no. 2 did not appear until Dr. Rogers' edition of the writings of John Shaw Billings in 1965.

The BULLETIN itself, though of exceptionally high quality, cannot be called a pioneering feat, but it has recorded the basis of this brief account, which is surely what Dr. Brodman recently well described as "a feat of ancestor worship, a glorification of the giants of the past," but it can serve also as a background for what she calls "a study of the culture and beliefs of the society it represents at a particular period of that society's development"[35]. In 1937 the Association was emerging from its first period, a period in which the bookish, scholarly physician dominated. The large libraries were chiefly collections made by practicing physicians and administered by medical societies. The contents of the BULLETIN for a decade continued to reflect these interests. Articles on the history of medicine appeared regularly. In January 1945, the editors announced that ninety-seven postcards had been received in response to their request for guidance in planning future issues. Of these, thirty-seven voted to continue the present policy of alternating historical and librarianship numbers; thirty-five wished each number to contain both in equal proportions; thirteen recommended less historical material; and two, less on librarianship. A frequent feature was the listing of current sale catalogs of antiquarian book dealers. The layman's needs were considered to the extent that a Committee was appointed to consider the compilation of a list of health works recommended for lay reading. In October 1938 two were published in the BULLETIN on diet and nutrition and on medical biography and history for the public. Four years later, the October issue included a bibliography of books by and about doctors, a layman's checklist for 1941. Occasionally a brief section of "Queries and Answers" brought forth questions on such varied themes as "The Handsome Men of Iowa" and "The Pearl of Allah." In contrast, there were but two historical articles in 1966 and no concern for the needs of laymen. Recent emphasis is on the demands of medical research and education and on the techniques of an electronic world, unthought of in 1937.

In these years the day of the devoted amateur passed, the trained medical librarian came into being and matured, and today we look to a future of information centers and networks manned by experts with varying skills. These changing trends and developments are clearly shown in the pages of the BULLETIN. Less obvious is their effect upon the Association's own role. Alfred N. Brandon's editorial in the January 1967 issue of the BULLETIN provides a clue. Commenting on "Continuing (or Discontinuing) Education," he writes that "it is necessary for the MLA to subsidize" that program. "Subsidize" is the important word, for the Association, ever increasing in size, and the programs developing from small voluntary efforts into highly specialized projects, has been faced with the necessity of providing funds. The operation of the Association's business became too unwieldy to be carried on solely by the voluntary work of members, and a Central Office came into being in 1961. Although the original aims of the Association still obtain, they are increasingly difficult to carry out without financial assistance. Federal support for training programs, surveys, statistical studies, are increasingly sought to further the obvious goals of the Association. A committee to outline future programs found no crystal ball. Happily, a glance at developments in past yeas indicates that members of the Association have been alert to point the way, and the uncertain future will surely bring the same response.

This, the first Janet Doe Lecture, is named for one who illustrates the best in medical librarianship, serving with scholarly distinction. It is a brief survey pointing to some of the Association's significant achievements during the years of Miss Doe's greatest activity, when she and her colleagues met their "Challenge of Change" with imagination, with argument, with hard work, and with persistence. Her own words, written in 1949, give evidence of the continuing collaboration which made their progress possible: "Libraries are born of mutual needs and mutual giving, and they continue to exist and grow largely through the same process. . . . Out of this have come not alone ever growing collections: these are but the outward and visible signs of a strong inward grace. Libraries have exemplified to an outstanding degree the inestimable value of generous and continuing assistance to one another"[36].

REFERENCES

1. Reports. Bulletin 26: 27-30, Oct. 1937.
2. U.S. Army War Department. Surgeon General's Office. Annual Report, 1938, p. 237-240.
3. *Ibid.*, 1941, p. 246-252.
4. Personal communication.
5. American Library Association. The National Medical Library; Report of a Survey of the Army Medical Library. Chicago, 1944.
6. Bulletin 49: 251-449, July 1961.
7. *Ibid.* 26: 25, Oct. 1937.
8. Personal communication.
9. Personal communication.
10. Walter, Frank K. Training for Librarianship at the University of Minnesota. . . . Minneapolis, University of Minnesota, 1942, p. 24-25.
11. Walter, Frank K. Training for hospital librarianship. Libr. J. 63: 579-583, Aug. 1938.
12. Marshall, M.L. Training for medical librarianship. Bulletin 34: 247-252, Oct. 1946.
13. metcalfe, k.d., and others. Program of Instruction In Library Schools. Urbana, University of Illinois Press, 1943.
14. Doe, Janet. The development of education for medical librarianship. Bulletin 37: 213-220, July 1949.
15. Abstracts of Refresher Courses to be Given May 31, 1958, *ibid.* 46: 122-132, Jan. 1958.
16. Continuing Education: Boston, 1966. *Ibid.* 53: 659-660, Oct. 1965.
17. Jordan, Mildred. Regional meetings for the Medical Library Association. *Ibid.* 35: 309-320, Oct. 1947.
18. Doe, Janet. The new venture: regionial meetings. Bulletin 38: 273-274, July 1950.
19. Wanted: a Clinical Abstract Journal. Bulletin 25: 146, Sept. 1936.
20. Cunningham, E. R. Problem of abstract publications in medical and allied sciences. Bulletin 26: 211-217, May 1938.
21. *Ibid.* 27: 63-65, Oct. 1938.
22. *Ibid.* 36: 391, Oct. 1948.

23. CUNNINGHAM, E. R. Looking forward. BULLETIN 25: 100-108, Sept. 1936.
24. A SYMPOSIUM ON MEDICAL LITERATURE. BULLETIN 27: 103-161, Dec. 1938.
25. LARKEY, S. V. Introduction to the problems of medical subject headings. BULLETIN 36: 70-81, Apr. 1948.
26. LARKEY, S. V. The Army Medical Library research project at the Welch Medical Library. BULLETIN 37: 121-124, Apr. 1949.
27. BRODMAN, ESTELLE. The Development of Medical Bibliography. Baltimore, Medical Library Association, 1954, p. 174.
28. BENNETT, M. A., AND LICHFIELD, D. H. Problems of microphotography. BULLETIN 28: 105-109, 114, Dec. 1939.
29. *Ibid.* 35: 274-275, July 1947.
30. *Ibid.* 36: 296-298, Oct. 1948.
31. CUNNINGHAM, E. R. Evaluation of a three-year program of international cooperation in medical librarianship. BULLETIN 39: 295-305, Oct. 1951.
32. Personal communication.
33. BULLETIN 28: 114, Dec. 1939.
34. Libr. J. 81: 1137-1138, May 1, 1956.
35. BRODMAN, ESTELLE. The special library, the mirror of its society. In: Marshall, J. D., ed. Approaches to Library History; Proceedings of the 2nd Library History Seminar. Tallahassee, Journal of Library History, 1966. 32 p.
36. DOE, JANET. Growth by gift. Academy Bookman 2: 5-9, Fall 1949.

Problems of Medical Subject Cataloging*

By Frank B. Rogers, M.D., *Librarian*

Denison Memorial Library
University of Colorado Medical Center
Denver, Colorado

ABSTRACT

The subject catalog of the University of Colorado Medical Center Library is examined in considerable detail. Annual revisions of the subject catalog required by annual revisions of the subject heading authority list used, NLM's *MeSH*, are analyzed in terms of man-hours required for the effort and the effect on the catalog's structure. It is contended that, in a divided catalog, changes of headings on a one-for-one equivalency basis are no more difficult than they would be in a computerized catalog, but that in many-for-one changes the manual catalog and the machine catalog face exactly the same dilemma and in the same magnitude, the only solution in either case being the reexamination of many entries. The proliferation of subheadings is shown to present particularly vexing problems in catalog revision. A plea is made to recognize the *MeSH* system for what it is, a legitimate compromise between the descriptor-oriented terms of a computer coordinate-indexing system, and the subject-heading-oriented terms of the conventional card catalog.

It is an honor to be asked to present the second annual Janet Doe Lecture. Janet Doe is a great figure in medical librarianship, a great contributor to the development of this field. I have had occasion in the past to seek her advice and help many times, and it was always given generously and wisely; there are many in this Association who would join me in that avowal.

Of Miss Doe's many interests, a special one is cataloging, and particularly subject cataloging. Our Association has not shown much interest in this area in late years, as if these problems were such that they could be left to others to solve for us. It is my hope that the emphasis on this subject in the program of the 1968 Annual Meeting of the Medical Library

*The second Janet Doe Lecture. Presented at the Sixty-seventh Annual Meeting of the Medical Library Association, Denver, Colorado, June 11, 1968.

Originally published in *Bulletin of the Medical Library Association*, Volume 56 (October, 1968), pp. 355-364. Reprinted by permission.

Association will serve to provoke a renewed interest in and attention to that technical area which, in my mind, more than any other tends to define and illuminate the special job and the special glory of the special librarian.

The charge given to the Janet Doe lecturer is that he speak on some historical or philosophical aspect of medical librarianship. My remarks may seem to fall short on this score, for what I have to say deals largely with description, in considerable detail, of an attack on an operational problem in a single library. I justify this by my feeling that the University of Colorado Medical Center Library is fairly typical, in most ways, of that group made up of about one hundred of the larger medical libraries of the United States. And I justify it, in a larger sense, by quoting the remark of Alvan Feinstein, who said that he doubted that it was the case that Isaac Newton sat down one fine evening and decided that he would posit the notion of gravity, and that he would then go outdoors the next day to see if any apples were falling. What I want to do first is to count some apples and see where they are falling. After this, it is unfortunately unlikely that I shall come up with any such elegant notion as a bibliothecal theory of gravitation. It is a regrettable but almost inevitable fact that, in this era of burgeoning social complexity, more and more the theoretician and the practitioner are no longer combined in a single person, but are different persons pursuing their disparate but equally important tasks. I take it that it is the duty of the practitioner to point out to the theoretician *where he should look*. Again, in the phrase of Dr. Feinstein, it is not the case that one fine day Linus Pauling decided to do some hemoglobin electrophoresis on the notion that it might have something to do with blood dyscrasias. Practitioners had told him where to look. They had identified the sickling trait, and Pauling's elegant work provided explanations which advance both theory and practice thereafter. The best I can hope to do here is to identify some of the sickling traits of subject cataloging.

The University of Colorado Medical Center Library holds upwards of 85,000 volumes, the greater portion of which are imprints of the last two decades. It has a divided catalog, for which I have my predecessor to thank, and I offer these thanks fervently. There is no doubt in my mind but that the separate subject catalog is preferable from the library patron's point of view, and highly preferable from the librarian-practitioner's point of view, in that catalog maintenance is greatly facilitated. In this subject catalog are represented imprints of 1946 or later date; we place our reliance on printed bibliographies, such as the *Index-Catalogue,* for imprints of an earlier date. And since studies have shown us that only 15 percent of the action in our Library concerns earlier materials, and that most of this concerns serials rather than monographs, we are content with this arrangement.

The separate subject catalog provides the opportunity to file subject cards behind guide cards which bear the subject headings. It is our practice to file subject cards in reverse chronological order, so that the latest work always first engages the attention. Only current editions are represented in our subject catalog; earlier editions are to be found in the separate author catalog.

In 1965, our subject catalog was thoroughly revised to accept the National Library of Medicine's *Medical Subject Headings (MeSH)* as the subject heading authority. In 1966, the subject catalog was again revised to reflect the introduction of standard subheadings into the system. We procured a set of these standard subheadings on preprinted center-cut guide cards to go with our left-cut guide cards bearing main headings. We adopted the forty-two topical subheadings then in the *MeSH* system and the four additional topical subheadings (e.g., *in infancy & childhood*) authorized by *MeSH* for book cataloging. We also adopted twenty-one of the form subheadings authorized, rejecting only a few, such as *juvenile literature*, as being unsuitable for the scope of our collection. At the same time, on a purely intuitive basis, we made the decision that we would divide main headings by either topical or form subheadings, placing them within a single alphabet arrangement, but that we would not subdivide a topical subheading by a form subheading, or vice versa.

There are two main reasons for adopting the *MeSH* system. First, maintaining a subject heading authority list is a task of a high order, requiring much skill and many man-hours of effort; we wished to take advantage of the effort already performed at the National Library of Medicine which we could not afford to duplicate even if we could muster the skill and resources. Second, we wished to take the greatest possible advantage of the centralized cataloging product of NLM, being made available in the *NLM Current Catalog*, for the same reasons.

Then in 1967, *MeSH* introduced 200 new main headings, and made slight changes of form in an additional fifty main headings, for a total new authority list of about 6,600 main headings. It also introduced eleven new subheadings to the apparatus. This called for another revision of our subject catalog, the third in what is now clearly an annual series. What I want to document for you is what happened in this third revision and what some of the implications are of the difficulties encountered.

I performed the revision of the subject catalog myself, and it required 240 man-hours, or six man-weeks. While I happen to find this kind of task congenial, I do begrudge the long hours involved. Because of the fact that this was a third revision, and because of certain peculiarities of our catalog, such as that the earlier subject cards do not bear subject tracings, something more than merely taking care of the new changes was involved, but I am unable to say just how much time these extraneous factors amounted to.

There is another possible circumstance which must be alluded to. In revising a subject catalog, one is dealing with a corpus that is fixed in size at that moment in time, and there is a danger that one will yield to the temptation of revising it as a fixed item, as one would index an individual book or arrange a one-time bibliography, rather than revising it prospectively with an eye to the next decade's library patrons. I strove to avoid this hazard, and some evidence that I may have succeeded in large measure is the fact that at the end of revision there were 882 main headings which held but a single entry behind them.

My method of work was crude because of the time limitations involved. My sources of information were limited to the title of the book, the tracings on the card, and the guide card heading under which it was filed. Seldom did I succumb to the longing to reexamine the book itself, which of course would have been desirable ideally.

I moved cards around at will, placing them under new headings and new subheadings. At the conclusion of the exercise, the entire subject catalog was filmed and reproduced on paper slips. A library assistant then spent seventeen weeks, first making the tracings on the slips agree with the actual point of filing, then rearranging the slips in call number order, and then transferring the new valid information to the shelflist. It was in the course of this exercise that the data to be exhibited were collected.

We found that the number of cards representing books was 21,600, pertaining to 16,000 volumes, but only 13,000 titles. (Cards under the subheadings *abstracts, indexes,* and *periodicals* are not considered in this study.) Considering the rate of processing, it is difficult to see how the job could have been done in a shorter period of time.

The average number of subject cards per title was 1.66. When single card titles are eliminated, the remaining titles show a representation by an average 2.55 cards, which happens to be identical to the ratio of the *Cumulated Index Medicus* of 1966.

Of the 21,600 cards, 17,600 were under undivided headings or "up front," and 4,000 cards were under subheadings. Of the 6,600 main headings available in the system, only 42 percent had been utilized, and of these, only one-quarter had been divided by subheadings.

The number of main headings used is neither surprising nor disturbing; the Colorado set is simply a subset of *MeSH,* a subset which may be enlarged as the need becomes manifest. The low proportion of use of subheadings is somewhat startling, but it must be remembered that to a certain extent this is an artificial situation, i.e., in editing the older material there may not be enough information available in title and tracings, unequivocally, to warrant assignment of subheadings.

TABLE 1

University of Colorado Medical Center
Subject Catalog 1946-1967

Total cards representing books	21,604
Total volumes represented	16,028
less multivolume works, duplicates, superseded editions	3,050
Total book titles represented	12,978
Librarian man/hours to edit (average 40 seconds per card)	240
Library assistant man/hours to post (average 3 minutes per title)	680

TABLE 2

Subject Cards per Title

Average subject cards per title	1.66
Titles represented by single card only	7,411
Titles represented by multiple subject cards	5,567
Cards representing multiple-card books	14,193
Average subject cards per multiple-card book	2.55

TABLE 3

Headings Used

Cards representing books	21,604
Cards—undivided headings or "up front"	17,637
Cards under subheadings	3,967
under FORM subheadings	1,318
under TOPICAL subheadings	2,649
Number of main headings used	2,772
Number of undivided main headings	2,058
Average card density per undivided heading (or "up front")	8.6

Table 4 displays subheading usage. It shows that the number of new "access points" created in the subject catalog was 629 with the use of eighteen form subheadings, and 831 with the use of fifty-seven topical subheadings. This tends to confirm what we might have expected in terms of proportional use. We may note that the inclusion of *history* under topical subheadings, rather than under form subheadings where it would have been just as appropriate, tends to distort the picture.

Table 5 summarizes the usage in the Colorado catalog. It shows that the use of subheadings has increased the number of access points by 50 percent, and has reduced the average density of posting under each access point from 7.8 to 5.1, a decrease of 35 percent.

Now let us recall that *MeSH* was created as a common subject heading authority list for indexing journal articles as well as for cataloging books. The rationale for this position is that it is too costly to maintain two separate authority lists, even if there were otherwise some positive reason for doing so, and that a single list facilitates the library patron's use of what is inherently a complicated apparatus. This position seems sound.

With this in mind, it may prove interesting to compare practice in the Colorado catalog with *Index Medicus* practice, using 1966 as an example. Table 6 gives the basic facts for the *Cumulated Index Medicus*, 1966.

These figures pertain only to the printed subject section for the year stated. The term "access point" is defined in the same manner as for the Colorado catalog earlier.

TABLE 4

SUBHEADING DENSITIES

Number of divided main headings	714
divided by FORM subheading only	234
divided by TOPICAL, or TOPICAL and FORM	480
Number of cards under FORM subheadings (18)	1,318
Number of MH/SH (FORM) combinations	629
Average card density per MH/SH (FORM) combination	2.1
Number of cards under TOPICAL subheadings (57)	2,649
Number of MH/SH (TOPICAL) combinations	831
Average card density per MH/SH (TOPICAL) combination	3.2

TABLE 5

ACCESS POINT DENSITY

Main headings available	6,600
Main headings used	2,772
"Access Points" used	4,232
Main headings	2,772
MH/SH combinations (FORM)	629
MH/SH combinations (TOPICAL)	831
Total MH/SH combinations	1,460
Average card density per "access point"	5.1

TABLE 6

Cumulated Index Medicus 1966

Total articles indexed	157,798
Total citations printed	402,908
Average citations per article	2.55
Number undivided or "up front"	186,139
Number subheaded	216,769
Total "access points" used	36,154
Average citations per "access point"	11.1

Table 7 juxtaposes the two sets of figures. First, one must adjust to the fact that the *Index Medicus* corpus is more than twelve times the size of the Colorado catalog, despite the discrepancy in number of years covered. One sees that the greatest disproportion occurs in the frequency of use of subheadings. One also sees that this indeed must occur, as the number of access points in the *IM* case exceeds the total number of cards in the Colorado catalog.

Table 8 compares catalog and index use of the body of forty-two topical subheadings available in 1966. Subheadings printed in capitals are those which fall in other percentiles in the opposite list. The two central columns indicate the number of times each subheading was used, with the figure for *IM* being derived by dividing the actual figure by a factor of a little more than twelve—in other words, the *IM* number is the number of times the subheading would have been used in indexing the same number of items represented in the Colorado catalog.

TABLE 7

INDEX USE AND CATALOG USE

	Index Medicus	U. Colorado
Articles indexed/Titles in catalog	157,798	12,798
Citations printed/Cards in catalog	402,908	21,604
Average citations/cards per article/title	2.55	1.66
Number undivided	186,139	17,637
Number subheaded	216,769	3,967
Total "access points" used	36,154	4,232
Average density per "access point"	11.1	5.1

Table 9 shows the other end of the line. Again, the subheadings printed in caps are those which do not match this percentile in the opposite list.

Table 10 shows where the widest discrepancies lie. It is easy to see why this should be so, considering the differences that naturally exist as between the two bodies of material.

TABLE 8

·HEAVY-USE SUBHEADINGS

Rank	U. Colorado	Times Used	Times Used	*Index Medicus*	Rank
1	HISTORY	549	1880	metabolism	1
2	surgery	274	1524	PHARMACODYNAMICS	2
3	therapy	165	1287	etiology	3
4	physiology	144	1257	diagnosis	4
5	diagnosis	110	1081	therapeutic use	5
6	metabolism	106	1066	surgery	6
7	therapeutic use	96	1030	COMPLICATIONS	7
8	ANATOMY & HISTOLOGY	95	861	drug therapy	8
9	NURSING	58	770	physiology	9
10	etiology	57	737	pathology	10
11	drug therapy	48	643	DRUG EFFECTS	11
12	pathology	46	523	therapy	12
12 subheadings—66 percent of all topical use			12 subheadings—71 percent of all use		

TABLE 9

LEAST-USE SUBHEADINGS

Rank	U. Colorado	Times Used	Times Used	*Index Medicus*	Rank
31	classification	7	103	RADIATION EFFECTS	31
32	ADVERSE EFFECTS	6	89	administration & dosage	32
33	VETERINARY	6	85	BLOOD SUPPLY	33
34	CYTOLOGY	5	83	isolation & purification	34
35	administration & dosage	4	71	poisoning	35
36	ENZYMOLOGY	3	70	congenital	36
37	injuries	3	58	pathogenicity	37
38	poisoning	3	47	injuries	38
39	COMPLICATIONS	2	41	INNERVATION	39
40	congenital	1	40	EMBRYOLOGY	40
41	isolation & purification	0	37	classification	41
42	pathogenicity	0	12	NURSING	42

TABLE 10
WIDE RANK VARIATIONS

Rank	U. Colorado	Times Used	Times Used	*Index Medicus*	Rank
1	HISTORY	549	1524	PHARMACODYNAMICS	2
8	NURSING	58	1030	COMPLICATIONS	7
22	PHARMACODYNAMICS	12	142	HISTORY	25
39	COMPLICATIONS	2	12	NURSING	42

TABLE 11
SUBHEADINGS INTRODUCED 1967

	Times Used at U. Colorado
analysis	12
blood	9
cerebrospinal fluid	0
chemically induced	1
diagnostic use	0
education	43
microbiology	0
mortality	0
radiography	120
rehabilitation	39
urine	3

TABLE 12
HIGHEST AND LOWEST USE—U. COLORADO

Highest		Lowest	
history	549	enzymology	3
surgery	274	injuries	3
IN INFANCY & CHILDHOOD	258	poisoning	3
ATLASES	234	URINE	3
NURSING TEXTS	217	complications	2
BIBLIOGRAPHY	193	CHEMICALLY INDUCED	1
therapy	165	congenital	1
physiology	144	CEREBROSPINAL FLUID	0
RADIOGRAPHY	120	DIAGNOSTIC USE	0
DIRECTORIES	115	isolation & purification	0
diagnosis	110	MICROBIOLOGY	0
metabolism	106	MORTALITY	0
therapeutic use	96	pathogenicity	0

It will be remembered that eleven new subheadings were introduced in 1967. Table 11 shows their use in the University of Colorado catalog.

The three new subheadings, *radiography, rehabilitation,* and *education,* are fairly useful. The remainder are of little help.

After the 1967 subheadings have been incorporated, and considering the use of form subheadings as well, the highest use and lowest use groups in the Colorado catalog appear as in Table 12. In the highest use group in the left hand column, note that the new appearances, signalled by capitalization, include six subheadings, one of which is a 1967 topical addition, *radiology*. In the lowest use group in the right column, note that there are six new members, all of which are 1967 additions.

TABLE 13

MAIN HEADINGS WITH HIGHEST POSTING DENSITIES—U. COLORADO

	Total Cards	Up Front	Number Subheadings	Density Per Subheading	Form Subheadings	Density Per Form SH	Topical SH	Density Per Topical SH
Biochemistry	169	158	5	2.2	4	2.2	1	1.0
Biology	86	58	9	3.1	7	2.3	2	6.0
Brain	108	28	8	10.0	1	19.0	7	9.0
Child Psychology	95	95						
Education	119	110	4	2.2	3	2.7	1	1.0
Education, Nursing	150	148	1	2.0	1	2.0		
History of Medicine	94	82	3	4.0	3	4.0		
Medicine	106	46	6	10.0	6	10.0		
Neoplasms	150	35	22	5.3	6	3.0	16	6.3
Nursing	126	103	7	3.3	7	3.3		
Personality	101	92	1	9.0			1	9.0
Pharmacology	92	69	5	4.6	4	4.5	1	5.0
Physiology	97	65	8	4.0	7	4.6	1	1.0
Psychiatry	195	156	11	3.5	8	2.1	3	7.3
Psychoanalysis	163	142	7	3.0	4	1.5	3	5.0
Psychology	91	64	5	5.4	4	5.5	1	5.0
Psychotherapy	141	139	2	1.0	1	1.0	1	1.0
Public Health	98	59	10	3.9	8	2.4	2	10.0
Science	111	27	8	10.5	7	4.0	1*	57.0
Surgery	144	75	9	7.7	6	3.7	3	16.0
Composite	122	88	6.6	5.1	4.4	4.0	2.2	7.0

* History.

Table 13 is a list of the twenty main headings with the highest posting densities in the Colorado catalog. The list holds no surprises, except perhaps for the inclusion of PERSONALITY. Note that many of these heavy-use main headings are themselves, in another incarnation, identical with subheading concepts. Recall that these twenty headings, and their 131 subheading combinations, represent only 3 percent of the total access points used but accommodate over 11 percent of the total catalog entries.

With this as background, I offer the following observations:

(1) The number of items cataloged for the *Index Medicus* being far larger than the number of items in the average library subject catalog, it is reasonable to expect that the library catalog may require a lesser number of access points than does the *Index* and that this smaller set may be a subset of the larger.

(2) When additions and changes are made to subject heading authority lists, as is inevitable, demands on the time of librarians, necessitated for revision of subject catalogs, is far from being negligible.

On this second point, there emerges another notion of great importance—the use of machine or computer systems has little or no bearing on the amount of librarian man-hours required for subject catalog revision. Consider the following instances:

(a) In the case of a new term, such as PARKINSONISM, being substituted in a one-for-one exchange for an old term, such as PARALYSIS AGITANS, there is no problem in either a machine or a manual system. In the machine, we simply substitute one code for another; in the subject portion of a divided catalog, we simply remove a block of cards from behind one guide card and place them behind a new guide card; and to me, there does not seem to be a requirement for modifying the shelflist records in such instances.

(b) But in the case of new main headings which do not have this one-for-one equivalency with the old, as for example, the new KIDNEY CORTEX NECROSIS and KIDNEY FAILURE, CHRONIC, which were formerly not differentiated from the broader term KIDNEY DISEASES, there is no solution possible except a reexamination of all of the material under the older term. In these cases, there is at least some comfort in the thought that only particular areas of the subject catalog, e.g., KIDNEY DISEASES, need be examined to establish which items are now to be cataloged under newly established headings, e.g., KIDNEY CORTEX NECROSIS.

(c) In the case of the introduction of additional new subheadings, however, in the majority of instances no such limitation of effort is possible. Often the entire file must be reexamined. All candidates for inclusion under the subheading *blood* are certainly not going to be found under the main heading BLOOD. And where, for another example, would one be expected to look for material now eligible for inclusion under the new subheading *diagnostic use*? The problem of dealing with new additions to a subheading list is far more severe than dealing with the problem of new main headings.

There is no question but that, to remain viable and useful, subject heading authority lists must undergo changes and must receive new additions from time to time. What I want to warn against is the easy and fatal assumption that massive proliferation of terms brings with it no penalties. It is understandable that the tired indexer or the tired subject cataloger or the tired reference librarian may at some particular moment long for the inclusion of a new and very specific term in the system because its presence would dispel the particular concern of the moment. Any coordinate indexing system, as Calvin Mooers pointed out long ago, must favor the descriptor end of the subject heading-descriptor continuum. The more minutely precise and limited and precoordinated are our terms, the further are we drifting from the principle of coordinate indexing and the less useful that mechanism becomes. As an example, I exhibit a partial list of some main subject headings suggested for addition to the *MeSH* list. These are in the field of alcohol studies (Table 14).

TABLE 14
SUGGESTED MAIN HEADINGS

Adaptation to alcohol
Alcoholic brain disease
Alcoholic hallucinosis
Alcoholic intoxication
Alcoholic paranoid states
Alcoholic psychoses
Alcoholism
Aversion therapy of alcoholism
Chronic alcoholic psychosis
Dependence on alcohol
Deviant drinking
Drinking behavior
Drinking pattern
Early skid career pattern
Endogenous alcoholic
Exogenous alcoholic
Hidden alcoholic
Lay therapy
Nonaddictive pathological alcoholic
Nonbeverage alcohol drinking
Pathological intoxication
Physiologic dependence on alcohol
Plateau drinker
Prealcoholic personality
Psychological adaptation to alcohol
Psychological dependence on alcohol
Remission of alcoholism
Research on alcoholism
Ritual drinker
Schizophrenic drinker
Situational drinker
Social drinker
Solitary drinker
Successfully arrested alcoholic
Symptomatic drinking
Teetotalism
Withdrawal syndrome (alcohol)

TABLE 15
NLM *MeSH* HEADINGS

Alcohol deterrents
Alcoholic beverages
Alcoholic intoxication
Alcoholism
Korsakoff's syndrome
Psychoses, alcoholic
Temperance

Actually, these suggested alcohol headings constituted 10 percent of the entire list of headings suggested by a group of behavioral scientists. The field of work of the most active member of this group is evident. He is thinking of a list of headings suitable for his private files of material, which contain nothing but alcohol studies. It would be fatal to adopt such a list as part of a general scheme. In contrast, I exhibit in Table 15 a list of the more descriptor-like subject headings now available in *MeSH*.

This is as it should be. While we are on the topic, I should like to allude to the problem of subject heading equivalency, the reduction of separate authority lists to an overall authority list. All studies in this area which I have seen are vastly oversimplified and contain many illusions when they imply that all that is needed for consolidation of lists is an act of will. Table 16 shows the list of current Library of Congress headings on this topic.

Surely these show that the Library of Congress and the National Library of Medicine have different fields of interest and that the search for subject heading standardization is going to be one of the most resistant areas to effective compromise in the entirely laudable efforts that are now underway to achieve greater cataloging standardization among the several national library systems.

TABLE 16

LC Subject Headings, Seventh Edition 1966

Alcohol in the body
Alcoholics
Alcoholism
Alcoholism and crime
Alcoholism and employment
Alcoholism and religion
Cocktails
Drinking and traffic accidents
Drinking in literature
Drinking on aircraft
Drunkenness (Criminal law)
Liquor laws
Liquor problem
Liquor traffic
Liquors
Prohibition
Punched card systems—alcohol
Temperance
Temperance and religion
Wine in literature

I have described the efforts required to conform to the 1967 changes in *MeSH*. Soon I shall have to tackle the problems, till now postponed, of 1968 *MeSH* changes. These changes are enormous, including main heading additions totaling more than 10 percent of the entire list, and including additional subheadings. The subheading changes are more numerous than the mere number of subheadings added; they embrace the extension of existing subheadings to additional categories. While the number of subheadings has increased by 46 percent in a period of two years, the available subheading-category combinations have increased by 76 percent. And when the 1968 revisions are completed, the 1969 changes will be at hand.

To my colleagues at the National Library of Medicine who are in charge of the *MeSH* operation, I would wish to say the following. I applaud the generally fine work which you have performed in keeping the *MeSH* list viable. I ask you never to forget that in adding new main headings to the list, one of the most important points is to establish the relationship of the new heading to the headings in the existing corpus. This implies especial care in establishing the cross-reference structure, which has negative as well as positive aspects.

Cross-referencing is inherently complicated enough without complicating it further with the addition of what I would call "gratuitous" cross-references. The first two examples in Table 17 are of this type. If this type of cross-reference is included—the gratuitous cross-reference of the type "Leukemia *see also* Anemia"—there is no limit whatsoever which can be imposed on the extent of the cross-reference system.

The third pair in Table 17 is an example on the other side. Great care must be exercised to provide crosses between closely related headings of this kind.

TABLE 17

CROSS-REFERENCE PROBLEMS

Thermography
XR Autonomic dysfunction
XR Body temperature
XR Paraplegia
Cystic fibrosis
See also related Sweating

Anoxia (C17)
Cerebral anoxia (C8, C10)

But the main thing I want to say to my *MeSH* colleagues is this—I plead for an early stabilization of topical subheadings. There is some evidence to suggest that the subheadings of maximal usefulness have already been discovered and adopted and that extensive further elaboration of the list is not warranted.

To my colleagues in the subject cataloging departments of the many medical libraries across the country and to my colleagues in reference services, I would like to say the following. Let us not lightly recommend changes in what is really a very delicate structure without realizing all the different aspects which are at stake. There is, for example, the problem of achieving indexer and system consistency, as well as the problem of trying to achieve instant user satisfaction in 100 percent of cases. Let us not naively imagine that parts of the system can be tampered with without causing reverberations throughout the system. Let us recognize and support the *MeSH* system for what it is, a legitimate compromise between the descriptor-oriented terms of a computer coordinate-indexing system, and the subject-heading-oriented terms of the conventional card catalog.

Finally, let us realize that we are up against some tough professional problems in the field of subject cataloging and that these problems are crucial to the nature and adequacy of the services which we can provide. Neither Billings nor Cutter found permanent solutions to these problems, nor do today's computer systems figure in any central way in their solution. We need new ideas, large and small and medium-sized. Perhaps, for example, we should probe further into the notion of time-segmentation of subject catalogs, it being evident that this is the factor which "solves" the situation for the *Index Medicus,* and is absent in large part from our library catalogs. But "time-segmentation" is just a phrase. What we need is to explore some possible operational systems, weighing what we must yield for what it is possible to achieve, and never being seduced into the notion that we can get something for nothing.

Meanwhile, my catalog is growing larger. In twenty more years, I expect it to be five times its present size.

Academic Status for Medical School Librarians*

BY ALFRED N. BRANDON, *Chairman*

Department of Library Science
Mount Sinai School of Medicine
New York, New York

ABSTRACT

Results of a survey conducted indicate that most medical schools grant academic status in some degree to their professional librarians. Faculty appointments and benefits are not always awarded. In order to upgrade the stature and effectiveness of the medical school librarian in relation to his institution and to the teaching faculty, his having faculty status is desirable. It is the medical school's responsibility to grant faculty status to librarians who possess necessary qualifications; likewise, it is the responsibility of the medical school librarian to merit faculty rank on a basis with other teaching faculty. In three new medical schools, the library is considered an academic department, and other schools are considering such designation.

DURING the past twenty-five years the inundation of medical literature, the search for adequate control of it, the development of new technologies, and the requests for greater services have created a pernicious demand for more qualified, capable, and well-trained medical librarians. In these post-World War II years, we have seen most of our older medical school libraries rebuilding physical quarters, updating and strengthening collections as budgets have skyrocketed, replacing and adding new staff, and restructuring library services. At least twenty new medical schools have been established during this period, thus further draining the channels of medical librarian recruits. To keep pace with the increasing demand for medical librarians, efforts have been made to upgrade positions and salaries to meet competition. Attracting desirable personnel entails more than just offering good salaries and challenging opportunities. Librarians from the college and university community are attaining faculty status and comparable benefits. Perhaps we should investigate

*The third Janet Doe Lecture, presented at the Sixty-eighth Annual Meeting of the Medical Library Association, Louisville, Kentucky, October 28, 1969.

Originally published in *Bulletin of the Medical Library Association*, Volume 58 (January, 1970), pp. 1-6. Reprinted by permission.

means whereby we can compete with this existing situation in our universities and colleges.

For several decades, college and university librarians have struggled to achieve faculty status. In his 1968 article on the status of academic librarians in retrospect, Robert B. Downs has indicated that librarians have in recent years made great forward strides in achieving improved status and that full faculty status and rank are being quite generally accepted today[1].

In a 1968 survey of eighty-seven major American academic institutions, Hintz stated seventy signified that their librarians had academic status in one measure or another[2].

A resolution adopted at the membership meeting on June 25, 1969, of the Association of College and Research Libraries states:

> Whereas academic librarians must have:
> 1. Rank equivalent to other members of the teaching faculty;
> 2. Salary equal to that of other members of the teaching faculty;
> 3. Sabbatical and other leaves;
> 4. Tenure;
> 5. Access to grants, fellowships, and research funds;
> 6. Responsibilities for professional duties only;
> 7. An adequately supportive non-professional staff;
> 8. Appointment and promotion on the basis of individual accomplishment and involving peer evaluation;
> 9. Grievance and appeal procedures available to other members of the academic community and involving peer review;
> 10. Participation of all librarians in library governance;
> 11. Membership in the academic senate of their institutions, or other governing bodies.
>
> Therefore, be it resolved that the Association of College and Research Libraries and the American Library Association adopt as their official policy the support of these standards for all academic librarians and the implementation of these standards by any and all appropriate professional means. . . .

The Academic Status Committee of the Association of College and Research Libraries specifies:

> Academic status for professional librarians may be defined as the formal recognition, in writing, by an institution's authorities, of librarians as members of the instructional and research staff. The recognition may take the form of assigned faculty ranks and titles, or equivalent ranks and titles, according to institutional custom[3].

The obligations that such status demands may well correspond to the librarian's responsibilities to his own profession which include: (1) continual intellectual activity and growth; (2) interest in research and publication; (3) active participation in professional organizations; and (4) attainment of the highest level of professionalism in performance of his duties.

Although the battle for complete recognition of the academic librarian as a teaching member of the faculty with all the rights and privileges appertaining thereto is not entirely won, the trend toward this ultimate objective is undeniably here.

We as medical school librarians can learn much from studying the library literature which traces the development of academic status for college and university librarians. Obviously, we are embarking—somewhat belatedly—on the same course which they began decades ago. It is essential that we be aware of the problems and challenges which confront us if we are to achieve significant advances toward this goal in the foreseeable future.

One of the most interesting and controversial statements contained in the 1967 report of the Library Study Committee of the Association of American Medical Colleges was that the medical school library should be accorded full academic partnership in the educational endeavor; that it be granted all the rights and privileges that other academic departments enjoy; and that it should be allowed to compete on equal terms with other academic departments for its share of the instructional budget[4].

This recommendation was predicated on the assumption that medical school librarians must embark on a very active period of research; that they should be willing to accept a greater teaching role than they have previously undertaken; and that they employ a new philosophy in public service.

To ascertain what progress is being made toward the goal of recognizing the medical school library as an academic department and granting the professional librarians academic status, a questionnaire was circulated to 101 medical school libraries in the United States. One result indicated that although it is not unusual for the library to be a separate *administrative* unit or department of the medical school, in only three institutions is the library established as a separate *academic* department. These libraries having such status were all established recently in new medical schools. Some older institutions are considering academic departmental status for the library, but there is nothing definite to report at this time.

The picture is significantly brighter when academic or faculty status for the professional librarians in medical schools is considered. Of the 100 reporting libraries, only twenty-seven give neither academic status nor faculty appointments to librarians. In twenty-nine institutions, all librarians have faculty appointments; in six others, some of the professional staff have faculty appointments; in eighteen schools, only the head librarian has been given a faculty rank; and in twenty others, librarians have academic status but no faculty appointments. (See Table 1.)

In equating the academic or faculty benefits that medical school librarians enjoy in comparison to those of other medical school faculty, the most noticeable difference is that of inequitable salary schedules. In only twelve institutions are salaries of librarians on a par with other medical school faculty. Generally the librarians are accorded the same holiday, vacation, and sick leave benefits as other medical school faculty; and in the majority of instances, they also have tenure. Sabbatical leave is granted librarians in thirty-seven schools. In only forty-six schools are any librarians members of committees (other than the Library Committee), or members of the Faculty Council. (See Table 2.)

In seventy-one schools the chief medical librarian is responsible to an administrative officer of the medical school or medical center; in twenty-four institutions, to the university librarian; and in five instances, to both officials.

Perhaps one of the primary reasons for the medical librarian's deficiency in academic respectability has been his failure to distinguish between the routine techniques and the professional, intellectual, and instructive aspects of his work. A clear delineation between subprofessional and professional duties is necessary. A well-trained medical library technician can effectively perform many jobs now undertaken by professional staff. Unless each of us is willing to forego routine clerical procedures and instead concentrate on true professional library endeavors, we cannot merit and should not expect faculty recognition.

A major stumbling block in the establishing of faculty status for all medical school librarians is the inequality in capabilities, education, and productivity of existing personnel. We have had to operate on shoestring budgets and pay inadequate salaries for so long that we have not always been able to attract good people with competent backgrounds for medical librarianship. In addition to salary inadequacies producing lack of interest, the shortage of librarians qualified for special librarianship has further complicated the problem.

Because of these existing circumstances, recruiters have all too frequently settled for incompetents, misfits, or castoffs and failures from other professions. No longer can we be willing to have this type of personnel blight the medical school library profession.

Better salaries, challenging jobs, and academic status must be offered so that the *best* of our library school graduates will be attracted to the medical school library field. Future recruiters will have to insist on paying competitive salaries thereby enabling us to hire the caliber of person who is best qualified to advance the goals of a teaching library department.

If the librarians in academic institutions are demanding academic status, then pressure must be brought by the profession upon library schools and their teaching programs. The schools should continue reevaluating their programs in order to ensure that students are taught more than routine techniques and impractical abstractions and are given more than a superficial exposure to a myriad of bibliographical and reference tools. More instruction in search techniques, personnel relationships, and administrative acumen are both needed and essential. Further specialization in our library school curricula—additional training for catalogers, acquisitions librarians, reference librarians, and administrators—is a vital necessity. The developing of a well-adjusted, capable, research-oriented library school graduate should be—but often has not been—the cardinal objective of every library school. Inferior output from library schools produces inferior librarians!

Within our own field, we should recognize our individual needs for specialization, and through workshops, institutes, library school seminars, or graduate study seek to develop ourselves more fully to meet the academic demands of our positions. We have standards for libraries and librarianship. These standards are but goals; excellence and perfection in our duties should be the absolute objective for which we aim.

For a moment, let us consider the position, impact, and stature of the medical school librarian as he or she relates to the overall academic atmosphere of the medical school. Can we describe this individual as a staid, elderly lady sitting behind a desk checking books in and out and fervently guarding access to the library's collection? Twenty-five years ago, this was perhaps generally an acceptable description and impression of the typical librarian. Unfortunately, even now the concept of the stereotyped librarian has not disappeared—certainly not from the medical field; recently our catalogers were depicted as "little old ladies with buns."

TABLE 1

FACULTY STATUS OF MEDICAL SCHOOL LIBRARIANS*

Librarians Have Academic Status but No Faculty Appointments	Only Head Librarian Has Faculty Appointment	Some Librarians Have Faculty Appointments	All Librarians Have Faculty Appointments	Librarians Have Neither Academic Status nor Faculty Appointments
20	18	6	29	27

* 100 out of 101 libraries reporting.

TABLE 2
FACULTY BENEFITS OF MEDICAL SCHOOL LIBRARIANS*

Given Tenure	Granted Sabbaticals	Represented on Faculty Councils or Faculty Committees	Same Holidays, Vacations, Sick Leave, Etc. as Other Faculty	Salaries Same as Other Medical School Faculty
64	37	46	66	12

* 100 out of 101 libraries reporting.

During the last two decades the typical librarian has indeed changed face and form, and librarianship has assumed its position among other professional groups in the United States and abroad. Today the typical medical librarian must be an administrator, educator, researcher, collector, public servant, fund raiser, accountant, architect, psychologist, and public relations expert. With this enlightened viewpoint in mind, I object to being classified as the stereotyped librarian of twenty-five years ago. I object to following outmoded policies and procedures. I object to the status quo attitude and lack of experimentation and desire on the part of some for improved methodology for librarianship. I do admit that the traditional, stereotyped librarian has not completely disappeared from our ranks, but I optimistically hope that in future years the medical school librarian will be identified as a fully qualified scholar in an academic setting.

To initiate the academic setting for the medical school library, its having an official department designation, comparable to the Anatomy Department or the Pharmacology Department, would be a significant development in this direction. Even though three schools have given their libraries official departmental status as the Department of Library Science, Department of Medical Library Science, and Department of Medical Communications, most medical libraries presently have various names, notably lacking departmental connotation. Results obtained from the questionnaire show the following names to be currently in use: Medical Center Library—nineteen; Medical School (or College) Library, and School (or College) of Medicine Library—twenty-three; Medical Library—thirteen; Biomedical Library—four; Health Sciences Library—nine; Health Center Library—three; Library of Medical Sciences, or Medical Sciences Library—three; Medical-Dental Library—three; other names—nine; and fourteen are named after individuals.

If we are to develop into academic departments of the medical school, the role of the technical service librarian, as well as that of the public services librarian, must be restructured. Personnel involved in acquisitions, cataloging, and serials control are to have an awareness of evolving techniques and aids which will assist in performing routine tasks more efficiently and effectively. The public services librarian should possess skills in search techniques which complement the faculty's expertise in literature research.

Marchant holds that greater opportunity should be provided for librarians to interact with each other[5]. The holding of regularly scheduled professional staff meetings where topics of immediate and long-range importance can be thoroughly discussed is one excellent method of achieving this type of interaction. As a result of this communicative means, each librarian develops a closer tie to the department and feels himself to be an integral part of the decision-making process.

I would like to pose the question: should we strive for academic or faculty status for all medical school librarians? Only if we are willing to accept the responsibilities that are inherent in such recognition must be *my* answer. Are we disposed and able to revise our procedures and policies to effect a better control of the medical literature and to facilitate the dispersal of information more rapidly? Are we ready to conduct library research and experiment with new methodologies, or are we too enmeshed in our everyday activities to be bothered with new ideas or suggestions for improvement?

Today we do have more personnel devoted to research and writing than ever before, but there are still many new technologies to investigate and adapt judiciously for our profession. Medical school librarians who have knowledge, time, and financial resources must volunteer to pursue research topics which will improve some of our outmoded procedures. We must be aware of new programs of information retrieval being developed and investigate in what ways our patrons can be benefited by them.

I am completely convinced of the desirability of being identified with the faculty rather than with service departments, the category in which libraries are sometimes classified. The only means of obtaining this identification for the professional staff is to be given faculty status. A close identification with the teaching staff may produce a better understanding of the educational role of the library itself as a teaching entity. Likewise, it may also encourage the faculty to cooperate with the library staff in developing the resources needed to meet their requirements. Faculty status improves the morale of the librarians and adds to the confidence of the general faculty in the library staff.

Again let me stress that I believe librarians should have faculty status only if they are fully worthy of it. They should in some sense be scholars and teachers comparable to the rest of the teaching faculty. Mere technical competence is not sufficient reason for granting them faculty status.

We should not endeavor to cheapen high standards for faculty appointments by recommending poorly-qualified staff members to such standing. Librarians must possess equivalent qualifications if they are to expect equivalent academic recognition.

A teaching program has to be developed by us within our own institutions which will be accepted by a curriculum committee as being important enough to medical and graduate students so that it can compete successfully for a place in the scholastic program. We should offer seminars for faculty and research staff that will inform them of information retrieval methodologies and research techniques.

We have to associate with our faculty and staff to ascertain their program plans and their needs for library services to support such plans. We cannot learn how to provide efficiently for patron needs unless we become involved in the total school endeavor and are able to communicate with other faculty members on an equitable basis.

While the medical school librarian assiduously buys, catalogs, and shelves the materials which he hopes will support the curriculum, often he fails to demand any part in the intellectual process which determines that curriculum. This situation is detrimental not only to the librarian involved but also to the institution involved. Unless he is full integrated into faculty planning, he cannot possibly build a collection which will most advantageously serve the needs of his institution. Developmental plans affecting library services should be determined with the counsel of the medical librarian; he should not be the last to hear about them.

If we are to take the position that the medical school librarian should be accorded full faculty status, a proposed policy statement based on one that Hintz suggested for university and college librarians might be appropriate to consider (2):

SUGGESTED POLICY STATEMENT

The medical school librarian should be granted recognition based upon his qualifications, experience, and responsibilities. He should hold a graduate library degree or an equivalent graduate degree, perhaps in a suitable subject field. His assigned tasks are to be of a professional nature, and he should be active in professional library associations. Faculty benefits and advancement policies should be on the same basis as for other medical school faculty.

Advancement for medical school library professional personnel is to be based on the following:

1. Effectiveness in instruction and teaching (group or individual).
    (a) Efficient use and development of library resources for enhancing the medical school's undergraduate, graduate, postgraduate, and research programs.
    (b) Competent performance in library technical service areas which add support to the research and teaching programs of the medical institution.
    (c) Opinions of clientele (students and faculty).
    (d) Opinions of supervisors and colleagues within the library.
2. Recognition for research and creative work.
    (a) Publication of books, articles, reviews, and reports of a scholarly nature.
    (b) High degree of proficiency in the use of various bibliographic resources.
    (c) Original creativity in experimenting with or using new methodologies or techniques.
3. Professional competence and initiative.
    (a) Dynamic participation in professional associations.
    (b) Knowledge of philosophies relating to librarianship, education, and administration.
    (c) Study in related pertinent fields and for advanced degrees.
4. Service to the medical school (involving committee and administrative activity).
    (a) Leadership and assistance in the internal affairs of the school in addition to the duties required by faculty position.
    (b) Demonstration of and capacity for administration as indicated by performance on councils and committees.
5. Service to the public at large.
    (a) Participation on statewide committees and various government committees and task forces.
    (b) Availability for consultation and community service.

Only when the medical school library is staffed with competent professional people who are involved in and devoted to developing new and innovative library services can we expect to receive academic status for the medical school library or for the medical school librarians.

We have made a beginning toward such recognition. Let us strive to swell the number of institutions recognizing the value and vitality of the medical school library and its librarians.

REFERENCES

1. DOWNS, ROBERT B. Status of academic librarians in retrospect. Coll. Res. Libr. 29: 253-258, July 1968.

2. HINTZ, CARL. Criteria for appointment to and promotion in academic rank. Coll. Res. Libr. 29: 341-346, Sept. 1968.
3. AMERICAN LIBRARY ASSOCIATION. ASSOCIATION OF COLLEGE AND RESEARCH LIBRARIES. ACADEMIC STATUS COMMITTEE. Status of college and university librarians. Coll. Res. Libr. 20: 399-400, Sept. 1959.
4. ASSOCIATION OF AMERICAN MEDICAL COLLEGES. LIBRARY STUDY COMMITTEE. The health sciences library: Its role in education for the health professions. J. Med. Educ. 42: 1-63, pt. 2, Aug. 1967.
5. MARCHANT, MAURICE P. Faculty-librarian conflict. Libr. J. 94: 2886-2889, Sept. 1, 1969.

The Pursuit of Excellence*

By Estelle Brodman, Ph.D., *Librarian and Professor of Medical History*

Washington University School of Medicine
St. Louis, Missouri

ABSTRACT

An attempt is made to define excellence and then to apply that definition to some of the problems facing medical librarianship today.

ALL those who have known Janet Doe intimately must have been touched with the spirit of greatness which is a visible and living aura around her. And yet to say that is to bring to mind the stained glass window and the hushed voice of sanctimony. Nothing could be farther from reality. The robustness of a love of good cooking and fine detective stories, and an extraordinarily acute sense of humor are characteristics in Janet Doe which belie the false image of the plaster saint.

And yet there remains the greatness; a greatness in which the attributes of scholarship, love of her fellow-man, and tolerance for small foibles are mingled with forthright condemnation of evil and dishonesty and inhumanity. More than anyone else I know she exemplifies the person who loves the sinner while hating the sin.

But neither do these excellences of heart and mind describe Janet Doe as the great medical librarian she is. What, I thought, when I was honored by being asked to give this Janet Doe Lecture on the History or Philosophy of Medical Librarianship, what has made her the great medical librarian, a person from whose strivings and accomplishments we all take inspiration?

It so happened that while I was pondering this, I was engaged, far from my normal habitat, in trying to explain to librarians, government officials, privy purses, deans, and directors of institutions in a land where medical libraries are a new phenomenon, what it is that a medical library could and

*Janet Doe Lecture in History or Philosophy of Medical Librarianship, presented at the Seventieth Annual Meeting of the Medical Library Association, New York, New York, June 1, 1971.

Originally published in *Bulletin of the Medical Library Association*, Volume 59 (October, 1971), pp. 549-554. Reprinted by permission.

should do, and a medical librarian strives for. Unless I could do so, I knew that the recommendations I might make would fail to be implemented, and my time and the dislocation of my life would have been for naught. The two needs came together, and this Janet Doe Lecture is the substance of my thoughts "on the pursuit of excellence in medical librarianship."

* * *

What is excellence, a term so hard to define, so difficult to agree on? Perhaps one can get some inkling of it by calling to mind some of its examples. For centuries, I mused as I stood looking at it, the House of Audience at the Red Fort in New Delhi, built by the same Shahjahan who erected the Taj Mahal in Agra, has moved men by its lines and its proportions. The early Cape Cod houses, so fitting for the conditions in the area, can stir one equally—as do the remains of the Parthenon or the great barrel-vaulted ceilings of the early cathedrals. They are right for their purposes, and bring with them a sense of rationality and understood use. They exude both honesty and imagination, and provide the viewer with an emotional experience which transcends the particular example he is observing. Or take the exhibit a few years ago at the Metropolitan Museum of Art—"In the Presence of Kings"; or the BBC's recent successful series on "Civilisation." Even in the proof of a Euclidian theorem: The *quod erat demonstrandum* at the end is a cry of exhilaration and victory that the logic of man's mind has solved a problem completely and without waste.

Let us not become too serious, however. Excellence is not only in great works visible to all. The President's National Advisory Commission on Libraries met many times in Washington, and frequently the members were luncheon guests at one of the great private clubs in the city. Because these were working meetings, the menus were always kept comparatively simple. But whether it was carrots or lamb chops, mushrooms or strawberries, each item had been chosen with care, cooked with respect, and served with an eye for how it looked on the plate—which caused one commission member to state despairingly that he only hoped the recommendations of the Commission would come up to the standards of excellence of its food!

Excellence, then, I concluded, must consist in "fittingness"—the solution must evolve from the terms of the problem. Secondly, it must contain proportions which, like the coda of a musical composition, give a sense of resolution and final ease. And lastly, like beauty, which (you remember) Wordsworth defined as emotion recollected in tranquillity, it must be a moving emotional experience long after it ceases.

If these are, indeed, the characteristics of excellence, how is it shown in the field of medical librarianship?

If the solution of the problems of medical librarianship must evolve from their terms, it follows that one must first understand these terms, study their backgrounds, ponder their constraints, and see them in relation to what follows from proposed solutions. Medical librarians who have been actively working with computers have learned (often the hard way) the necessity for this study before even approaching the machine, but not all are equally successful in comprehending its universal importance.

As I see it, the problems of medical librarianship relate to the goals of medical libraries, the willingness or ability of society to provide the means to reach these goals, and the effectiveness of medical librarians in devising the best methods to reach these goals. To slight any of these facets makes it impossible to achieve the excellence which all sentient workers must wish to see in their results. For, as Disraeli put it, "it is a wretched thing to be gratified with mediocrity, when the excellent lies before us." It is the realization of the necessity for taking into account all these things which leads Indian librarians to accuse American librarians of paying great attention to techniques without considering the philosophy of librarianship behind them; while American librarians retort that it does little good to devise esoteric philosophies of librarianship (complete with gurus and their disciples), if a reader cannot get the information he needs. Behind this name-calling lies the ancient dictum that form must follow function.

Medical libraries are the recorded experiences of mankind in its attempt to study and take action on the problems of health and disease. Their purpose is to bring the information gathered in the past to bear on the questions of the present and the future, and thus to break down the barriers of time and space. Notice that there are two components to this: gathering the recorded experiences, and bringing them to bear on the problems. It is in these two things that the expertise of the medical librarian resides.

Neither of these is easy to do. Take acquiring the records. From one end of the world to the other, I have heard medical librarians complaining that they have too few resources to acquire all that they wish to put in their collections. And yet, is that not to be expected? All societies, even our comparatively rich American one, have a sense of unfulfilled needs, an inability to do everything desirable, a list of priorities on which they will spend their resources. The difference between the rich and the poor nations is merely the size of the gap between what they wish to do and what they can do—and as a member of a more favored nation, I can only say thankfully, *"Vive la difference!"* (And we can all hope that the present economic recession is merely a short-term aberration from our normal situation.)

Priorities, however, are set by each society in terms of what it thinks will yield the best returns on its investment. In the past eight to ten months we have seen how little our government thinks it obtains for its grants for research, education, and libraries, as the always meagre sums devoted to these things were pared still further. In many countries where medical libraries have just been established, there is nothing on which the society can base a judgment on the value of such institutions. When people are starving, when over a million people in your largest city have no homes, but live on the pavements, when unemployment is causing riots, the needs of new medical libraries must take a back seat. The few such institutions which are set up are not only starved for funds, but their keepers are paid pittances, are of generally marginal education and ability, and are hemmed in with all sorts of restrictions, which make it almost impossible for them to obtain the information needed to bear on the problems of their society. And so, by a sad circle of events, the medical libraries are not very helpful to society, and the society does not place them high on the list of priorities.

But even if money were plentiful, obtaining the records of medical endeavors is not easy. The National Library of Medicine has as its objective the acquisition of all substantial medical publications from all countries, in all languages, and of all times. Moreover, it has a quite substantial budget. Yet the difficulties it encounters in tracking down and physically obtaining everything, with the startling and inexplicable gaps which occur in spite of its valiant efforts, is a lesson to all that even abundant funds may bring their own problems with them.

Obtaining literature—even large amounts of it—is, however, no guarantee that the information in it will be brought to bear on the problems. Indeed, if all one does is to pile one's acquisitions in great bins, literally or figuratively, it can hardly do anyone but the builders of warehouses much good. To make literature useful it must be presented in some ordered manner, so its contents are known and so its physical containers can be retrieved when its contents are deemed pertinent to the solution of a problem. More acquisitions require more people to handle them, and more space in which to store the physical objects, and anyone (like the oriental professor-librarian I met last year) who thinks only of acquiring items and not of the people or space required to make them useful is not building a library but a mausoleum. It takes excellence of judgment to decide where is the optimal point on the continuum between few books and journals, well-mined and presented to users promptly, and large acquisitions backlogged for use, or only superficially described and shelved. Such judgments must be based on a study of all the alternatives and their consequences, and must contain the elements in right proportion.

But adding books and journals cannot mean adding more staff proportionately, while continuing to do the same things in the same way that one did before. If it teaches us nothing else, a study of the history of the world empires which have risen and fallen over the centuries shows that only those had any chance of surviving whose founder realized that a large empire could not be governed in the same simple, personal way that had sufficed for the conqueror's original tribe or kingdom. A large state is not merely the sum of many smaller ones, but a new entity which requires new forms and new bureaucracies to govern it. The medical librarian of today, dealing in larger quantities than his predecessors ever dreamt possible, must also realize that the methods of the past must be transformed into entirely new ones to handle the problems of his larger kingdom. The pursuit of excellence here consists in the search to devise that system which accomplishes the goals in the best, fastest, and cheapest ways—and note that I have put "best" first. By "best," of course, I mean that which will bring the librarian closest to his *raison d'être,* the use of the information in his store for problem-solving; for what availeth speed and small cost if the result misses the ends of the library altogether?

Perhaps an even more striking example of the necessity of proportion—of making "the punishment fit the crime" as Gilbert and Sullivan would have put it; of making the solution of a problem evolve from the terms inherent in it—can be found in classification in medical libraries. Is classification an end in itself or a means to an end? Stated so baldly, all medical librarians will readily answer that of course it is the latter, the means to an end. But what is the end, and is classification the only or best way to reach it? Imagination is needed to see that in today's larger medical libraries, classification is only one way of physically ordering the containers of knowledge, and that the subject designations of the contents of the containers might conceivably better be reached in another way than in classifying the physical book; and then they might come up with an alternative solution.

Indeed, almost without realizing it, we have seen at least part of such a change in medical libraries in the past generation, just as probably William Rufus and Charlemagne and the Emperor Ashoka were not aware they were making a change to independent and continuous and impersonal rule through a civil service, until it was all over and someone looked back. Medical librarians of my age can remember when journals were as likely as not to be classified by subject; yet in the thirty-five years of my professional career, I have seen the dichotomy of physical volume on one hand and intellectual content on the other emphasized more and more. As a result, almost everywhere today medical journals are arranged on the shelf by an external criterion—the alphabet—while their contents are made known by subject approaches in depth indexes and detailed abstracting tools. As Popsy Welch is supposed to have said about the building of the old Army Medical Library, "That isn't the library. The library is inside."

The need to classify is, of course, a fundamental one for anyone trying to bring order out of chaos. One can almost imagine God looking at his first week's handiwork and saying, "I will call this thing night and what I separated from it day; this will be the water and that the land; and what I will give man dominion over I will classify as the beasts of the field, the birds of the air, and the fish of the sea." To understand a series of complex situations one must have the imagination to extract from them the essential likeness contained in their outward diversity.

No science could exist without classification. But classification is not science, nor book classification library science. Both exist to make possible the handling of groups of items, thus cutting down on the time and effort required to think of each one singly. At the most, book classification is a rough approximation, and the fact that there are so many schemes of classification extant shows that none is so superior to all the rest that it has overshadowed all its rivals. Moreover, the fact that our standard medical library classification schemes used different bases for categorizing medical knowledge leads inevitably (at least to me it is inevitable) to the conclusion that there are several equally valid axes by which to orient one's view of health and disease.

Since this is so, should we spend so much time in book classification? In the large, closed-stack library, would not John Shaw Billings's simple scheme of one hundred large subject groups, with books in each subject shelved alphabetically by author, work just as well? If the NLM returned to some such system, or to using a simple accessions register, how many man-hours could be diverted to the more useful task of indexing the chapters or sections of the chapters of these books? What would be lost in such a switch? What effects would this system have on the smaller, open-stack browsing medical library, and where is the cut-off point? In the pursuit of excellence it is necessary to ask such heretical questions, and to ask them at intervals, as the size of the problem and the emergence of new machinery change the "givens" in the particular situation.

How important it is to examine our problems regularly to try to devise solutions which fit the time is shown by the recent history of many of our library groups, including the American Library Association and the Medical Library Association. The classic disturbances which hurled empires and institutions to their doom in the past have caused stresses and strains in our professional organizations recently which must end in either one or another resolution. We struggle on the same shaky battlefield which brought ruin to Tamerlane and Louis IX, and success to Elizabeth I and William the Silent. How we will resolve the situation (or whether the recession we are entering will resolve it for us) only time can tell—and I can hardly wait for next year or ten years hence to learn the results.

The classic disturbances I have just alluded to include the enlargement of numbers of members of the group, with its natural result of impersonality in group action. My compeers can remember when annual meetings of the Medical Library Association turned up sixty or seventy participants, and where the Special Libraries Association might muster 400, instead of the thousands we now expect. (I meander now, like an old gaffer reminiscing of the "good old times.") Personal rivalries could be—and were—satisfied by appointing or electing everyone to positions in the group, either in tandem or seriatim, as the situation made it desirable. The stakes were not high, the voices low in debate, and if one lived long enough and were so inclined, one expected rightly to go through the whole *cursus honorum* from dogcatcher to president. Business meetings were held without benefit of microphones, and were somniferous intervals between technical papers and tea time. Indeed, the main purpose of these meetings was to give and listen to such papers—on a new circulation system, recently published reference tools, simplified binding, or the handling of duplicates—and to get to know others working in one's own field.

There was a world outside, of course. The depression had cut deeply into library budgets and staffs, and apple-sellers were on many streetcorners. Hitler was sending refugees to all countries willing to accept them, and strikes and strike-breaking occurred in Ford's River Rouge plant and at the pitheads of the Pennsylvania coal fields. Later there was Senator McCarthy and his red-baiting, and bombs on Hamburg and Canterbury. But these things were not something about which a library association took direct action, for its sphere of influence was thought to be in librarianship, not politics. How to obtain German periodicals in spite of the blockade and the embargo was seen to be its province, but not how to stop the war which caused the blockade.

Moreover, by and large the country was peaceful internally, and generally unified in purpose. Students were swallowing goldfish instead of burning university buildings, and the confrontation of citizen versus government had not begun. The sense of guilt of a nation betrayed into ignoble actions, at home in its treatment of its minorities and abroad in indefensible and interminable wars, had not yet reached many people, to force them into actions of emotion instead of reason. Minorities then either had no hope or too much hope to revolt and forcefully bring their plight to everyone's attention.

Today, all these conditions have changed. I have no illusion we can bring the old back—nor would I wish to do so. Large library associations now spend less of their time on professional and technical subjects and more on procedural matters meant, out of guilt and fear, to redress past wrongs, and on politicking of the kind which used to be considered the special province of the local ward-heeler. "Is member A or B fit for the office?" is less frequently asked than "Is he a member of this or that group?" Large library organizations have seen takeovers of their meetings by militant groups who, by playing on the deep-felt shame of the majority, and by using tactics of disruption and physical violence learned from Hitler's Nazis, Cromwell's dissolution of Parliament, or the last days of the Roman Senate, have been able to change the entire direction of these organizations. All of us who have taken part in faculty meetings have observed the same phenomenon, though library groups have not yet been physically threatened by the militant outsiders which some university faculties have had to face.

Under these conditions: impersonality, guilt, lawlessness, and the substitution of force for reason by embittered people within and without the professional organizations, the pursuit of excellence, I fear, is likely to be abandoned in favor of the pursuit of power. In some cases, of course, redress of grievances can only be brought about by powerful groups using that power. But let us also consider that the disgruntled never accept defeat gracefully: from time immemorial the cry of the poor player who has lost the game has been, "I was cheated." Perhaps some who wish to change our professional organization into bloc-groups have been cheated—though if so, I suspect they have been cheated by sins of omission rather than those of commission. But if they have been cheated, in whatever way, we are all the losers, for no society can afford the luxury of not using all its members to their fullest capacities.

The world is not a pretty place, and I am as guilty as are all of my generation that we did not start earlier and work harder to right the wrongs. But guilty as I feel, and as I suspect most of us feel, I do not consider it a necessary result that I should therefore approve our Samson's bringing down the edifice we have built up over the years, as we cry with him, "Oh Lord God, let me die with the Philistines." We must not allow adults to act like children.

What we need here as in all our endeavors, is to try to follow the rules for the pursuit of excellence, which I have tried to derive earlier in this talk. What are the terms of the problem? Does the proposed solution encompass them and flow from them? What consequences will the proposed solution bring in its train? Is it an efficient solution, or does it leave unanswered aspects of the question or require complicated methods to accomplish simple things? Is the *quod erat demonstrandum,* which leaves us with a sense of rightness and completeness, inherent in it? And above all, in this time of economic distress in libraries, are we acting cravenly, out of fear for our jobs, or honestly and forthrightly?

To some I may be putting too many obstacles before the process of change. The pursuit of excellence, however, is not an easy thing, nor do excellent results descend upon a person as a gift from the gods, without his having to do any work himself. "Badness you can get easily and in quantity," said Hesiod. "The road is smooth and it lies close by. But in front of excellence the immortal gods have put sweat, and long and steep is the way to it." Some people may understand the essentials of a problem more easily than others, see possible solutions more quickly and more imaginatively than others, or extrapolate results more certainly. But all must think and consider and ponder and often be frustrated and unhappy. There is no quick and easy way to excellence, and the sooner we acknowledge that fact, the more likely are we not to waste our energies in day dreams and in devising turns of the wheel to determine our future.

All institutions should change—must change—to meet changing conditions, or they die. But let us think about our changes. If the kind of professional association which has come down to us since its burgeoning in the past century is not needed today—is not "relevant" as our students put it—then it should and must be transformed or done away with. Perhaps the burning issue of our time *is* redressing the wrongs of our minority groups or getting out of a degrading war, and such inconsequential matters as bringing the past knowledge of health and disease to bear on present problems is unworthy of our energies. If so, let us strive, not for the pragmatic solution, not for the agreement based on the fear of noisy disruptions of those who prefer force to reason, but for the best solution which our best minds can conceive. Can we not think together, even if we dare not pray together?

For the pursuit of excellence is a statement of faith in ourselves and our abilities and our minds to reason. Just as Thomas Aquinas could fearlessly pursue whatever avenues his logic took him to, secure in his belief that it would lead ultimately and only to a knowledge of God himself; so should we as fearlessly pursue professional excellence, secure in the belief in our capability for solving problems, trusting in the honesty and good will of our colleagues, and thinking always to advance that high calling which we profess. "And when at some future date the high court of history sits in judgment on each of us . . . our success or failure . . . will be measured by the answers to four questions. First, were we truly men of courage . . . Second, were we truly men of judgment . . . Third, were we truly men of integrity . . . Finally, were we truly men of dedication?"*

*John F. Kennedy. Speech at Massachusetts State Legislature, January 9, 1961.

The Way of the Innovator: Notes Toward a Prehistory of MEDLARS*

By Scott Adams

Biological Sciences Communication Project
The George Washington University
Washington, D.C.

ABSTRACT

The concept of MEDLARS as a publication/retrieval system was the product of several forces operating during the fifteen years prior to 1961. These included the overriding imperative of medical index publication, the Welch Medical Indexing Research Project, a drive to master the theory of medical subject headings, the innovative impact of coordinate indexing, and the confidence produced by the success of the Index Mechanization Project. By virtue of this experience, MEDLARS became a prime example of a well-understood enterprise seeking a computer application, a circumstance which augured of its success.

GERTRUDE Annan, who honored both us and her distinguished predecessor at the New York Academy of Medicine with the first Janet Doe Lecture in 1967, established the theme which I propose to follow today. Addressing the topic, "The Medical Library Association in Retrospect," she chose to signalize those individuals who singlehandedly pioneered professional advances in medical librarianship. Thus, in our traditions she searched out innovation.

So today, as I respond to your invitation to address "an historical or a philosophical topic," I choose to pursue the same paradoxical course of searching out the seeds of today's innovation in yesterday's history. The complete title of my lecture is: "The Way of the Innovator: Notes Toward a Prehistory of MEDLARS." In it I wish to record my own observations, as a

*Janet Doe Lecture in History or Philosophy of Medical Librarianship, presented at the Seventy-first Annual Meeting of the Medical Library Association, San Diego, California, June 13, 1972.

Originally published in *Bulletin of the Medical Library Association*, Volume 60 (October, 1972), pp. 523-533. Reprinted by permission.

bystander, of the events, forces, benchmarks, and breakthroughs of the fifteen-year period which preceded the award of the MEDLARS contract. Because I was an observer, and not a participant, I have entitled my lecture "*Notes* Toward a Prehistory." The history itself is still to be written, hopefully by those who participated in it, and if the errors of fact and the misassessments I may make by reason of my secondhand knowledge cry aloud for corrective retribution, or if the National Library of Medicine can be persuaded to update the Rogers-Schullian history, I shall have been amply repaid for my effort.

The late Ralph Esterquest once paid tribute to MEDLARS: "The impact of MEDLARS on the medical library world is not that of the familiar metaphor—the pebble dropped into the pond, casting concentric circles that reach many points on the shore. The impact is no pebble for sure. It is a mighty rock. The waves it will cause will surge and splash for a long time to come. MEDLARS is the great bibliographical breakthrough of our generation"[1].Let me say "Amen!" to that. Not only in the world of medical libraries, but in that of research libraries, of information science, of information systems nationally and internationally, MEDLARS was the rock which raised the level of the ocean.

Whatever may have been, and indeed still are its shortcomings, MEDLARS has grown to be one of the largest openly available information retrieval systems in any field of science in the world. This alone merits an enquiry into its genesis.

The systems conceptualization and basic design of MEDLARS were fundamental to its success. The understanding of the job to be done, in all of its ramifications, culminated in the technical specifications mailed to the systems industry in February 1961, and there my story will end. The completion of the MEDLARS contract, the continuing effort to improve *MeSH*, the decentralization, first nationally and later internationally, of the MEDLARS search capability, the conversion to an on-line system and to a national service network: all these highly significant accomplishments I commend to the historical attentions of others.

I am concerned here with an exploration of the infrastructure of MEDLARS, the intellectual and managerial foundations, whose firm placement resulted in the later success. The late Verner Clapp stated that the reason for the success of MEDLARS was that it represented a classic example of a well-defined job seeking a technology, rather than the technology seeking an application[2].

We owe this understanding of the job to be done to a group of pioneers. You will note that I say "group." Dr. Frank Bradway Rogers, who led the group, will be the first to admit that, however pervasive his leadership role may have been, the inputs into the continuing effort which became

MEDLARS were many. Indeed, Janet Doe herself contributed to the modernization of the library's indexing program, first as a member of the Survey team assembled by the American Library Association, later as a member of the Committee of Consultants on Indexing, and finally as a member of the Armed Forces Medical Library Advisory Group. The concept of publishing multiple specialized indexes from a common data base, which came to fruition in the MEDLARS recurring bibliographies, can be traced to her suggestion[3].

I have divided my lecture into the following sections:

(1) The Publication Imperative, in which I find the basic motivation which was to drive the National Library of Medicine to MEDLARS;
(2) The Eel of Science, which will concern itself with the pursuit of that slippery and elusive aspect of MEDLARS: the subject indexing of medical papers;
(3) Commotion in the Wings, the offstage background of contemporary noise, without which an understanding of MEDLARS is incomplete; and
(4) The Index Mechanization Project, wherein the publication imperative, the new-found intellectual control, and the contemporary technology were all conjoined for the first time, leading to MEDLARS.

THE PUBLICATION IMPERATIVE

The history of MEDLARS does not begin, as do so many other aspects of the modern National Library of Medicine, with the 1944 Report of the Survey of the Army Medical Library. The Survey did call for renewed effort to rationalize the functions of the three existing bibliographic services: the *Index-Catalogue*, the *Quarterly Cumulative Index Medicus*, and the *Current List of Medical Literature*, a recommendation which was to be translated into a major program objective of the Army Medical Library. Tacitly, the Survey recognized an assumption of earlier origin: a principal, if not a primary function of the library, was to publish an index to the journal literature of the medical sciences.

The annual reports of Librarians of the Library of the Surgeon General's Office may seem to us now like battle reports from tribal chieftains to the Merovingian kings. A constant theme, however, is their sense of responsibility for continuing the indexing traditions laid down by John Shaw Billings. Indeed, their reports are occupied either with proud statements of *Index-Catalogue* volumes achieved or with apologetic statements for nonpublication. "The clerical force is adequate to keep current work up to date," Col. Percy Ashburn reported successively and without alteration in 1928, 1929, 1930, and 1931, "but there is a great accumulation of back work which has lain dormant for many years"[4].

The indexing must go on, and it must be published. The mission formulated by Billings to acquire, to catalog, and to index the literature of the medical sciences endured long after his departure. When, therefore, the ALA surveyors explored the library, they did not question the library's responsibilities for publishing indexes to the literature of medicine. Index publication must continue, and the library must find a solution to the unification of bibliographic services in medicine[5].

It is significant that one of the first responses of the library's new administration was entitled "The Army Medical Library's Publication Program." In this paper, Dr. Rogers and I traced the long history of indexing publication in the library and concluded with the announcement that the Committee of Consultants for the Study of Indexes to the Medical Literature had recommended the cessation of publication of the *Index-Catalogue* and the substitution of a current index to current publications[6].

The appointment of this Committee of Consultants was a major event in the library's history. The Survey Committee had recommended that the library establish an advisory committee on the *Index-Catalogue*, with representatives from the American Medical Association, the Medical Library Association, the Bibliographical Society of America, and the National Research Council. In May 1947, Col. Joseph H. McNinch, then Director, proposed the creation of the Committee, and it was established formally on July 7, 1948.

To provide the Committee with an operating arm, which might concurrently investigate problems of priority concern, Col. McNinch arranged a contract through the Army Research and Development Board with the Johns Hopkins University. The contract of Nov. 5, 1948, established the Welch Medical Indexing Project, under the direction of Dr. Sanford V. Larkey one of the first government-sponsored research projects in the field of information science. It investigated, on behalf of the Committee, the size of universe of biomedical literature, and the extent of its coverage by the existing services, the common and disparate features of subject-heading among the services, and the application of machine methods to medical indexing. It is worthy of note that Dr. Larkey hired a young chemist, Eugene Garfield, to head this last-named activity.

The Committee of Consultants for the Study of Indexes to the Medical Literature met many times between its establishment in 1948 and its discharge on May 1, 1952. It addressed a series of questions relating to the publication of medical indexes, including the following:

—What are the indexing requirements of modern medical science?
—Does the *Quarterly Cumulative Index Medicus* meet these requirements? Does any one of the three indexes in existence, or all of them?

—What modifications of existing publications are necessary to meet these requirements?
—What are the characteristics of a good index, with reference to subject headings, with reference to periodicity, with reference to cumulative issue, with reference to format and printing characteristics?
—What are the possibilities of using mechanical devices to accelerate indexing?

These were both urgent and practical questions relating to the library's traditional responsibility for publishing an index.

For the library in 1945 had taken over the responsibility for the publication of the *Current List of Medical Literature*, which Dr. Atherton Seidell had developed and supported with private funds as a means of announcing the availability of free microfilms. It had done so without adequate calculation of the manpower resources and organization required for its production.

By May 1949, when the Medical Library Association met in Galveston, the weekly issues were a month behind schedule, and the monthly indexes were a year behind. Emergency assignment to the Catalog Division, and a tripling of the staff, were successful in eliminating the backlog, but even as the Committee of Consultants were debating the form of a future index, the fate of the one already undertaken by the library was in doubt. Small wonder that the dominant consideration, becoming at times almost an obsession, was the library's responsibility successfully to publish a current medical index.

Seymour Taine became the Editor of the newly reconstituted *Current List* in August 1949, and the library dedicated itself to a course which was to lead through many vicissitudes to the Index Mechanization Project of 1958-60, and to MEDLARS.

This is not to suggest that the course of the *Current List* was tranquil. Indeed, in 1953 and 1954, Rogers and Taine, with the support of members of the AFML Advisory Group, had to fight for its life against conditions and restrictions placed on it by the Bureau of the Budget and higher echelons within the Department of Defense. This dramatic episode, in which for a time all appeared lost, served but to strengthen the library's dedication to index publication.

"I believe," wrote Rogers to members of the Advisory Group, at the time of crisis, "that the *Current List* has the greatest and most immediate social usefulness of all the activities of the library, in proportion to dollar expenditure"[7]. The *Current List* survived the crisis. The *Index-Catalogue* was brought to a successful, albeit truncated, conclusion, and the *QCIM* was terminated. In the final resolution of the duplication of index-publication functions between the library and the American Medical Association,

Rogers achieved a cooperative agreement for the latter to publish the annual cumulation of the new *Index Medicus* from copy compiled by the library.

This has been an abbreviated record of the enormous preoccupation of the library with its responsibility for publishing an index to the medical literature of the world. This preoccupation was a principal force leading to MEDLARS. It accounted, in the Index Mechanization Project, for the priority, assigned to the publication system over the retrieval capability, and in MEDLARS itself for the unit record concept, and for the library's requirement for graphic arts quality computer printout, which led to the development of the Zip Photon. It led also to the exploitation of MEDLARS power to produce specialized recurring bibliographies, and it is still a prime dynamic of MEDLARS.

The Eel Of Science

How index learning turns no student pale,
Yet holds the eel of science by the tail.
Alexander Pope

A second theme in the prehistory of MEDLARS is that of the library's long and still-continuing occupation with the theory and practice of subject controls for the literature of biomedicine. Harold Bloomquist has provided us with an excellent review of the attention given to subject cataloging by medical librarians generally[8]. Within the National Library of Medicine, there was a special concern for subject controls by virtue of the library's index and catalog publication responsibilities. Anecdotal material, sometimes apocryphal, from the life of John Shaw Billings usually serves to illustrate this traditional concern.

I choose to dip into the library's more remote past for only one passing reference to Billings. Dr. Silas Newcomb, the famous American astronomer, and Dr. Billings were selected to represent the United States at the conference convened by the Royal Society of London in 1896 to plan the *International Catalogue of Scientific Literature.* Otlet and La Fontaine, representing Belgium at this Conference, vigorously proposed the use of the newly elaborated Universal Decimal Classification as the basis for organizing the *Catalogue,* and Billings just as resolutely opposed them, arguing for indexing under subject rubrics. "But," interposed LaFontaine, "the French do not have a word for 'indexing'. It will be necessary to invent one. Let us call it 'l'indexation' "[9].

Billings prevailed, and the Royal Society developed a classification for the *Catalogue* independent of Dewey and the U.D.C., a circumstance which Bradford, writing nearly fifty years later called "the worst of the calamities" to befall the U.D.C.[10].

At the 1896 conference, Billings offered the following conclusions from a lifetime of medical indexing: "The scientific relations of any subject extend not merely in space of one dimension, but in all the varieties of space of three dimensions, and no possible linear arrangement that can be made will suit the wants of a great majority of enquirers. The scientific investigator is always seeking to make new combinations; he will not be satisfied with any arrangement, nor can any arrangement be made in science, that will be at all permanently satisfactory"[11].

In the years prior to the Survey of 1944, the *Index-Catalogue* had become the bibliographic tail which wagged the library dog. The surveyors were hypercritical both of the internal inconsistencies in the organization of the *Index-Catalogue*, and of its indifference to a standard list of subject headings for medicine. In what is perhaps one of the more simplistic of statements made about a complex intellectual function, the surveyors called for such a standard list, and proposed that "headings chosen should be those most commonly known and used in this country, and adequate cross references should be provided to round out the system"[5]. They proposed further that "the list of subject headings that has been worked out by the *Quarterly Cumulative Index Medicus*" be taken as the basis of the new list. Parenthetically, it might be noted that the *QCIM* Authority List, dating to 1935, is one of the earliest examples of a thesaurus for an indexing system.

For a library which had never had a book classification, the Surveyors recommended the development of a modern scheme "to be based (hopefully) on a thorough revision of the Library of Congress schedules for medicine, with certain basic ideas drawn from the Cunningham classification"[5]. Mary Louise Marshall of the Survey team was given a contract to develop this new classification.

A preliminary version of the new classification was delivered to the library in 1948 and was promptly referred by the library's Director, Col. Joseph H. McNinch, to Dr. (then Major) Rogers, working on his master's degree in library science at Columbia University. Dr. Rogers's introduction to the subject control of library materials was thus far from academic; with his extraordinary ability to organize masses of detail, he inundated the library with a spate of revisions, which were incorporated in time for a first edition of the *Classification* in September 1949.

In the meantime, even prior to Dr. Rogers's involvement with the *Classification*, the library had taken a preliminary step to implement one of the Survey's recommendations. On December 12-13, 1947, the library conducted a Symposium on Medical Subject Headings for the dual purpose of addressing the questions: What principles may be found for developing subject heading terminology in the medical sciences? and What are the recognizable differences in principles to be applied to the subject heading of monographic and periodical literature?

Janet Doe presented a paper "A Critical Review of Existing Medical Subject Heading Lists," and Sanford Larkey, soon to contract with the Army Research and Development Board for the Welch Medical Indexing Project, a paper on "Introduction to the Problems of Medical Subject Heading." An extracurricular activity of this symposium, however, is particularly prophetic. The minutes of the Symposium contain this note: "During the recess before discussion, Col. McNinch led a group through the Medical Statistics Division, Office of the Surgeon General, where the IBM punch card machinery was in operation. Possible application of punch card controls for medical bibliography was suggested"[12].

The 1947 symposium came at the low point in the library's indexing fortunes. The backlog problem had in fact become so acute that the MLA meeting in Galveston in April 1948 took formal action to urge the library to catch up. Volunteers were welcomed at that time, with Helen Bayne preparing the May 1948 and Mary Louise Marshall the June 1948 subject indexes to the *Current List.*

By heroic efforts, the indexing backlogs were reduced by the time Dr. Rogers became Director of the library on October 21, 1949. Seymour Taine had been made Acting Editor on August 19 of that year, and the staff of the *Current List* had been considerably augmented. With the major work of the revision of the classification behind him, Dr. Rogers could devote time to the stubborn intellectual problems of subject headings.

The Welch Medical Library Indexing Project had as one of its objectives exploration of "The theory and practice of subject heading (nomenclature) and classification (coding) as they concern medical literature." Helen Field, Williamina Himwich, and Sanford Larkey, working on the Project, had explored the principles underlying the subject heading practices of the *Index-Catalogue* and the *Quarterly Cumulative Index Medicus.* They found the categorization of the terms used convenient for purposes of analysis, and created sixteen categories, a prototype of the *MeSH* categories[13].

From the outset, Dr. Rogers was confronted with the necessity of solving problems of subject heading in two separate, but related contexts: that of providing a subject catalog for the library and that of creating a subject indexing authority list for the *Current List.* The problem had many interesting ramifications. Not only were there differences of traditions of library cataloging and scientific indexing; there were also fundamental differences in user groups and their purposes, and in the characteristics and forms of the literatures.

The revitalized *Current List* had depended on the *QCIM* list for its subject heading authority. This list needed updating and was not suited to the new indexing style of the library's "Index." It became imperative to implement the Surveyors' recommendation and to develop an authority list proper to the *Current List.*

The theoretical work done on subject headings in the Welch project was discontinued, and a team including Dr. Rogers, Mr. Taine, Mrs. Gertrude Butler, and Miss Helen Field undertook a crash effort to produce on 6335 IBM cards, by October 1951, the list which became the first *Subject Heading Authority List(SHAL).* The Field categories again proved useful in dividing up the work.

With this introduction, both practical and urgent, Dr. Rogers set for himself an intellectual challenge which has occupied his professional career—to master the principles underlying the construction and use of formal systems of subject headings in the medical sciences. I need only remind you that the subject of his own Janet Doe Lecture in 1968 had to do with the impact of changes in *MeSH* on the subject catalog of his library.

Dr. Rogers's first conclusions were published in a collection edited by his Columbia mentor and colleague, Dr. Maurice Tauber, *The Subject Analysis of Library Materials*[14].

Noting that subject control of the periodical literature is a preeminent requirement in science, Dr. Rogers proceeded to analyze the likenesses and differences between subject headings for periodical indexes and book catalogs. He concluded that the similarities were basic (a conclusion which was to lead later to the use of *MeSH* for both the *Index Medicus* and the *NLM Catalog*), and that the principal differences arose from the need for topical subdivision in indexes, as well as a more intensive degree of subject analysis. This theme and its variations were to preoccupy Dr. Rogers until he resolved the conflict by creating *MeSH* (or *MSH*, as it was initially known) as a combined indexing and subject heading authority list in 1959.

In the meantime, a new and a very powerful influence on the library emerged. Dr. Mortimer Taube, after serving as Chief of the Science and Technology Division, Library of Congress, and Deputy Chief for Scientific Information of the Atomic Energy Commission, had established Documentation, Inc., as a vehicle for expounding, marketing, and further developing his revolutionary concept of coordinate indexing. Many of us on the Washington scene were fascinated with the simplicity of Taube's concept of posting items on subject terms, instead of subject terms on items, as we had been taught. We watched with great interest his installation of Uniterm indexing at the Armed Services Technical Information Agency (ASTIA) and read avidly his *Studies in Coordinate Indexing.*

Dr. Rogers became one of the staunchest interpreters and defenders of Taube in the library profession. His two reviews of Taube's work showed him not only to have mastered the implications of Taube's original thought but also to be an active champion for Taube, seeking to stir up the library community to this powerful new idea. Rogers did not follow Taube blindly, however. As friends who had taken each other's measure, they must have argued long over the principles underlying Uniterms. "What was and is essentially wrong with the Uniterm system," wrote Rogers in his staunchest exposition of Taube's work, "is not its unusual posting system, and certainly not its central coordinate indexing concept, but its employment of article-derived catchwords in preference to a carefully chosen controlled vocabulary of terms"[15].

Rogers's philosophy of medical subject headings, which he had worked out through wrestling with might and main with this most challenging and elusive of topics, is best expressed in the prefatory matter to the first edition of *MeSH*, 1960. Subject cataloging and periodical indexing are, in their major dimensions, identical processes, and a single authority should be used for both. Headings should be considered as pointers, not as descriptive labels. Topical subheadings, as substitutes for phrase headings, can be standardized, and should be, in contrast to specific main headings that generally represent broad concepts.

It is interesting to note, in the 1960 Preface, the influence of the coordinate indexing concept: Subject headings, being pointers, "the intersect of two or more such pointers will define a very specific subject"[16].

The second edition of *MeSH* was prepared specifically in anticipation of its use in the search operations of MEDLARS. Winifred Sewell joined the library in May 1961 as the first full-time editor. The sixty-seven subheadings of *MeSH* 1, in combination with the main headings, exceeded the estimated capability of the developing system, and after test with a more finite set of subheadings had failed, it was decided to abandon topical subheadings and to substitute where practicable precoordinated terms. The categories were thoroughly reviewed, and authoritative nomenclatures checked for the most generally accepted terminology.

Over the years immediately preceding MEDLARS, much effort went into the preparation of the *MeSH* vocabulary for machine retrieval. *MeSH* was evolving into a controlled list of descriptors, and away from a list of conventional subject headings. "The new subject heading," said Rogers in reporting on computer developments to the Board of Regents, "says in effect, 'There it is, right there'. Two or more of the new subject headings will indicate a precise point most satisfactorily, as by an intersection of vectors. What is more, they lend themselves more readily to adequate control, and maintenance of consistency in the retrieval vocabulary is a necessity"[17].

Thus did the library prepare itself intellectually over the years, through trial and error, theory and practice, for the advent of MEDLARS. Since

Billings, the vocabulary had been built laboriously from the living literature; the structure had been evolved through both trial and error and theory.

Despite this long record of experience, the testing of the vocabulary under operating conditions showed need in many areas for improvement. The need continues, as evaluation and testing have shown. But the main outlines and structure of *Me*SH have survived, a credit to the effort which Dr. Rogers expended on this most intractable of problems.

Commotion in the Wings

This is not the place, nor do I have the time, to describe at any length the onrush of contemporary events in the world of information retrieval, yet no discussion of the prehistory of MEDLARS can be complete without an understanding of the frenetic environment in which the library's concepts matured. Memex, Vannevar Bush's electronic adaptation of the World Brain proposed by H. G. Wells, had captured the imagination of all. With the creation of ENIAC and SEAC, the electronic revolution was upon us, and the computer age had been born. Imaginations were unbridled; potential applications to bibliographical management proliferated; initiatives abounded, and research and development funds flowed freely.

Rapid and spectacular as was the growth of data processing capability and systems technology during these years, the growth of projects conceived to apply them to the "information problem" was even more dramatic. Industry aided and abetted academic enthusiasts; information processing technology was overadvertised and oversold on every hand. At dozens of meetings and symposia, and at industrial tutorial retreats, statements descriptive of potential applications of mechanized information handling were presented in the declarative mood, rather than in the more correct subjunctive. These were indeed exciting, if frustrating, times.

One can even be nostalgic about some of these developments. Where are the systems of yesteryear? A review of the National Science Foundation's publication *Current Research and Development in Scientific Documentation* for these early years reveals dozens of names, once billed as universal solutions, now fading into history. Documentation, Inc., produced COMAC, Kodak developed MINICARD, while Magnavox worked on MAGNACARD. The CIA engaged in Product Walnut. The National Bureau of Standards perfected a "peek-a-boo" system for controlling the literature of basic instrumentation. The National Research Council organized the Chemical Biological Coordination Center for punched card control of information on the biological action of chemical compounds. Western Reserve promoted "semantic factoring" as the ultimate intellectual control over information and constructed the WRU Searching Selector to use it. The Zator Company developed Zatocoding, while George Washington University worked out Tabledex.

There were claims and counterclaims, rivalries and polemics, and one scarcely knew whether to place bets on a sure thing, or whether to play the field.

The first Sputnik added greatly to the confusion. Politicians rapidly convinced themselves, not without help from American information specialists, that the spectacular Soviet success was due to a superior scientific and technical information service, and charted a course of national competition to catch up with, and then best, the Soviets. The management of scientific and technical information programs by federal agencies came under the critical scrutiny of both houses of Congress; oil was poured on the fires of competition, and technological confusion compounded with political commotion.

The National Library of Medicine inevitably drew the attention of Senators and Congressmen who, on more than one occasion, expressed their impatience with the library's inability to match some of the more imaginative solutions to the science information problem then being proposed by the library's contemporaries in academia and industry.

But during these years the overbearing problems of the library were not technical ones relating to information retrieval. As a responsible operating agency with publication deadlines to meet, the library's problems were concerned with getting the work done and on time. They were major organizational and management ones: the interagency struggles, as well as those internal to the Department of Defense, for the stewardship of the library; resistance to the transfer of the library to Chicago, the drafting and passage of legislation establishing the National Library of Medicine; and, above all, that supreme imperative, the new building.

Inevitably, Dr. Rogers and his associates were involved in the new information technology as critics and advisors. They attended the documentation and information science meetings and symposia and served as consultants on such projects as the Cardiovascular Literature Indexing Project of the National Research Council. They were in the world of systems, and yet not quite part of it. As a responsible and overburdened manager, Rogers was appalled by the nonsense and waste which he identified in so many of these efforts to reinvent wheels, and made no bones about saying so. This experience not only kept him and the library currently aware of the developing technology; it sharpened his judgment and firmed his convictions on what would or would not work.

The Index Mechanization Project

The new *Current List of Medical Literature* had begun its publication under Seymour Taine's editorship in 1950 in three separate sections: the article registry, and the subject and author indexes. A serial numbering device was used to link the two indexes to the full citation found in the registry. In nine years of successful production, the index had seen a steady growth; journals covered had increased from 1,225 to 1,600, and articles indexed reached 110,000.

But a 1957 survey by Estelle Brodman and Seymour Taine for the International Conference on Scientific Information had estimated the current world production of medical papers at 220,000, and the NLM was under compulsion to increase its coverage. However, the larger the issues became, the more cumbersome the process of referral and rereferral between the index sections and the article registry. Clearly a new format was essential.

This practical problem led to a decision to undertake a development project to apply the best of the current information processing technology to the production of the *Current List*. An application for $73,800 to support a two-year developmental project was submitted to and approved by the Council on Library Resources in the Spring of 1958[18].

Index publication was still the imperative. The project's objectives were those of "developing and demonstrating in the field of medicine improved methods for the rapid and efficient publication of comprehensive indexes to the literature of broad scientific fields, with simultaneous provision for meeting the requirements of specialties within these fields, making use of hitherto unutilized mechanical applications"[19].

It might be noted that the secondary objective, the "simultaneous provision" was conceived of in terms of "encoding unit-citation cards . . . to make them immediately available for whatever limited indexes that might be desired (for example: cancer chemotherapy listing; cardiovascular drugs listing)." The objective was closer to what Janet Doe had proposed in 1952 and to the recurring bibliographies of MEDLARS than it was to bibliographic search on demand. In passing, it may be noted that an Advisory Committee to the project included both Dr. Eugene Garfield and Dr. Sanford Larkey, a provision for continuity between the Welch Project and the library's new venture.

The published report of the Index Mechanization Project is generally conceded to be one of the more candid records of the successes and failures of an information systems development project ever written. The operational history, demonstrating the almost daily operation of Murphy's Law (if anything can go wrong, it will) has been the envy of many report writers.

The project accomplished its primary objective brilliantly, and the published *Index Medicus* from 1960 through 1963 is its monument. It failed in its efforts to achieve the type of subject retrieval that would permit the publication of specialized bibliographies.

But, as Dr. Rogers stated in his *Annual Report* for 1960, "As for the ill-fated bibliographic retrieval system—despite the negative outcome, much valuable experience and knowledge has accrued which may well be of greater significance in the long run than the successful publication program. . . .NLM received the impetus for further investigation of the application of more sophisticated mechanized techniques, which will continue to influence the library in the future"[20].

I believe this conservatively worded forecast of things to come owes its origin to an educational event which occurred in the fall of 1958. The Central Intelligence Agency had sent Joseph Becker to UCLA to study information retrieval and to familiarize himself with the advances made by the Southern California computer industry. Foster Mohrhardt, then with the National Agricultural Library, at Becker's suggestion, persuaded Dr. Rogers and Verner W. Clapp to pay Becker a visit. The four friends visited many California firms, discussed information retrieval systems, and argued over a ten-day period.

Dr. Rogers had gone to California a skeptic, believing without doubt that the California systems approaches were no better and no worse than those he had criticized on the East Coast. He returned a changed man, with a new set of convictions. As in the case of subject headings, he had wrestled the problem to the mat and won. He had met the computer, and had become its master. Indeed, so thoroughly had he mastered the principles of the computer that he presented to the NLM Board of Regents at the instigation of Dr. Michael DeBakey, then Chairman, a tutorial on the "Consideration of the Use of Computers in Bibliographical Tasks"[21].

I can hear him now as he elucidated programming to the Board members. "If we want to tell a clerk to put a letter on the table, we can say, 'Put this over there'. But suppose we have to instruct a mechanical robot to do the same thing. We would give him a long sequence of minute instructions: 'Extend right hand. Open fingers. Accept letter. Close fingers. Lower arm. Turn 180 degrees. Place left foot ahead of right foot. Place right foot ahead of left foot. Etc. Etc. Halt. Extend right arm. Open fingers. Turn. Etc.' "

This was what the computer business all boiled down to: detailed instructions to accomplish a predetermined objective. And meticulous attention to detail and to accuracy is present both in library cataloging and in computer programming. Medical indexing and the computer obviously were made for each other.

This new-found confidence in the library's ability to understand and utilize the computer was added to the earlier foundations: a long and successful record in the management of indexing and of index publication, a hard-earned mastery over the principles of subject heading, an enthusiasm for the philosophy of coordinate indexing, and an outstanding success in the Index Mechanization Project. All the preconditions necessary to MEDLARS were here but one, the necessary financial resources.

These came from a quite unexpected source. The law establishing the National Heart Institute within the National Institutes of Health authorized the Surgeon General to "establish an information center on research, prevention and treatment of heart disease." In an effort to secure guidance on what he might do most effectively to implement this statutory responsibility, Dr. James Watt, Director of the National Heart Institute, in January 1960 commissioned a study. Mr. J. Douglas Knox, the contractor-investigator, noting the scope of the library's coverage of the biomedical literature, the success of its Index Mechanization Project, and its interest in further developmental work, concluded that "establishing an effective flow of scientific communications is a problem of documentation which logically suggests a collaborative effort with the NLM." He recommended that the National Heart Institute establish a joint working group with NLM to explore advanced techniques for information retrieval[22].

The Knox Report is amazingly prophetic. Knox proposed "a collaborative plan with the National Library of Medicine, whereby NLM would be responsible for the mechanized storage of the world's biomedical literature, and selective retrieval geared to the needs of the cardiovascular scientist; and whereby the National Heart Institute would be responsible for planning utilization programs for the basic bibliographical and documentary data produced automatically by NLM, with servicing of requests from regional centers by an electronic network joined with the master center at Bethesda, from which current lists, abstracts and facsimile documents could be rapidly disseminated."

The Knox Report led to negotiations between the library and the National Heart Institute, and at its fall meeting in 1960 the National Advisory Heart Council approved the transfer of $500,000 from NHI to NLM for the purpose of initiating the development project.

The fall months of 1960 were spent in drafting the technical specifications for MEDLARS. The necessary arrangements were made with the Public Health Service contracting officials for advertising for bids.

It has been stated that in the Index Mechanization Project the library had as its objective the development of a publication system from which a retrieval subsystem might be derived. The serial search of the million punched cards produced annually, however, made the subsystem impractical.

In contrast, MEDLARS was conceived of as a system based on individual machine-readable citation records from which both a publication system and a retrieval system might be elaborated with equal facility. This is evidenced in the primary objectives associated with the statement of specifications, which included among the desiderata not only an increase in the volume and speed of indexing publication, but also "the prompt and efficient servicing of relatively complex demand requests for bibliographic information, and recurring bibliographies on such topics as 'diseases of the cardiovascular systems.' "

On Feb. 2, 1961, the technical specifications, accompanied by invitations to submit proposals, were sent to forty selected commercial and nonprofit organizations. The word spread throughout industry, and before the deadline for submission of bids arrived, some seventy-two companies had indicated their interest. Twenty-five proposals in all were received by the deadline, April 24, 1961[23]. It is worthy of note that the industry was highly complimentary over the thoroughness, the precision, and the clarity with which the specifications were drafted, a circumstance which paid tribute to the library's comprehension in detail of the job to be done, and of the ability of the computer to perform it.

It has been fashionable to comment that while John Shaw Billings conceived the *Index Catalogue* in 1876 and the punched card in 1883, it took over eighty years before the two were successfully married. For those who may believe that successful information retrieval systems are products of instant parthenogenesis, I wish it noted that even after the punched card technology and medical indexing were introduced to each other in the Welch Medical Indexing Project, it took ten years of ardent and arduous courtship before the union could occur.

REFERENCES

1. Esterquest, Ralph T. Discussion of paper presented by Taine, Seymour I. Bibliographic data processing at the National Library of Medicine. In: Clinic on Library Applications of Data Processing, University of Illinois. Proceedings of the 1963 Clinic. Champaign, Ill., The Illini Union Bookstore, 1964. p. 124-125.
2. Clapp, Verner W. Personal communication.
3. Doe, Janet. Methods for medical indexing. Bull. Med. Libr. Assoc. 39: 23-27, Jan. 1951.
4. U.S. Army. Surgeon General's Office. Annual reports, 1928, 1929, 1930, 1931.
5. Metcalf, Keyes D. [and others]. The National Medical Library; Report of a Survey of the Army Medical Library. Chicago, American Library Association, 1944.
6. Rogers, Frank B., and Adams, Scott. The Army Medical Library's publication program. Texas Rep. Biol. Med. 8: 271-300, Summer 1950.
7. Rogers, Frank B. Memorandum to Members of the AFML Advisory Group, 5 Jan. 1954.
8. Bloomquist, Harold. Cataloging and classification of medical library materials, 1946-1956. Ten years of progress and problems. Bull. Med. Libr. Assoc. 47: 28-47, Jan. 1959.

9. INTERNATIONAL CONFERENCE ON A CATALOGUE OF SCIENTIFIC LITERATURE. Report of the Proceedings . . . July 14-17, 1896. London, The Royal Society, 1896, p. 27.
10. BRADFORD, S.C. Documentation. London, Crosby, Lockwood & Son, 1953, p. 140.
11. *Op. cit.*, p. 78-79.
12. Symposium on Medical Subject Headings. Minutes of the Symposium . . . Dec. 12-13, 1947. Washington, Army Medical Library, 1947, p. 3.
13. FIELD, HELEN G. [and others]. Final Report on Subject Headings and on Subject Indexing. Baltimore, Welch Medical Library Indexing Project, The Johns Hopkins University, 1955.
14. ROGERS, FRANK B. Application and limitations of subject headings: the pure and applied sciences. In: Tauber, Maurice F., ed. The Subject Analysis of Library Materials. N.Y., Columbia University School of Library Service, 1953.
15. ROGERS, FRANK B. Review of Taube, Mortimer. Emerging solutions for mechanizing the storage and retrieval of information. (Studies in Coordinate Indexing, vol. 5) Coll. and Res. Libr. 21: 489-492, Nov. 1960. See also, Rogers, Frank B. Review of Taube, Mortimer. Studies in coordinate indexing. Bull. Med. Libr. Assoc. 42: 380-384, July 1954.
16. NATIONAL LIBRARY OF MEDICINE. Medical Subject Headings. First Edition. Washington, Government Printing Office, 1960. p. i-xix.
17. ROGERS, FRANK B. Consideration of the Usė of Computers in Bibliographical Tasks. Unpublished abridged version of a paper presented at the Meeting of the National Library of Medicine Board of Regents, April 11, 1960.
18. TAINE, SEYMOUR I. New program for indexing at the National Library of Medicine. Bull. Med. Libr. Assoc. 47: 117-123, Apr. 1959.
19. NATIONAL LIBRARY OF MEDICINE. Index Mechanization Project, July 1, 1958—June 30, 1960, Bull. Med. Libr. Assoc. 49, no. 1, pt. 2. Jan. 1961.
20. NATIONAL LIBRARY OF MEDICINE. Annual Report for the Fiscal Year 1960. Washington, National Library of Medicine, 1960. p. 41.
21. ROGERS, *op, cit.*, p. 6-7.
22. KNOX, J. DOUGLAS. Report of a Study on Collection and Dissemination of Heart Research Information. Bethesda, National Heart Institute, 1960.
23. NATIONAL LIBRARY OF MEDICINE. Annual Report for the Fiscal Year 1961. Washington, National Library of Medicine, 1961. p. 27-29.

The View Behind and Ahead: Implications of Certification*

By Louise Darling, *Librarian*

Biomedical Library
Center for the Health Sciences
University of California, Los Angeles

ABSTRACT

The Medical Library Association's certification plan, never of real significance in employment and promotion practices in health sciences librarianship, does not reflect the many changes which have occurred in swift progression since adoption of the code in 1949. Solutions to the problems which have accumulated since then are sought in a brief examination of trends in credentialing and certification in the health professions and in the library field, both general and special. Emphasis is given to the historical development of provisions in the MLA Code for the Training and Certification of Medical Librarians, the limited opportunity for practical implementation of most of the provisions, the importance of the code in stimulating the Association's educational programs, the impact of the Medical Library Assistance Act, Regional Medical Programs, and increases in demand for health information on manpower requirements for health science libraries, the specific dissatisfactions MLA members have expressed over certification, and the role of the Ad Hoc Committee to Develop a New Certification Code.

OUR Association has been talking about education, standards, and certification for medical librarianship for most of its life. At least a half million words and probably a good many more must have appeared in the *Bulletin* on this complex of topics. What more can there possibly be to say? Why then choose certification on this for me once in a lifetime occasion? The reasons are many. First, the charge to the Janet Doe Lecturer is to speak on a philosophical or historical aspect of medical librarianship. Certification nicely combines both aspects and thus seemed to me appropriate for the Medical Library Association's seventy-fifth anniversary.

*Janet Doe Lecture in History or Philosophy of Medical Librarianship, presented at the Seventy-second Annual Meeting of the Medical Library Association, Kansas City, Missouri, May 29, 1973.

Originally published in *Bulletin of the Medical Library Association*, Volume 61 (October, 1973), pp. 375-386. Reprinted by permission.

Second, certification has a direct-indirect relation to the theme of this conference, "Are health science librarians prepared to meet the challenge of their jobs?" Further, though there may be nothing very new or revolutionary to say about certification, the subject is in many ways once more as far from being settled as it was in 1946 when Mary Louise Marshall introduced it at the Association's first post-World War II conference. The lack of definitive action on revision of certification policy is holding up a good deal of Association business. Currently affected are questions before the Committees on Membership, Curriculum, Internship, Medical Library Technician Training, Continuing Education, Central Office, Finance and, of course, Certification. Finally, and of special significance to me, certification was and is a subject close to the heart of Janet Doe herself whose ideals and ambitions for the Association in combination with her practical understanding of and gentle sympathy for the professional problems of all its members we pay homage to in this annual lecture. The original Code for the Training and Certification of Medical Librarians was adopted during the year of her presidency of MLA at the Annual Meeting of 1949 in Galveston.

In the time allotted I want to say a few things about certification in general and its impact on librarianship and the health professions, make a few observations on the course it has run within the Medical Library Association, then discuss our current problems and a few of the solutions which have been suggested.

Occupations are generally classified as professional, technical, managerial, clerical, sales, skilled, semi-skilled, and unskilled with endless subdivisions into particular occupations[1]. The strong trend toward upward career mobility results in shifts not only of individuals from one occupation to another, but also in the effort of occupational groups to move from one classification to another toward eventual professional status. Boundaries of the professions are thus fluid and indistinct and there are many borderline groups whose professional status is equivocal, but the generally recognized core criteria are these: (1) formal technical training which aims at mastery of a generalized cultural tradition in a manner emphasizing its intellectual components and development of skills in some form of its application, (2) an institutionalized mode of validating the adequacy of training and the competence of trained individuals, and (3) institutional means of making sure competence will be put to socially responsible uses[2]. (The tedious question of whether librarianship is a profession is not at issue here; the Association assumes it is in its definition of active membership.)

The efforts to validate training and competency and to safeguard society have led to accreditation, licensing, certification, and registration. The

National Commission on Accrediting defines these terms as follows:

> *Accreditation* is the process by which an agency or organization evaluates and recognizes a program of study or an institution as meeting certain predetermined qualifications or standards. It shall apply only to institutions and their programs of study or their services. [MLA has been using this process to approve medical library courses in American Library Association accredited library schools.]
>
> *Licensure* is the process by which an agency of government grants permission to persons meeting predetermined qualifications to engage in a given occupation and/or use a particular title or grants permission to institutions to perform specified functions.
>
> *Certification* is the process by which a nongovernmental agency or association grants recognition to an individual who has met certain predetermined qualifications specified by that agency or association. [It may be more or less mandatory for the group or voluntary as in MLA.]
>
> *Registration* is the process by which qualified individuals are listed on an official roster maintained by a governmental or nongovernmental agency[3].

These definitions are not, however, universally followed. For example, state and local governments certify school and public librarians.

Regulation of the professions began early in America with a major emphasis on the field of education where certification made its first formal appearance in the Massachusetts Education Act of 1654 which provided for letters of approval for prospective teachers who passed an oral test of religious and political orthodoxy. Armed with the letter of approval, the candidate next presented himself to the town council, whose prime requirements generally were strength of arm and will, for the man without them ran the risk of a beating by the students he sought to teach. County certification of teachers began in 1825 and led later to local certification of librarians whose functions were linked with those of teachers in the public mind[4]. There were also varying degrees of state control of medical practice from colonial times onward, but licensing in the modern sense did not begin until the latter part of the nineteenth century. State legislatures tended to have considerably higher regard for examination and degree from the early medical schools than for apprenticeship and public examination. As the country expanded and proprietary schools sprang up to meet the need for doctors, the standards of medical education became very heterogeneous and in many instances markedly inferior. However, with the founding of the American Medical Association (1847) and the strengthening of key state associations pressures again developed for state legislation to regulate the practice of medicine so that by 1895 all the existing states had established procedures for examination and licensing of physicians[5]. The latter half of the nineteenth century also saw other health professions organizing on a national basis to set standards for education and practice, e.g., the American Dental Association in 1859, the American Veterinary Medical Association in 1863, and the American Nurses Association in 1896.

The proliferation of associations since then has been second only to the proliferation of new journal titles. Occupational groups of every size and variety are organized into societies which seek to raise standards, presumably in the public interest, engage in programs to forward the field, specify and maintain control of education for entry into the group, and gain recognition and economic betterment for members. Credentialing is obviously a direct avenue to most of these objectives.

A great deal of attention is at present focused on licensing and certification in the health professions because of the effects of these procedures on the management of health manpower, as many of you are well aware. Not surprisingly, many of the problems are similar or contiguous to our own; some of the solutions being tested certainly merit our careful study.

There are close to 200 separate health occupations which can be identified now by distinct job title, with a forecast for 20 to 25 supportive personnel for each physician alone in the near future[6]. As knowledge is extended into more scientific areas, specialization of personnel grows more pronounced as well as specialization in functions created to provide services from the new knowledge. This means more categories of positions and classifications. New classifications, in turn, promote organizations of people to share common interests and to gain common goals, economic, political, social or professional in nature. The organizations push toward recognition by licensure or at least certification and in the process develop restrictions on who can and cannot enter the field and what duties are appropriate to it[7]. This fragmentation of the field keeps pace with the ever expanding demand for health care and simultaneously contributes to inflating costs, all at a time when a national health insurance system has become one of the country's top priorities. Problems of licensure and certification are obviously only a part of the health manpower crisis, but they are among the more serious ones. It is no wonder then that health leaders are calling for a moratorium on licensure and certification of new ancillary occupations while ways are sought to revamp old provisions so that there is greater flexibility in modes for entering an occupation or profession and in the duties which are regarded as proper to it. In revising licensure laws affecting the primary providers of health care (the physician, dentist, nurse, etc.) the chief need is seen as provision for more delegation of routine procedures so that full advantage can be taken of nurse practitioners, physicians' assistants, vocational nurses, nursing assistants, etc. In both ancillary and primary areas requirements for initial testing of competencies need to be made far more relevant to the jobs to be done, while the rapid obsolescence of information makes it essential that there be rigorous standards for making sure competencies are kept up-to-date. Also, to counterbalance the guild-like orientation common to many licensing and certifying bodies, there should be representation on them not only of practitioners from the occupation involved, but also of members who reflect the interests of consumers, educators, other health care providers, and related occupational groups[6].

Though credentialing problems are still to be solved on a broad scale, recommendations growing from numerous conferences are under study by health professions associations, and possible solutions are being tested in limited areas. Proficiency testing is under development in both the primary care area, e.g., in orthopaedic surgery and pediatric cardiology, and the ancillary areas, e.g., medical laboratory work, physical therapy and occupational therapy, as validation of educational requirements and evidence of the individual's ability to perform at a certain level. Equivalency testing, designed originally for universities and colleges to use in granting academic credits for off-campus learning, should prove widely valuable for health science employers and certifying bodies to use in equating nonformal study and on-the-job learning with the kind of job preparation expected from formal programs.

There has been widespread consideration by professional societies of ways and means to implement continuing education programs but, as we know from MLA experience, truly successful programs require great effort, money, and long refining. Thus far only a small number of national organizations have continuing education requirements for renewal of certification, among them the American Academy of Family Practice, American Dental Assistants Association, American Dietetic Association, National Board for Certification in Dental Laboratory Technology, and American Registry of Clinical Radiography Technologists. At the state level the Oregon Medical Association led the way in 1968 with a C.E. requirement for membership renewal, a pattern a few additional states have followed and more are pondering. The American College of Physicians has offered its members voluntary, self-administered examinations, and the AMA has its Physician Recognition Award for 150 hours of continuing education courses in a continuous three-year period. Many associations, of course, sponsor courses for their members and potential members. There is less activity in the licensing area though state boards are also moving by various routes in the direction of C.E. requirements for relicensing[8]. Three major questions for either recertification or relicensing are how to evaluate C.E. requirements, how, in the interest of mobility and reciprocity, to attain more nationwide uniformity in requirements, and how to make requirements fair and meaningful for health professionals in geographically remote or isolated places.

The parallels of MLA certification problems with those in the health professions at large do not need belaboring. I want to refer to them again in the last section of my remarks, but before then let us take a quick look at certification efforts in the rest of the library world.

Library associations have always agreed that promoting the qualifications of their members through education and training programs is a major objective; they have disagreed on the best ways to lead them to it. The two main approaches have been by accrediting institutions on the one hand, by certifying individuals on the other, though no association has followed either way exclusively[9]. The organization which has come nearest to doing so is the Library Association in Great Britain where certification by examination is specified in its charter. The Library Association grants certificates of competence at two levels: the A.L.A. (Associate of the Library Association) for those who meet the educational qualifications, are members of the Association, pass a set of examinations, and complete three years of experience in approved libraries; and the F.L.A. (Fellow of the Library Association), which requires five years or more of approved experience plus submission of a substantial thesis judged to merit publication. The A.L.A. is the career degree and now may be obtained through various combinations considered equivalent to the requirements just noted. The combinations include a university degree and/or full-time tuition at one of the several Schools of Librarianship which have been established in more recent years[10]. The flexibility in certification requirements exemplified in the regulations of the Library Association is what a number of MLA members have requested.

In the United States we have followed the course of accrediting training institutions through standards set up by the American Library Association. Probably the alternate course of certifying individuals would never have worked in a country as big as ours and one where credentialing has traditionally occurred at the state or local level, with nothing equivalent to the British Ministry of Education. One of the problems in our system, of course, is that request for institutional accrediting is voluntary and lack of ALA approval cannot be blanketly interpreted as failure to meet standards, another point of controversy in existing MLA certification policies.

The American Library Association early in its history and at various times since has also been interested in certification of individuals and has had great influence on the institution of state certification which is now almost universal for school librarians and widespread for public librarians. For school librarians, though certification is mandatory (required by law), authority for fixing professional and educational requirements, regulations for issuing and renewing certificates, etc. are delegated to state boards of education. For public librarians certification may be mandatory, permissive (sanctioned by law but not compulsory), or voluntary, the latter usually developed and administered by state library associations and/or state library agencies. Mandatory certification is generally for minimum requirements. Examinations are often not required except to determine equivalencies for those who are not graduates of ALA approved library schools. Grade levels are frequently provided in state certification plans (but not often where certification is mandatory) and grandfather clauses are usual. Permissive and voluntary plans usually include academic librarians, but mandatory plans almost never[11].

The most important and far-reaching development in general library education in recent years has been the ALA Policy Statement on Education and Manpower adopted in 1970[12]. As you know from Lester Asheim's paper at the New York MLA meeting two years ago and from many other sources, the main tenor of the statement is that "the demands of the position should be the test of professional quality, and not the diploma held by the applicant." In support of this thesis four levels of classification are endorsed: the Library Technical Assistant, the Library Associate, Librarian, and Senior Librarian and along with them equivalent classes for related nonlibrary specialists whose skills are increasingly necessary in libraries. Classification is based on requirements for education and experience with the suggestion that until examinations are identified that are reliable tests of equivalent qualifications, education is the single best criterion[13]. All in all it is an admirable policy statement, with the kind of flexibility that makes it as applicable to the special fields of librarianship as it is to the general field.

To turn now to the special fields, the Special Libraries Association has appointed committees in the past to study certification but, as most of us are well aware, has elected to raise professional standards through membership requirements, though this decision does not, of course, rule out certification at some later date. The qualifications officially adopted in 1959 for both Associate and Active membership were based on various equivalent combinations of education and/or professional experience, at least a part of the latter having to be in special libraries. The primary difference between the two classes of members was that the Active member, regardless of education, must have at least three years of special library experience. A grandfather clause covered all who were members at the time the membership qualifications were adopted. Institutional membership, incidentally, was dropped because there was no effective way to control who would serve as the institutional representative[14]. However, subsequent amendments to SLA bylaws have watered down requirements considerably. "A serious interest in the objectives of the Association" is now the only stated qualification for Associate status and the experience requirement has been lifted from the Active member category for those with the requisite education[15].

The American Association of Law Libraries (AALL) decided in 1960 on a certification plan similar to MLA's in preference to more rigorous membership standards. Their code differs from ours in the following respects: only members can apply for certification, there is a minimum experience requirement, provision for appeals is made, and equivalencies are established for requirements in terms of a point value system for education and experience. For example, law school and fifth year library science degrees count for two points each, AALL approved library courses one point each, professional law library experience one point for each year and so on. There is no provision for certification by examination, but continuing education approved by AALL carries credit toward certification. The AALL's three grades of certification are also based on the point system[11,16].

The Medical Library Association certification program, now about to enter its twenty-fifth year, was conceived as a kind of system to: (1) assist in improving the quality of medical librarianship, (2) establish minimal educational and training standards, (3) determine whether applicants have received adequate training, and (4) certify competence of those who meet the requirements[17]. The system provided for a strong recruitment effort, for graduate education in librarianship and in medical librarianship through Association approved courses, practical but truly professional level experience through internships, and at the top level, two years or more of graduate work in library science and in appropriate subject fields, correlated if possible, and leading to a higher degree. There was also the usual grandfather clause providing for charter certification for the five-year period 1949-1954. Certification furnished formal evidence of having entered the system at some point, ideally, but not necessarily, progressing from I through III. System management was the responsibility of the Committee on Standards for Medical Librarianship assisted by the four Subcommittees on Recruitment, Curriculum, Internship, and Certification. Rather curiously there was never any attempt to attach the continuing education program directly to the system.

The history of the certification program has been ably chronicled by Mildred Jordan and more recently by Miriam Libbey[18, 19]. I intend therefore only to select a few items from our past which seem to have bearing on the current dissatisfaction with the way our system has functioned—or more often not functioned.

In 1946 the Committee on the Training for Medical Librarianship surveyed the membership to determine Association views on what kind of training should be sponsored. Five criteria were proposed—academic training, professional library training, medical training, experience, and personality qualifications. Library training ranked highest, experience second, medical training third, but academic training and personality qualifications were considered the most basic. The difficulty of grading the last two, however, made them impractical for criteria.

During the final discussion of the certification code in Galveston in 1949, Sanford Larkey, representing the small minority who were opposed to formal certification, spoke in this vein:

> We must realize that this will not be an experiment. Once we have adopted certification, we are more or less committed to it.
>
> A good deal has been said about the advantages of certification. The case for it has been well presented. But I question whether certification will achieve the desired ends; namely, higher prestige and standards for the Association. We think of ourselves as a learned profession and here our position will depend on educational competence and proved ability and not on certificates. Our training programs, internships, and conferences are great steps along these lines[20].

Dr. Larkey had other fears, which proved groundless, but he was certainly correct in the views just quoted. We are indeed committed to certification, for we have certified some 1,200 people to date. For this reason, if no other, the Association is unlikely to abandon the basic concept of certification in the foreseeable future, certainly not until it has tried harder and longer to make it work. True, we are judged as a group by the degree of proved ability and educational competence shown by our individual members; these are what determine our prestige, not the 1,200 certificates issued. Standards, however, *have* been significantly raised by the educational components of the MLA training program, I believe. Even the existence on paper of those standards we have had most trouble realizing have been valuable as focal points, as desirable if not mandatory goals. Whether they needed to be reinforced by certificates is, of course, another matter.

In reviewing what has been accomplished since 1949 we must think back to the situation described by Janet Doe in her presidential address. She said on training for medical librarianship:

> Education has been almost wholly the old apprenticeship method of learning on the job, until within a very few years. Medical libraries seem to have existed apart from ordinary library currents almost up to the present

time, and are only just beginning to be drawn into the main stream. The cause lies probably in the difference in the evolution of medical librarians and of general librarians[21].

She goes on to point out that in medicine book collections began as the private possessions of physicians who gradually pooled their collections into libraries for medical societies and hospitals. Physician-librarians were the titular heads but their secretaries and technical assistants did most of the work. As collections grew large, physicians stepped out of the library but became the employers of library staff whom they usually continued to recruit from the auxiliary medical services with whom they worked. Thus, at the time certification was approved by the MLA, a fair number of the members had never had formal training of any kind. That they went along with the new standards so wholeheartedly tells us a great deal about their generosity of spirit as well as their dedication to the progress of medical librarianship. We cannot appreciate the significance of the requirement for a fifth year library degree from an ALA accredited school except against this background. It was the really important qualification for Grade I certification, so far as professionalism is concerned, rather than the medical library courses. The latter were innovative, to be sure, and milestones in the movement for specialization in library education which began about this same time, but the great need then was to establish a basic professional education requirement. We are only now at the point where it is practical to press for specialization in education for librarianship on a broad scale; though medical librarians have been pushing in this direction longer than most, full success for whatever we undertake is bound to be tied to progress in the field as a whole in the long run.

As courses in medical librarianship began to multiply, so did the problems of the Subcommittee on Curriculum, which has the task of reviewing new courses and recommending them for approval or disapproval. When the first statement on standards for the courses was drawn up in 1950, the only course offered was the one at Columbia University. The first statement, five lines long, merely indicated in a general way what course content should be—an introduction to medical literature and each of its specialties plus special problems of organization, administration, and techniques in medical libraries[22]. The prescription is essentially the same today, but qualifications of instructors, eligibility of students, methods of instruction, more specifics about course content and related matters have been added. The latest revision of *Minimum Standards for Training of Medical Librarians* was in 1964. As early as 1955 questions were arising about the length of time allotted the courses in the library school curriculum, the relations of the schools to the MLA, the wide difference in the backgrounds and experience of the students, and the superficiality of the work because of the breadth of content to be covered[23]. The problems have not changed in nature but they have in degree, for there were four courses in 1955, 19 today with a 20th pending and more on the way; and the course content specified, difficult enough to cover then, is impossible to cover in two or three courses today. The teachers of the courses, most of them practicing medical librarians and Association members, have been convened for advice on a few occasions and from time to time they have been drawn on for membership on the Committee, but for the most part remarkably little input has been sought or received from them. Perhaps it is because so many of them are not certified. Still, despite the problems there has been an astoundingly good response from the library schools over the years to adding courses on medical librarianship to the curriculum. We do have a strong base for strengthening education for our field in a meaningful way. From this point of view, the specialty requirement for Grade I certification can be regarded as a resounding success.

The Grade II requirement for internships has presented a different set of problems. The chief difficulty has been the scarcity of programs. There were never more than two available from 1949 until 1961 when NIH made awards to support pilot programs at Emory and UCLA. With the passage of the Medical Library Assistance Act, additional programs were funded but there have never at any time been more than seven open at once, i.e., places for twenty to twenty-five in the peak years. The scarcity is due, of course, to the cost of internship training in terms of trainee stipends and staff time; it really is impossible to support training of this kind without extra funding over and above regular operating budgets. A proper internship is a practical education experience which works to best advantage in institutions where medical library staff and facilities are above average and where opportunity is available for additional academic work related to medical librarianship. These requirements cut down the number of potentially suitable institutions still further.

Grade III requirements have produced the biggest block of all to the functioning of the system. First, there were and are no existing two-year academic programs "correlating work in library science, medical library work and medical subject work leading to an advanced degree" as prescribed in the original code[24]. Reading through the *Bulletin* on the early years of certification, one comes across a few hints and promises from institutions that such programs would be given, but none materialized. The closest thing is the new two-year master's level programs which allow for specialization in the second year.—twenty years too late. The alternative of "graduate work in library science and in medical and related subject fields, leading to an advanced degree" was too imprecise to be very useful.

Consequently, in 1956 Grade III requirements were changed to a doctor's degree in librarianship, but that did not help much, as the record shows.

By 1964 it was clear that our certification system had never operated beyond the Grade I level except on a token basis. It was given a fairly thorough overhauling at that time, not so much with the idea of updating it but rather in order to implement fully what we already had[17]. Medical library courses were still very limited in number and the provision for special certification for those with unusual credentials not very satisfactory; so the taking of an examination geared for the Grade I level was introduced in lieu of special certification and as an alternative to the course. It has been difficult to devise valid examinations, but the concept itself, I believe, is a good one. Grade II was broadened by making an appropriate subject master's degree and one year of professional medical library experience an alternate to internship. Grade III was liberalized to permit meeting the requirement for a doctor's degree in librarianship with a doctor's degree in any appropriate subject area providing the applicant also had a fifth year library degree from an ALA accredited school and five years of experience. These changes kept the original concepts fairly well intact except that they further weakened the idea of each grade building on the qualifications of the one before. The innovation was the experience requirement for Grades II and III. The pity is that it was not added for Grade I at the same time and some experience equivalency worked out for the course requirement. In any case, we now can boast that of the 1,200 MLA certified librarians around 100 are at Grade II and 9 at Grade III. Some 300 received charter certification prior to April 13, 1954 and the rest are at Grade I.

The only change of any moment since 1964 was the abolishing of the Committee on Standards for Medical Librarianship and the raising of the subcommittees to full committee status. This revision makes more direct and hence faster action possible, but coordination of efforts is more difficult. In 1967 the MLA Board of Directors requested the Committee on Certification to make recommendations on changes needed in the code and in 1969 appointed an Ad Hoc Committee to Develop a New Certification Code. Its membership was altered somewhat in 1971. In 1972 the new committee, chaired by Martha Jane Zachert and Joan Titley, came up with a proposed new code which the Board gratefully received but decided would be too costly and complicated to implement. Now the Board has appointed a new Ad Hoc Committee to Develop a New Certification Code.

Though the code has not been revised since 1964, in the intervening years medical librarianship has itself gone through a sea change. In the short time left me I want to note some of the elements in this transformation which will most affect any new code we may devise, mention some additional dissatisfactions members have expressed about certification, and list some of the changes which have been recommended.

The Medical Library Assistance Act and, in their heyday, the Regional Medical Programs have been of enormous importance in enhancing the status of medical librarianship and in improving both quantity and quality of training through the financial support they have made available to libraries and library schools. Particularly pertinent to certification have been the policies on and provisions for training programs and for regional medical library networks.

The National Library of Medicine, in presenting its Extramural Program objectives to the Medical Library Association in 1966, stated that serious as the quantitative problems were, simply adding more schools with courses in medical bibliography would not solve the more far-reaching qualitative problems. Most needed were training programs going beyond the basic traditional training in library science to provide the student with a combination of further theoretical depth and either research or practical experience directly related to the problems of medical science[25]. Acting on this policy, NLM funded, in addition to the internships to which reference has already been made, master's programs in medical librarianship designed on a new pattern. They aimed, in Alan Rees's words, to "represent a specialization in health sciences librarianship within the master's curriculum offering the student an integrated program rather than a single course. Formal course work is supplemented by field work, site visits and seminars in health sciences librarianship. An attempt is made to explicate the environmental, sociological, and other factors peculiar to the health sciences"[26]. These courses usually require at least an extra summer session to complete and clearly fall between the present Grades I and II as is also true of the two-year master's program with specialization in the health sciences. The current manpower situation and the phasing out of federal support for training can certainly be expected to lessen enrollments in these programs temporarily, but they appear to be here to stay and to multiply.

The networks, in an effort to bring library services to all health professionals in their respective geographic areas, have promoted a regular schedule of technician level workshops and institutes for nonprofessional level hospital health science librarians all over the country. The American Hospital Association and the Catholic Hospital Association have continued their good work in this area and have furnished models for the newer endeavors. There is growing evidence that this has been an effective measure in utilization of interlibrary loan service, MEDLARS, and

MEDLINE and in bringing a new awareness of health information sources and services to the health sciences community at large. Most importantly, networking has also brought libraries of all sizes into a much closer partnership to achieve common goals. However, in the wake of these developments have come two more problems for certification. Technician level personnel, whether products of the new library technician training courses in the junior colleges or of on-the-job learning, are becoming interested in certification. If they work in health sciences libraries, they naturally look to the MLA for this, but thus far the Association has not indicated whether it considers this within its province. Certainly we must come to grips with the problem in devising a new code. The technician question raises, too, what is to me an even more serious problem. Some—a minority, I believe—of the library school qualified hospital librarians feel that training directed to raising the competency of nonqualified personnel is a disservice to the qualified and a distinct handicap to the development of good library service nationally. Understandably, they resent the recruit from the medical records department or the doctor's office taking the title of librarian and they point out that many library school graduates are now available on the job market, so the plea of scarcity is no longer valid. Should technician level MLA certification be developed, it might very well tend to aggravate further this dissension. On the other hand, we must keep in mind findings from health sciences library manpower surveys of recent years. Among the conclusions Rees, Rothenberg, and Denison drew in 1968 in their study of library education in the United States in relation to the qualifications of medical library manpower, were that there is no universally accepted standard of educational preparation for work in medical libraries, that an increasing number of untrained personnel will continue to be employed in medical libraries, that many of them have and will have sole responsibility for these libraries and that appropriate educational programs must be designed specifically for them[27]. In the large scale "Investigation of the Education Needs of Health Sciences Library Manpower" it is stated again that there is no clear agreement on standards for hospital libraries or on how they should be staffed[18]. However, with more than 50 percent of the 6,018 hospitals in the American HospitalAssociation survey of 1968 apparently without libraries of any kind and only 12 percent reporting librarians at the master's degree level, it seems obvious that the first job is to establish some point in each institution where service through the medical library network can begin. The investigation suggests that for library programs in smaller hospitals which cannot develop viable service programs on their own, we need to develop cooperative arrangements for services in order to make best use of available talents, a suggestion that has been tested here and there with encouraging results.

If I seem to be dwelling overlong on this problem in hospitals, it is because certification is much more important there than in the academic health sciences library. As we have seen, many categories of hospital personnel are licensed or certified. Because hospital personnel administrators are accustomed to thinking in terms of certification, there is a good possibility of making MLA certification a meaningful, if not mandatory, requirement. In the academic library, on the other hand, administrators think in terms of academic degrees and academic achievement. There are usually well-defined criteria for hiring and promoting personnel. They may apply to whole university library systems, including some that are statewide. As faculty or equivalent status becomes increasingly widespread, these criteria will take on added importance while MLA certificates, never recognized to any appreciable extent, are likely to become at best but added ornaments of no special significance in curriculum vitae folders.

The increases projected in the number of health care institutions, in the schools preparing personnel for them, and in the continuingly accelerated production of scientific and technical information assure us that need for health sciences library personnel at all levels will also grow apace despite the current slump. In what ways should a meaningful certification program attempt to accommodate to the size and diversity of this population? Should we again adopt a graded system, including this time nonprofessional levels, or should we concentrate on a single minimum standard for professional personnel only or something in between? What about the changing patterns in general library education? Should we, for example, prepare for the ALA suggested new classification of Library Associate? What do we do about the 1,200 people already holding MLA certification if we go to a radically new plan? With all the current emphasis on continuing education, should we stay with lifetime certification or do we plan for recertification despite the complications it introduces? Is it necessary for us to continue to review approved courses formally every five years or shall we count ALA accreditation as sufficient for our purpose since we accept it for all the rest of the curriculum? If so, can we sell ALA on MLA representation on accrediting committees? Is it wise to ask associations which are responsible for accrediting health science schools and hospitals to make MLA certification of librarians a requirement? And would they? What about certification criteria? Do we need to add or substitute such qualifications as experience, equivalency of experience, and education, evidence of continuing education? Many members think these are basic for any plan. Or should we toss out all criteria except for minimum standards of education and experience and rely on written examination alone? Many members favor this option. Can we work out any system whose costs will not exceed the values received? Most critically, are we able to identify with any precision what are the competencies medical librarianship requires? These are the primary issues, but committees and individual members have identified a number more.

A recurring theme is the unfairness of requiring that either the M.L.S. degree or the medical library course must be taken at only ALA approved schools—especially when the school is later approved. Another is that long and/or high-level experience should be an alternate for the course and examination. Some go further and claim experience should be an alternate for the basic fifth-year degree or even the college bachelor's degree. There is unhappiness over the lack of meaningful recognition of MLA certification by employers, including Association employers, and recommendations that MLA do better by its own program, e.g., require certification of its officers. The unhappy ones suggest that certification ought to bring job preference and pay increments. Several members have altruistically complained that teachers of approved courses cannot be certified unless they can meet the paper qualifications. As one of these people pointed out, in most cases the teacher is at least as qualified as the student.

A number of different criteria have been suggested as additions or alternates, usually in combinations, to existing criteria: membership in the Association, active participation in Association affairs, job analysis, performance evaluation, professional contributions and achievements, and various kinds of continuing education. All kinds of grade combinations have been proposed, as already indicated, with abolishment of Grade III and more alternatives for Grade II being most frequent. However, only a limited number of members in relation to the size of the Association have spoken out on any phase of certification. When the Ad Hoc Committee on the New Certification Code mailed invitations to the entire membership in 1971 to make written statements on their views or to appear in person before the committee at its August special meeting, no one appeared and only 28 sent statements—18 from hospitals, 7 from academic centers, 2 from large societies, and one from a library school faculty member. This small return may in itself be indicative of lack of very vital concern on the part of most of us, yet there have been 1,200 certificates granted and the idea of certification is interwoven with much of our organizational activity.

Perhaps the difficulty is that there are too many diverse opinions on what should be done to set off the groundswell of conviction necessary for sound restructuring of our present scheme. The 1971 Ad Hoc Committee on Certification tried very hard to be sensitive to as many of the membership's expressed views as they reasonably could. In the end they came up with something which approximates the ALA policy statement but includes a number of additional details. The chief obstacle to its implementation, I think, is that a policy statement is like a guideline; it has a great flexibility which is almost impossible to put into a certification scheme where the administrators of the scheme must have specific directives. For this reason my one and only recommendation at this point is that we devise a fairly simple new code that will require a minimum amount of interpretation.

I have not gone into the pertinent recommendations of the Ad Hoc Committee to Review the Goals and Structure of the Medical Library Association which appear in Part I of its Report[29] first, because most of you have probably read them and second, they are largely covered in what I have already said. You will recall that the emphasis is on raising standards, not seeking for the lowest common denominator, on flexibility and on the continuous adjustment in our educational programs to the theoretical and technical developments in the information field.

I am afraid that I have told you more about certification than most of you ever wanted to know. I did so because the committee on the new certification code desperately needs to learn—and quickly—what the main number of you want in the code. At the moment the only point I feel certain we all agree upon is that the true status of medical librarianship rests most on the character and ability of its practitioners, what they bring to the field, and what they leave there. And this brings me back full circle to Janet Doe, who has left us so much.

REFERENCES

1. Form, William H. Occupations and careers. In: International Encyclopedia of the Social Sciences. 17 Vols. New York, Macmillan, 1968. Vol. 9, p. 245-253.
2. Parsons, Talcott. Professions. In: International Encyclopedia of the Social Sciences. 17 Vols. New York, Macmillan, 1968. Vol. 12, p. 536-547.
3. National Commission on Accrediting. [Definitions.] In: Study of Accreditation of Selected Health Educational Programs. I. Staff Working Papers. Accreditation of Selected Health Educational Programs. Washington, Study of Accreditation of Selected Health Educational Programs, 1971. p. ii.
4. Shuman, Bruce. Patterns of American Library Certification. Unpublished Master's paper, Graduate Library School, University of Chicago, 1965.
5. Derbyshire, Robert C. Medical Licensure and Discipline in the United States. Baltimore, The Johns Hopkins Press, 1969. p. 2-8.
6. Egelston, E. Martin. Licensure—effects on career mobility. Am. J. Pub. Health. 62: 50-53, Jan. 1972.
7. Selden, William K. The dilemmas of credentialing: SASHEP looks at forces affecting health. J. Am. Diet. Assoc. 61: 22-25, July 1972.
8. U.S. Department of Health, Education and Welfare. Office of Assistant Secretary for Health and Scientific Affairs. Continuing education. In: Report on Licensure and Related Health Personnel Credentialing, June 1971. Washington, 1971. (DHEW Pub. no. (HSM)72-11) p. 57-63.

9. SHORES, LOUIS. Qualifications of personnel: training and certification. Libr. Trends. 3: 269-278, Jan. 1955.
10. Royal charters and bye-laws of the Library Association: membership and registration. The Library Association Yearbook, 1972. p. 40-43.
11. MORTON, FLORRINELL F. Librarians, certification of. In: Encyclopedia of Education. 10 Vols. New York, Macmillan, 1971. Vol. 5, p. 511-516.
12. Library education and manpower. Am. Libr. 1: 341-345, Apr. 1970.
13. ASHEIM, LESTER. Preparation and use of library manpower. Bull. Med. Libr. Assoc. 60: 288-291, Apr. 1972.
14. SASS, SAMUEL. The Special Libraries Association takes a step forward. Law Libr. J. 52: 397-405, 1959.
15. Special Libraries Association Bylaws. Article II: Membership. Spec. Libr. 63: 14s-15s, Aug. 1972.
16. Certification of law librarians—AALL. Law Libr. J. 60: 434-435, Nov. 1967.
17. Code for the training and certification of medical librarians. Bull. Med. Libr. Assoc. 52: 784-789, Oct. 1964.
18. LIBBEY, MILDRED HAWKINS. MLA certification: the certification program and education for medical librarianship. Bull. Med. Libr. Assoc. 55: 5-8, Jan. 1967.
19. JORDAN, MILDRED. Events in the development of education for medical librarianship in the last decade. Bull. Med. Libr. Assoc. 45: 351-360, July 1957.
20. LARKEY, SANFORD. Remarks against certification. Bull. Med. Libr. Assoc. 37: 296-298, Oct. 1949.
21. DOE, JANET. The development of education for medical librarianship. Bull. Med. Libr. Assoc. 37: 213-220, July 1949.
22. MEDICAL LIBRARY ASSOCIATION. SUBCOMMITTEE ON CURRICULUM. Report. Bull. Med. Libr. Assoc. 38: 346-348, Oct. 1950.
23. STEINKE, ELEANOR G. Our standards dilemma. Bull. Med. Libr. Assoc. 45: 587-588, Oct. 1957.
24. Proposed code for the training and certification of medical librarians. Bull. Med. Libr. Assoc. 37: 350-352, Oct. 1949. [Adopted April 13, 1949]
25. WILSON, MARJORIE P.; DOUGLASS, CARL D.; AND KEFAUVER, DAVID F. Extramural programs of the National Library of Medicine: program objectives and present status. Bull. Med. Libr. Assoc. 54: 293-310, Oct. 1966.
26. REES, ALAN M. [and others]. Certification reform. Bull. Med. Libr. Assoc. 58: 601-602, Oct. 1970.
27. REES, ALAN M.; ROTHENBERG, LESLIEBETH; AND DENISON, BARBARA. Professional medical library education in the United States in relation to the qualifications of medical library manpower in Ohio. Bull. Med. Libr. Assoc. 56: 368-379, Oct. 1968.
28. KRONICK, DAVID A.; REES, ALAN M.; AND ROTHENBERG, LESLIEBETH. An investigation of the educational needs of health sciences library manpower. VII. Summary and conclusions. Bull. Med. Libr. Assoc. 60: 292-300, Apr. 1972.
29. MEDICAL LIBRARY ASSOCIATION. Ad Hoc COMMITTEE TO REVIEW THE GOALS AND STRUCTURE OF THE MEDICAL LIBRARY ASSOCIATION. Report. I. Bull. Med. Libr. Assoc. 60: 236-246, Jan. 1972.

Library Cooperation: Wave of the Future or Ripple?*

BY JACQUELINE W. FELTER, *Director*

The Medical Library Center of New York
New York, New York

ABSTRACT

Little of the literature in library cooperation applies specifically to library service for the health sciences. Based on experience in and observations of the cooperation of health science libraries, this short lecture reviews aspects of general library cooperation, networks, and consortia. The effects on library operation of several cooperative activities are enumerated and cooperation management is discussed briefly.

I CHOSE cooperation among libraries as my subject for the simple reason that it is the field in which I have worked for the past ten years. I thought, too, that there might have been little written about it in comparison with other aspects of library management and service. On the contrary, quite a lot has been written about it. For example, a selection of both papers and pertinent excerpts from books on cooperation written between 1948 and 1972 make a book nearly 400 pages long[1], with a considerable number of papers, monographs, and conference proceedings left over. Nevertheless, little of this spate of publications applies specifically to the health sciences, and I think this is an appropriate time to review the subject. Besides, a lecture on cooperation offers a tempting opportunity to make observations on practically any aspect of library operation.

What makes the time right? Cooperatives are proliferating, for one thing. And the cooperatives are forming associations with other cooperatives. Because it appears that joint action may be more effective than individual action, libraries form cooperative groups which in turn look to

*Janet Doe Lecture in History or Philosophy of Medical Librarianship, presented June 4, 1974, at the Seventy-third Annual Meeting of the Medical Library Association, San Antonio, Texas.

[1]The exact quotation is "cooperation has gone as far as it can due to localism." Libr. J. 98: 2237, 1973.

Originally published in *Bulletin of the Medical Library Association,* Volume 63 (January, 1975), pp. 1-6. Reprinted by permission.

other groups for ideas about solutions to common problems and goals to be achieved. This "layered look"—to borrow an expression from the clothing industry—bewilders me, and I suspect that, as in the world of fashion, results depend on how skillfully the layers are laid on. Finally on top of it all, in its draft of a "New National Program of Library and Information Service," the National Commission on Libraries and Information Science (NCLIS) views local cooperatives as "stop-gaps," and proposes "a total system rather than a collection of separate parts"[2]. Closer to home, our own National Library of Medicine looks upon regional plans and multilibrary enterprises as the methods of choice, rather than stop-gaps, for more effective use of library resources. Unfortunately the NCLIS draft program seems not to recognize the progress of the National Library of Medicine and its Extramural Programs toward a total system.

Then there is the terminology. Library cooperation has long been a familiar term applied to all or various, and presumably beneficial, library relationships. Networking—that term has been around for a while, too—connotes participation in and commitment to a system, library interaction rather than just action. Now there is a new term, consortium, as yet not precisely defined for libraries. It suggests a joining together for a common purpose, a union stronger than mere library cooperation.

In the articles in the literature the guidelines put forth are mostly extrapolations based on surveys of current practice. So I propose that although we proceed along paths already trod, we examine the present state of library cooperation with open eyes and minds, a reflection of Szent-Györgyi's comment, "Discovery is seeing what everybody has seen and thinking what nobody has thought." My observations or impressions are largely personal, without reference to the participants of any particular group or locality. My remarks pertain to libraries serving the medical community. And inasmuch as the Janet Doe Lecture is traditionally a philosophical exposition, I am not addressing myself in great detail to the financial aspects of various kinds of cooperation, although they influence the extent of an institution's participation and cannot be ignored. So much for the caveats.

Cooperation

In a report of a session at the ALA meeting last year in Las Vegas, Kenneth Beasley was quoted as saying that "cooperation has gone as far as it can go"[3]. This comment is out of context; I do not know what else Beasley said. To me, however, it is unthinkable that it should mean that cooperation is "out," and highly individual, independent operation is "in." Rather, I assume, it means that the cooperation of the old days has gone as far as it can go.[1]

What was it like in the old days? Cooperation was something one engaged in or not, as convenient, a moral rather than contractual obligation. It had various configurations. It began as the large library helping the smaller one. In the really early days, when MLA was young, a few medical libraries of great stature served *in loco parentis* to the young upstarts. These distinguished libraries took their moral obligation seriously, donating to their foster children their classification schemes, the advice of their librarians, and interlibrary loan. You notice that I said "donating"; it was all gratis. Over the years this kind of patronage continued—mostly in one direction, from large to small, usually without charge, dispensed sometimes grudgingly, but more often altruistically. Many libraries, particularly those in hospitals, could not have gotten off the ground without such help, but it has had adverse effects as well. For one thing, librarians of small libraries turning toward large libraries, as if to Mecca, formerly overlooked the opportunities to help each other, and thus become more self-sufficient. On another hand, institutional administrations, especially in hospitals, took free assistance for granted, and tended to value the librarian according to his ability to provide library service at little or no cost.

Of course, more recently the picture has changed. In every community now there are a greater number of libraries similar in resources and mission in each size category. Within their group these libraries are capable of reciprocal cooperation, dependent on one another rather than on the largest library in town. But although groups form, based on geographical propinquity or some other affinity, cooperation continues to be principally a one-to-one relationship, voluntary, and gratis, often following the channels of personal friendships among the librarians and justified to the administrations as furtherance of knowledge. Cooperation of this sort may have been acceptable in times of library affluence when there were light service loads, and when costly equipment like computers had not yet been introduced into libraries. In reality, however, it is, as Dagnese says, "at best a very tenuous idea, one which succumbs easily to the exigencies of self-interest and fiscal retrenchment"[4].

Networks

In contrast to participation in this desultory kind of cooperation, a library that becomes a member of a network participates in a system. A network improves the direct interaction between libraries by providing a switching center which can marshall the force of the group to fulfill the needs of one member. Library A may make a request that is filled by a combination of assistance from Library B and Library X, as arranged by the center; in this case Library A is obligated not to the assisting libraries, but to the center and pays a fee-for-service or accepts responsibility for honoring the request of Library Z, which also is a participant in the network. Libraries B and X, on the other hand, are compensated for assisting Library A by receiving assistance from Library Y. If the word "assistance" is translated to interlibrary loan, the verbal diagram becomes more clear. Or, as the Regional Medical Libraries do it, the old progression is reversed, and loans climb up a hierarchy from small to larger library. Network assistance, however, has other faces—shared data bases for producing catalog cards, for example, and union catalogs, sometimes linked to serials control systems.

Networks have other characteristics that make them different from the older form of library cooperation. Network participation is overt acknowledgment of the inadequacy of solo operation and the need for interdependence, whereas in old-fashioned library cooperation the admission of inadequacy was tacit. The need for expensive equipment, like computers, gave network development its impetus. Up to now, at least, libraries have been willing to admit all of them do not have their own computers. And in a network a library fulfills its needs from the resources of the membership as a participant rather than as a mendicant, because in some way, either in currency or in services, it pays its own way. In summary, networks are a business, not charity.

That brings us to money. Networks are likely to be fee-structured. If the members are the same size and all use the same network services, it is easy to set the fee. One simply divides the agreed-upon budget evenly. If the libraries are of different sizes, the fair allocation of cost is more complicated. The ideal would be to separate the network services into units, analyze the costs of each, and set unit prices. The participants could elect all, or some, units and pay accordingly. In such a network, the small library should come off rather better than it does in unstructured cooperation; it is not a "poor relation," but rather pays its own way. Many of us are still inexpert cost accountants, however, and instead of basing fees on cost analysis of segregated units, we base them on ability to pay. Thus the large libraries carry the load; the small ones ride half-fare, more or less; and the relationship of patron and dependent is not really changed.

Consortia

Since the word *consortium* came into vogue, the dictionary pages on which it is defined have been well thumbed. In addition to giving the business and banking derivation, the dictionary obliges with the broad definition of "an association for a common purpose." The broad definition is good enough for us, for, if we follow the precedents set by "library cooperation" and "networks," the term will be given substance according to the way it is applied to library practice. The difference is that, while we have inherited "library cooperation" and some of us are young enough to have inherited "networks," all of us are starting at the beginning with "consortium" and have the opportunity to shape the connotation of the word.

Cuadra and Patrick, reporting on the Survey[5] which produced, among other things, their excellent book, *Guidelines for the Development of Academic Library Consortia*[6], equate consortia with networks, but their characterization that "members share system planning and development resources, as well as operating responsibilities and functions," is good advice for any group, however small, however simple the program. Paraphrasing the criteria in the "Survey of Academic Library Consortia in the U. S." the following are applicable to any type of library group:

The cooperative must be organized voluntarily to pursue activities of benefit to the participants.
The participating institutions must be autonomous.
Two or more libraries must be involved, with activities extending beyond traditional interlibrary loan.
If the library cooperative is part of a higher level, multipurpose consortium, it must be a separate entity with the goal of improving library service.
The consortium must have developed beyond the exploratory stage; in other words, the group must have declared itself a cooperative entity and must be planning joint activities.

The *Guidelines* go on to consider administrative structure appropriate for programs of different complexity and to suggest a modular approach to consortium development. The design is flexible; the modules can be manipulated like building blocks. "Not all steps are necessary for every consortium; steps may be used in different sequences; several steps may be performed simultaneously; and steps tend to reiterate"[5]. With such a rational design, and perspective on past cooperation, consortia should develop, not "just grow."

Now some brief observations about some of the activities in which cooperatives engage. In the literature there are descriptions aplenty of the implementation and effectiveness of specific programs.

Interlibrary Loan

The first activity that comes to mind, of course, is interlibrary loan. It is the oldest tangible cooperation. For the *donor* library, it is also the easiest, or it was until library funds began to shrink. In the donor library interlibrary loan does not alter the familiar patterns of library service; no new techniques are required. It is, moreover, very gratifying to be able to play Lord Bountiful to one's neighbors. The institution's primary clientele is not inconvenienced, in fact, is scarcely aware of the library's lending function. Before networks, the *borrowing* library had a harder time of it, deriving satisfaction only at the end when the book was finally in the hand of the reader. In between, under the old pattern, the borrowing library was a suppliant, seeking its item by way of random requests and repetition. "If at first you don't succeed, try, try, again," is an old ILL adage.

Networks and their accessory, the union catalog, have improved the lot of the borrowing library. Networks have made borrowing, of uncommon journals, at any rate, a business, orderly and legitimate. Familiarity with library resources disclosed in union lists reduces, if not eliminates, the number of fruitless requests. In some networks interlibrary loans can be expedited through prearranged channels from library to library. Donor libraries are compensated for accepting responsibility for lending.

Union Lists and Catalogs

Union lists and catalogs are products of cooperation. They were almost lost in limbo until computer technology brought them back to life. Their cost effectiveness is often questioned, for they are expensive to maintain, but their usefulness, it seems, is never in doubt. In the words of the *Analysis of the Midwest Medical Union Catalog: Progress Report No. 1,* "There is no longer the undaunted enthusiasm for union catalogs that there used to be . . ."[7]. Yet whenever libraries form a group to provide better service for their clientele and their community, the first thing they plan is compilation of a union catalog of their holdings. The librarians in New York are no exception; after ten years, they are still calling for a union catalog of monographs, a companion piece for the *Union Catalog of Medical Periodicals*. SERLINE is NLM's current nod in the union list direction. Overall, we look forward to the completion of the Midwest RML Analysis for some sound conclusions. Possibly union lists have more validity as by-products of shared cataloging and shared serials systems than as independent projects. It may be damning with faint praise to add that, at any rate, union lists are another cooperative activity that does not essentially disrupt so-called "normal" operations in the participating libraries.

Shared Cataloging and Centralized Card Production

It is regrettable that cooperative cataloging and centralized card production have come on so slowly in health science libraries, regrettable because their missions are so similar and such quantities of their collections are identical, and because, seemingly, such small differences are deterrents to collective operation. In public library systems, the similarity of the branches and the duplication of books purchased make centralized card production an economical function. If we could look at all the health science libraries in a community as parts of a system, benefits would accrue from shared cataloging and centralized replication of cards, if not computer output in some form.

Even acknowledging the fact that there are some individual differences in libraries, it is hard for me to accept the necessity and justify the cost for the minute differences in handling the bibliographic elements and the subject control of the literature that so intrigue catalogers. I doubt that the library's patrons are aware of them, as long as they can find the book. Of course, NLM's *Current Catalog* and CATLINE and, for some, the MARC tapes serve as common denominators, and by standardizing many details go a long way toward speeding production and decreasing cataloging costs. Exquisite additions to the standard product are, I think, lost to all but the expert cataloger. Is it perhaps an effort to make something creative out of a rather dull job? As for typing and reproducing catalog cards, the photocopier and the MAG CARD have reduced the time and the dull routine, but wouldn't it be better if in some central location it could be done once for all?

Shared Resources

There are two facets to shared resources, sharing what one already has and coordinating the acquisition of new materials. The rationale for both is to provide maximum adequacy of resources without duplication and wasteful expenditure. The ideal is a well thought-out plan with input from every participant and latitude to accommodate individual library requirements. It isn't always so orderly, however.

Let's take the retrospective material first. Especially, if there is separate housing for the shared-use collection, each participant hastens to deposit what he needs least. Given the good judgement of librarians, a surprisingly good collection may accrue. Nevertheless, there will be gaps to fill from other sources, and there are some practices against which safeguards are necessary. After the first rush, subsequent deposits will produce a lot of duplicates, so it is necessary to tell the donors what they should *not* send, lest the depository staff spend all its time, and everyone's money, sorting out and disposing of unwanted copies. There must be guidelines for the kind and time-span of drug house organs and news sheets to avoid swamping the collection with ephemera; decisions about the extent of responsibility for local news publications, like county medical society bulletins; and directives about the retention of current awareness services of limited currency. Steps must be taken to prevent doctors who clean house or the libraries they shuttle through from unloading on the depository. Refusal of out-of-scope material is mandatory. A few participants are disgruntled when they find that the depository will not take the junk they cannot bear to throw away, but by and large the participants are understanding and cooperative. Shouldn't they be? After all this shared-use collection is the one they will depend upon.

Separate housing for depository collections is expensive to acquire and maintain. A less expensive alternative for a cooperative is the allocation to each participant of responsibility for retaining a designated segment of the literature. Assignments should be consonant with the special programs of each institution. This plan works well if there are firm ground rules: someone responsible for its continuing regulation; each participating library able to commit itself in perpetuity to its retention responsibility and willing to disengage from its collection the volumes that are held by someone else to make room for those it promises to keep. This kind of shared-use program has another advantage—each participant has to dispose of its own duplicates and "junk" publications.

Coordinated current acquisitions programs are another activity which has come on slowly. Apparently it is easier to pool the materials one has owned, used, and no longer needs urgently, than it is to share those not yet acquired. There seems to be apprehension that one's colleague, or his subscription agency, will not deliver the journals he is responsible for. One feels much more secure with his own subscription even when he has to claim missing issues. I cannot judge from experience the success of coordinated acquisitions programs. Most of us consider them last-ditch efforts to combat adverse fiscal conditions. It is unfortunate that we are forced by circumstances into programs that would succeed so much better on real enthusiasm. I hope that the composite records of current journals that are by-products of network-operated serials control systems will change the picture. Union lists are mainly retrospective and rarely up to date. Current serials control provides up-to-the-minute records which will, I trust, provide a safe and sound foundation for what I consider a provident program.

Undermining shared-resources programs is the fallacy that the size of a library collection is a measure of its importance. Until availability abroad as well as quality at home becomes the measure of library status, the odds will be against the sharing of resources.

This has been a once-over-lightly summary. There are other activities that cooperating libraries can enter into—a central circulation bank which would both reveal at a glance the immediate availability of any book anywhere in the system and spin off records, such as overdue notices, for each participant; a universal identification card which, geography permitting, would enable readers to move freely from library to library; shared MEDLINE service. As I have had no experience with these, I cannot speak of them with authority.

Nor have I specifically mentioned joint use of computer technology. The need to own and use a computer has indeed brought libraries together, but computer technology is a tool which can implement any of the cooperative functions that I have mentioned. The libraries in a group would make a grave mistake if they said "Let's get together and lease a computer," and then decide what to do with it. It should be the other way around.

How to Succeed in Library Cooperation

I have not had a heart-to-heart talk with Secretary-General Waldheim about this, but I suspect that library cooperatives are similar to the United Nations. Both depend for success upon the delicate balances between preservation of individual prerogatives and relinquishment of some of the prerogatives for the achievement of the common good.

Olson places responsibility upon the leadership for the failure of library cooperation[8]. The directors, he says, like participants who do not make waves. The directors would counter, I suspect, with the reply that no leader can make progress if he has to push, pull, prod, or pacify his co-workers, or cajole them into changing their behavior patterns. Certain facts must be recognized and dealt with. People are naturally competitive; librarians are dedicated to their institutions—or at least know who butters their bread; their libraries are reflections of their initiative, ingenuity, expertise, and professionalism; they frequently are bound by legal constraints, especially when public funds support them; they are sometimes loath to change comfortable behavior patterns and tend to have more confidence in themselves than in their peers. Cooperative programs thrive best, of course, on mutual respect and enthusiastic commitment of both participant and director.

At first glance it would seem that libraries of the same size and similar mission would make the best cooperative. Certainly it is somewhat difficult to plan programs for those of different size and requirements. Libraries too much alike, however, tend to be competitive. On reflection I think the best "mix" is of libraries oriented in different, but allied disciplines. They would then complement each other.

Now to answer the question posed in the title of today's lecture—is library cooperation a ripple or the wave of the future? It has been a ripple long enough, but I am not sure that a wave would be beneficial. Waves are sometimes rough and tumble, impelled by forces beyond one's control. I would prefer library cooperation to come on as a strong, steady tide. Ebb and flow is to be expected; the period of the ebb used for reflection and evaluation so that the flow will be more effective. I believe that cooperation by whatever name is viable and necessary. Only irreversible circumstances prevent me from continuing to be part of it.

REFERENCES

1. (a) Reynolds, Michael M., ed. Reader in Library Cooperation. Washington, D.C., NCR Microcard Editions, 1972. 398 p. (b) Stenstrom, R.H. Cooperation between types of libraries, 1940-1968: An annotated bibliography. Chicago, American Library Association, 1970. 159 p., Supplement, 1969-1971, by M.E. Gilluly and L.M. Wert. Ill. Libr. 54: 385-400, May 1972.
2. National Commission on Libraries and Information Science. Draft: A new national program of library and information service. Spec. Libr. 64: 583-590, Dec. 1973.
3. Beasley, Kenneth. Cited in Localism in Las Vegas. Libr. J. 98: 2231-2242, Aug. 1973.
4. Dagnese, Joseph M. Cooperation between academic and special libraries. Spec. Libr. 64: 423-432, Oct. 1973.
5. Cuadra, Carlos A., and Patrick, Ruth J. Survey of academic library consortia in the U.S. Coll. Res. Libr. 33: 271-283, July 1972.
6. Patrick, Ruth J. Guidelines for the Development of Academic Library Consortia. Santa Monica, Calif., System Development Corporation, 1971. (TM4597/005, Nov. 1971) 200 p.
7. Olson, Paul E. and Pletzke, Chester J. Analysis of the Midwest Medical Union Catalog; Progress Report No. 1. Chicago, Midwest Health Science Library Network, The John Crerar Library, May 1974, 25 p.
8. Olson, Edwin E. Interlibrary Cooperation. Washington, D.C., U.S. Office of Education, Bureau of Research, 1970. 139 p.

The Medical Librarian as Manager; or the Fruits of Fadism*

By Harold Bloomquist, *Librarian*

Francis A. Countway Library of Medicine
Harvard University
Boston, Massachusetts

THANK you, Dr. Brodman†, I appreciate your kind introduction. It is an added pleasure because, though I did not meet you personally for some years later, you had been one of my early heroines of medical librarianship since I first became embroiled in scientific and medical libraries in the early fifties. My admiration was based on your contributions to the literature and your reputation as an awesome intellectual. I have never been disappointed in these judgements of mine over the past twenty-five years.

I am also deeply moved to be able to honor Janet Doe, for whom these lectures are named. It occurred to me as I was preparing this talk, that, as I plunge faster and faster into middle age, not so many years from now there will be a Doe Lecturer who probably will never have had the opportunity to have met or known Miss Doe. And that is a pity.

I first met Miss Doe when I was a library school student in New York, but even as a student I got around to professional meetings, and even a rare and exciting reception at the fabulous New York Academy of Medicine Library of which she was Librarian for so many years. Not so long after Miss Doe's retirement in 1956, I was lured to Boston by the late Ralph Esterquest of Harvard University. In my title, as Assistant Librarian, lurked the formidable and mysterious words, "Resources and Acquisitions." In any case at that time, this included cataloging—never to this day my forte.

As Ralph and I perused the instrument that had developed as the library's

*The Janet Doe Lecture on the History or Philosophy of Medical Librarianship, presented June 2, 1975, at the Seventy-fourth Annual Meeting of the Medical Library Association, Cleveland, Ohio.

†Mr. Bloomquist was introduced to the audience by Dr. Estelle Brodman, Director, Washington University School of Medicine Library, St. Louis, Missouri.

Originally published in *Bulletin of the Medical Library Association,* Volume 63 (October, 1975), pp. 359-365. Reprinted by permission.

card catalog over fifty-some years, we decided that we were well over our heads in knowing what to do to bring things into consistency with our vision for the tool needed in the then proposed Countway Library. The answer: Consultant! I will not repeat the cogent details of Miss Doe's career which are set forth so lovingly by Thomas Keys in the April 1975 *Bulletin*, but suffice it to say that she was not a difficult consultant choice to come up with. Miss Doe and Miss Susan Haskins of the Harvard College Library did survey the catalog and came up with the principles that we are still using today in Countway.

What astonishes me even today was the clarity and incisiveness of Miss Doe's recommendations: such things as "divided catalog," "new classification scheme," "redefinition and declassification of serials." Some of these concepts bring gasps, polite but audible, from catalogers today—and this from a "librarian emerita."

Janet extended warmth, good New England common sense, and an infectious enthusiasm that made me really want to be a good librarian.

Miss Doe is now a lady of some years and in happy retirement; let us hope that we can keep her and her spirit alive for many years to come.

My third introductory remark is less serious and more personal: it deals with that aberrant year, referred to by Dr. Brodman, when I interrupted my thirty-two-year unbroken romance with libraries to go to work for a trucking company. In simple fact, I was saving money after college to go on to graduate school. It was a wretched year—although not without its lessons—and not without its moments of black humor. In spite of my fancy title, Assistant to the Superintendent of Transportation, I was a dispatcher. In the interstate trucking business, the dispatcher's role is to monitor the progress of those huge trucking rigs from their starting point to their destination, for, among other variables, punctuality was paramount. This was and is done by having the trucks stop at intermediate stations along the way and report in "pony express style," at which time a teletype message was sent from the way-station to headquarters in Grand Rapids (a now somewhat more famous city than then for totally other reasons).

The dispatchers had huge pads of ruled paper on their desks on which they kept track of the progress of these trucks across the verdant or icy countryside. If a driver should be careless enough, or if a mishap occurred, and he did not meet his ETA (to you layfolk, Estimated Time of Arrival), then all hell broke loose in our office.

I guess (in fact I am sure), it was because I was a "college graduate," that I was given a specialist's job. I monitored a particularly important species of cargo, known to us in the trade as "hot loads." "Hot loads" were those shipments which, because of their physical nature, or the customer's whim, had to be delivered on an unwaveringly rigid schedule (and at an unwavering surcharge). Most of these were perishables, so the need was obvious. They were transported in refrigerated trailers (known again, to us in the trade, as "reefers"). Now, if I discovered that a hot load was not meeting its checkpoint ETA, I made this known, and the office would suddenly become tense and quiet. The chief dispatcher's brow would furrow, and one imagined the headquarters of Scotland Yard or Interpol as he mobilized his interstate forces to "find that truck!" It was high melodrama.

One of the company's best, most regular, and lucrative customers was The Upjohn Company in Kalamazoo.Our job was to get truckloads of fresh codfish livers from the eastern United States to Kalamazoo where magic pharmaceutical fingers transformed the gooey mess into that favorite child's nostrum, cod liver oil. These were always refrigerated hot loads, and therefore in my province. Only twice during my one year of service did a mishap befall a load of livers, but the memory is unforgettable. Since it was *not* among my duties to put into effect any of the tracing and maintenance and rescue procedures, I could sit back and watch the drama unfold, with vivid pictures of a broken-down truck somewhere in Pennsylvania or Ohio and those *tons* of cod livers either freezing into a disgusting mass, or sizzling and baking in the noonday sun.

You may wonder what this bizarre chunk of autobiography—this piece of pentimento—has to do with medical librarianship. I assure you that it has none. And yet is that true? Are we not ourselves in the business of delivering loads of bibliographic data and printed facts to our customers—and are not some of these loads "hot loads" that are perishable if not delivered on time? And do we not adopt a James Bondian mien if the postal service fails us, although we seem to be pretty powerless to do much about that except to switch to UPD or some alternative? There *is* a tenuous connection.

The title of my lecture this morning, and it is printed in your programs, is "The Medical Librarian as Manager." This would seem to be a perfectly topical and timely subject for a talk—but would it fall into the definition of "history or philosophy of medical librarianship"? I think not.

There is a subtitle to my lecture that is not printed in your program—and that is "The Fruits of Fadism."

Dr. Frank Rogers, that most Dostoevskian of medical librarians, made a statement some years ago, and it has stuck with me; I paraphrase him, "In this imperfect world, it is tempting to think of a single, perfect solution to a problem." And so it is and has been since the great leap forward of librarianship that followed on society's discovery that scientific information can be usefully applied to current scientific problems.

I am not a historian, but let me go back in my "clearly selective" memory of twenty years or so and pick out some of the discoveries or proposals that, at the time, seemed tempting as really solid answers to our problems. Many of our problems at that time fell under the phrases, "bibliographic control," and "information retrieval," and, oh, there were some ingenious ones. Vannevar Bush's MEMEX made everyone's head snap up with the pioneer vision of the black box that would contain and spell out on command information of any sort. Bush's vision was prophetic, but it led to decades of questions of what some of us call the "Sunday Supplement" type of user expectation—"Why not store it all in a machine?" ("all" is never very clearly defined in these questions). And questions persist in spite of the advances that have been made over these decades. Indeed, we do come closer to the vision.

There has been fun along the way: to be nostalgic, remember coordinated indexing, Mortimer Taube, and edge-notched cards, somewhat like IBM cards in appearance, but coded around their periphery with holes to be notched to stand for certain subjects, names, dates, or whatever? A processed deck of cards was placed together, and needles (not unlike acupuncture needles) were inserted through the holes to match up the various elements to be coordinated in the search. Needles in place, the deck was shaken vigorously, and those cards having the same notches, and presumably the same characteristics, would fall out of the deck. Voila!

Again, being nostalgic, remember Ralph Shaw and the Rapid Selector, a mechanical device. I recall Mortimer Taube's statement—and perhaps "Taube's Law" that the shorter the input time into a retrieval system, the longer the retrieval time—and the corollary: the quicker the retrieval time from a system, the longer (and perhaps more expensive) the input time.

My personal favorite at that time was the "Peekaboo" system, in which holes were made in cards to code information, and then the deck was held up to the light and if one could see through, he knew he had a match. I do not recall how one got the matches out of the deck, but it was an ingenious system, and lots of fun.

There were many, many more such proposed systems. But they were very personal systems: good for a scientist's reprint collection, or for the circulation system of a small library. After all, how many edge-notched cards can one acupuncture, and how many peekaboos can one efficiently make to get an answer? They were faddish, to be sure, but there was no bandwagon effect in libraries. There were *uses*—but not *abuses.*

Some of the theoretical work, however, was having an effect on what was about to emerge. The systems above depended on a "yes"-"no" theory. If a card was edge-notched and it fell out, it was a "yes"; if it did not, it was a "no"; in "Peekaboo," if you saw light, it was a "yes," if you did not it was a "no."

Enter IBM and the punched card! In a card, a coded punch would be a "yes" and no punch at all would be a "no"—not unlike the now "quaint" systems I have mentioned—except that it was *mechanized*! That meant speed, the ability to handle larger decks of cards, and the lack of error in processing what had been put into them. Suddenly, the keypunch, the sorter, the verifier, and the accounting machine became household words in libraries, librarians went to school to learn how to "wire the boards" of these "infernal machines," and guided by the altruistic hands of IBM, librarians began encoding all kinds of data—and getting out all kinds of products. Here was data-processing equipment: national availability, pushed by a hugely successful company, and somewhat satisfying to the library user who was looking for the black box.

Then came the computer!

But let me backtrack a little for the sake of nostalgia. Concurrently with what we have been talking about there was the miniaturization phase in libraries. Microfilm was surely the answer to the problem of libraries generally. Why, you could get the contents of a huge and costly library into a nine by twelve room and retrieve it with ease. There was, of course, the microcard (both opaque and transparent), and there was microfiche. You could actually get the text of Gray's *Anatomy* into a microdot the size of the head of a pin! Some of these efforts are still with us in one form or another, and probably rightly so.

Let me pause in this Proustian stream of consciousness for a moment and tell you what I am getting at, because history it certainly is not. I have subtitled this paper "The Fruits of Fadism." Webster's Third, while confessing that the origin of the word "fad" is unknown, defines it as "a practice or interest followed for a time with exaggerated zeal." I shall let you decide for yourselves which of the systems I have touched on so far have been, or still are, fads.

And I would like to mention a few more and get a little closer to *medical* librarianship: book catalogs, core lists, union lists, audiovisuals, AIM/-TWX, hospital library consortia, MEDLINE, *Abridged Index Medicus*, storage libraries, computer-assisted instruction, regional library networks, xerox copying, management by objectives, and specialized information centers. Again, I shall allow you to decide for yourselves which of these were, are, or will be fads. Remember, the key phrases in the definition of fad are: "followed for a time" and "exaggerated zeal."

Now, lest you think me arch or oracular, let me say that I believe *fads* belong in *fashion*, not in professionalism, and not in medical librarianship. Fad deals with the length of a woman's skirt or the height of a man's heel; it is what the grille of the newest Pontiac will look like. It has to do with music, with theater, with vacation spots, and with sexual behavior. Fads are for the delight and titillation of the crowd; they provide fodder for small talk; and they keep busy people who have no inner resources or talent for anything more profound.

In professionalism, and in medical librarianship specifically, fads are expensive, transient, frequently iatrogenic, distracting from one's goals, and disillusioning. Question: How does one tell a fad from a real breakthrough? Do all advances go through a "fad stage"?

This was entirely true of X ray in 1896; within a year there were popular and utterly useless books on X ray published for a clamoring public; this seems to be true of acupuncture (which I sopke of irreverently earlier). I wonder if the part of "fadism" that so obviously offends me is the exploitation and hucksterism that accompany the discovery of a new idea or technique?

Let me talk about MEDLARS for a few moments. Several paragraphs back I paused in my nostalgic reverie with the arrival on the scene of the computer. Just as data-processing equipment was not designed for the use of librarians, neither was the computer. Bright minds in the library field, however, wasted little time in devising uses for them. Especially with the computer, the speed, storage capacity, and flexibility of products dazzled the imagination, and it was too tempting not to try to do something with it.

The death of manual indexing in our field came with the end of the [sic] *Index Catalogue*, when the backlog of unprocessed entries exceeded all of the published entries in all of the published volumes of that *Index*. Clearly something had to be done—or "bibliographic control," as we called it, in medicine would die. Again, to simplify vastly the historical record, the National Library of Medicine began to use the computer as an aid to publishing its bibliographic products, to speed them up—to preserve bibliographic control. At the same time the concept of computer storage and retrieval came to light—and after an agonizing birth, MEDLARS came to life. Subject searches with the capacity for many variables could be logically formulated and run against the computer's memory bank of bibliographic entries, and a search was produced. It worked!

Although MEDLARS I and its successors have progressed in a relatively orderly continuum, following (and sometimes aiding) technology, there have been moments of hucksterism—and even faddish elements. NLM obviously wanted to publicize a good thing—and clearly NLM officers had to rationalize within the bureaucracy the enormous research and development costs. Because it was something new, and because it came even closer to the idealistic "black box" that the public, both lay and scientific, yearned for, MEDLARS took on a kind of aura—arcane and fabulous. It was not aided by the early search specialist team, then being trained and regionally deployed who, without really intending to, became sibyline creatures whom one approached with hesitancy and awe.

A next technological step was the idea and the development of searching a computer data base by remote terminal. There were others toiling in the vineyards at this time: Frederick Kilgour and what was to become OCLC; the State University of New York and Irwin Pizer's SUNY System. Bureaucratic and technical problems beset NLM in its efforts, but one of the most ingenious and elegant solutions to the probably-carping bureaucracy, was AIM/TWX. Here was a small data base, relatively easy to handle, which could be queried by machines that either already existed locally or could be obtained at small cost.

In AIM/TWX, however, were the seeds of fadism. Despite its ingenuity, it was built on an inferior data base (*Abridged Index Medicus*), and it certainly had the characteristics of hucksterism (for whatever reasons), and there was a widespread "bandwagon" reaction. I heard, during this period, in Bethesda, a highly-placed officer of NLM (no longer with the library) say informally to a group of people, "You know, I was playing with AIM/TWX the other day, and I asked for citations on 'histopathology of the thymus,' and by God I got citations on 'histopathology of the thymus!'" I waited for him to finish his sentence or his story—but it seemed that that was the end of it. And I asked, "Were they the right citations? Were there enough citations from which a reader could make an intelligent choice? Were they the latest citations?" My questions were met with a look of obvious hauteur. The *process* had clearly become the Lord of the *intellect*.

In spite of the proven success of MEDLARS and its antecedents, they have been the products, or victims, of oversell, or overkill, from the beginning. The earliest search strategists constituted an elite corps—they were usually paid more than journeyman reference librarians, and yet they were making use of only a single bibliography, whereas the "regular" reference librarian was left to cope with *Bulletin Signalétique* and *Meditsinskiĭ Referativnyĭ Zhurnal*, not to mention *Chemical Abstracts*, *Biological Abstracts*, etc., when doing manual searching.

A generation of health scientists is growing up believing that a search of *Index Medicus* or MEDLINE constitutes a comprehensive search of the literature, when clearly hundreds of quality journals germane to medicine are not indexed because they are actually, or probably, indexed in other reference tools. And I continue to be really concerned about that "hopefully rare" character, probably in a hospital library, who conceives of a search in *Abridged Index Medicus* as a quality search of the literature—or who believes that some incredible genius tucked away in a corner of NLM has selected the "best and the brightest" articles for inclusion in AIM. I can only hope that there is a sharp hospital librarian on hand to set him straight.

Now, with the proliferation of machine-readable data bases covering closely-related subject areas, and the probability of compatability, these dangers recede more and more into the background.

Let us turn for a moment to citation indexing: a truly unique idea, one that lent itself beautifully to computer processing, and one that disgorged from the machine a product that we had never seen before—and that could never have been duplicated manually—a true child of the machine. The professional literature was full of papers on citation indexing, but it took the acumen of Eugene Garfield and his Institute for Scientific Information to get a useful product into the libraries. There was a real fad quality about the process: exaggerated zeal, hucksterism, and exploitation. But the system worked and weathered the storm. The reference librarians at the Countway Library keep *Science Citation Index (SCI),* along with *Index Medicus,* closest to their desks—for two reasons, I believe: one, that to the uninitiated, *SCI* is difficult to learn to use and requires help; and two, that the librarians use it themselves as an important tool of choice.

Some of the more recent claims that *SCI*'s use in the selection or promotion of faculty members is the product of an overzealous imagination, and one quite naive in the sociology of scientists. The ability of *SCI* to predict Nobel Prize winners is pushing a good thing to its outer limits.

I do not wish to belabor this point further. Fadism does exist in all areas of our profession: from NLM to the smallest community hospital library. This phenomenon grows from pressures outside the institution, or pressures within the institution itself, or the overzealousness of individuals with faulty perspective and judgment.

I want to make it clear that I am not confusing "experimentation" with fadism. I have a perfect example of the value of the trial and error of experimentation on the stage with me right now. Dr. Brodman and her staff, who have never ceased experimenting with the use of computers in the middle-sized medical library, wondered if a computer-produced book catalog with its ability to be distributed rather widely throughout her community would be a useful addition to her library service. She tried it, evaluated it, and learning that its usefulness was limited, stopped doing it.

Fadism in librarianship drains us uselessly of energy that could and should be put to better, sounder use. We *must* be aware of new ideas and their possible implications for our libraries—but we must use our professional intelligence: experiment, watch, perhaps wait a little while before putting all our eggs in one basket—the specter of our new Ohio State Medical Library looms large in my mind (not because of the failure of the system, but because of the fiscal naiveté among the University administration).

I remember a remark of Dr. Rogers again—not long after he had left

NLM and gone to the University of Colorado. He said, "I understand now why librarians are so reluctant to make major changes overnight in their card catalogs or classification systems." And of course Rogers is right: faddish changes in a library (and it takes time to separate the wheat from the chaff), not only "box you in" yourselves—but box in your successors, frequently in perpetuity. This way of approaching library problems is not "ultra-conservative," it is not "backward," it is not "negative"; it is simple prudence in a profession whose practitioners are duty bound to preserve a scholarly continuum, and exaggerated zeal should be studied with enlightened skepticism.

I seem to have taken up an inordinate amount of time talking about my unprinted subtitle: dealing with fadism; I should get on with the printed main title of my paper, "The Medical Librarian as Manager." No doubt you have guessed by this time the approach that I am going to take toward "management" in libraries.

Let me tell you at this juncture that so far I have done a little bit of warping of history to suit my purposes. I intend to play the devil's advocate to a degree, but by no means entirely. At the Countway Library we have several projects going that are based on modern management techniques, if one must call them that, and that within the next few weeks I shall be writing a foreword for a fine new book on modern management in libraries. So, take me seriously—but remember that I do not always practice what I preach.

First of all, I abhor the words "manager" or "management" as applied to libraries. It is at best a business term probably snuck in the back door via special libraries, which being largely business-oriented, toss these words around with abandon. Indeed, being in business, special libraries do have a concern with management, for they are the bosses, and employees are expected to earn their keep in their special libraries. What happens to the librarians under this set of circumstances? Frequently he or she become "information specialists," or some such thing to avoid what appears to be the odious term: "librarian." (This is the "camouflage" approach.) Another approach to maintaining identity is the "if you can't beat them, join them" tactic; I recently saw, on the ballot for the election of officers of the Special Libraries Association that the title of one of the candidates for President is "Libraries Manager."

May I return to Webster's Third to see exactly what we are talking about. The verb "to manage", the infinitive, is both a transitive verb and an intransitive verb. As an intransitive verb it means basically "to direct or carry on business or affairs." It is a reasonable definition of what many people do; there are certainly synonyms for the process, but neither the synonyms nor the word itself seem to make much sense to me as the activity that librarians perform. There must be motives behind this substitution, and we shall attempt to examine them.

First, however, let us look at the definition of the word "to manage" as a transitive verb: "handle, control; to make and keep submissive; to alter by manipulation." I, for one, think that there has been a subtle merging of the relatively benign (if unnecessary) definition of directing work or business—and the definition suggesting submission, control, and manipulation.

In a medical journal recently, my eye caught an advertisement for a tranquilizer. Glancing over the text, I saw the following phrase: "in large doses (*x* number of milligrams) useful for the *management* of the schizophrenic patient." I thought long and hard about that phrase: here was an ad designed, specifically and expensively, by ad men who make a career of understanding what will attract the attention of special kinds of people—and here was an ad aimed at doctors, that most human of professional groups, extolling the virtues of a drug that would control, keep submissive, and manipulate other human beings. Be it my own naiveté or an unbalanced sense of the need for human compassion, particularly for those with serious problems, I was grossly offended by the advertisement and its message.

It is distinctly possible that the librarian has reached something of an identity crisis. There are certainly today machines and systems that allow the librarian to assign tasks previously done alone to assistants. Does this relative freedom of time mean "time on my hands" for the librarian? And is he or she searching for things to do to fill it? If so, this is a malaise that bears a great deal of examination. I cannot discuss cures for such a malady here. But I do believe that an answer lies in the honing to greater excellence those things that librarians do well and have done well for centuries:

1. Selecting, acquiring, and acting as custodian of the record of man's accomplishments.
2. Organizing this record in a logical and understandable way so that desired pieces of it can be retrieved at a later time.
3. Retrieving portions of the record for a person who wishes to use it—and delivering it to him when and where he wants it and in the form he desires.

There is plenty of room for improvement in the efficiency and effectiveness with which these tasks are performed, and there is no reason in my mind why these tasks cannot be performed by "librarians." "Librarian" is a worthy title, and I can see no improvement to the librarian or to the users of our services by calling ourselves "managers." Indeed, I think of a manager as a manager of a vegetable concession in a supermarket —or the manager of a heavyweight boxer or a football team.

Librarianship has been through one stage in recent memory in which it sought to improve itself by grafting on the language of the so-called documentalists, and there were some intriguing "buzz words" circulating for awhile. Where are they now? Are we better off for having confused ourselves?

I feel the same way about "management science." In our dilemma about who we are, are we turning to the field of business, and are we fashionably merging that field's vocabulary with our own—and to what purpose? Are we improving our lot by blindly turning to the world of business, whose goals of profit making are so antithetical to our own? Are we really better off by studying the "determination of market segments and segment psychographics"?

I can remember years ago sitting in a colleague's room in Philadelphia and two of us reading to each other the abstracts of papers being presented at the American Documentation Association meeting downstairs in that hotel—and roaring with laughter at the pomposity of the language being used. I think the one that turned us on the most at that time was "heuristics" as applied to machine systems. Where is "heuristics" now?

I think that we were dealing then—as we are now—with a situation of fadism—it would seem to have all the characteristics: exaggerated zeal, bandwagonism, and exploitation (how many of you see the glossy advertisements put out by the American Management Association?) Only time will prove the last criterion, "a practice *followed for a time.*" But I will lay odds on it.

Surely there is no harm in looking into the methodologies of other groups to discern whether or not we can learn a technique that will help us in our own field. However, the grave seriousness with which these forays are taken disturbs me. Are our most precious resources: creativity and enthusiasms, being drained off by peripheral interests? Is a librarian-supervisor sitting in his office contemplating "market segments" rather than being out on the library floor nurturing his own staff members in how to serve the library's users? Are the persons that we attract to this newer, "jazzed up" version of librarianship the ones that we want to be the leaders of librarianship tomorrow?

Librarianship is an ancient and honorable profession. Its practitioners, "librarians" are honorable people. Through whatever permutations we go in the near or not so near future, we are likely to continue to exist. Let us make the best use of our time and minds while we are the active practitioners.

Thank you.

Now, if I have succeeded in irritating anyone in this audience, if I have made anyone angry, I consider this effort successful. If, on the other hand, I have raised latent questions in your minds, or possibly stretched your imagination, then I shall feel very successful indeed.

On the Uses of Diversity*

By David Bishop, *Director*

Library of Medicine
University of Nebraska Medical Center
Omaha, Nebraska

ABSTRACT

An examination is made of the uses of diversity in medical library activities and personnel. This concept is extended also to the broader field of librarianship and to some forecasts of future directions for medical libraries.

It is an honor to stand before this association to present the Janet Doe Lecture for 1976. It is also an honor to be introduced so warmly by a colleague whom I have so long admired.† I have never known how to respond to this type of introduction, to this mixture of biography and flattery. I thought it was time I learned how. In search of an answer, I went, by devious routes, to the writings of a seventeenth-century Spanish Jesuit, Baltasar Gracián y Morales.

Here is what old Baltasar (as I've come to think of him) has to say in one of his maxims:

> *Never talk of yourself.* You must either praise yourself—which is vain—or blame yourself—which is little-minded. It ill beseems him that speaks, and ill pleases him that hears. And if you should avoid this in ordinary conversation, how much more ...in public speaking, where every appearance of unwisdom really is unwise...[1].

Heaven forbid that I should give any "appearance of unwisdom" before this audience. We will speak no more of my biography and background. I

*The Janet Doe Lecture on the History or Philosophy of Medical Librarianship, presented June 15, 1976, at the Seventy-fifth Annual Meeting of the Medical Library Association, Minneapolis, Minnesota.

†The speaker was introduced by Scott Adams, a former President of the Medical Library Association.

Originally published in *Bulletin of the Medical Library Association*, Volume 64 (October, 1976), pp. 349-355. Reprinted by permission.

hope you will bear with me, though, if an occasional personal note does creep into this Janet Doe Lecture.

This year of 1976, as we all know almost *ad nauseam*, is one of great symbolic importance in the history of the United States, and in the history of librarianship in this country. In our own smaller world, it is also the tenth year of the Janet Doe Lectures on the History or Philosophy of Medical Librarianship. History is rampant. I hope, then, that I will be forgiven for focussing more on some philosophical aspects of our present and our future than on our past. In the spirit of the times I will try, at least, to put my reflections in a historical context.

To begin, I thought it might be of passing interest to you to know *how* one goes about giving a Janet Doe Lecture. First, of course, one is asked to. One's immediate reaction to this invitation—or mine at least, and with all respect to my predecessors—was "Dear God, I've joined the dinosaurs." Well, perhaps so. It happens that when I had this reaction, I was trying (unsuccessfullly) to read James Michener's *Centennial.* This documentary novel, as many of you know, sets its roots way back in time, and Mr. Michener had this to say of dinosaurs:

> Long after they disappeared . . . it would become fashionable to make fun of the great reptiles. . . . The lumbering beasts would be held up to ridicule as failures, as inventions that hadn't worked. . . . Facts prove just the opposite. The giant reptiles dominated the earth for 135,000,000 years. . . .[They]remain one of the most successful animal inventions nature has provided. They adjusted to their world in marvelous ways and developed all the mechanisms required for the kind of life they led . . .[2].

This may not be an *exact* description of Doe Lecturers, but it will suffice. It also takes care of the first reaction. Unfortunately, a second reaction closely follows. It is a cry from the heart: "But I have nothing to *say*." I wish I were a match for Jacob Bronowski's ideal person, the one with the creative mind, the habit of truth, and a sense of human dignity[3]. He or she would have much to tell us. But most of us mere mortals, faced with the injunction to *say* something, stand ingloriously mute.

But again, my peculiar reading habits came to the rescue. In the proceedings of a symposium on the creative process I ran across the following anecdote[4]. Albert Einstein and the French poet Valéry both found themselves at a reception in Paris. Valéry seems to have had a consuming interest in the process of intellectual creation, and buttonholed Einstein immediately. How, he wanted to know, did Einstein go about this work; please tell him about it. Einstein was rather vague, mentioning that he did start every day by going out in the morning for a walk. Ah, pounced Valery, and of course he took a notebook with him so that he could jot down the ideas that came into his head. Well, no, Einstein admitted, he didn't. Valéry was crestfallen. "You don't?" "Well, no," said Einstein, "You know, an idea is so *rare*."

And indeed it is. But with James Michener and Albert Einstein behind one, how can one say "No"? So one becomes a Doe Lecturer. And must then find a topic. The limits are set. The topic must be on the history or philosophy of our profession. If one is not a historian—as I am not—one must willy-nilly become a philosopher.

IN PRAISE OF DIVERSITY

My topic itself was chosen in a fit of pique. At the time, I was annoyed with some of our friends at the National Library of Medicine. I thought they were attempting to impose a needless uniformity on one aspect of the healthily diversified regional medical library programs. As it happens, I was mistaken. But my question to myself—"Don't they know the uses of diversity?"—stayed with me, and grew. Here, at last, was a topic, one on which some reflection might well profit us all.

But would it fit? Consider the Doe Lectures we have had: Annan on our history, Rogers on subject analysis, Brandon on academic status, Brodman on excellence, Adams on innovation and MEDLARS, Darling on certification, Felter on cooperation, and Bloomquist on fadism. Here is diversity enough to make the very word the hallmark of the lectures.

And would it honor Janet Doe? The time has already come, foreseen by Harold Bloomquist just last year, when "there will be a Doe Lecturer who probably will never have had the opportunity to have met or known Miss Doe"[5]. I shook her hand but once and know her not at all. But from all that I know *of* her, I know her talents to have been as diverse as her thoughts are incisive. Reflections on the uses of diversity do no dishonor to her legacy.

I must establish right away that I am not setting up a straw man whom it would be easy, but no honor, to knock down. I am sure we are all convinced that we approve of diversity among ourselves, that we would scorn a narrow uniformity. Total sameness—"library cloning," if you will—would be dull at best. Our work takes us close enough to biology to see the dangers of cloning. We can agree that "if we have learned anything from studies on evolution, it is that a highly varied gene pool confers adaptability and survival value upon a species. One of the effects of . . . cloning would. . .be reduction of the variability of the. . .gene pool"[6].

Ah, yes. We all favor plenty of variability in the library gene pool. But we must, of course, strive for, say, cost-effectiveness. And if a cost-effective procedure is demonstrated by one, then it should be adopted by all. And if a "core list" works in Long Island, it must of course work in San Mateo. And if "measurable learning objectives" are a retrieval dimension needed by some, they may as well be used by all. Or if, in the world of interlibrary loans, "hierarchical referral," seen large, is most effective, then it will be most effective, too, of course, seen small.

Of course we approve of diversity. We just don't want to practice too much of it. Fortunately, we're a lethargic group on the whole and we don't take action against the not-*too*-diverse. Oh, the bookmen mutter about audiovisuals, and the AV-types talk of "media" and sometimes forget that print is a medium too. But they live in semiharmony, or at least in contiguity. So, too, the computer people may scorn the scribblers, while the conscientious reference librarian worries over the mistaking of a limited computer-based file for the dawn of universal bibliography. But they work side by side.

The hospital librarian calls for recognition of the value of her or his role; the academic medical librarian nods agreement and ponders the criteria for academic promotion. But they work together. The clerk at the circulation desk wonders what on earth the regional library office does; the regional director gives little thought to the irate nursing student gloriously cursing the missing issue. But together, these librarians deliver documents.

Sometimes, the diversity appears to get out of hand and threaten an accepted unity. Then we do take action, if only by setting up a committee to study the "problem." We can set up all the committees we wish to see if that group is good for the MLA, or this group is bad for the MLA. But people are going to do what they feel they need to do. If a group of catalogers entranced by OCLC terminals—or a group of uncategorized librarians as worried about population graphs as about Bradford curves—wants to get together, they will, and there is nothing that can be done to stop them.

So we may as well make a virtue of it. And, in fact, there is virtue in it. For, in truth, in diversity lies unity, and the only true unity is in diversity.

I am not propounding anarchy. Diversity within a profession is variety within a framework. We cannot be all things to all men, but medical librarians must be many things to many people before our course is run.

Medical Libraries: Historical View

Let us consider our roots. We are an old profession, but a new specialty within it. The libraries of ancient and not-so-ancient times served only an elite. Only the elite, after all, could read. Then there came, in this country, the Jacksonian revolution: the franchise was extended to the workingman (provided, of course that workingman meant man, and not woman, and, of course, that he was white). There came, too, at this time the workingmen's libraries of Manchester and Boston. Only then did libraries, however hesitatingly, enter the world of the common people.

When our own specialty was begun, it too began as libraries for an elite—the physicians and surgeons of our society, who had a smattering of poor Latin but a groping towards a scientific basis for their calling. We perhaps forget how recent we are, yet as late as 1887, John Shaw Billings could say:

> ...we are all learning gradually how to use medical libraries, and in a few years more I predict that the wonder will be how we ever got on without them[7].

A good prediction. Yet we all know that it was not until 1937 that medical bibliography courses were begun for librarians, and not until 1942 that the first professional librarian was hired to work at the National Library of Medicine[8]. No wonder, then, that our own Jacksonian revolution—our own diversification of medical libraries beyond the elite—is a thing of living memory and present debate.

And what diversification we are seeing! Some of the great private libraries, both society and academic, have survived, generally by broadening their base to serve more than the doctor of medicine. New academic libraries have been founded, almost all of them including more of the health sciences than medicine alone. "Doctors' libraries" in hospitals, many with long histories of their own, have become or are becoming hospital libraries serving the whole gamut of health-care personnel.

It is hardly surprising, then, that we have seen diversification too, among ourselves. We have still the one-person library where the sole librarian must try to give "primary care" across the whole range of our services. (What an unsung hero or heroine he or she is, manning these outposts, meeting those needs that can be met from limited resources, sending for reinforcements when necessary—and, as a group, forestalling an invasion by information-hungry hordes before whom the larger centers would quickly crumble.) At the other end of the spectrum is the research librarian whose expertise is in toxicology and the manipulation of TOXLINE, subspecializing in the area of on-line bibliographic services, itself a subspecialty of medical reference work, itself a subspecialty of medical librarianship, itself a specialty within the library profession.

There is an obvious danger here. Too narrow a specialization could lead to what Lee Thayer bitingly attacks as "the functions of incompetence"[9]. Yet specialization is a rational response to complex needs. The answer is to see our specialization as being part of and within a unified whole. The things we do—select, acquire, record, organize, store, preserve, retrieve, and disseminate—are simple enough to list. But they are complex to do. To carry out this complexity of activities for a multiplicity of clienteles, it is no wonder that we have diversified, nor that we shall diversify further as complexity increases.

It is my thesis that health-information services *will* grow more complex, that even greater diversity will be needed among us in our future.

Medical Libraries: The Future

Let's try to see part way into that future. If the past is prologue for our present, our present is prologue for the future. It is not difficult to foresee some continuity. I have, for example, little patience with those who speak of the death of the book. It isn't dead, and it isn't dying. It's a very resilient and, indeed, rather remarkable technological invention. In serving three functions, as a mechanism for specific information recall, as a source for guided learning, and as a stimulus to thought and reflection, it is a hard tool to beat. It got beaten, of course, as a carrier of *new* information, by the codex-format journal, which for centuries now has taken pride of place as the source of the latest information. And it has been joined, in these past few decades, by another dimension in guided learning, the whole complex of audiovisual instructional aids. But these three live, it seems to me, in a healthy, if evolving, symbiosis, without mutual threats of extinction.

I have little patience, too, with those who, suffering from historical myopia, speak of the present time as the post-industrial era, or even the Age of Information. We still are very firmly within the Industrial Revolution. The application of science and technology to our daily lives has not ceased; we have not yet finished establishing the unity of nature, let alone the family of man. Nor does our society, present or immediate future, run on information systems. It runs on the extraction of wealth from the land and the sea, and on the processing or manufacture of that wealth, on its transportation and its commerce. Formal information systems are indeed one of the lubricants for the complex machine that society has made of these processes and their attendant human needs. But they are not the machine itself, and it behooves us to remember what a small part we play.

In case we should be feeling too uppity, remember these chilling words from Albert Szent-Györgyi:

> I am very ignorant of scientific literature and so, in an hour's time spent in the library, I could find more knowledge that is new to me than I can find at my workbench in a month or a year. All the same, most of the time I sit at my bench and not in the library. It is not knowledge, but new knowledge which attracts me, creating something that was not there before[10].

In his recent book on science and society[11], John Ziman helps put this in perspective for us. He agrees that new *ideas* come only from *individuals*—mulling over old concepts, reassessing the known in the light of the unknown. But for the three uses of scientific knowledge—the creation of new knowledge, the social use of physical resources, and the solution of social problems—for all of these, information is useless, Ziman reminds us, unless it is *communicated.* There, and there only, is the heart of our profession.

With these caveats in mind, let us look at where we are going. I take it as established fact that our society and its information needs are growing ever more complex. The Industrial Revolution grows in technologic complexity: it does not become simpler. I take it as an equally established fact that many people feel alienated by this technology: they wish for individual needs and worth to be recognized, for this technological complexity to be somehow brought to human scale, for man, not the machine, to be the measure. Our society is bearing these two seemingly conflicting trends into its future, and our profession is carried with them.

What is also being carried is the seemingly endless growth of scientific information. Our stacks and ourselves are already groaning under its weight. Is there no end in sight? Certainly, it has become commonplace to speak of the exponential growth of scientific information. And in that very phrase some have found hope. After all, exponential growth cannot logically continue forever: it should sweep gently into a nice logistic curve with a flattening of growth and eventual saturation. Derek Price, among others, has expressed the opinion that we are now in the flattening-out stage[12].

But it seems not to be so. In his OECD report, *Information in 1985*[13], Georges Anderla demonstrates that the growth curve is as steep as ever. This report has engendered furious debate, but its major qualitative findings have not been refuted. Scientific information, according to Anderla, is indeed growing exponentially, and will continue to do so as long as it is fed by the continuing diversification of the sciences, of which there is no end in sight. Anderla draws yet other conclusions: the greater the quantity of information, the greater its use. That is to say, the supply of information creates a demand for information. And the rate of growth of the supply is almost exactly matched by the rate of growth of the resultant demand.

Improving Access to Information

We will not only have to handle more information, we will have to handle more demand for it. Can our current mechanisms stand the strain? I don't think so. But I think we will have new mechanisms that can. Our current carrier of this ever-increasing new information is the journal. I doubt that it can continue in this primary role. It is fast becoming an uneconomic and inefficient means of transferring new information, and the resources to support an ever-increasing population of journals simply do not exist.

Once again, technology to the rescue? Yes, I think so. I happen to agree with those who say that "...unless technology, clearly understood, is systematically evaluated with each application...it carries with it a propensity to fail. The existence of technology is not a valid reason for its application"[14]. But in this instance, I see no reason why, at this moment, journals should continue in their present format. For those publishers who can afford it, editing and layout are already being done on video display tubes from manuscripts (!) already converted into computer-readable form. It will seem ludicrous to future generations that this computer-based information is then once more put back into print format for distribution.

The National Science Foundation has already issued guidelines[15] for proposals for what it calls an "Access Improvement Program," which is bureaucratese for just such computer-readable information-transfer systems. In their study[16] for the NSF on publisher-library relationships, Fry and White give serious consideration to the future electronic storage and distribution of the kind of information currently published in journals.

It will not happen overnight, but it will happen: in the future many a scientific article will not be published at all. Rather, through some device, probably an automatically produced alerting system, the information seeker will be led to key-in his need at a remote terminal, perhaps scan an article on a CRT, command its delivery to him (probably in computer-output microform, or perhaps in electronic transfer to his local computer bank), and no doubt be billed automatically for the service.

This tale of the future need not alarm us. The technology is already familiar to us, and we don't have to leap ahead to the development of high-density photo-optical systems with laser scanners; I'll let some future Doe Lecturer comfort us with those. We can take some comfort from the past. Among its other distinctions, 1976 is the 350th anniversary of the death of Francis Bacon, and it was this great believer in natural philosophy who warned us that "... he that will not apply new remedies, must expect new evils"[17]. And there is comfort, too, in the present. One of my favorite contemporary novelists, Ursula LeGuin, in one of her tales of the future, has her characters use a moving bedtime invocation: "Praise then darkness, and Creation unfinished"[18]. In this I find the artist telling me that all information is imperfect, and that if it were not we would need to strive no more.

In a lighter vein, I am reminded of an occurrence some years ago in Kew Gardens in London. A large Cockney family was enjoying an outing, having brought with them their very old grandmother. She had not, I gather, been often away from her own city neighborhood. Spying a very beautiful sundial, she wanted to know what it was. Her grandchildren explained in detail how it worked. Beaming with delight, the grandmother could only say, "What will they think of next!"

Future Role of Medical Libraries

But back to the medical library, now that "they" have thought of the on-line journal. What has become of the medical library with its great store of medical journals and its bibliographic retrieval systems? It has become one site, and one only, of the remote terminal. At least in the major centers its journal-reading clientele is sitting at its own terminals getting its own materials directly, at its own cost. The library will still have its review journals and some journal-compendia. There must be a digestive system between the issuance of new knowledge and its absorption into the teaching corpus of books and audiovisuals and the other instructional aids that the library still will retain. But the medical library will not be the primary source for journal-article dissemination that it is today.

What then will it disseminate? The answer is *information*. This is already the thread that ties us together with all of our diversity, from the smallest one-person library to the behemoth that is NLM. It will become an even stronger thread as the diversifying sciences cause us further to diversify among ourselves. For, while on-line systems can be made fairly simple to operate, they cannot be made to simplify the content of their materials. As our knowledge and information increase in complexity, so does the need increase for people trained to thread their way through this maze of information, to find what is pertinent, combine it with what is related, merge it into what is needed. There is a need, in brief, for what Estelle Brodman calls the "information synthesizer."

Nor must we wait for the on-line journal, or the use of an in-house mini-computer as a Mixmaster. Already there is an area of need evident between the formal state-of-the-art review and those address lists of information that we call bibliographies. This is the area of need for analyzed, synthesized, packaged information.

Our society has entered a phase in the evolution of health care that requires such a service. The allied health professions are proliferating almost as quickly as is new information itself. A concerned public will not much longer be content with home medical encyclopedias. In a survey conducted for NLM, the Association for Hospital Medical Education reported that "...rather than instantaneous computerized generation of a bibliography, interviewees [in community hospitals] indicated a greater need for some meaningful assessment for the contents of the articles that might be in such a bibliography"[19].

The journal-article bibliography, the full-text document, or even the on-line data bank will not answer these groups' needs. An information center dispensing *information* will. I do not know where these information synthesizers will come from. I think I know where they will most effectively *be*—in the medical library.

And I hope you realize what they will be doing: giving individualized service in response to need, and using technology as their tools-in-trade. Nor, despite my examples of the allied health professions and a concerned public, will this somehow be a less sophisticated service than some others we profess to. (I must digress here to say that I am always saddened that in a democracy a writer of "popular" scientific articles is somehow considered to be of lesser stature. The only answer I know to Jefferson's noisome "aristocracy of the intellect" is Bronowski's "democracy of knowledge"[20].)

All health professionals will need information as they struggle with the never-ending task of continuing education, whether self-inspired or socially required. There will be many support services for continuing education outside the purview of the medical library, and in the future these will include the individual's own computer-terminal access to primary resources. But there will remain that intermediate need, the development of *individualized* packages from the enormous stock of information, selected, retrieved, and put together. If medical librarians do not do this, I do not know who will.

Diversity and Unity

Throughout this journey into our possible future, we have travelled two main tracks: the increasing impact of technology and the increasing need for personalized services. I think we have found that these two seemingly conflicting trends have a high degree of complementarity.

They will certainly have a profound impact on the practice of our profession. The world we have been talking about is the world of scientific information, not that of the humanist tradition of our great scholarly libraries. If information services in the health sciences develop even roughly in the way I foresee, the gap between medical librarianship and general humanistic librarianship will grow even wider. We may well be seen as *too* diverse a specialty within librarianship, and find ourselves cut adrift. Our historical collections and rare-book colleagues may keep us attached for a while, but they are a fragile connection. Already, if I read correctly between the lines of the reports of the National Commission on Libraries and Information Science, we are considered pesky nuisances who don't really fit.

Yet it is as necessary to meet the future information needs of the health sciences as it is to meet society's needs in general to learn from our great humanist traditions, from those works so carefully preserved in our scholarly libraries. Our diversity as medical librarians is necessary if we are to continue to work for the health of mankind. But the unity of all librarianship is necessary to continue the advancement of all learning.

Within our own specialty of medical librarianship we have seen the future bringing us yet further diversity. The "firing line" library will not disappear: the immediacy of working information is too important. Yet how different will be the core collection librarian of the future—with how qualitatively different a core from our present concepts—from the information synthesizer working with his or her computer banks in the area, say, of environmental carcinogenesis. And how different will the monograph cataloger feel—still, in Robert Merton's phrase, "converting the tacit empiricism of lists into the analytical rationalism of categories"[21] —from the media librarian discussing curriculum design with the biomedical communications specialist and the director of continuing education.

Yet these, and many others, will be the diverse members of the profession of medical librarianship. Our strength, our ability to disseminate medical information effectively, will depend on this diversity. But there is danger too: will we become too dissimilar and too removed from our humanistic roots, to form a unity? Can we continue down this road of diversification, at the same time taking aboard colleagues from biomedical communications, computer sciences, management studies, operations research, and Lord knows what other disciplines, and still retain our colleagueship?

The question is not one that applies to a profession alone. Mankind itself seems cursed with a need to distrust, or even hate, that which is too divergent from its immediate group. Our society struggles to find an answer that will let all men live together in peace and dignity, yet it is deeply afflicted with the foul disease of racism. There is a recent work on racism[22] that casts aside pious hopes and gives instead some practical recipes for actions that may help bring us together. We, facing our own group interactions in divisive circumstances, might learn from it.

Five conditions are set for a favorable outcome to interactions for reducing prejudice. First, there must be positive interdependence in meeting broad goals that are held in common. Second, those working together must have equal status. Third, there has to be a social climate favorable to the goals. Fourth, those working together must do so with a high degree of intimacy. And finally, the outcome should be rewarding.

I do not know how well or how broadly this prescription will work in our society at large: the roots of racism are deep and multiform. But I cannot come up with a better prescription for a Medical Library Association threatened by diversification and disunity. We must all, indeed, recognize our interdependence as we try in common to make available the information of the health sciences. We must recognize the equality among us: we are all colleagues. We ourselves must set our standards so that they are favorable to our goals. We must indeed work closely together, one with another; none of us can stand alone. And for a rewarding outcome, what could be more rewarding than the realization that we have helped to improve the health of mankind?

Diversity among us is essential if we are to continue our work effectively. Unity among us is essential if our work is to be worthwhile. Let us have both.

REFERENCES

1. Gracián y Morales, Baltasar. The Art of Worldly Wisdom, transl. from the Spanish by Joseph Jacobs. London, Macmillan, 1930. (Reprint of 1st ed., 1892.) Maxim no. 117.
2. Michener, James A. Centennial. New York, Random House, 1974. p. 63-64.
3. Bronowski, J. Science and Human Values. New York, Harper, 1959.
4. Krebs, Hans A. and Shelley, Julian H., eds. The Creative Process in Science and Medicine. Amsterdam, Excerpta Medica, 1975. p. 3.
5. Bloomquist, Harold. The medical librarian as manager; or the fruits of fadism. Bull. Med. Libr. Assoc. 63: 359-365, Oct. 1975.
6. Dodson, Edward O. Further thoughts on molecular biology and metaphysics. Perspect. Biol. Med. 18: 306-312, Spring 1975.
7. Billings, J. S. Methods of research. In: Rogers, F. B., comp. Selected Papers of John Shaw Billings. Chicago, Medical Library Association, 1965. p. 198-206.
8. Annan, Gertrude L. The Medical Library Association in retrospect, 1937-1967. Bull. Med. Libr. Assoc. 55: 379-389, Oct. 1967.
9. Thayer, Lee. On the functions of incompetence. Perspect. Biol. Med. 18: 332-344, Spring, 1975.
10. Szent-Györgyi, Albert. On scientific creativity. Perspect. Biol. Med. 5: 173-178, Winter 1962.
11. Ziman, John. The Force of Knowledge: The Scientific Dimension of Society. Cambridge, England, Cambridge University Press, 1976.
12. Price, D. J. de S. Little Science, Big Science. New York, Columbia University Press, 1963.
13. Anderla, Georges. Information in 1985. Paris, Organization for Economic Co-operation and Development, 1973.
14. Taub, Arthur. Electrical stimulation for the relief of pain: Two studies in technological zealotry. Perspect. Biol. Med. 19: 125-135, Autumn 1975.
15. National Science Foundation. Office of Science Information Service. Guidelines for preparation of unsolicited proposals for the Access Improvement Program. Inf. News & Sources 7: 259-263, Nov. 1975.
16. Fry, Bernard M., and White, Herbert S. Economics and Interaction of the Publisher-Library Relationship in the Production and Use of Scholarly and Research Journals. U.S. National Science Foundation, Office of Science Information Services, Nov. 1975. (PB 249 108.) (Synopsis in: Inf. Hotline 8(3): 17-21, March 1976.)
17. Bacon, Francis. The Essays or Counsels, Civil and Moral, of Francis Ld. Verulam. . . . Mt. Vernon, New York, Peter Pauper Press, n.d. p. 96.
18. Le Guin, Ursula K. The Left Hand of Darkness. New York, Ace Books, 1973. p. 232.
19. Association for Hospital Medical Education. Role of Community Hospitals in Continuing Education of Health Professionals; Final Report. Contract no. 1-LM-4-4732, National Library of Medicine, Arlington, Virginia, 1975. (PB-243 986.) p. 63.
20. Bronowski, J. The Ascent of Man. Boston, Little, Brown, 1973. p. 435.
21. Merton, Robert K. Thematic analysis in science: notes on Holton's concept. Science 188: 335-338, Apr. 25, 1975.
22. Katz, Phyllis A., ed. Towards the Elimination of Racism. New York, Pergamon Press, 1976.

Foundations of Medical Librarianship*

By Erich Meyerhoff, *Librarian and Assistant Dean for Information Resources*

Cornell University Medical College
New York, New York

ABSTRACT

The development of medical librarianship during the last forty years is examined as reflected in the changes of its resources, technology, education, and knowledge base. A shift from historical to scientific inquiry constitutes the direction of medical librarianship. Its nexus is the gathering of information and the transfer of knowledge. The social and human resources for this ongoing change and the basis for a quest for excellence is seen in the pool of talent represented by hospital librarians and the aspirations of the women's movement for equality.

BEFORE you stands a reluctant Janet Doe Lecturer, uncertain in purpose, of limited vision, and feeling unequal to the task with which you have honored him. David Bishop, my immediate predecessor, wondered about his mission and whether the call had already placed him among the ancients, among the dinosaurs whose faulty adaptation led to extinction. Diplomatically and with witty assurance, however, we were reminded of the dinosaurs' hardiness and on the authority of one of our successful contemporary novelists, of their millennia-long rule of the earth. Ambiguity seemed evident in the presentations of the two lectures which preceded that of David Bishop. The late Jacqueline Felter asked whether cooperation was a wave of the future or a ripple. Harold Bloomquist, ever so incisively, looked at fads and fashions in the management of medical libraries in a somber, introspective appraisal. How different in approach and feeling from Scott Adams's "The Way of the Innovator," a celebration of the achievement of Frank Rogers in transforming the form and function of the

*The Janet Doe Lecture on the History or Philosophy of Medical Librarianship, presented June 14, 1977, at the Seventy-seventh Annual Meeting of the Medical Library Association, Seattle, Washington.

Originally published in *Bulletin of the Medical Library Association*, Volume 65 (October, 1977), pp. 409-418. Reprinted by permission.

National Library of Medicine; Estelle Brodman's affirmation of intellectual excellence; Alfred Brandon's review and support of faculty status for librarians; Louise Darling's examination of certification; Rogers's analysis of a runaway *MeSH*; and Gertrude Annan's review of the association's history from 1937 to 1967.

Doubt rather than affirmation has characterized the intellectual and artistic analysis of our times and my own beginnings in the profession in the fifties. Auden[1] spoke of the Age of Anxiety; 1984 became the catchword for the dehumanization and harsh conformity of our society in Orwell's[2] apocalyptic vision. Hannah Arendt[3] could speak of the banality of evil in describing Eichmann, a bureaucrat who managed the unprecedented extermination of several million human beings.

In our own field the past fifteen years have been a period of immense growth of ideas, resources, and services. It was a period of marvelous advances which conferred professional satisfaction on those who came into the field as well as the older, established practitioners. Yet the temper of our times no longer equates change with progress, and buoyant notions of abundance are challenged by admonitions of physical and personal limits in a new age of scarcity. "Are we really on the threshold of a renaissance for the library profession, or are these the long days of a twilight in which libraries continue to be exhausted by budget cuts and abandoned by their constituencies?. . ." Nina Matheson[4] asked, examining the future of our profession. This is also the uncertainty that I bring to the task. Change has been the most prominent characteristic of the immediate past and a personal experience. To stand at the end or close to the end is neither tragic nor unpleasant.

I would like to bear witness, then, to some of the changes in our profession, its resources and services, its education and its knowledge base as they occurred in the United States of America. In this review persons and contributions serve as types and illustrations. Exhaustive attribution to all who may have been involved has not been attempted. The title of this paper then is a little high-flown and unfortunately pretentious. My reach was so much higher than my grasp.

Resources

The growth and development of resources, technology, and services in all medical libraries is an astonishing achievement. In 1898 a total of 48 libraries were recorded in the February issue of *Medical Libraries,* the predecessor of the *Bulletin.* In 1940, 842[5] and in 1973, 2,984[6] were listed. In 1940, 5 million[5] bound volumes constituted total holdings. There were more than 30 million in 1973[6]. Susan Crawford[7] has just documented an even greater growth of the resources of medical school libraries. She reported average library budgets of medical schools in 1960/61 as $57,471 compared to $328,093 in 1973/74. Bloomquist[8], in his survey of medical school libraries, reported a median of 992 current serial titles held in 1960, while in 1975 the median was 1,942, according to Hendricks[9]. A threefold increase in the number of professional librarians occurred in the fifteen-year period following Bloomquist's[8] findings in 1960, and eighty-six new library buildings were constructed between 1966 and 1975[7].

The acceleration of change after the implementation of the Medical Library Assistance Act of 1965 is so marked that a causal relationship appears self-evident. Of the appropriated funds, $11.8 million or 29% were expended for the improvement of resources during its first five years[10]. These funds were used mainly for the purchase of journals and books in medical school libraries. Not only did the library collections show growth in their book and periodical holdings but with the advent of self-instructional materials, audiocassettes, tape-slides, and videocassettes were acquired at a time when this educational technology was still undergoing rapid changes in format and was extremely costly. Computer-assisted instruction became another library-based dimension of new modes of learning. Libraries accepted these new materials easily as part of their acquisition and dissemination function.

Crawford[7] suggests that the rise in the rate of development of resources in medical school libraries has come to an end. The resources for health care institutions directly concerned with patient care, however, must expand. To meet information needs in the community, hospitals, and other health care establishments, support is provided by consortium resource grants from the National Library of Medicine. The development of library-based patient education programs is beginning to add a new and exciting dimension to library service in hospitals and health care centers.

What is the relationship of resource development to the growth of the biomedical literature? Corning and Cummings[11], in a cogent review of the development of biomedical communications in the United States, found that of the 19,000 periodical titles received by the National Library of Medicine in 1974, 6,318 are included in SERLINE because they are deemed sufficiently important to be part of this on-line location service, and 2,244 of these are indexed in *Index Medicus* because they are substantive journals. Current subscriptions in the libraries reported in Hendricks's[9] survey varied from 6,836 at the Biomedical Library of the University of California, Los Angeles, to 520 at the newly established Wright State University in Ohio. The median number of subscriptions was 1,942. Thus 50% of the libraries surveyed were not receiving all of the journals indexed in the *Index Medicus*. To attain subscriptions to all journals covered by this index was once a prominent goal of collection development in medical school libraries, just as the magic one hundred titles in the *Abridged Index Medicus* became a convenient goal for smaller collections.

Inflation, the devaluation of the dollar, and the sharp curtailment of funds in the health sector of our economy suddenly put a halt to the euphoric hopes of continuous resource development. Instead, desperate measures became commonplace. Some libraries placed a moratorium on new subscriptions. Five hundred or even 2,000 titles were discontinued in some larger libraries. Unable to hold what was useful, libraries had to define what was necessary. Not all were equally affected and we need to assess again the quality of resources and their distribution.

To deal with these adverse economic conditions by discontinuing all journals published in languages other than English, for example, as Truelson[12] suggests, implies an unfortunate parochialism and intellectual isolation. Our troubles had the salutary effect of beginning an examination of the rationale of our acquisitions policies. It also emphasized how much we have indeed become part of a national medical library system which so far has had an enviable success in reaching the goal of equality of access to biomedical information. The provision of sufficient resources and the viability of the system is, and remains, a national responsibility. Only on the basis of continuing and adequate government funding can our network retain and improve its reliability.

Technology

Times when automation consisted of punched cards, a sorter, and an accounting machine are beyond the recollection of some of us because the one central element of technology applied to medical library practice has been, and continues to be, the computer. While the *Index Medicus* was fashioned in 1960 with the use of punched cards and the step and repeat camera, the capability of automating the arrangement of citations to make these searchable by the computer was achieved in 1964 through the Medical Literature Analysis and Retrieval System at the National Library of Medicine. The National Library of Medicine led not only all other libraries, but the country, in the development of a large-scale computer-aided indexing and information retrieval system.

Especially noteworthy was Rogers's insistence that the bibliographic integrity of the record should not be sacrificed to the limitations of the machine, as was frequently the custom when "quick and dirty" often characterized computer-produced bibliographies. The controlled indexing vocabulary of *MeSH* became what is to date the last major effort by a librarian to cope systematically with the organization of information in medicine. Large-scale data systems in biology, psychology, chemistry, and engineering, which developed subsequently, either abandoned the effort or never attempted it and left us with some of the vagaries of free text searching. MEDLARS developed into an international biomedical information system. Another of its major accomplishments was the significant enlargement of the productivity of librarians in providing bibliographic information. Manual literature searches were then and continue to be performed in libraries, and complete literature searches require them. But the number of searches which could be performed by journal scanning and the use of printed indexes and abstracts was so time-consuming that such a service was offered in few libraries. Computer-assisted searching satisfied the real and immediate demand for this service. Librarians trained in search formulations acquired a unique expertise which could be learned by others devoting sufficient time and practice to it, but it compared to other analytical skills found in a medical setting, best left to those with the training and experience to perform them. No small part of the professional recognition of librarians may be attributed to the use of this new and needed technology.

With the support of the National Library of Medicine a burst of experimentation in computer applications to medical library tasks ensued. At the University of California, Los Angeles, under Louise Darling, and at Washington University, under Estelle Brodman, to name two prominent examples, applications were made to circulation, cataloging, production of book catalogs, and serials control. At Washington University this last developed into the PHILSOM network. The late Jacqueline Felter developed a computer-assisted union catalog at the Medical Library Center of New York and its programs spawned other union catalogs in many regions.

These are only instances, as the list of librarians who have made productive use of these new resources is long and many of them are known to you. Perhaps the most fruitful applications have been those which provided centralized services for many, especially smaller, libraries. The Medical Library Center of New York, for instance, provides a catalog card procurement service through its access to the Ohio College Library Center System. The inclusion of the current catalog data in OCLC will increase the utility of this system for medical libraries.

The new technology has increased labor productivity by the reduction of clerical routine. Reliable controls and ready access to management data which are crucial to planning have become readily available. The advent of the minicomputer has marked the beginning of a cost reduction of this equipment, and the expansion of the shared use of computers will make their use in smaller libraries economical and desirable.

Services

As resources expanded so did services. Document delivery and interlibrary loans increased steeply with the operation of the Regional Medical

Library Network. The 108 institutions, nearly all medical schools, in Hendricks's[9] survey for 1975/1976 lent nearly 925,000 items, while they borrowed only 180,000. They lent five times the amount borrowed. The beneficiaries were hospitals with small or no collections. The availability of computer-assisted searches and a federally supported system of document access and delivery suddenly brought journals and books easily within the reach of practitioners. Libraries were making significant progress in replacing the "detail man" as a source of reliable information. The change which transformed medical libraries from information sources to information agencies has been going on since the founding of the association but came into prominence in the last fifteen years.

Ralph Shaw[13], in his recommendation for the National Institutes of Health Library, suggested long ago that in addition to look-up services for facts in standard sources, a "bibliographic intelligence" be manned by subject literature specialists with advanced education to provide services tailored to the needs of the investigators, including state-of-the-art reports and evaluative information. These proposals were realized in part in the information centers established by the National Institute of Neurological Diseases and Stroke. Their rise and fall was reviewed by Darling[14]. Today only the Brain Information Service at the University of California, Los Angeles, and the Clinical Neurology Information Center at the University of Nebraska remain.

The manual bibliographic search service and the routing of journals have been superseded by computer-aided searches and selective dissemination. The circulation of tables of contents of journals, initiated by the late J. Alan MacWatt, librarian at Lederle Laboratories, has become a vast commercial success through *Current Contents*®.

Clinical librarianship broke completely new ground in bringing information and librarians to the bedside. Gertrude Lamb initiated this service at the University of Missouri and has continued it at the Hartford Hospital in Connecticut. It is a mode of service which promises to establish once again a close and systematic relationship between physicians and librarian.

The Regional Medical Program funded many library-based information and document delivery services. Many have continued because the medical community found them essential and was willing to fund them.

We are still at the watershed but the issues are joined and it is my own bias that we must be accepted not for the volumes on our shelves but for the information needs to which we can professionally respond. To be sure, this calls for subject expertise, which many already possess. The main problem is not one of preparation and direction but, at least in academic institutions, the demonstration and acceptance that librarians are far better than others, including graduate students, at information gathering.

Education

Medical librarians today have completed far more formal education than had practitioners in the fifties. Nearly all have a master's degree from an accredited library school, many have degrees in a subject specialty, and increasingly heads of medical libraries have doctoral degrees. Whether we are better educated than Janet Doe, who did not attend a library school, or James Ballard of the Boston Medical Library who was superbly self-educated and unencumbered by any academic scrolls, is questionable.

In ever-increasing numbers we attend continuing education courses offered by the association at annual meetings and locally in our regions. We have attested to the seriousness of our purpose by employing a full-time director of education, and under this professional leadership the syllabi of the continuing education courses have been revised, improved in content and appearance, and directed toward defined educational objectives. An evaluation of the quality and effectiveness of this effort, however, is needed.

Mary Louis Marshall established a twelve-month residency at Tulane's Rudolph Matas Medical Library in 1941 and Eileen Cunningham followed in 1944 at Vanderbilt. Both ladies were endowed with formidable personalities, as those here who remember them may attest. It is perhaps for this reason that these programs did not survive their departures. In conception and content these were vigorous, dedicated, but still searching efforts to acquaint librarians with the unique features of a specialty as practiced in the libraries where the training took place. With the funding of training by the National Library of Medicine these programs took on a new and sophisticated dimension. Specialized instruction, for example, in computer applications to medical library problems was offered at Washington University, in administration and the history of medicine at Johns Hopkins, and in several specialties at the University of California, Los Angeles. The careful selection of participants to involve those most likely to benefit from and to succeed in the program, a choice of academic courses to provide an underpinning of their practical training, the evaluation of the program, and the progress of the participants characterized these efforts. They ended when training grants were discontinued as part of a general reduction of support of all federally funded training programs in the health sciences.

The training coordinator at the Biomedical Library of the University of California, Los Angeles, commented (on the end of its federally funded training program which began in 1961 and continued without interruption for thirteen years to 1974) that forty-six young librarians had passed through the programs and that more than 80% of them had remained active in the field. She believed, and with justification, that the impact of the program had been felt throughout the library community.

Indeed, centers of excellence with good training facilities had developed and the trainees of these programs were desirable recruits for positions in other libraries. Often several positions were available to them even under the adverse job market conditions which have prevailed these last long years[15]. An analysis of all programs and their description was undertaken by Fred Roper[16]. Their discontinuance is a political fact and a contemporary tragedy.

Courses in Medical Librarianship

A course in medial literature at Columbia University's School of Library Service in 1939, and taught by Thomas P. Fleming, began formal education in our field. These courses have proliferated. Julie Virgo[17], in a full-dress review of medical library education, noted that in 1975, thirty-seven out of sixty-two accredited library schools in the United States and Canada offered such courses. With some exceptions, they are taught by part-time faculty, often the chief librarian of the medical school of the university with which the library school is associated. In the early days following the Columbia University model, an introduction to the bibliography of medicine was taught in one semester. Today, a more general approach to content is common, with emphasis on the unique aspects of medical library practice, biomedical communication, and information retrieval. Research, a basic function of university graduate programs, with some notable exceptions, for example the work of Chen at Simmons, Rees and Cheshier at Western Reserve, and Crawford when she was at Columbia, has not developed. A compilation of doctoral dissertations in library science accepted between 1925 and 1972 at American universities lists only seven dissertations related to medical librarianship out of a total of 660[18]. The absence of organized research at library schools constitutes a serious obstacle in the development of our discipline and its knowledge base.

A significant educational effort, especially related to the utilization of computer-assisted information retrieval from different data compilations, takes place completely outside the above mentioned channels. The National Library of Medicine, of course, is a primary site for such instruction. However, the Biomedical Communication Network, when it functioned as part of the State University of New York, the Bibliographic Retrieval System, Inc., Lockheed, and other commercial distributors of data systems provide learning opportunities for their users.

Although attempts were made to develop library school programs with special options in medical librarianship, only at Case Western Reserve has such a program remained viable. An integral part of its curriculum is a unique work-study program developed jointly with Cleveland Health

Sciences Library. As training for specific skills in library schools has given way to instruction of concepts and the rationale of practice, the need for supervised work situations has become essential.

While educational opportunities have increased, the dilemma which Estelle Brodman[19] posed in 1954 remains unanswered: "What is needed and has not yet been attained is a clear knowledge of the goals and philosophic aims of medical librarianship. Until the profession as a whole has decided what its functions are . . . any system of education can only be the teaching of limited techniques with a limited view. The challenge of education for medical librarians today is not the *how* but the *why* of medical librarianship, and unfortunately very little has been done to answer this basic question." What appears to emerge as the nexus of our concern is communication, information, and its mode of transfer. We need to return to this in examining our knowledge base.

Knowledge Base

In recognition of a profession, its unique contribution to a segment of knowledge or the possession of specialized training and techniques is essential. The description of books, manuscripts, the bibliographic organization of their contents and those of journals was central to our endeavors and formed a close link with academic scholarship. George Sarton[20] *states, "The main point to emphasize . . . is that accuracy is as fundamental in the* historical field as in the scientific one, and that it has the same meaning in both fields." With this observation he introduced the need to investigate carefully evidence for the time of occurrence of historical events, the sources of errors in dates in tombstones and books, and the problem of periodicity in history. It parallels our concern with the establishment of the main entry, the authenticity of the document, pseudonymous authors, dates of birth and death, the succession of editors in journals, the careful collation and detailed description of books, and their provenance. If the historian's task was to write history as it really occurred, then the need for the careful establishment of the authenticity of documents and the objective evaluation of evidence was a mandate for librarians. Janet Doe, herself, personifies this approach, and her *Bibliography of the Works of Ambroise Paré* embodies this knowledge base. In the chapter "Paré, author or plagiarist, a weighing of the evidence," she carefully establishes the authenticity of the works. But beneath the careful scholarship and attention to detail, her heartbeat is heard in every sentence. She characterizes the ninth to the thirteenth editions of the collected works of Paré as the "Lyons malprints." She gives us a preview of her deep feeling about the thirteenth edition in her introduction: "And in 1685 the last, the unlucky thirteenth, came out, to fall into an oblivion deserved by its wretched typography, worn wood blocks, and sleasy paper"[21]. Describing the book later in detail she concludes, "This edition is the most detestable of all. The pages have been compressed into eighty-five lines each, the paper is wretched, and the typography more vicious than in any of the preceding....All the Lyons ones, beginning with the ninth edition in 1633, are abominable: the paper is inferior; the text continues, and even adds to, the indefensible alterations; and typographical errors abound. The plates for the illustrations, recut in 1633, are not so good as the originals, and have grown worn and broken by the time of the last impression of 1685. In fact the farther from the source, the poorer the editions become"[22]. Certainty of judgment is expressed in vigorous declarative sentences. Doe dares to be righteous because she knows. Janet Doe used Geoffrey Keynes's bibliography of William Harvey[23] as a model for her own method of presentation. Keynes, a surgeon and brother of Maynard, the economist, was already acknowledged as a modern bibliographer. The meticulous description of books and journals, their bibliographic, classificatory, and subject analysis formed an identifiable foundation of knowledge and expertise for medical librarianship. It formed not only the base of a common interest but a bond of mutual respect between physicians and librarians. Corning and Cummings in the previously cited review summarized this relationship thus:

> One of the most exciting aspects of library development and organization at the end of the nineteenth century and the beginning of the twentieth was the close collaboration of physician and librarian. As the issues being discussed became more related to classification, union catalogues, and cooperative sharing, however, the management and organization of medical libraries no longer commanded the attention, much less the full support, of the medical community. The librarian began to carry the burden of seeking funds, of management, and of providing service. The intellectual bond between the medical and library communities began to weaken[11].

From a long list of physician-bibliographers some representative instances may suffice. Sir William Osler[24], a founder of this association, not only brought together one of the great collections of books illustrating the history of medicine but began their bibliographic description and annotations. Harvey Cushing[25] found time for the *Bio-Bibliography of Andreas Vesalius*, and John F. Fulton[26] of Yale published his study of the *Great Medical Bibliographers*. Their books reflect the relationship with librarians, Osler and Marcia Noyes, Fulton and Helen Bayne and Madeline Stanton. Librarians in turn contributed to the history of medicine. Thomas Keys collaborated with Willius[27] on *Cardiac Classics* and wrote the *History of Surgical Anesthesia*[28]. William Postell[29] contributed a classic review of the health of slaves in the antebellum South. David Kronick[30] wrote a history of the scientific and technical periodical now in its second edition, Myrl Ebert[31] a definitive paper on the rise and development of the American medical periodical, Estelle Brodman[32] the history of medical bibliography, James Ballard[33] of the Boston Medical Library compiled a list of its incunabula, and Leslie Morton[34] has guided "Garrison and Morton," a key to the history of medicine and a boon to historians, librarians, and auctioneers, through its third edition.

CLASSIFICATION

The arrangement of materials as well as their classificatory organization also formed part of the central interest. The *Bulletin of the Medical Library Association* published many classification schemes. The association, no doubt in a moment of utter abandon, even adopted the Boston Medical Library Classification as its official classification in 1921 only to retract by silence after Ballard had revised the classification scheme without prior notification to the association. John Shaw Billings had a scant interest in classification and one of the major recommendations of the survey of the Army Medical Library in 1944[35], with Janet Doe as a leading participant, was the development of a new medical classification. After Rogers developed the National Library of Medicine Classification the problem came to rest and he never returned to it. Recently a large-scale revision of it, to be carried out by Emilie Wiggins, has been announced. The classification schemes of the Library of Congress and of the National Library of Medicine gained greater and greater predominance since they provided libraries with complete cataloging information, especially with the advent of the *Current Catalog*. One by one special classifications were discontinued; that of the New York Academy of Medicine and even the established Boston Medical Library Classification and the Cunningham Classification succumbed. The Bellevue Nursing Classification still survives in isolated instances. The problem of classification then was simply abandoned in the health sciences.

Subject analysis remained an active issue. Rogers's unorthodox insistence on analyzing information in books and journals with the same indexing vocabulary raised questions which quickly subsided because practice proved him correct, and the inclusion of monographs in the *Index Medicus* foreshadowed by Irwin Pizer's[36] original program for the Biomedical Communication Network at the Upstate Medical Center of the State University of New York was consistent, logical, and inevitable. The development of a new subject headings list for the production of the *Index Medicus* in 1960 and its adaptation by Sewell for the hierarchical arrangements in *MeSH* was a necessary and sufficient prerequisite for the development of the machine manipulation of citations in MEDLARS. Revised and enlarged, it remains one of the most useful and best controlled indexing languages available today. In spite of the agitation and excitement which prevailed around the construction of thesauri, my limited search for a serious critique of *MeSH* has only revealed Rogers's concern about the too free addition of terms in his Janet Doe lecture of 1968. With the firm establishment of a national system of medical classification and subject headings the concern with the development of such systems in individual libraries atrophied. The Ohio College Library Center and the computer-aided catalog of the University of California, Los Angeles all give promise to a vast improvement in access to books and monographs and present a viable base for resource sharing. The organization of knowledge in the health sciences, however, remains an important unsolved problem, worthy of our best minds and their best efforts.

Emerging Scientific Inquiry

The strength and appeal of the humanistic, historical foundation of medical librarianship is profound and continues into our times. As late as 1949 Janet Doe[37] concluded her presidential address on the development of education for librarianship with a long and affectionate review of Osler's knowledge and appreciation of medical librarians and their work. A change in the direction of library education away from training and day-to-day practice to the principles underlying practice and to a critical and experimental point of view had taken place at the Graduate Library School of the University of Chicago under the direction of Lewis Round Wilson in the 1930s. Waples, Butler, and Wilson[38] applied the methodology of the social sciences, the use of survey questionnaires and sampling statistics to the study of library users, reading and reading habits, libraries, and communication, including radio and cinema. Somewhat later, experimental inquiry was employed in medical librarianship. Estelle Brodman's[39] master's thesis at Columbia University, "Choosing physiology journals," was published in the *Bulletin of the Medical Library Association* in 1944. It was a carefully designed study testing the validity of the Gross and Gross[40] method of journal selection on the basis of the frequency with which they were cited. She compared a list of titles derived by the Gross and Gross method with a listing based on ratings of faculty experts. No correlation was found between the rank order of the list based on expert opinion and that established by citation count. William Postell[41] was so excited by the approach that he tested the results by an analysis of journal use in his library and found further support for Brodman's conclusions. Her findings and methodology are still germane today when citation counts are proferred as a rational method of selecting the best and most useful journals.

Research Efforts

Fact-finding studies became more frequent and attained an increasing degree of sophistication. Kilgour[42] at Yale studied the use of books and journals at his library to determine an arrangement which would best suit the needs of users so that the most frequently used journals would be placed in the most accessible locations. He confirmed Bradford's law of scattering. A relatively small number of titles commanded high usage while the largest number were moderately or little used. For comparative purposes the same study was conducted at Columbia University[43] with the same results.

At the National Library of Medicine the first full-scale analysis of interlibrary loans was accomplished by Kurth[44]. The geographic distribution and the characteristics of the requesters, as well as the materials requested and the frequency of the requests were studied. Among many important findings was one, surprising at the time, that the bulk of the journal requests were for commonly available titles and not for esoteric journals. *Lancet*, *British Medical Journal*, the *American Journal of Physiology*, and the *JAMA* were in the first four positions of the most frequently requested journals.

Support for research provided by the National Library of Medicine in the late sixties and early seventies accelerated the research effort. At the Medical Library of Wayne State University, Pings[45], an intellectual gadfly and iconoclast, unleashed a series of studies ranging from the effectiveness of the operation of the Regional Medical Library which he headed, to assessments of training programs, the coverage of nursing literature in MEDLARS, and an examination of the medical library as a social institution.

The first comprehensive census of health sciences libraries and their resources was conducted by Susan Crawford[46] and provided the factual basis for planning. She has continued these surveys and her most recent study of medical school libraries has already been cited. At a time when uncertainty existed about the manpower needs for health sciences librarians, when little was known about their training, academic preparation, educational attainment, and needs, David Kronick[47] headed an investigation which gave the answers. The survey was carefully planned with the prominent help of Rees and others of the Library School of Case Western Reserve. These efforts approached a program of research in medical librarianship. While more limited in scope, programs of research had also been begun at Yale on the use of library materials and at the University of California, Los Angeles, and Washington University in computer applications.

The entire biomedical communications process and its relation to libraries was examined by Richard Orr and others[48]. At a later time he and his associates developed a new set of methodological tools to measure various library services. Users' services offered in medical school libraries were not only systematically described for the first time but were subjected to a comparative analysis derived from a national survey.[49].

To give one last example, let me cite the work of Ching-chih Chen[50] on the use of monographs at the Francis A. Countway Library of Medicine at Harvard. The study tests whether the mathematical techniques used by Phillip Morse at the Massachusetts Institute of Technology to predict library use are applicable in other libraries. The evaluation of her argument requires a knowledge of mathematical statistics which I do not possess but which more and more librarians will have. What is important is the approach, the careful development of the study, the sample selection, its justification, and the attempt to validate it by comparison with data obtained in this instance by Robert Cheshier of the Cleveland Health Sciences Library. The *Bulletin of the Medical Library Association,* especially during the past five years, is replete with good investigations and its editorial direction contributes significantly to the enlargement of the scientific base of our profession. Medical librarians, then, are moving towards the scientific investigation of their field and are developing methodologies comparable to the scholarly, analytical skills of Janet Doe.

Conclusion

"The prospect of fundamental theories of information phenomena is not on the horizon," Vladimir Slamecka[51] says in a recent assessment of the state of information science. He continues: "The information research community should, as soon as possible, shift from a preoccupation with document housekeeping and delivery mechanisms to the related, but much broader, problem domain that is based on the need to discover the principles of (and to develop the means for) the optimal husbandry of one of man's key resources, knowledge."

A theory of medical librarianship also has not yet been developed. We are beginning, however, to study systematically, and with increasing sophistication, the facts and processes of our field. We are aided in this by an influx of those who have pursued scientific careers in other fields before becoming medical librarians. We are on the way to a new self-consciousness and to a better understanding of our purposes and functions. These are clearly in the area of communication and the transfer of knowledge to researchers, teachers, students, the sick and the healthy.

The detailed knowledge of bibliography and the organization of books and journals also formed the basis of peer group formations. When collections and staffs were small they did not require the administrative expertise demanded in the management of large aggregates of people and services. Those heading libraries knew them in all their aspects and the quality of this knowledge served as a measure of a practitioner's standing. Specialization has replaced this system in our libraries. At one time it seemed relatively easy to obtain a consensus as to who were our most able librarians, persons of great productivity, the intellectually keen, good organizers, and those with charisma.

Those who have led us through this enormous expansion are leaving and a new leadership has not quite emerged. I think that two elements may clear Nina Matheson's cloudy crystal ball. First, the development of libraries in hospitals and other health care centers, and the emergence of hospital librarians as a creative and productive group of practitioners with professional strivings and close relationships with their clientele represents a pool of talent which has already begun to make its mark. Second, as members of a profession composed overwhelmingly of women we will gain from the drive for equality and recognition of excellence which will continue to affect our political and social life in the foreseeable future.

THE 1977 DOE LECTURE: A CLARIFICATION

To The Editor:

This is likely to be the first time in the history of the *Bulletin* that a Janet Doe lecturer (BMLA 65: 409-418, Oct. 77) has written to correct an error. I sent Janet Doe a copy of my talk about the time I gave it. On July 25 she wrote a gracious letter in which she pointed out two errors. One is an unforgiveable error of fact. She writes. "You may want to make a few corrections of fact before the paper gets into print. I did attend the Library School of the NYPL which later merged with Columbia." The other is an error of interpretation. It refers to my comment that one of the major recommendations of the survey of the Army Medical Library of 1944, chaired by Keyes Metcalf, was the development of a classification scheme for the literature of medicine. I also stated that Janet was a prominent participant of the survey. She writes as follows: "...In the matter of the NLM classification, I was not a 'leading participant' in its production, but merely on the committee responsible and did its index. Its conception and development in detail were the work of Mary Louise Marshall, and it was a tremendous task. After it was put into use, Brad Rogers made revisions where practice showed need. She deserves credit for its birth, form and connection with the LC classification."

The misfortune of this Janet Doe Lecturer has at least provided an opportunity to recall one of the many contributions Miss Marshall made to the development of the Medical Library Association and to our profession. I hope that Janet Doe will forgive me.

ERICH MEYERHOFF
New York, New York

REFERENCES

1. AUDEN, W.H. The Age of Anxiety. New York, Random House, 1947.
2. ORWELL, G. Nineteen Eighty-Four. New York, Harcourt, 1949.
3. ARENDT, H. Eichmann in Jerusalem. New York, Viking Press, 1963.
4. MATHESON, N.W. The clouded crystal ball and the library profession. Bull. Med. Libr. Assoc. 65: 1-5, Jan. 1977.
5. DOE, J., ed. A Handbook of Medical Library Practice. Chicago, American Library Association, 1943, p. 8-9.
6. CRAWFORD, S. Survey of health sciences libraries in the United States, 1965-1975. In: The Bowker Annual of Library & Book Trade Information. 21st ed. New York, R.R. Bowker, 1976. p. 112-118.
7. CRAWFORD, S. Medical school libraries in the United States 1960 through 1975. JAMA 237: 464-468, Jan. 31, 1977.
8. BLOOMQUIST, H. The status and needs of medical school libraries in the United States. J. Med. Educ. 38: 145-163, Mar. 1963.
9. HENDRICKS, D.D. Medical Library Statistics 1975-1976. Dallas, Library, University of Texas Health Science Center at Dallas, 1977.
10. CUMMINGS, M.M., AND CORNING, M.E. The Medical Library Assistance Act: an analysis of the NLM extramural programs, 1965-1970. Bull. Med. Libr. Assoc. 59: 375-391, July 1971.
11. CORNING, M.E., AND CUMMINGS, M.M. Biomedical communications. In: Bowers, J.Z., and Purcell, E.F., eds., Advances in American Medicine: Essays at the Bicentennial. v. 2. New York, Josiah Macy, Jr. Foundation, 1976. p. 722-773.
12. TRUELSON, S.D., JR. Selecting for health sciences library collections when budgets falter. Bull. Med. Libr. Assoc. 64: 187-195, Apr. 1976.
13. SHAW, R.R. A Medical Intelligence Program for the National Institutes of Health. Bethesda, Maryland, National Institutes of Health, Jan. 1961.
14. DARLING, L. Changes in information delivery since 1960 in health sciences libraries. Libr. Trends 23: 31-62, July 1974.
15. CAMPBELL, C. Graduate training program in medical librarianship. In: Annual Report for the Biomedical Library 1972-1973. University of California, Los Angeles, 1973. p. 36-37.
16. ROPER, F.W. Special programs in medical library education, 1957-1971. Bull. Med. Libr. Assoc. 61: 225-227, Apr. 1973; 61: 387-395, Oct. 1973; 62: 397-404, 405-412, Oct. 1974.
17. VIRGO, J.A. Education of medical librarians. In: Encyclopedia of Library and Information Science. v. 17. New York, M. Dekker, 1976. p. 342-378.
18. SCHLACHTER, G.A. AND THOMPSON, D. Library Science Dissertations, 1925-1972. Littleton, Colorado, Libraries Unlimited Inc., 1974.
19. BRODMAN, E. Whither education for medical librarians? Stechert-Hafner Book News 8: 61-62, Feb. 1954.
20. SARTON, G. The Study of the History of Science. Cambridge, Harvard University Press, 1936. p. 10-11.
21. DOE J. A Bibliography of the Works of Ambroise Paré. . . Chicago, University of Chicago Press, 1937. p. 93.

22. ———— Ibid. p. 142.
23. KEYNES, G. L. A Bibliography of the Writings of Dr. William Harvey, 1573-1657. 2d ed., rev. Cambridge, England, Cambridge University Press, 1953.
24. OSLER, W. Bibliotheca Osleriana. Oxford, The Clarendon Press, 1929.
25. CUSHING, H.W. A Bio-Bibliography of Andreas Vesalius. New York, Schuman, 1943.
26. FULTON, J.F. The Great Medical Bibliographers, a Study in Humanism. Philadelphia, University of Pennsylvania Press, 1951.
27. WILLIUS, F.A. AND KEYS, T.E. Cardiac Classics. St. Louis, Mosby, 1941.
28. KEYS, T. E. The History of Surgical Anesthesia. New York, Schuman, 1945.
29. POSTELL, W.D. The Health of Slaves on Southern Plantations. Baton Rouge, Louisiana State University Press, 1951.
30. KRONICK, D.A. A History of Scientific and Technical Periodicals. New York, Scarecrow Press, 1962.
31. EBERT, M. Rise and development of the American medical periodical. Bull. Med. Libr. Assoc. 41: 243-276, Jan. 1953.
32. BRODMAN, E. The Development of Medical Bibliography. Baltimore, Medical Library Association, 1954.
33. BALLARD, J.F. A Catalogue of the Medieval and Renaissance Manuscripts and Incunabula in the Boston Medical Library. Boston, priv. print., 1944.
34. MORTON, L.M. A Medical Bibliography (Garrison and Morton). 3d ed. Philadelphia, J.B. Lippincott, 1970.
35. METCALF, K.D., et al. The National Medical Library; Report of a Survey of the Army Medical Library. Chicago, American Library Association, 1944.
36. PIZER, I.H. A regional medical library network. Bull. Med. Libr. Assoc. 57: 101-105, Apr. 1969.
37. DOE, J. The development of education for medical librarianship. Bull. Med. Libr. Assoc. 37: 213-220, July 1949.
38. SHERA, J.H. The Foundations of Education for Librarianship. New York, Becker and Hayes, Inc., 1972. p. 244-249.
39. BRODMAN, E. Choosing physiology journals. Bull. Med. Libr. Assoc. 32: 479-483, Oct. 1944.
40. GROSS, P.L.K. AND GROSS, E.M. College libraries and chemical education. Science 66: 385-389, Oct. 28, 1927.
41. POSTELL, W.D. Further comments on the mathematical analysis of evaluating scientific journals. Bull. Med. Libr. Assoc. 34: 107-109, Jan. 1946.
42. KILGOUR, F.G. Recorded use of books in Yale Medical Library. Am. Doc. 12: 266-269, Oct. 1961.
43. FLEMING, T.P. AND KILGOUR, F.G. Moderately and heavily used biomedical journals. Bull. Med. Libr. Assoc. 52: 234-241, Jan. 1964.
44. KURTH, W.H. Survey of the Interlibrary Loan Operation of the National Library of Medicine. Washington, D.C., U.S. Department of Health, Education, and Welfare, Public Health Service, 1962.
45. Wayne State University School of Medicine Library and Biomedical Information Service Center Reports 1-62, Jan. 1964-June 1973.
46. CRAWFORD, S. Health sciences libraries in the United States: a statistical profile. Bull. Med. Libr. Assoc. 60 (Suppl.) 1-56, April 1972. SCHICK, F., AND CRAWFORD, S. Directory of Health Sciences Libraries in the United States. Chicago, American Medical Association, 1976.
47. KRONICK, D.A., REES, A.M., AND ROTHENBERG, L. An investigation of the educational needs of health sciences library manpower: I. Bull. Med. Libr. Assoc. 58: 7-17, Jan. 1970; II. Ibid. 58: 510-520, Oct. 1970; III. Ibid. 59: 21-30, Jan. 1971; IV. Ibid. 59: 31-40, Jan. 1971; V. Ibid. 59: 392-403, July 1971; VII. Ibid. 60: 292-300, Apr. 1972.

48. ORR, R.H. Communication problems in biochemical research: report of a study. Fed. Proc. 23: 1117-1191, Sept.-Oct. 1964.
49. ORR, R.H., et al. User services offered by medical school libraries in 1968: results of a national survey employing new methodology. Bull. Med. Libr. Assoc. 58: 455-492, Oct. 1970.
50. CHEN, C. Applications of Operations Research Models to Libraries. Cambridge, The MIT Press, 1976.
51. SLAMECKA, V. Pragmatic observations on theoretical research in information science. J. Am. Soc. Inf. Sci. 26: 318-320, Nov./Dec. 1975.

II
THE PROFESSION

Introduction

> Medical librarianship deserves respect because it is a worthwhile and an important job. Medical librarians deserve respect because their skill is the resultant of years of training and experience [and] because they are purveyors of an indispensable commodity—Information.... Professionalism implies the firm establishment in its own right of a vocation that is neither subservient nor dependent. Librarianship defines its own frame of reference, its own standards, its own achievements, and its own aspirations. The challenge of professionalism resides in the ability to enlarge its frame of reference, to raise its standards, to multiply its achievements, and to fulfill its aspirations[1].

Early Spanish explorers searching for cities of gold in New Mexico commemorated the adventure by carving their names and the phrase *Pasamos Por Aqui* ("We passed by here") in what is today known as Inscription Rock. These proud records are still visible nearly 500 years later. What of the memorials for medical librarians and their profession? The papers in this chapter, coupled with those in Chapter I, the "Janet Doe Lectures," register the history of this profession. Achievements, problems, and concerns are discussed. In addition, several of the papers reflect something of the character of individual practitioners as well as involvements of the transmuters.

Sir William Osler, in an address at the opening of the Summer School of Library Service of the University of Wales at Aberystwyth on July 31, 1917, gave valuable advice about the training of librarians and the conduct of libraries. The most important portions of his address appear in our reprinted selection for this chapter.

William Postell discusses and compares the arts of librarianship and scholarship. His message is that scholastic accomplishments, technical abilities, and a professional attitude are inextricable components of true librarianship—and that they must be in happy balance with one another.

Certification and its advantages for medical librarians are outlined by Mildred Jordan. She notes the evolutionary stages of professionalization and the progress of the Medical Library Association.

The historical articles by James Ballard and Margueriete Prime, together with those in the first chapter, flesh out the narrative of our association's "roots," years of infancy, developments, labors, and achievements.

For nearly 40 years, Dr. Thomas Keys gave service of mind and heart to medical librarianship. The concept "The College of the Medical Book" uniquely epitomizes a lifetime of study, thought, and writing directed to the problem of how one should master a learned discipline like medical librarianship. This is an idea to provoke introspective thought on the part of a truly devoted philobiblist.

REFERENCE

1. LONG EC: Professionalism in the Library. Bull Med Libr Assoc 50:203-206, 1962.

"THE SCIENCE OF LIBRARIANSHIP."

By

Sir William Osler, M. D.

Foreword—The (English) "Library Association Record" for August-September, 1917, prints an address made at the opening of the Summer School of Library Service of the University of Wales at Aberystwyth, on July 31, 1917, by Sir William Osler, Bart., M. D., F. R. S., Regius Professor of Medicine, Oxford, a Curator of the Bodleian, and President of the Bibliographical Society. Those who remember the great interest he took while in Baltimore in the Libraries of the Johns Hopkins Hospital and of the Medical and Chirurgical Faculty will not be surprised that he has continued that interest and that his advice is valuable as to the training of librarians and the conduct of libraries. The most important portions of this address are as follows:

"Within the last few years the work has been so organized that we may speak of a science of librarianship. The old rule-of-thumb order which each custodian of a collection of books adopted, as his own knowledge or ignorance suggested, is giving place to carefully thought-out methods of arrangement designed to make the books of greater service, and more easily accessible. The librarians of today, and it will be true still more of the librarians of tomorrow, are not fiery dragons interposed between the people and the books. They are useful public servants, who manage libraries in the interest of the public. The old notion of the right person to have charge of books is going, but by no means gone; the sooner it goes the better for everybody. Many think still that a great reader, or a writer of books, will make an excellent librarian. This is pure fallacy. . . . .

"Between the years 1855, roughly, and the present, there has grown up in Britain and America libraries of a type altogether different from anything existing before—the libraries of the people, public libraries, sometimes miscalled free libraries, brought into existence by the will of the people, maintained by funds derived from the rates. These libraries are firmly established as a factor in promoting education and culture, besides serving many other useful purposes. They are in many places highly organized contributors to the general welfare, but their potential place in the scheme of things intellectual has not been grasped as yet in Britain. Perhaps it is because too much has been done for the people, who have not in this matter worked out their own salvation. Mr. Carnegie and his Trust have spent on library buildings in the United Kingdom more than two millions sterling. In America the function of the public library is better understood than it is here. Why is this? . . . .

"America has gone further than we in the matter of technical training. Library schools have been in operation for many years, and their graduates in large numbers have found employment. In this country the Library Association has laboured with praiseworthy zeal to set up standards of proficiency, to establish classes for instruction, and to test by means of examinations the qualifications of candidates. . . . .

"Let us glance for a moment at the subjects. What librarian or assistant can hope to deal with books without a good knowledge of literary history, not merely of his own, but of other countries? . . . .

"Bibliography, next in order, is sub-divided by the Library Association into Historical Bibliography, Practical Bibliography, and Book Selection. How many people would be able to pass even an elementary test in either of the first two sub-divisions, or even to define them. Many cataloguers (of sorts) describe themselves as bibliographers, thereby displaying their ignorance of terms, and of the whole subject.

Bibliography deals with the history of printing, the evolution of the printed book from the manuscripts, paper, bookbinding, book illustration, authors, publishers, booksellers, the collation and description of books, the various methods of book production; while book selection is concerned with the type of books suitable to the needs of the people who are to use the library. To do this efficiently requires wide knowledge of books of reference—bibliographies—practical experience, and sound judgment. . . .

"Next in order is Classification, the application of which to collections of books is comparatively recent, and the outcome of modern experience. By it the library is made an organized instrument of service, like a well-trained and disciplined army. For just as hundreds of thousands or even millions of men without proper organizations form a mere mob, so a library without classification is nothing more than a mob of books. Catalogues lessen the confusion, but every catalogue is out of date as soon as it appears, and the reader becomes dependent upon his own and the librarian's memory for the latest books on his subject. With classification, however, this difficulty disappears. The books are sorted to their proper place as they come in. If one wishes to study 'Cancer,' for example, or 'Poultry-keeping,' or any other subject, a properly classified library would be of infinitely greater help than any catalogue, and more expeditious. . . .

"The Library of Congress started reorganization some years ago, a heroic thing to undertake with such large collections, and the re-classification has occupied a special staff for over seventeen years. It is now approaching completion, and incidently has produced the soundest and most practical scheme of classification yet given to the world, known as the Library of Congress Classification. . . .

"Following the subjects in the order of the Syllabus of the Library Association we come to Cataloguing, an important branch of the work, but not, as many people suppose, the most important. The widely prevalent idea that library work is made up of cataloguing and that beyond compiling catalogues the staff is mainly engaged in reading and writing books is very wide of the truth. Valuable as is a catalogue it can be of little use unless the books have first been arranged in an order which will enable them to be found when called for, and returned to their places when done with. The classifier in fact must precede the cataloguer, or the labor will be wasted. . . .

"At this point we take leave of the Syllabus of the Library Association and come to two branches of a librarian's equipment which have been rather neglected in this country. On the Continent the Archivist is an important personage. He is going to be important here. We welcome, therefore, the addition of Archives as a subject for study in this Summer School. . . .

"The course of instruction in bookbinding will be a useful auxiliary to the study of Archives, as in addition to bookbinding in its usual forms, instruction and demonstrations will be given in cleaning, repairing, and preserving documents, rare books and valuable manuscripts.

"It is not a little strange, it is indeed a singular anomaly, that our universities, whose chief function is to train men to influence others, do little or nothing directly for the education of those great teachers of the nation, the masters of the elementary schools, and the purveyors of knowledge called librarians. . . . .

"A collection of books is, as Carlyle says, a university, and a custodian of books is necessarily a teacher. Post-graduate education is largely in the hands of libraries. Take in illustration my own experience of the past ten days. In a complicated and unusual type of war-shock case, about which I asked my own books in vain, the answer was easily found in the Royal Society of Medicine Library. About a Cambridge University medical diploma, 1683, I bothered my teachers at Bodley, at Cambridge, and at the British Museum. An early, possibly unknown, edition of the "Malade Imaginaire" led me far afield beyond the Taylorian Institution. The British Museum and Bodley are themselves Universities as great as Oxford and Cambridge. The London Library possibly helps the education of more people than London University. . . .

"The Library is everywhere becoming one of the great factors in our educational system, and the director is perforce a teacher of wide and critical influence. How shall he be trained so as best to utilize his opportunities for the public good? No man in the community requires a more comprehensive and thorough education. All knowledge is his province. A common tap for the waters of wisdom, he should not perhaps know everything, but he should know where everything may be found. The parson, the doctor, the lawyer, the engineer, the farmer, the worker in every craft should be able to go to him with full assurance that he will be able to help. The Apocalyptic literature, the recent theories of immunity, the law of war claims, submarine engineering, the chemistry of dyes, the metallurgy of nickel steel, the story of aviation, the laws of trajectories should be as familiar to him as the 'best sellers' among the novels or the most popular of the war poets. He is the badly salaried intellect of the community and, if fortunate enough to be able to suffer fools gladly, he leads a life of surprising usefulness. And let us not forget other important qualifications—an ability to manage a business as complicated as a department shop, and a knowledge of men and a gift of manners that will enable him to drive his Committee or Council without strain on bit or rein. As Mr. Tedder remarked in a recent address, 'The Librarian in Relation to Books,' 'The model librarian must be two-sided—at once a man of business, and a man of learning and reflection.'

"I should like to see added to the schools of at least one University in each division of the Kingdom a School of the Book, in all its relations historical, technical and commercial—every aspect of bibliography, every detail of typography, every possible side of bibliopoly. And the Press should be included, as the daily paper is nothing but a glorified broadside. The opportunities exist, as the great library furnishes a laboratory, the college with the library staff supervise the courses, and a University Press subserves the typographical side of the training. . . . .

"In America the Library School has been a great boon, and has been the means of furnishing highly trained men and women who have, within my knowledge, completely changed the atmosphere of the libraries. I have seen the Surgeon-General's Library, the College of Physicians, Philadelphia, the Boston Medical Library, the McGill Medical Library, to mention only those in which I have been personally interested, grow from small beginnings to collections of national importance. The most striking bibliographical contrast in my own collection is the tiny octavo of 32 pages, the first catalogue, 1865, of the Surgeon-General's Library, Washington, alongside of the 36 folio volumes of the first and second series just completed. The stimulus of trained specialists has been a potent factor in this development. . . .

"Modified to meet local conditions the scheme of the National School would be as follows:

I. Organization—Control jointly by a Committee representing the Library, the Press, the University, and the Colleges.

II. Staff—(a) Permanent. The heads of the Library and of the Press, and the assistants in special departments, who would supervise the technical work.

(b) Lecturers on library economics, history, bibliography, publishing, binding, etc., chosen partly from the library, partly from the college staffs.

(c) Special lecturers from outside, as you have arranged for this Summer School. Publishers, manufacturers, printers, and inventors would be asked to give special lectures.

III. Students—(a) Ordinary undergraduates, who would be given instruction in (i) the use of the library; (ii) the elements of bibliography; (iii) palaeography.

(b) Special students: (i) in library work; (ii) in newspaper work, printing, publishing, binding and illustrating.

The school in these departments would offer practical training quite as important as in other technical subjects. For a time at least the courses in library economics may have to be given in a Summer School, but to fit men for the higher library posts we should look forward to an advanced course of two years' post-graduate work.

(c) Research students. One of the chief functions of the school would be to train men and women in methods of literary and historical research. Tutorial classes and private instruction should be offered in all departments. The National Library with its unique collections should become the Mecca for Celtic students from all parts of the world for whom skilled assistance should be provided by the best scholars.

IV. The Public—The classes in bibliography should be open. Anyone desiring special instruction in any matter relating to a book from the preparation of manuscripts to the designing of a book cover, should be able to find it at the school. In the great working centres of South Wales extension classes would be held for working men dealing with the book as a tool of the mind.

"And in connection with the Press there would be organized a typographical museum in which would be displayed by models, etc., everything relating to the art of printing—a place in which the historical evolution could be 'studied from the Chinese movable type to the latest linotype machine." . . .

"Your business is that of purveyors, universal providers of the mental food of the public; and not only are you caterers but you will often be called upon to do the work of cooks and doctors. The majority of mankind, as Burke says, providence has doomed to live on trust, a trust less in you, I fear, than in the ephemeral literature of the day. It is not often that one has a vivid, enduring impression of a newspaper article; but one day in October, 1872, in a Tottenham Court Road tea-shop, I read in 'The Times' a statement of Ruskin to the effect that no mind could resist for a year the dulling influence of the daily paper. Doubtless as an exclusive dietary the press and the magazine do lead to mental conditions the counterpart of what we know in the body as the deficiency diseases, scurvy, rickets, etc. The Library through you supplies the vitamines which counteract the mental lethargy and anaemia which come from too exclusive use of Northcliff and other patent foods."

W. R. S., Hartford, Conn.

The Art of Librarianship

By William Dosite Postell, *Librarian*

School of Medicine
Louisiana State University

It has been rather crudely put that the difference between man and animal is that man has access to libraries while animals do not. Man can take advantage of the experiences of his fellowmen. Animals must rely on instinct. It is rather interesting to compare the state of culture achieved by man throughout history with his libraries and the skill of the librarians in bringing together man and his works. In the past a well equipped and organized library has connoted a high state of culture and some degree of skill in practicing the art of librarianship.

In the year 1850 there was excavated at Nineveh a number of clay tablets covered with cuneiform characters. On further examination these tablets proved to be the remains of a library which seems to have been methodically arranged and catalogued. Probably this is one of the earliest references to a collection of books organized for the use of the public. History has recorded the state of culture reached by the inhabitants of the Tigris-Euphrates valley. Their achievements were great. Undoubtedly the librarians were more than custodians. They practiced the art of librarianship, if one is to judge by their results.

In classical Greece, there were many who were collectors of books, among whom were Pisistratus, Polycrates of Samos, Euclid, Nicocrates, Euripides, Aristotle, and Plato, but nowhere is the art of librarianship mentioned. It is not until the organization of the Alexandrian library under the Ptolemies that once again is there mention of libraries and their work. The organization of 700,000 (some estimate) rolls called for skill so that the library could be utilized by scholars and students. With the state of learning prevailing in Alexandria it must logically be assumed that the scholars assembled there had access to an excellent and well organized library. But again, of the art of librarianship little is known, except the account of the organization of the library in separate buildings and the compiling of catalogues of their contents. There have been preserved the names of the first five librarians who were all scholars. They were poets, gram-

Originally published in *School and Society,* Volume 61 (June 30, 1945), pp. 419-421
Reprinted by permission.

marians, mathematicians, and literary critics, and their writings covered a wide range of subjects. Undoubtedly, the arts of librarianship and scholarship were very closely related.

The renowned library of Alexandria excited the admiration of the kings of Pergamum who vied with the Egyptian kings in their encouragement of literature. Despite the embargo placed by the Ptolemies upon the export of papyrus, the library of Attali attained considerable size, and when it was transferred to Egypt it numbered 200,000 rolls. The name of only one librarian has been preserved, that of Euphorion of Chalcis, a grammarian and poet.

The early Romans were too warlike and practical to be interested in books, and it was not until the last century of the republic that there is mention of libraries. The first books brought to Rome were spoils of war, and soon it became fashionable for men of wealth to collect books. Finally the Roman emperors adopted the policy of establishing libraries for the public until the number had grown to 28 by the fourth century. Of the art of librarianship little is known. The structural plans of the libraries at Ephesus and Timgad in Algeria have been preserved. Caesar entrusted Terentius Varro, a poet and writer of note, with the task of collecting and arranging books for a system of public libraries of which only a few works have been preserved. The position of librarian was held in many cases by slaves or freedmen; only the names of a few men are known who served as librarians. Among these were C. Hymenaeus, physician and librarian to Augustus, Dionysius, an Alexandrian rhetorician, and C. Julius Vestinus, former tutor to the Emperor Hadrian.

The period that followed the fall of the Roman empire marked a low ebb in the promotion of learning and scholarship. Books sought refuge in the monasteries where they were patiently copied and stored. With so few books there was probably little need for any one to practice the art of librarianship, and no doubt those in charge of the books served as little more than custodians. However, it is to the religious orders that we owe the beginning of modern library methods. The Benedictines introduced the first library practices. The library was housed in a separate room in charge of a librarian. The Carthusians were perhaps the first to lend books away from the monastery. The Augustinians formulated rules for binding, cataloguing, and arranging the books by the librarian, as well as the policy of borrowing books from elsewhere.

As colleges and universities developed, they fitted out their libraries much on the same plan as the monastic libraries. Books were placed in a separate room on desks to which they were attached by chains. Later they were placed on shelves along the walls, but in many cases they still continued to be fastened by chains until the early part of the 18th century.

With the revival of learning, interest began to be shown by others besides the religious orders in collecting books. In France, beginning with Charles V, many of the kings were very much interested in building up their libraries. In Italy, the Italian princes were disposed to encourage literature and in England and other countries of Europe, the same trend showed itself.

The names of a few librarians are known. Claude Mallet, the first librarian and cataloguer of Charles V, is known to have compiled a catalogue of the library. Laurent Paulmier served as librarian under Louis XI. Jacques Amyot, a French writer and translator of merit, was also librarian of the Bibliothèque. Under J.A. DeThou, noted historian, this library was greatly enlarged. However, it was the 16th century that produced the greatest librarian since antiquity, Gabriel Naudé, organizer of the Mazarin library. The accomplishments of this great man were amazing. He was a physician, editor of nearly a hundred books, collector and organizer of a library of over 40,000 volumes for Cardinal Mazarin. His concept of librarianship as shown by his book, "Avis pour dresser un de bibliotheque," was sound and surprisingly modern. He has been rated the first to co-ordinate the science of books and to set proper standards for it.

Libraries from then on continued to grow and expand, and almost from necessity something had to be done to organize the libraries so they could be used. Libraries had outgrown themselves. The development of library techniques became essential if libraries were to become little more than storerooms for books.

Prior to 1876, very little had been accomplished in the way of a scientific classification of books, but in that year Melvil Dewey issued his classification system which soon became widely used. When Dewey established his School of Library Economy in 1887, the library would set out to catch up with the technical side of library work, and has succeeded almost too well, so that for the past fifty years the art of librarianship may be referred to as the "era of techniques."

Warnings have been issued repeatedly against this overemphasis of techniques by leaders in the profession. In 1898, Daniel C. Gilman, president of Johns Hopkins University, wrote that the librarian would be the better administrator if he cultivated his own special study (3: 255), and Sydney B. Mitchell also expressed the opinion that a librarian should be an administrator and scholar with emphasis on the latter (5: 69).

William S. Learned expressed himself as follows (4: 17):

The outstanding need in library education is the identification, selection, and stimulation of a type of mind that knows books comprehensively in a given field, or in given fields, and is able effectively to recognize and minister to the needs of individuals or groups in the use of these books. Library technique is a necessary but minor part of this equipment.

Lucy E. Fay, in an excellent article[2], expressed the opinion that the weakest element in librarianship today is the lack of a solid foundation of human learning. As an example of true librarianship she cited the work of three librarians; Gabriel Naudé, Henry Bradshaw, and Justin Winsor. Each at an early age showed a keen interest in books, a desire to search for the truth, which resulted in important contributions to the fields of bibliography, paleography, cartography, and history. Although their specialties were not in the field of science, their methods of work were the methods of science, and finally the specialties of each were closely integrated with the technical library processes each was developing. As Miss Fay expressed it: "Their scholarship was not divorced from their librarianship, a thing apart, but was the very foundation of it. The results of their librarianship fulfilled Mr. Bay's definition of librarianship, 'human enlightenment in a historical continuity.'"

Probably the most significant discussion of what has happened during the past fifty years in the field of librarianship was an article by J. I. Wyer[9], who severely criticized the scholastic accomplishments of librarians. To his statement that librarians do not read, he added evidence that they do not write. He compiled a list of 64 librarians who had made some literary contributions and classified them into four groups. Group one, 35 librarians with no formal training for library work, who wrote books in other fields while actively engaged in library work, yet with whom writing was secondary and subordinate; Group two, 12 librarians who were made librarians after, and in some cases solely because, they had written books; Group three, 10 librarians who followed formal training for the profession, became good librarians, and have written creditable books on other subjects; Group four, 7 librarians, authors who are rumored to have been librarians, but who appeared unwilling to acknowledge it in standard reference books.

In articles by Frank K. Walter[8] and G. B. Utley[7], some additional names were added bringing the total in group one to 62, "the old fashioned librarian" as Dr. Wyer referred to them, and group three to 16. Mr. Walter made the additional comment that Dr. Wyer had assembled conclusive evidence that the growth in size, scope, and use of libraries had been accompanied by a decline in "creative scholarship."

In order to verify Dr. Wyer's statement as to the amount and kind of professional writing of librarians which he refers to as "casual," 1,371 articles appearing in professional journals were examined and roughly grouped in the following classes: those dealing with library economy, 974; original contributions to librarianship, 243; and descriptive material (libraries), 154. Obviously there are amazingly few articles in the professional literature which may be considered as making an original contribution to the art of librarianship. The large majority add little to what has not been discussed time and time again.

There is probably another implication that can be drawn from this overemphasis on techniques: the lack of a professional attitude on the part of librarians. The "Statistical Abstract of the United States" lists 36,347 librarians in the United States (6: 75), while only 16,000 belong to the American Library Association. Likewise membership in the Medical Library Association is only 188 out of approximately 500 workers.

If there is one group of workers who need to read it is librarians. The problems arising in library procedures cannot as a rule be empirically verified as they can in the pure sciences. In library science, one is dealing essentially with rationable conditions, and as a result, there never seems to be an end or a clear-cut decision in the solution of any problem. That probably accounts for the large amount of repetition in the professional literature. From the nature of their problems it would appear as if the greatest tool librarians have at their command is logical thinking. Centuries ago the Greek philosophers learned that the more facts one had at one's command the better one could rationalize. Likewise it is with librarians. Librarians will obtain their facts and ideas from reading good literature. The classics are never old. Ideas expressed centuries ago are in many cases just as applicable today. Then, too, there is never any final solution to library procedures. There is always the possibility that they can be done better. In any attainment there is always the inspiration for a fresh approach.

As Miss Fay expressed it (2: 516):

> Without this improvement in the scholarship of librarians the library will lag behind in the intellectual and moral progress of education. We must recover for all professional levels of librarianship the "general corpus of human learning" and put it to work in providing more adequate book and periodical collections for existing needs; more expert service; more sympathy for an intelligence about research problems. The librarian will then be a scholar in his own right and the library a vital force in educational progress.

REFERENCES

1. "Encyclopedia Britannica," 11th ed., 1910-11. 29 v.
2. FAY, L.E. "The Librarian as Scholar,".SCHOOL AND SOCIETY, 37: 511-516, April 22, 1933.
3. GILLMAN, D.C. "University Problems in the United States," Century, 1898. 255 pp.
4. LEARNED, W.S., as quoted by Munn, Ralph. "Conditions and Trends in Education for Librarianship." Carnegie Corp. of New York, 1936. 49 pp.
5. MITCHELL, S.B. The Academic and Professional Education of College Librarians. ALA *Bulletin*, 30: 69-74, February, 1936.

6. "Statistical Abstract of the United States." Government Printing Office, 1942. 1,097 pp.
7. Utley, G.B. "Librarian Authors." *Library Journal,* 64: 766-767, October 15, 1939.
8. Walter, F.K. "It Might Be Worse." *Library Journal,* 64: 666-667, September 15, 1939.
9. Wyer, J.I. "American Librarians as Writers." *Library Journal,* 64: 584-587, August, 1939.

Certification: A Stage of Professionalization

By Mildred Jordan, *Librarian, A. W. Calhoun Medical Library, Emory University, Georgia*

Fifty years ago medical librarians entered the first stage of professionalization by organizing in Philadelphia the Medical Library Association. They were ably aided and abetted by several far-sighted and outstanding members of our brother profession—the physicians. One of these, Dr. Browning, reminisced twenty-five years later: "At this first session there were eight (8) participants, certainly not a large number, yet quite enough. Had there been more we might not be organized yet."[1] Since that time, when so few accomplished so much, we have come far in our professional development, but several stages in our growth are still necessary before we can achieve the real professionalization begun a half-century ago.

The evolution of a profession has been outlined as follows:

Preprofessional stages

1. A social need arises.
2. Interested persons try to meet this need.
3. These persons talk or write about their work among themselves and with others who are interested in this or similar work.
4. These individuals find themselves set off from other groups because of the specific functions which they perform and the specific problems which they try to solve, and they are also drawn together because of these common interests. Because of these two forces, differentiation and specialization, a group consciousness develops.
5. As the social need for the skill and knowledge of this differentiated-specialized group increases in amount and complexity, the group develops an increasing need for a common basis for standardizing its skills and for adequate preparation among its members in order to meet these needs. This phase in its evolution takes the group from preprofessional to professional stages.

Originally published in *Bulletin of the Medical Library Association,* Volume 36 (April, 1948), pp. 108-116. Reprinted by permission.

Professional stages

1. An organization is formed as the most efficient means of exchanging ideas, discussing problems, formulating policies. It builds up its membership by being helpful to that membership in three ways: (a) increasing the members' functional effectiveness; (b) furthering the objectives of the profession; (c) helping members to better their social and economic status.
2. General meetings are held for the membership, bringing ideas, procedures, techniques into wider circulation, clarifying aims and objectives for the guidance of the profession and determining its relationship to its social milieu.
3. A publication becomes necessary for the wider discussion and dissemination among the membership of the proceedings of the meetings; to give wider currency and permanent printed form to all matters which concern the profession. It becomes a "binder" of first importance in holding the membership together.
4. Curricula are developed to give the special training necessary to those people who perform the special functions of the profession. The amount of specialized literature grows for and through those who are so trained.
5. The organization sets up professional standards for the education of its members, the conditions under which its members shall work, and in accrediting practices, brings pressure to bear upon society to see that these standards are met. It brings its forces to bear upon the making of public policy in the fields which impinge upon its members and their institutions.
6. As the parent organization grows, those members engaged in specialized phases of the profession tend to repeat the evolutionary phases outlined above. These further specialized groups may continue to have varying degrees of organic relationship with the parent organization, from informal discussion groups within the parent organization to completely autonomous organizations with no connections. The degree of separateness will depend upon the differentiation of and complexity in functions and techniques, and also in the tolerance of the parent organization towards change and its ability to develop co-operative techniques in preference to domination.[2]

It is with the higher stages of our professional development that the Medical Library Association is now struggling. The proposed program for achieving stage four: "Curricula are developed to give the special training necessary to those people who perform the special functions of the profession," has not only been enthusiastically received and heartily endorsed by the members of the Medical Library Association, but some very real progress has been made toward its achievement. It is with the fifth stage of our professional development, on which the success of the fourth stage depends in part, that the members of the Medical Library Association show, shall we say, something less than complete unanimity:

"The organization sets up professional standards for the education of its members, the conditions under which its members shall work, and in accrediting practices, brings pressure to bear upon society to see that these standards are met. It brings its forces to bear upon the making of public policy in the fields which impinge upon its members and their institutions."

Even in our internal disagreements concerning the establishment of standards, we repeat the history of other professional groups who have achieved this stage in their evolutionary development. Neo-natal emergence as a profession is a birth pain that apparently has to be endured by each group. It would seem, however, that we might alleviate our pain by a liberal assimilation of the experience of other bodies in their struggle for professionalization.

"The mind," says Wilfred Trotter, "likes a strange idea as little as the body likes a strange protein, and resists it with a similar energy."[3] However, the underlying idea back of certification is not new—it is almost as old as civilization. By the Middle Ages it was part and parcel of the social fabric. Not only were standards for groups definitely established in this period, but the two methods of achieving regulation of personnel that are used currently were instigated then. The hewers of stone and carriers of water banded together in workers' associations known as craft guilds. These guilds, forerunners of our modern labor unions, were self-regulating bodies. They established standards of training, working conditions, and wages. They controlled the entrance to the trade. Other groups, largely of an academic nature, did not fit into these workers' organizations but were organized as professions with their standards established for the most part through educational institutions.[4]

The medical profession (only recently physicians and surgeons within one organization) offers an interesting example of these two approaches to standards and of the two types of bodies who conferred their standards. The surgeons of those medieval days were craftsmen and as members of a vocational group were organized in a craft guild. The guild set up the standards by which surgeonhood was achieved. In contrast, the physicians, with their higher educational requirements, were certified by the medical faculties of the various universities. The physicians, needless to say, were accepted by the public as a professional group much earlier than the surgeons. In England to this very day the surgeons are still addressed as "Mister" as opposed to the "Doctor" accorded the physicians. From certification as a craftsman by the guild, to certification as a specialist by the American Board of Surgery is a long, long journey. The journey has been made, stage by stage, through the establishment of standards and their continuous revision.

The story of medical licensure and certification in the professionalization of medicine is much too long and generally too well known to medical librarians to repeat here, even though its history is and has been the one to which all groups aspiring to professionalization have turned. Contributing to the advances in medical standards have been the strong support and occasional pressure of the public. The public, while interested in the establishment of standards for personnel in any group, is slow to support the establishment of such standards in those professions that it does not see clearly as contributing directly or immediately to its life or welfare. Consider the slowness of the public in becoming aware of the all but disastrous situation that has been allowed in our public schools because of inadequate or poorly enforced standards of personnel.

The earlier attitude of the public toward public health is a further example of this general apathy, although public health admittedly contributes vitally to our collective well-being. On the other hand, the recent progress in public health is a good example of how much can be accomplished through the support of an interested public when that public finally becomes aware of its personal interest in the establishment of personnel standards for such a group. The immediate interest to us, though the ultimate value of the lesson of educating the public to know and to insist on standards for medical librarians should not be ignored, is that the public health personnel is becoming professionalized rapidly. A further point of interest to us is that, despite the fact that the American Public Health Association celebrated its 75th Annual Meeting this past October, "it is only in recent years that the crystals of professionalization have begun to appear in the amorphous mass comprising the personalia of public health."[5] As long as any group fails to have minimum standards of personnel the result will be an "amorphous mass" in which the professional individuals will be lumped.

From the timely story of "The Professionalization of Public Health," the following excerpt seems highly pertinent:

> It is interesting to observe the developmental steps common to all learned professions and to compare these with the evolution of the public health profession. Usually, a profession first organizes to protect its members against unfair competition. Next, it proceeds to improve relationships between members of the profession. Next, it attempts to establish educational qualifications for admission to practice. Throughout the evolutionary process, public needs are

placed above professional desires. Professional development in public health has followed these stages, always devoting itself to public needs first. Only relatively recently has it attempted to protect the profession from injustices.

The effort to improve educational qualifications for admission to practice, characteristic of the evolution of all professions, is one of the most recent developments in our Association. It dates back to a Committee on Training and Personnel appointed in 1931 and consisting of representatives from each of our sections. That Committee pointed up its objectives as follows:

1. Equal academic standing of public health workers with other professions.
2. Progress through evolution without discrediting present workers.
3. Keeping a suitable list of candidates.
4. Recognition of experience as well as training.

They recommended the following:

1. Definition of the different types of public health workers.
2. Registration of workers now in health service.
3. Setting up definite standards for future reference.
4. A campaign of popular education for better tenure, adequate salaries, and appointment of trained workers in the future.
5. Development of suitable licensure legislation to necessitate the appointment of trained individuals.[6]

In relation to our own proposed program which is voluntary rather than legal, it is encouraging to read further:

The objective 'Development of suitable licensure legislation to necessitate the appointment of trained individuals' has become less urgent than it was in 1931. The alacrity with which appointing bodies throughout the country have accepted American Public Health Association educational qualifications is as gratifying as it is unexpected. If this continues, licensure legislation with all its cumbersome machinery and shortcomings may be unnecessary.[7]

In the library field, as long ago as 1919 an effort was made by certain distinguished members of the American Library Association to establish a National Board of Certification for Librarians. The committee report of 1920-21 "National Certification and Training" bears the name of C. C. Williamson as chairman.[8] In that report and in the chapter "Standardization and Certification" of his *Training For Library Service* are to be found the most comprehensive and reasonable arguments for a certification program.[9]

Ten years earlier the first step in compulsory certification for librarians had been taken in California as a result of teacher certification. Since that time a great deal has been done state by state to further the certification program. Its growth is shown conclusively by a comparison between the number of states included in the most recent *Certification of Librarians*[10] compiled by the A. L. A. Board of Education for Librarianship and any earlier edition of this geographic summary. While the standards still leave much to be desired at least there is a minimum standard and in many states this minimum has been raised. Conditions in the general library world are infinitely better than they were before the inauguration of the certifying program.

Certification for Medical Librarians

Certification, whether legal or voluntary, is but a method of establishing minimum standards. Its purpose is to improve the standards of education and training of the group, thus assuring a higher level of service to the public, but also resulting ultimately in benefits to the group through increased prestige and social and financial status. Its corollary is to circumvent the undermining of the group's standards by preventing the acceptance of unqualified persons into the field. This phase of its purpose lies in the future, because one of the basic principles of the proposed voluntary certification program for medical librarians is the protection of those of us already in service by charter certification. This underlying principle of protection of workers already in the field, in which experience is accepted in lieu of formal academic and professional education, is inherent in and characteristic of programs of other professional bodies seeking the establishment of minimum personnel standards. The improved standards are for future reference. Although undoubtedly desirable, it is not suggested that any of us go back to school or become "interns" or "externs." Just by being or continuing to be, for all practical purposes, we receive charter certification. Death will eventually remove our individual deficiencies from the professional program. But until we start the program, even death cannot help. Certification is the first collective step of the group in its forward march to the goal of a level of education and training, below which no person may be accepted as a member of the group. No certification program of or by itself claims or promises to raise the status, standards, or prestige of a single individual, but it does raise the level of the group and as this level is raised to a professional status, the prestige inherent in any recognized profession cloaks the individual member. Modern Harveys and Listers, modern Deweys and Putnams, however, are as always a measure of the heights to which the individual can and will go, and not of the level of the group.

From the report of Charles C. Williamson's *Training For Library Service,*[11] published in 1923, to that of J. Periam Danton's *Education for Librarianship: Criticisms, Dilemmas and Proposals*[12] published in 1946, the underlying deficiency of librarianship is found to be a basic lack of education. "Education," said Ray Lyman Wilbur in discussing the medical profession, "has really provided the basis for the present status of our professions. Recognition of education through processes of licensure . . . made it possible to get expert service of a professional character in almost all parts of our nation."[13] While the establishment of minimum standards of education through certification is but one phase of the whole forward push toward professionalization and professional recognition, it is a fundamental one laying a stout flooring upon which a more respectable and respected educational edifice can be built by medical librarians.

By our failure as an organization to establish standards we are permitting others to assume our prerogatives. In connection with this the following should be considered thoughtfully:

1. Although the American Library Association has to a certain extent defaulted, its proposed National Certification Plan was "based fundamentally on the principle that it is not only the right but the duty of the American Library Association to formulate standards of fitness for professional library work."[14] Other professions have assumed that "right" and that "duty" and their national councils of certification have been influential.

2. According to the history of medical certification and licensure, it would not seem desirable for the library schools to assume responsibility for certification. When education as well as certification and licensure were in the hands of the medical schools, diploma mills and such flagrant abuses resulted that finally certification and licensure was taken over by state boards. This division of responsibility was followed by the establishment of the National Board of Medical Examiners.

By our failure as an organization to establish standards we are permitting other agencies to establish them for us. In connection with this the following should be considered thoughtfully:

1. By having no formulated standards of fitness for professional medical library work, we have failed and are failing as an association to influence Civil Service standards. This is of particular interest to us as medical librarians because of the number of librarians connected with the Veterans' Administration and the Army Medical Library.

2. Some form of standardization is implied in the dictum "a trained librarian" of the American Medical Association and of the American College of Surgeons. The hand writing on the wall is there. In case you have forgotten, it still means weighed in the balance and found wanting.

3. Because we have no recognized standards, in a sense each medical library is of necessity establishing its own standards no matter how much

of a compromise they may be, but such standards are both local and individualistic and can be ignored or abandoned at any time.

4. Because standards have not been established some librarians are becoming impatient and are joining labor unions in the hope of obtaining certain benefits. This undermines our claims to the time honored method of standardization on a professional level through certification as opposed to standardization through labor or trade unions.

Certain Advantages of Certification for Medical Librarians

1. The experience of other professions shows that this evolutionary steps has redounded to their own advantage as well as that of the public.

2. Certification would help to mark the boundaries of the profession. It would help to delineate the face of the profession so that the public would be able to tell the difference between a librarian and a person who works in a library and eventually the difference between a refugee from some other profession and a librarian. What shall it profit a man if he prepare himself for a profession and there be no recognition of the difference between him and others?

3. Certification would also help establish in the minds of the administrators of the institution of which the library is a part, and of the administrators of the library itself, the difference between a page boy and a librarian, a secretary and a librarian, and any other non-professional worker and a librarian, although all may work in the same library. The administrators of libraries must differentiate more clearly between professional and non-professional work. Even where it is almost impossible, because of the smallness of the staff to differentiate in actuality, it is essential that the Librarian be keenly aware of the necessity for striving toward this goal. The lack of distinction between manual, clerical, and professional activities contributes to the profession's loss of superior personnel, to the uneconomic use of trained librarians, and to the proverbial low salaries. Standards of service are inseparable from standards of training.

4. Certification, of course, would benefit most the younger librarians. Those just beginning their professional careers would enjoy the full developments of the slow ripening fruits of improved status, tenure, and prestige. For the older librarians some satisfaction should be derived from Bacon's statement: "I hold every man a debtor to his profession; from the which as men of course do seek to receive countenance and profit, so ought they of duty to endeavor themselves, by way of amends, to be a help and ornament thereunto."

5. Certification would also have a protective value to the medical librarians should economic history repeat itself in a depression.

6. Certification, at this particular time, would act as a stimulus to the various curricula that are being proposed and even adopted by the various library schools. These schools, in response to the demand for higher standards of education for librarians, are struggling with the revision of their curricula. They might receive some support and some guidance through our establishment of standards of personnel.

7. Certification, at this particular time, would help the recruitment program that is being pushed by all library organizations. It would indicate to those potential librarians whom we would like to have in the medical library field that we are becoming professionalized as a group and would be an inducement to them to meet our educational requirements. It might further attract desirable candidates who would not otherwise enter the library field at all.

Finally, as Phelps states:

> . . . the stablization of minimum qualifications for professional employment, is a major factor in the economic well-being of any group. In the long run, it is the decisive element in the determination of salaries and conditions of work.[15]

Cogently, he summarizes our needs:

> No short-run program of amelioration will be very effective so long as the boundaries of the profession are poorly defined, standards are low, and the general public remains uneducated to the need for trained and competent personnel in the acquisition, housing, managament, and distribution of the accumulated knowledge of the race. What is equally important, no *long-run* program of amelioration is likely to progress far unless sponsored and led by a tightly integrated, nation-wide organization capable of speaking authoritatively for the profession as a whole.[16]

REFERENCES

1. Browning, W., The development of the Association of Medical Librarians, Bull. M. Library A. n.s. 9:1, July '19.
2. American Library Association, College and university libraries and librarianship, Chicago, A.L.A., 1946, pp. 89-90.
3. Trotter, W., Has the intellect a function? Lancet 1:1424, June 24, '39.
4. Sigerist, H., The history of medical licensure, Diplomate 7:229-236, Nov. '35.
5. Shepard, W. P., The professionalization of public health, Am. J. Pub. Health 38:146, Jan. '48.
6. *Ibid.*, p. 147.
7. *Ibid.*, p. 152.

8. Williamson, C. C., National certification and training, American Library Association, Annual Reports 1920-21, pp. 78-89.
9. Williamson, C. C., Training for library service, New York, Carnegie Corp., 1923.
10. American Library Association. Board of Education for Librarianship, Certification of librarians, A.L.A., 1945.
11. Williamson, C. C., Training for library service, New York, Carnegie Corp., 1923.
12. Danton, J. P., Education for librarianship: criticism, dilemmas, and proposals, [N.Y.] Columbia University School of Library Service, 1946.
13. Wilbur, R. L., Professional education and licensure, Federation Bull. 27:282-283, Sept. '41.
14. Williamson, C. C., National certification and training, American Library Association, Annual Reports 1920-21, p. 79.
15. Phelps, O. W., Organizations of employees, in Martin, L., Personnel administration in libraries, Chicago, University of Chicago Press [c1946] p. 109.
16. *Ibid.,* p. 110.

The Past History of the Medical Library Association, Inc.*

By JAMES F. BALLARD,
Librarian, Boston Medical Library

THE Medical Library Association is celebrating its fiftieth anniversary appropriately in the city where it came into existence in 1898. The College of Physicians of Philadelphia, its learned librarian, and the other medical libraries participating as hosts at this anniversary session deserve the heartfelt thanks of the Association for their unselfish assumption of such a great burden.

In addressing you at this time, it seems appropriate to discuss briefly the early history of the Association on the assumption that this period would prove interesting to the newer members of the organization, both libraries and individuals.

I have been, at least, an eye witness to the whole span of the existence of the Association over its fifty years, as I was a member of the staff of the Boston Medical Library for six years when the Association was organized at Philadelphia in 1898 with the Boston Medical Library participating as a charter member. Dr. Edwin H. Brigham attended the first meeting as the representative of Dr. J. R. Chadwick, who generously paid the expenses of the trip, while I was left at home to help mind the Library.

My personal interest may be said to have begun in 1914 when I presented a paper entitled: "Some problems in the administration of a medical library," at the annual meeting at Atlantic City, and since then I have been more or less interested in and identified with the Association, and have held many offices and appointments, from the highest to the lowest, if there is any low appointment.

A group of persons interested in medical libraries met in Philadelphia

* Presented at the annual meeting of the Medical Library Association, Philadelphia, May 28, 1948.

Originally published in *Bulletin of the Medical Library Association,* Volume 36 (October, 1948), pp. 227-241. Reprinted by permission.

FOUNDERS OF THE MEDICAL LIBRARY ASSN.

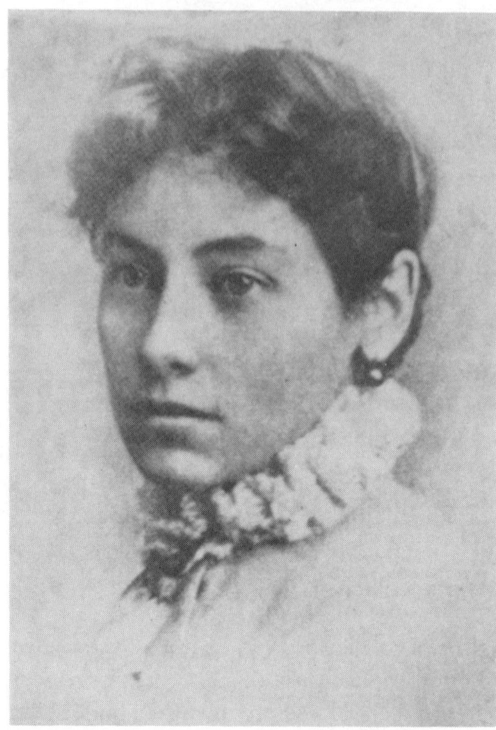

MARGARET CHARLTON
Librarian, McGill University Medical School
Montreal, Quebec, Canada

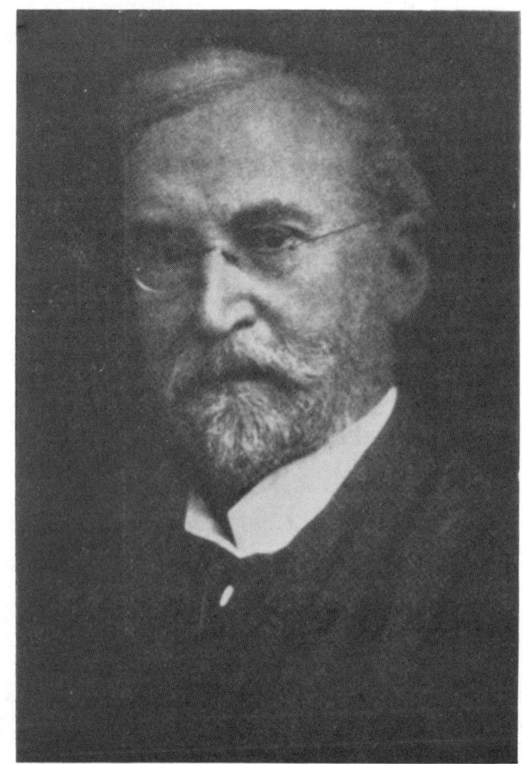

GEORGE MILBRY GOULD, M.D.
Philadelphia Physician

on May 2, 1898 in the office of the *Philadelphia Medical Journal* on the invitation of Dr. George M. Gould, the editor of the Journal. The meeting was called for the purpose of organizing a medical library association. Invitations were sent to prominent medical libraries in the United States and Canada. The following persons attended the meeting:

Dr. Edwin H. Brigham, Boston Medical Library.

Dr. William Browning, Kings County Medical Society, Brooklyn, New York.

Miss M. R. Charlton, McGill University, Montreal.

Charles Perry Fisher, College of Physicians of Philadelphia.

Miss Marcia C. Noyes, Medical and Chirurgical Faculty of Maryland.

Dr. J. L. Rothrock, Ramsey County Medical Society, St. Paul, Minnesota.

Miss E. S. Thies, Johns Hopkins University Medical School.

Dr. George M. Gould.

Seven libraries were represented. A number of letters were received from physicians, including Drs. Adami of Montreal, Osler of Baltimore, and Spivak of Denver, who were unable to attend the meeting; expressing the belief that an organization of medical libraries was needed and promising their co-operation. It is well known that this co-operation was rendered a hundred fold.

It is well corroborated that the original idea was Miss Charlton's, and that she approached Dr. Gould, as he was in a position to further the project. Miss Noyes told me this a number of times and no one knew more about the early years than Miss Noyes, who was deeply interested in the Association and in close contact with its affairs from its foundation until near her retirement. It is regrettable that Miss Noyes was unable to write her history of the Association, a project dear to her heart.

Dr. Gould was appointed temporary chairman and read a paper entitled: "The work of an association of medical libraries."[1] In this paper was outlined eight projects to be carried out by committees of the proposed association. These proposals embraced the procurement of material, a union catalog of rare books, an abstracting and reference service, and general library administration.

Following Dr. Gould's address, it was decided to organize as he proposed and under the name of the "Association of Medical Librarians." Dr. Gould was elected President; Dr. J. L. Rothrock, Vice-President; Miss M. R. Charlton, Secretary; and Dr. William Browning, Treasurer. These

[1] Medical Libraries, 1898, 1: 15-19.

four officers were designated an executive committee to carry on the business of the association during the ensuing year and to arrange for the next meeting of the organization.

On June 6, 1898, at the time of the meeting of the American Medical Association in Denver, a meeting of medical librarians was held in response to an invitation of a local committee, for the purpose of aiding the newly formed Association of Medical Librarians. Dr. C. D. Spivak was a member of the local committee. Twenty-five physicians, representing nearly as many medical libraries, attended the meeting, at which Dr. Gould spoke on the objectives of the new Association of Medical Librarians. He outlined his plan for the establishment of an exchange for medical duplicates and suggested that it be located in Philadelphia. A letter from Melvil Dewey, at the time secretary of the A. L. A., was read, concerning possible affiliation with the A. M. A. or the A. L. A. Dr. Gould was appointed a delegate to the A. L. A. meeting in Chatauqua, July 5, 1898. Dr. Gould attended the A. L. A. conference and read a paper entitled: "The union of public and medical libraries."[2]

Dr. Gould likewise proposed the following resolutions to the Executive Committee of the A. M. A., which endorsed the resolutions, and then were passed unanimously by the A. M. A.:

"WHEREAS, The establishment, organization, and filling of public medical libraries is a means of vast and increasing importance both for the preservation of medical literature, and the progress of medical science; and,

WHEREAS, There are at present but very few such libraries in the United States, and of these the great majority are in a sad state of imperfection and inefficiency; and

WHEREAS, Most valuable literature is wasted because of the non-existence and imperfection of such libraries; it is therefore,

RESOLVED, That the American Medical Association unanimously approves of any ethical and legitimate methods of encouraging the organization, perfection and support of public medical libraries in all the cities, towns and villages of the United States, and earnestly urges the members of the association to aid in the formation and organization of such libraries; also

RESOLVED, That the *Journal of the American Medical Association* be sent gratis to the membership libraries of the Association of Medical Librarians, or to other libraries that may be recommended by the Executive Committee of said Association."

It is to be noted that Dr. Gould did not waste any time in placing the matter before the medical library profession of the country.

[2]Phila. Med. J., July 30, 1898, p. 237.

Dr. C. D. Spivak of Denver, was a pioneer in the promotion and expansion of medical libraries and he wholeheartedly supported the new association. He established and edited a small bi-monthly periodical that he called *Medical Libraries*. It began publication in February 1898 and ceased publication in December 1902, succeeding the *Monthly Bulletin of the Colorado Medical Library Association,* published previously in five numbers. His program as outlined in number one was as follows:

"OUR AIM.

First—To encourage founding of Medical Libraries and Medical Departments in Public Libraries, wherever the medical profession is fairly organized.

Second—To encourage the compilation of union catalogues of medical books and periodicals of private libraries, as outlined in our pamphlet, "How Every City May Secure a Medical Library."

Third—To further the project proposed by Dr. M. Gould of Philadelphia of organizing a Medical Librarians' Association and the perfecting of plans whereby the wasted medical literature all over the world may be utilized.

Fourth—To gather statistical data, publish reports, news and historical sketches of public and private medical libraries and biographies, of medical librarians and book lovers."

It is evident that Dr. Spivak was very active in the fostering of medical libraries, as he lists eight papers of his published in medical and library periodicals during 1897 and 1898 before the establishment of his *Medical Libraries,* and that he had the strong support of the medical profession of Denver and Colorado.

He gave considerable space in his periodical to the new Association of Medical Librarians. In its volumes are found reports of the organization and early meetings of the Association, Dr. Gould's paper read at the organization meeting of the Association of Medical Librarians, and papers presented at the meetings. It was the official organ of the Association until 1902, when the Association published its own Bulletin.

The Colorado bulletin was originally published in the *Colorado Medical Journal,* beginning in September 1897, and ending in January 1898. The first issue was not dated or numbered, but thereafter the bulletins were numbered and dated. Numbers three to five were reprinted and issued separately. This data is compiled from a letter of Dr. Spivak to Dr. J. R. Chadwick, dated March 10, 1900, and is in Dr. Chadwick's *Medical Libraries,* volumes one and two, along with the three reprints of the Colorado bulletin and other publications of Dr. Spivak.

Dr. Spivak in January 1899 wrote a valuable paper of fourteen pages, and three double-page charts entitled: "The medical libraries of the United States." In addition to listing the medical libraries of the country and extensively analyzing them, the author discusses important topics relating to the improvements and expansion of medical libraries under the headings: "Suggestions for the improvement of existing libraries; make better use of existing libraries, and revive the libraries which are in a state of syncope; how to organize new medical libraries; the union catalogue." Dr. Spivak advocated the advisability of having one large medical library in one city, and stressed the idea of a union catalogue of private resources of a locality. The doctor was years ahead of his time. At this time there were 120 medical libraries in the country and 165 medical colleges. The publication of *Medical Libraries* by Dr. Spivak must have been a labor of love as the yearly subscription price was only one dollar and he depended to a large extent on private donations to carry on his work. The cessation of his journal was without notice in 1902 and evidently due to a sudden decision on his part, as in the last number he states in a notice that after January 1, 1903 it would be issued from a new address in Denver. It is probable that he believed that the new bulletin of the Association of Medical Librarians would take the place of his journal and therefore felt secure in abandoning a liability. Unfortunately, the Association could not carry on the bulletin and likewise it ceased with 1902.

The second annual meeting of the Association was held in Philadelphia on October 5, 1899. At this meeting a constitution of thirteen articles was adopted:

"1. This Association shall be called the Association of Medical Librarians.

2. The object of the Association shall be the fostering of Medical Libraries and the maintenance of an Exchange of medical literature among its members."

The officers were re-elected and a planning committee of five (four physicians and Miss Charlton) was appointed by the President.

The third annual meeting was held at Atlantic City on June 4, 1900. At this meeting it was proposed that only one library from a city or town or foreign country be admitted to membership in the Association. After discussion this proposal was withdrawn and the second member library from Chicago was accepted. The officers were continued in office, except for the Treasurer, where Dr. George D. Hersey of Providence succeeded Dr. William Browning, resigned.

The fourth annual meeting was held in Baltimore on May 25, 1901. At this meeting a resolution was passed limiting membership only to librarians representing medical libraries of not less than 500 volumes and with regular library hours and attendance.

Dr. Gould gave up the presidency because of press of work and Dr. William Osler was elected President and Dr. Gould, Vice-President, and Dr. Hersey and Miss Charlton were re-elected Treasurer and Secretary respectively. It was also proposed that future meetings be planned to coincide with the meetings of the American Medical Association. At this time the membership represented 34 libraries and there were 26 affiliated members (physicians).

The fifth annual meeting was held at Saratoga Springs, New York, on June 10, 1902. Dr. Osler, Dr. Hersey and Miss Charlton were re-elected to their respective offices. Dr. Robert Fletcher became Vice-President, succeeding Dr. Gould.

ORGANIZATION.

In 1928 it was voted to revise the By-Laws completely, and a special committee was appointed for the purpose, consisting of Mrs. Rosa M. Hibbard, Chairman, Miss M. Edna M. Poole, Miss Elisabeth M. Runge, and Miss Eva M. West. The meeting voted to add the Executive Committee to the By-Laws Committee: James F. Ballard, Chairman, J. C. Harding, and Miss Louise Ophuls. This was an important committee, as it proposed a number of drastic changes in organization and administration. The proposed changes were brought before the annual meeting in 1929 at Cleveland and all the changes except those relating to the distribution of materials by the Exchange and the limitation of officers to professional librarians were accepted, the two last named proposals being defeated. The membership was reclassified into three classes: library members, supporting members, and professional members. The qualifications for membership were defined with dues for each class and the voting power for the first time was established. The classes were: "A. Library members. Medical libraries and allied scientific libraries of not less than 500 volumes, with regular hours and attendants shall constitute the voting membership of the Association. Each Library member shall be entitled to two voting representatives at business sessions of the Association. B. Supporting members. Any person interested in medical and allied libraries, except those professionally engaged in library work, shall be eligible to supporting membership. C. Professional members. Any person actively engaged in library work shall be eligible to professional membership. The power to vote shall be vested solely in the library members and exercised by their official representatives." This change, by the addition of "allied scientific libraries," broadened the scope of membership to include dental, veterinary, biological, psychological, and like allied libraries. The individual members, mostly physicians, were definitely separated from the libraries and set up as a new class of supporting members, at the same annual dues of $5.00. The new class of professional membership was limited to persons actively engaged in library work and the annual dues for this class was fixed at $2.00.

The voting power was established in the member libraries, and each library was limited to two voting representatives. Other major changes included the establishment of a Nominating Committee, and the provision for voting by mail, thus giving all library members a voice in the election of officers; the establishment of Standing Committees; increasing the Executive Committee to five from three, with a three-year term of office; the determination of the place of the annual meeting by the Association instead of the Executive Committee; and perfecting and safe-guarding the presentation of amendments to the By-Laws.

A new method of distribution of materials by the size of libraries was proposed and defeated. A new amendment limiting the officers to professional librarians also was defeated. This was the first step towards a professional association but the members were not ready to divorce themselves from the physicians who had held major offices, particularly the presidency, from the beginning of the Association.

The meeting of 1929 was a very important meeting and was held at Cleveland as a central point in the country, although two invitations had been received from the Pacific Coast. The attendance was fifty-five, representing 49 libraries. At the previous conventions in New York, in 1928, 47 libraries were represented, and in 1927 at Washington 45 libraries were registered. These figures emphasized the importance of the meeting to the membership. The first mention of incorporation was in the minutes of the 1931 (New Orleans) meeting. Although these minutes are fragmentary it is evident that a special committee on incorporation was appointed consisting of Miss Sue Biethan, Chairman, James F. Ballard, Mrs. Rosa M. Hibbard, and Miss M. Myrtle Tye, and this committee reported to the Association at San Francisco in 1932. The matter was deferred for further study until 1933. In 1933, it was voted to authorize the Executive Committee to proceed with incorporation and make such minor changes in the Constitution as were required by the chartering state and presented to the meeting at that time. In 1934 The Association was incorporated in the State of Maryland. In the charter the Association was given the power to hold real and personal property. The principal office of the corporation was established in Baltimore at the Library of the Medical and Chirurgical Faculty. The governing body, the Executive Committee, and the membership of four classes: library, supporting, professional, and honorary, with their definitions, were included in the charter. The only change in membership from the previous By-Laws was the inclusion of the class of honorary members. In 1946 the constitution was amended to provide for a physician as Honorary Vice-President, the office of the President and all other offices to be held by professional librarians in active work. A Vice-President, to be President-Elect, was set up as a new office. In 1947, the Constitution and By-Laws were revised to set up the Constitution separate from the By-Laws. The important major changes were to reduce the voting representation of library members from two to one representative, to re-define the qualifications of professional membership, and to establish a Committee on the Exchange and a Finance Committee with definite powers.

At Newark in 1939, the Association revised its Constitution by increasing the admission qualifications for libraries to 1000 volumes and increasing the annual dues of Library members to $15.00 and professional members to $3.00 with the Bulletin.

NAME.

The organization was first named *The Association of Medical Librarians* and was composed of individual members with annual dues of five dollars. At the seventh annual meeting in 1904, the By-Laws were amended and two classes of membership were formed, libraries and individuals, with annual dues of $10. and $5. respectively. At the tenth annual meeting held at Atlantic City, June 3, 1907, the name of the Association was changed to the *Medical Library Association*. At that time the international scope of the association was recognized for the first proposal for a change in name was the American Medical Library Association.

In 1920, it was proposed to change the name of the Association and a special committee was appointed to consider the matter. In 1921, the committee recommended that the name be changed to Medical Library Association of America. A motion was duly carried to that effect but under the Constitution and By-Laws had to go over until the next annual meeting. In 1922, the motion was put before the Association and the amendment was lost on a vote of 12 to 9, and the original name of Medical Library Association retained.

AFFILIATION.

In 1898 the question of affiliation with the American Library Association or the American Medical Association was considered at the Denver meeting of librarians, but evidently this idea was not received favorably by the founders of the Medical Library Association. In 1923 there was a proposal to affiliate with the Special Libraries Association, but likewise this did not meet with the approval of the membership.

PRESIDENTS.

From the beginning until 1933, the office of President was held by prominent physicians interested in medical libraries. In 1933, Miss Marcia C. Noyes was elected President, thus breaking the line of medical succession. She was followed during the next year by Charles Frankenberger of Brooklyn. Then Dr. W. W. Francis, of Montreal, was President for two years, and James F. Ballard, of Boston, for two years, followed in succession to the present by professional medical librarians.

MEETINGS.

In 1928 it was formally proposed that, if possible, the Association should hold its annual meetings in a city extending a formal invitation to the Association, and should not impose itself upon a library or a community.

Also it was urged strongly that libraries should recognize the importance of the Association and include in their annual budgets travelling expenses to send their librarians to the annual meetings. It was suggested, because of the widespread membership, that regional meetings of the Association might he held in the Middle West, the Far West, and the South.

The attendance at meetings in the early years was small, ten or fifteen at the most, but has gradually increased until we now have large numbers at the annual meetings. The establishment of the professional class of membership has helped the attendance, as it has made available to librarians, not representatives of libraries, the advantages of the meetings.

MEMBERSHIP.

In the beginning the membership was constituted of physicians and librarians, representing libraries or interested libraries. In the Constitution and By-Laws of 1922, Art. I, Chapter 3, the membership was defined as follows:

"Medical libraries of not less than 500 volumes and with regular hours and attendance, medical librarians, and other persons interested in medical libraries shall be eligible to membership."

There was not any breakdown into classes. Dues were $10. for libraries and $5. for individuals.

The membership has gradually increased over the years until the total as of May 1, 1947 was 701, made up of 288 libraries, 282 professional members, 126 supporting members, and 5 honorary members. If new supporting members are desired it is logical to suppose that at least one physician from each member library could be persuaded to join the organization. This should be a fertile field for the membership committee to cultivate.

About 1933, the dental libraries became quite active in the Association, and about 1937 the hospital libraries likewise became a recognized group in the Association.

PUBLICATIONS.

As previously noted *Medical Libraries,* Denver, v.1-5, 1898-1902, was the official organ of the Association. In 1902, the Association published its own *Bulletin* for that year. In 1903, the *Medical Library and Historical Journal,* Brooklyn, edited by Albert T. Huntington, Librarian of the Medical Society of Kings County, became the official organ. This periodical lived for five years, 1903-1907. Volumes one and two carried on the title pages the designation, "Official Organ", and gave considerable space to the doings of the Association and printed lengthy lists for the Exchange. With volume three the designation, "Official Organ", was dropped from the title pages, as well as the exchange lists, although space was given to reports of the annual meetings. There was evidently a rift in the lute somewhere that the old-timers in the Association may remember and wish to forget. After the death of the *Medical Library and Historical Journal,* there was a gap in official publications until the Association began the new series of its BULLETIN in July 1911. The BULLETIN had passed through many vicissitudes, but has survived to reach its thirty-sixth volume for the year 1948. The BULLETIN has improved in content and publishing, until today it is a good professional periodical.

MANUAL.

A medical library manual was originally proposed in 1920 and was considered as late as 1929 when it occasioned considerable discussion at the annual meeting, where the membership voted to continue the project. The special problem at the time was the financing of its publication. In 1940 Miss Janet Doe reported for the Committee on the Medical Library Handbook that progress was being made on the expansion and development of Miss Irene Jones' manuscript. A committee of twelve members was appointed in 1939. Further progress was reported in 1941 and early publication was hoped for. In 1942 the Committee reported that the manual had been completed and that the manuscript was in the hands of the American Library Association, who had agreed to publish it on a subsidy basis. The Handbook was published in 1943 and has been very successful.

THE EXCHANGE.

The Exchange is the soul and heart of the Association. It is our Rock of Gibralter, the life-line of our existence. Without it, the Association would become moribund. Conceived in the highest spirit of altruism, it has maintained this spirit through all the years of its existence. Much of its success is due to the unselfish loyalty and labors of Dr. Gould, Miss Noyes, Miss Lawrence, other exchange managers, and our present incumbent, Miss Naylor.

In the address given by Dr. Gould at the organization meeting in 1898, *The Work of an Association of Medical Librarians,* he advocated the assignment of various activities to special committees. First on his list was the exchange of duplicates between libraries. In the first Constitution, Article two, following the name of the association, concerns the fostering of medical libraries and the maintenance of an exchange of medical literature among its members. The operation of the Exchange in the beginning was financed by voluntary contributions. The first headquarters was established in Philadelphia and Mrs. E. R. Clifton was engaged to carry on the work. Operations began on December 1, 1899. The method used at that time was three fold: the reception and allocation of material, the reception of lists of duplicates, and wants from libraries, and direct exchange between libraries. The first report, six months' work, shows that 1782 items were received and 813 items distributed to fifteen libraries. It is interesting to note that 76 books were sold for $16.64, the cost of the bindings. In the early days publishers of some of the American medical periodicals sent complimentary copies to member libraries as a contribution to the work of the Association. Exchange between libraries was encouraged, and the reports of the Exchange give some figures of the number of volumes involved in this exchange of material.

On December 1, 1900, the Exchange was moved to Baltimore under the management of Miss Noyes, and housed in the building of the Medical and Chirurgical Faculty of Maryland. In 1902 the manager of the exchange (Miss Noyes) was sent to New York and Brooklyn for ten days to examine the duplicates which the New York Academy of Medicine and the Medical Society of the County of Kings had offered to the Association. In 1905 the Exchange was moved to Brooklyn and Mr. Albert T. Huntington was made manager. This move was necessitated because of lack of room in Baltimore.

In July, 1909, the Exchange again moved back to Baltimore, with Miss Noyes as manager, and an assistant was provided to work for the Exchange only. The Medical and Chirurigical Faculty provided space in its new building. In November, 1914, the method of mimeographing exchange lists was inaugurated by Miss Noyes, and five lists averaging eight pages were issued up to July 1915. Practically every item on these lists were asked for by members of the Association. Previous to this time lists had been published in the organs of the Association. The mimeographed lists were successful beyond anticipation and much superior in results obtained to the printed lists in the BULLETIN and elsewhere. Material was received at headquarters and the lists were made up from the material. In the report for the year ending June 1, 1917, there is reported a distribution from headquarters, of a total of 3433 items, and in addition there was a direct exchange between libraries of 1892 items. Also, the Exchange received a number of duplicate and want lists from member libraries. Despite the problems engendered by World War I and the necessity of cancelling one annual meeting, the work of the Exchange did not falter but was carried on at its regular rate of accomplishment.

In the By-Laws of 1922, Article IV is devoted to the Exchange.

Chapter 1. Provides that the management and location of the Exchange shall be determined by the Executive Committee who shall have the direction of its affairs.

Chapter 2. Says that libraries shall be given precedence in the disposal of the material in accordance with their size, the largest library being given first choice.

Chapter 3. Prohibits the requesting of material duplicated in the requesting library, subject to the penalty of expulsion for violation of this rule.

Chapter 4. Provides for distribution to individual members after all libraries have been satisfied.

Chapter 5. Prohibits sale of material until after it had been offered to all members.

In April, 1923 the suggestion was made that a small service fee should be assessed for each item distributed, but this idea was abandoned as working a hardship on the small library least able to pay such a fee. At the 1923 meeting, problems concerning the Exchange were discussed and it was suggested that a Committee on the Exchange be appointed to consider matters relevant to the Exchange. During these years the financial support for the Exchange was a serious question and kept recurring at meetings and in the pages of the BULLETIN. As early as 1925, there had been some concern about the method of distribution as provided for in the

By-Laws. At the Atlantic City meeting in 1925 there was considerable discussion on the management of the Exchange and Miss Noyes pointed out the difficulty occasioned by the requests of many libraries for the same item, and also stated that some libraries took but did not give material. This last inequity was remedied later by the regulation that a library must submit material at least once in two years in order to receive material. At this meeting, Mr. Ballard requested that a special committee be appointed to work out the problems of the Exchange and suggested that the By-Laws might be amended to change the priority of distribution. This Committee was authorized by the meeting, and the President appointed the Committee: Dr. B. Gilchrist, Miss M. C. Noyes, Miss M. M. Loomis and Miss E. B. Lawrence, later to become Manager of the Exchange. The Committee was intrusted to report to the Executive Committee during the year and that report was to be submitted to all members. This special committee reported as directed, submitting a plan for re-organization based on operating upon a cash basis. The report was considered by the Executive Committee and discussd by the conference of medical librarians held at New York in March, 1926. The plan was found too complicated and expensive to operate, although containing many good ideas.

In 1926, Miss Noyes reported that her organization could not retain the Exchange in Baltimore after June 1, 1926, because of existing conditions. The matter was referred to the Executive Committee and a special conference of medical librarians was called at New York, on March 22nd, to consider the crisis confronting the location and operation of the Exchange. There was a prolonged general discussion on all phases of the exchange work. Dr. Frederick Tice of Chicago, President, remarked that the Exchange was the heart and life of the organization. "When that goes the Association is dead." At least three locations were mentioned and the Exchange was moved to Ann Arbor with Miss Sue Biethan as Manager.

In 1927, the key list of libraries, arranged alphabetically by states and cities, was originated and it was proposed that lists should be broadcast from early September until May. Miss Biethan, in her first report, stated that eight lists had been broadcast and cleared, and that the ninth list had been sent out just before the meeting. Likewise, the lists were made longer as the work progressed. Miss Biethan requested that libraries asking for volumes for second sets should note that fact on their requests and not ask for second set material without indicating that it is for that purpose.

In 1928, at the New York meeting, there was a round table discussion on the Medical Library Exchange conducted by Mr. Frank Place of the New York Academy of Medicine. Miss Noyes spoke on the early history,

Miss Biethan on its operation, and Mr. Ballard outlined his plan of designating large regional libraries throughout the country to serve as repositories for all medical literature, to which state libraries would be subordinated. The working collections of hospitals, clinics, government offices and medical schools would be subordinated to the state libraries. Mr. Ballard explained the By-Law concerning the distribution of material to libraries in order of their size. He stated that the rule is based on the reasonable theory that the larger the library, the less material it requires, and the smaller the library, the more it takes from the Exchange, and that if the large library is to receive anything it must have first choice of material and likewise, should normally give at least ten times what it receives.

In the same year Mr. Ballard read a short paper before the Special Libraries Association on the Exchange, and the feasibility of the S.L.A. organizing an exchange. At this time, in addition to maintaining headquarters at Ann Arbor, a depositary was maintained in New York for eastern libraries where material was received, listed, and distributed on assignments by the Exchange Manager.

In 1928 the broadcasting of lists was standardized. They were sent out at six weeks' intervals. In this year the Chairman of the Executive Committee journeyed to Ann Arbor to consult with Miss Biethan on the Exchange and to try to persuade Miss Biethan to retain the managership for at least another year, as she had expressed her intention of relinquishing the work at the next meeting of the Association. The same year the Chairman made a number of visits to Eastern and Western libraries in the interest of the Exchange. Miss Ella B. Lawrence of St. Louis took over the management of the Exchange from Miss Biethan in October, 1928, and in 1929 Miss Lily Hanvey became associated with Miss Lawrence in operating the Exchange.

In 1929 when the By-Laws were completely revised it was proposed to give the Executive Committee, at its discretion, the power to put in operation a new plan of distribution in which the libraries would be classified into six groups according to size:

Group 1. Libraries over 100,000 volumes.
2. Over 50,000 and under 100,000.
3. Over 25,000 and under 50,000.
4. Over 10,000 and under 25,000.
5. Over 5,000 and under 10,000.
6. Under 5,000.

The priority of distribution would be by groups, all libraries in group one receiving consideration before those in group two and so on through the groups. The libraries in each group were to be arranged in strict numerical order according to size, and distribution within a group was to be rotated with each successive list. The members at the meeting considered the plan too complicated and the testimony given by the small libraries made it quite evident that there was not any need of a change on their part. The small libraries were greatly pleased and satisfied with the material they received. There was not any complaint concerning the conduct of the Exchange. The meeting decided to retain the old method of distribution of the largest library having priority. In 1928-29 the Chairman of the Executive Committee made visits to New York to confer with the President, to Chicago to consult with the Treasurer, to St. Louis to see Mrs. Hibbard, Chairman of the special committee on revision of the By-Laws, and to Cleveland and Detroit concerning the annual convention. On his travels he obtained large quantities of good duplicates for the Exchange and located other large accumulations of good material.

In 1930 Miss Lawrence reported to the Association that the new By-Law, compelling libraries to send lists of duplicates to the Exchange, was beginning to have its effect, and pointed out that this change greatly increased the work and would eventually lead to higher costs of operation. In 1931 sixty-eight libraries, out of a total membership of 176, sent in lists, seventeen sending in two or more lists. In 1932-33 Miss Lawrence and her assistants, Miss Hanvey and Mrs. Hennessey, were so swamped with lists that sixty libraries listed and distributed their own material. In 1931 Miss Lawrence reported that the publication of "want lists" had become a serious problem. In 1932 at San Francisco a paper of Dr. Archibald Malloch, entitled "The Medical Library Exchange—Why not play the game?", was read in his absence, in which he opposed the practice of direct exchange by libraries, although this method had been used and encouraged from the beginning of the Association. He likewise deplored the sale of duplicates to dealers, except in special limited classes, of rare and expensive works, material paid for by the libraries, and material left over from exchange lists. This was a reversal of the original policy advocated by Dr. Gould and the first group of charter members. In 1937 the President stressed the need of funds to carry on adequate operation of the Exchange for the 220 library members of the Association, and suggested a membership drive for new supporting members.

Following the resignation of Miss Lawrence in 1942, after a remarkably successful term of fourteen years as manager of the Exchange, headquarters was transferred to the Army Medical Library with Dr. Atherton Seidell as manager. After one year it again was transferred, this time to New Orleans with Miss Alice Rogers as Manager. It began to travel again after a short period and located itself in Newark under the able management of Miss Naylor in 1945.

The Exchange was a perpetual source of discussion at every annual meeting from the beginning until the present. Likewise every volume of the Association's official publications contains material on the Exchange.

During the past twenty-five years the Association has been assuming progressively a professional status, working on medical library problems through special committees and co-operating with national and international bodies on problems relating to medical library work. All of us look forward to its future growth.

The Medical Library Association: Aims, Activities, and a Brief History*

BY L. MARGUERIETE PRIME
Librarian, American College of Surgeons, Chicago, Illinois
President, Medical Library Association

I THINK of the Medical Library Association as being woven of three main strands of interest, each colorful in itself, each made up of many threads varying in length and composition. The first of these main strands has to do with organization and survival and goes back to 1898 when our Pilgrim fathers, so to speak, assembled in Philadelphia to consider the possibility of establishing a medical library association. The American Library Association was then 22 years old and Miss M. R. Charlton of Montreal had found that "their problems were not our problems. . . . She felt lost and that the time was wasted." She had therefore suggested to Dr. Osler that it would be a fine thing if the medical libraries could form an organization of their own, similar to the American Library Association. Hence this meeting in the editorial office of the Philadelphia Medical Journal on May 2, 1898, of eight founding fathers: four medical men, one male librarian, and three women. Montreal, Boston, St. Paul, Brooklyn, Baltimore, and Philadelphia were represented. One of the physicians, Dr. Gould, whose hospitality made the meeting possible, became the first president, serving for three years. Doctors Osler and Chadwick who were unable to be present were keenly interested in the new Association of Medical Librarians and became the second and third presidents, respectively. Dr. Rothrock was the first Vice-President; Miss M. R. Charlton, Secretary, and Dr. Browning, Treasurer. Any survey of the Association leads to an appreciation of the contributions made by interested members of the medical profession not only at the time of founding, but down through the years.

Still within the strand of organization, it is interesting to see how the Association has broadened. The first organization provided for a primary member-

* Read at meeting of Midwest Regional Group, Medical Library Association, North Chicago, Illinois, October 6, 1951.

Originally published in *Bulletin of the Medical Library Association,* Volume 40 (January, 1952), pp. 30-36. Reprinted by permission.

ship of individual librarians representing medical libraries having 500 or more volumes. This was changed in 1904 to a primary membership of medical and allied libraries. In 1904 also two classes of members were set up, one for libraries, the other for individuals, with annual dues of $10.00 and $5.00 respectively. At the Cleveland meeting in 1929 revision of the By-laws provided for the broadening of the field of membership so as to permit the admittance of allied scientific libraries, such as dental, veterinary, biological, psychological, zoological, and the like libraries, and for the reclassification of membership and the establishment of the new class of Professional membership for library workers. The voting power, however, was in the Library members each of whom might have 2 voting representatives.

The Constitution and By-laws under which the Association was incorporated in 1934 established four types of membership, viz.: Library members, Supporting, Professional, and Honorary members.

In 1946 the Constitution was amended to provide for a physician as Honorary Vice-President, the office of the President and all other offices to be held by professional librarians in active work. In 1947 the By-laws were revised to reduce the voting representation of Library members from two to one representative, and a further revision in 1950 provided also for voting by each Professional member (then classified as Active). A new class of membership was established in 1948, the Sustaining members with dues of $100.00. I am delighted to be able to tell you that we now have seven such members, an addition of four in the last two months.

Early annual meetings were held in conjunction with meetings of the American Medical Association and the Congress of Physicians and Surgeons in order to assure a good attendance and to interest other physicians in the Association. With the tremendous growth in the attendance at such large society meetings, this became impossible although as recently as 1947–48, meetings were held preceding or following those of the American Association of the History of Medicine, a smaller group with many interests in common with our own. In recent years we have endeavored to keep in touch with kindred souls in the medical profession by requesting their cooperation as speakers and in 1946 (as above stated) by the provision in the Constitution that the Honorary Vice-President shall be a member of the medical profession. In the mean time our own growth has been such that eminently successful annual meetings have been held in various parts of the country, in Richmond, Boston, Portland, Galveston, and Denver for example.

Finally, as you all know, within the last three years has come recognition of the need for Regional Meetings and provision in the By-laws for such meetings. Two years ago it was my privilege to serve as liaison officer with the groups then in the process of formation. As a result of those contacts the importance of the groups has been borne in upon me. I hope in requesting Mr. Postell, our present Vice-President, to act as liaison officer, a precedent may have been established which will be effective in future years, i.e., that the Vice-President may always carry that responsibility. I trust that the steering committee of the Midwest Regional Group will send him frequent progress bulletins. The main purpose of the regional group, we must always remember, is to acquaint junior staff members with the Medical Library Association and to encourage the attendance and participation of those members.

At the second annual meeting (1899) the objectives of the Association were made to read: "The object of the Association shall be the fostering of medical libraries, and the maintenance of an exchange of medical literature among its members."[1] As an editor, Dr. Gould knew "that absolutely tons of really good things were being discarded and felt that the time was ripe for everyone to begin to conserve."[2] Accordingly the Exchange was opened in Philadelphia in December, 1899. The Exchange was at the beginning so much the *raison d'etre* of the Association that, in my mind at least, it is closely interwoven with the organizational strand. For many it is, even at the present time, "the magnet which is steadily increasing the library membership."[1] I will not attempt to trace the history of this very effective voluntary activity of the Association. Those who knew the work of Marcia Noyes and Ella B. Lawrence in this field need not be reminded. Adequate description to newcomers would be difficult. In January 1945 the Exchange came to roost on the doorstep of its present manager, Miss Mildred V. Naylor, who has carried on the work very satisfactorily on a full time basis. It has been, through the years, the means of husbanding our resources to our mutual advantage. It has required generous sharing and has permitted individual gain. If it has not represented daily bread for our libraries, it has, at least, included some much desired loaves from time to time—and many generous slices.

The BULLETIN is the bright thread which runs through all our strands. It links bit to bit; it catches and reflects all our activities. As its beginnings were among our early efforts we will discuss them here.

"The first reports and news of the Association," according to Mr. Ballard, "were printed in *Medical Libraries*, Denver, 1–5, February 1898–December, 1902."[1] In 1901 it was agreed to publish a quarterly *Bulletin* to be conducted by Miss Noyes, Dr. H. N. Hurd of Baltimore and Mr. John S. Browning, librarian of the New York Academy of Medicine.

In 1902 the BULLETIN was discontinued in order to effect a collaboration with the new *Medical Library and Historical Journal*, an arrangement which later proved unfortunate. In 1911, the BULLETIN again came to life as a new series under the editorship of Dr. John Rührah, the Treasurer, and Miss M. C. Noyes, the Manager of the Exchange, a combination which remained in effect for 15 years.

Many persons have contributed to the success of the BULLETIN since that time. We will not attempt to list them. You are all familiar with this very fine publication of today; it has presented our problems, and recorded our wit, our disagreements, our progress through the years; it is a source of justifiable pride to all of us and probably our ablest emissary to foreign lands.

The work of the Committee on Periodicals and Serials, in my thought, represents the closing of one era within the Association and the beginning of another. It represents the insertion of another strong strand, the international interest. In 1924 this Committee proposed resolutions disapproving of the unfair discrimination of the German publishers against American subscribers and urging the Library and individual members of the Association to discontinue the purchase of German medical books until such time as German publishers adopt a more equitable policy toward American subscribers. The campaign instituted at that time was carried on successfully until the Second World War. It presented a united front economically and is still our watch dog. It marked the entry of the Association into the international picture. The Committee is still active.

Side by side with its entry into the international field came an added emphasis upon professional growth. We were beyond the early period which represented the struggle for survival. We were ready for the third of the interests which is so strong a factor in the Association: conscious professional development. Accordingly *A Handbook of Medical Library Practice*, which had been contemplated for more than 20 years, was in 1941 undertaken in earnest under the editorship of Miss Janet Doe. In 1943 it was published. It has gone through four printings—an indication of the need for such a publication and of its adequacy.

As far back as 1939 a Committee on Standardization in the Field of Library Work and Documentation (Z39) under the auspices of the American Standards Association was established. The Medical Library Association was one of eleven library associations to participate actively in this program, a program which continues to the present time.

The Second World War emphasized the need for more trained medical librarians. Though no national meetings were held during the War years (1942–1945), the Association was not dormant. The Committee on Medical Library Service for the Armed Forces did its part, as did each individual library, and when we emerged from that period, our able president, Miss Mary Louise Marshall, issued the clarion call at New Haven in 1946 for the training and certification of medical librarians. In accordance with the wishes of the members in attendance, the incoming president, Mr. W. B. McDaniel, 2d, appointed a committee to study a "Training Program for Medical Librarianship." The results of that study were presented at Cleveland in 1947; a further study was made during the following year, not only by the Committee, but by the entire membership. A program for training was adopted at Philadelphia in 1948 and one for certification of medical librarians in 1949 at Galveston. The Code for the Training and Certification of Medical Librarians was accepted at Galveston also.

In accordance with the program planned by the Committee on Standards a six weeks' summer course was resumed at Columbia University in 1947, 1949, 1950, and 1951. An additional course was presented at Emory in 1951. Two scholarships were offered by M. L. A. for each of the courses in 1951 and will be again in 1952. To meet the needs of the Veterans Administration, similar, but more concentrated 3-week courses were given in 1949 at the library schools of the University of Southern California in Los Angeles, the University of Chicago, the University of Illinois in Chicago, and Columbia University in New York. The course was repeated at the University of Illinois in 1950. These courses were approved by the M. L. A. under Grade I.

The program of Certification is well on its way; the applications of some 156 persons were reviewed and 56 evaluated and sent to the Standards Committee for final action during the Association year, 1950–51. The questions of internship and recruitment of librarians are likewise being worked upon.

Not only have standards for librarians held the interest of the Association as exemplified by the steps taken in providing training and certification as noted above, but committees are at work in providing Standards for Hospital Medical and Nursing School Libraries, Criteria and Standards for Medical School Libraries, Criteria and Standards for Pharmaceutical Libraries. We are at that stage of our professional development where a need for standards is being felt—and we are looking toward our membership to provide them.

At the same time we are working with other library associations to improve standards for librarians in general. Under the auspices of the Council of National Library Associations, Miss Marshall and Mrs. Cunningham are serving on the Joint Committee on Library Education and Miss Marshall on the Subcommittee for Special Librarianship. Other responsibilities in the Council are carried by M.L.A. members. Dr. Larkey is the present chairman; Miss Doe has served as Secretary. Each year the President of M.L.A., the immediate Past-President or representatives chosen by them, serve as delegates to the Council.

Then again there is the international phase of our activities. The Committee on International Cooperation in 1948 was headed by Miss Janet Doe. More recently Mrs. Eileen Cunningham has served as Chairman. This committee has been awarded funds for 3 successive years with which to finance traveling Fellowships for 3 foreign medical librarians each year. That appropriation this June was renewed on a three-year basis. This bespeaks the confidence which the Rockefeller Foundation has in the program of the Medical Library Association in this field and of its great success. As you know, Fellowships have been awarded to three librarians from Chili, to one from Cuba, one from Brazil, one from Uruguay, one from Ireland, one from Austria, and one from India. Plans for the coming year have been made. This program has called for an unbelievable amount of work on the part of the Chairman, staunch support from committee members, and a great deal of cooperation from the librarians in each city visited by the Fellows. It is a program with far reaching benefits to the Fellows and to the Librarians participating in it.

We joined the International Federation of Library Associations in 1934 and were represented at its second annual meeting in Spain by Miss Darrach and Mrs. Cunningham. Other work of international scope is that of Mrs. Cunningham in connection with the program of UNESCO. She is currently attending the conference on Coordination of Medical Abstracting Services in Paris called by the Natural Science Section of UNESCO and this year will represent the Association at the meetings of the International Federation of Libraries and the International Federation of Documentation in Rome. At the last named session, she is likewise the representative of the American Documentation Institute through the appointment of Mr. Luther Evans, Librarian of Congress and Chairman of the Institute.

It is impossible in this brief period to tell of all the activities of the Association. Since 1945 we have had a Committee on Placement headed by Mrs. Breed Robinson. Each annual meeting includes a Program and Hospitality Committee. The former endeavors to strike the key note of our interests at the time and the latter furnishes the many touches which make the gathering the especially delightful affair it always is. Individuals and round tables discuss subject headings, classifications, and other technical problems. Breakfast and dinner meetings are supported by subject groups. Reports are prepared, read, and discussed. Our members participate and lead in the work of the joint committees sponsored by the Council of National Library Associations and the American Library Association. While Mrs. Cunningham flies to Paris and Rome, other members carry on with both routine and especially assigned tasks. The Secretary, the Treasurer, the Membership Chairman—each makes a considerable contribution to the work of the Association.

A glance through the BULLETIN at the record of achievement down the years leaves one impressed with the number of jobs which have been carried on to a successful conclusion. Tasks have not just been proposed. They have been studied, rounded out, in some cases fought for, and finally proudly presented as a completed job. The whole picture is that of a handsome fabric. The three main strands are there for those who wish to see: organization, professional development, and international cooperation. Each is intertwined with many smaller fine threads bespeaking service to the organization and to the individual.

As this is something of a historical presentation, I should like to quote from

W. B. McDaniel, 2d, Past President of the Association, as he wrote of the then forthcoming 50th Anniversary of the Medical Library Association:[5]

"We owe much to the past, but more to the future. While we are in Philadelphia, commemorating the past, deeply involved with the present, planning for the future, let us recollect that, even as there is no such thing as a bystander, so we today are, in a sense, founders of this Association. It exists only through us and will be only what we make it. It is not wise to regret ever what a small part of time we play. All that matters is to make the small part count, and in as creative a way as possible. That is to say, we must give as well as take."

BIBLIOGRAPHY

1. BALLARD, J. F.: President's Address. BULLETIN, 27: 3–17, 1938.
2. NOYES, MARCIA C.: Presidential Address. BULLETIN, 23: 33–4, 1934–35.
3. FRANCIS, W. W.: Margaret Charlton and the Early Days of the Medical Library Association. BULLETIN, 24: 58–63, 1936.
4. BALLARD, J. F.: The Past History of the Medical Library Association, Inc. BULLETIN, 36: 227–241, 1948.
5. MCDANIEL, W. B., 2D: 50th Anniversary of the Medical Library Association. BULLETIN, 36: 124–5, April, 1948.

The College of the Medical Book*

By Thomas E. Keys, MA, *Librarian*

Mayo Clinic
Associate Professor of the History of Medicine,
Mayo Graduate School of Medicine
(University of Minnesota)
Rochester, Minnesota

"Only one who is able to couple thought with scholarship is a really educated man."—Confucius: (The Wisdom of Confucius, Ed. and Tr. with notes by Lin Yutang. New York: Modern Library, Inc., 1943, p. 205.)

As a medical librarian, I am most appreciative of this opportunity to address you on *"The College of the Medical Book."* Perhaps some of you are not aware of Doctor George Dock's keen interest in medical libraries, and by implication, in the subject of my address. Indeed, Doctor Dock was President of the Medical Library Association from 1906 to 1909; and, as further pointed out by Suzanne Fallot:[1]

> From the beginning of his medical studies, he was keenly interested in medical libraries. He knew and understood library problems, and did much to promote and support the profession. A man of erudition, he was possessed of a vast knowledge of medical and non-medical books, authors and libraries of the whole world.

Some of Doctor Dock's interest in books and libraries stemmed from his contacts with Sir William Osler. Graduating in medicine from the Univer-

*George Dock Lecture on the History of Medicine, sponsored by the Los Angeles County Medical Association, Los Angeles, California, March 31, 1966.

Originally published in *Bulletin of the Los Angeles County Medical Association,* Volume 96 (December 1, 1966), pp. 16, 24-25, 31, and (December 15, 1966), pp. 23, 26-28. Reprinted by permission.

sity of Pennsylvania in 1884, where Osler was one of his teachers, Doctor Dock spent three years in Europe acquiring a knowledge of clinical and laboratory research in pathology and bacteriology. He returned to the University of Pennsylvania to become Assistant Pathologist under Osler. His skill caused Doctor Osler[2] to refer to Doctor Dock as "a man who knows more about clinical laboratory procedures than anyone in the United States." A prominent influence in Doctor Dock's frequent later visits to Europe was the internationally distinguished cardiologist and clinician, Doctor Karel Frederik Wenckebach[3]. No doubt because of Wenckebach's stimulus, Doctor Dock[4] in 1896 published the first American account of a case of coronary thrombosis diagnosed during life and confirmed by necropsy findings. Dock's study is referred to in James Bryan Herrick's[5] classic account of this disease published in 1912.

Doctor Dock became Professor of Pathology at the Texas Medical College and Hospital in 1888. He left this post in 1891 to become Professor of Theory and Practice of Medicine and Clinical Medicine at the University of Michigan. Here he remained until 1908, when he began two years of service in a similar capacity at Tulane University. He then was appointed Professor of Medicine and later Dean of the Washington University Medical School, in St. Louis. After retirement in 1922, he moved to Southern California, where he was active in the affairs of the newly reorganized Medical School of the University of Southern California and was an Honorary Professor of Medicine.

Throughout his long and useful life, Doctor Dock received frequent academic recognition. He was granted honorary degrees by Harvard, Pennsylvania, and Southern California. Among many other honors, he received in 1944 the American Medical Association's Distinguished Service Medal and Award "in recognition of his outstanding work in the field of Internal Medicine and Pathology with a particular citation in regard to his research in hookworm."[2]

As mentioned by George Blumer[6], Doctor Dock was especially interested in the literature of medicine. Here in Los Angeles, he concerned himself with the library organized by Doctor W. Jarvis Barlow, and was its President for a number of years. Later, when this became the Library of the Los Angeles County Medical Association, he served as a member of the Library Committee. Not only was he a constant library user, but he donated over 1,500 volumes to the library, several of them early imprints of great rarity. When the Walter Jarvis Barlow Society of the History of Medicine was organized in 1940, coincidentally with the celebration of his 80th birthday, Doctor Dock gave the first of the George Dock Lectureships on the History of Medicine.

An honor especially appropriate to this physician and lover of medical history was given him by the Department of Internal Medicine at the University of California Medical School, San Francisco, in presenting him a replica of the famous original "Gold-Headed Cane" carried by Doctor John Radcliffe,[7] the great British physician, and passed on to several other distinguished members of the profession in London.

The Librarian in Medical Education

What, now, is the role of the librarian in medical education? Traditionally, the librarian is concerned with the collection and the distribution of the printed word. His task is to gather—and thus preserve—reading matter, and then to aid in making it available to the hoped-for user. This second function is becoming more and more formidable with the enormous proliferation of the literature of medicine and allied sciences, which presently exceeds our ability to index it suitably—even with the use of the computer and other electronic devices.

But in addition to the preservative and interpretative functions of traditional librarianship, the third vital function is teaching. How do we, specifically as librarians, perform as teachers also? First, we teach by helping the reader find what he needs. This entails not only instruction in using the indexes to the literature, such as *Index Medicus* and *Science Citation Index,* and the special index files of the library, but also cultivation of judgment in selecting from the mass of seeming possibilities what is relevant to the need. We teach when we enhance a student's overall conception of the importance of the printed word. We teach when we emphasize the importance of the historical approach to the study of medicine. We teach when we point out the primary accounts of medical discoveries. We teach when we emphasize the ethical imperative of giving credit to original contributors and when we help the reader locate such contributions. Some librarians and physicians with educational and historical perspectives also collaborate in the editing and republication of medical classics in many fields. How much better to read descriptions in their original wording or in a translation of the original paper than to read a secondary interpretation of a classic work! We teach when we prepare bibliographies of special subjects of interest to our readers. And we teach when we prepare exhibits that awaken the interest of our readers in special resources of the library.

One way that I have found useful and that I am sure other librarians have employed is the "book walk." It is customary in our institution to have Tuesday night seminars. The surgeons have their seminars, the ophthalmologists theirs, and the radiologists theirs, for example. One of these may be devoted to the library. For the book walk in radiology I put out on the tables the historical publications on radiology—the first

Roentgen papers, the first Curie papers, the first Kelvin papers—with the latest textbooks and a recent issue of each journal in radiology the library receives. The examination and discussion of these volumes makes for an interesting and informative evening.

Likewise, the historical clubs of medical institutions can flourish under the auspices of the library. For instance, I am indebted to your Librarian, John Connor, for the pleasure of being with you this evening. Our own Mayo Foundation Society for Medical History, of which I happen to be President, has a membership of nearly 200, of whom more than 100 belong to the American Association for the History of Medicine. The officers of the national organization have accused me of blackmail! They think I won't let our readers take books out unless they "join up!" Our meeting each quarter is prefaced by a tasty buffet supper, after a modest draught or two from Ponce de Leon's fountain; and the conversation that precedes the meeting is delightful to hear! I would hate to think that our members come just for the free dinner, although the Mayo Foundaton House is considered the town's best restaurant! I know this can not be the only attraction, for thus far we have never lacked for good papers with an interesting historical treatment and we manage to keep the programs scheduled at least a year ahead.

History of the Proposal for the College of The Medical Book

The subject which I wish particularly to explore with you this evening is *"The College of the Medical Book."* There are many reasons for my interest in this topic. I should point out to you the origin of this interest. Five years ago I wrote a paper[8] pertaining to Sir William Osler's enthusiasm for and encouragement of those dedicated to the work of medical librarianship.

In gathering material for this study I naturally read everything I could find about Osler and medical librarianship. In Cushing's[9] life of Osler was a mention of some unpublished writings of the beloved master physician and a brief account—which fascinated me—of one of them, an unfinished paper entitled *"The College of the Book."* Cushing assigned it to 1907, and he quoted Osler as follows:

> There should be a college where men could learn everything relating to the Book, from the preparation of manuscript & the whole mystery of authorship, to the art of binding; everything from the manufacture of paper to the type with which the book is printed; everything related to the press & to the mart; everything about the history of printing from Gutenberg to Hoe; everything about the precursors of the printed book; the papyrus, the rolls, the parchment & the vellum, even about the old writing on the burnt bricks of Nineveh; everything about the care of books, the Library

lore, how to stack & store books; how to catalogue, how to distribute them; how to make them vital living units in a community; everything that the student should know about the use of books, his skilled tools in the building of his mind. That there should be such a College & that it should be at Oxford is evident to anyone who knows the Bodleian Library & the Clarendon Press. Here is a unique opportunity—let us see how it can be utilized."

Osler then suggested that there be four great divisions of this college: (1) The School of Library Economics, (2) The School of Bibliography, (3) A School of Publication, and (4) A School of Printing. Included in this manuscript is a suggestion of a lecture list to cover several courses on libraries, ancient and modern; the book itself and its make-up; other courses to cover copywriting, publication, reviewing, selling, auctions, and all other aspects.

Osler referred the manuscript to Doctor D.C. Gilman, President of Johns Hopkins University, and accepted his suggestion for improving it. Serious enough to want financial backing, Osler thought of Andrew Carnegie, saying: "A big scheme might, of course, appeal to Mr. Carnegie, and the question is, who would be the best person to present it if put together in an attractive form."

The inspiration did not strike fire, however; and the appeal for funds was not attempted. But 10 years later Osler[10] again referred to this subject as follows:

I should like to see added to the schools of at least one University in each division of the Kingdom a *School of the Book*, in all its relations, historical, technical, and commercial—every aspect of bibliography, every detail of typography, every possible side of bibliopoly.

These remarks were included in his address given at the opening of the Summer School of Library Service, Aberystwyth, Wales, on July 31, 1917. Lacking the impetus of the earlier manuscript, it was devoted more to what over the years, especially in the United States and Great Britain, has passed for library science—and was for the most part dull, probably on that account.

Reading Osler's publications and getting to know him through his writings and those written about him initiated me in the College of the Book, but I have another reason for my own interest in all phases of the subject. It has to do with the lack of status of librarianship. The need for librarians is acute. Yet there is a very little interest on the part of young people in librarianship for a career. In project Talent[11], recently conducted by the University of Pittsburgh, about 440,000 students in 1,353 high schools in the United States completed a questionnaire. One part was to select a vocational preference from a list of 122 different occupations. Among the boys, none chose librarianship; and among the girls of grades

11 and 12, it was not recorded in the top 20 choices. Under a title that mixes amusing and pathetic implications, *"Little Girls Don't Play Librarian,"* Jesse Shera[12] has discussed the shortcomings of present-day librarians.

Thus, in the late nineteenth century, librarianship came to be regarded as a kind of consolation prize for matrimonial disappointment. Girls chose careers as teachers, nurses, social workers, secretaries, because for one reason or another they were attracted to those professions; they became librarians because they couldn't think of anything better to do. From such roots has grown modern American librarianship, stigmatized by futility, frustration, and the appearance of inactivity, in a world where activity, any kind of activity, is applauded.

Donald F. Strout[13] has attributed the shortage to many causes, such as muddled administrative thinking, the librarians' unfavorable image, failure of library schools to make a successful impact even on their own campuses, and lack of attention to recruiting problems. In other words, there is a general failure to attract young people to this basic and challenging field.

To be sure, librarians and scholars finally are gaining attention to their plight. The Higher Education Act of 1965 recently signed by President Johnson contains a library-aid section that suggests $150,000,000 in grants for books and audiovisual aids to universities. An additional $45,000,000 is suggested for the training of librarians for research and demonstration projects to improve libraries. Another bill with special interest for medical librarians, the Medical Library Assistance Act of 1965, was signed by the President on October 22, 1965. It should be noted that at this time no monies have been appropriated to implement these acts, but the appropriations will be considered by the present Congress.

Even with government aid, though, how are we to interest desirable candidates in librarianship? Many suggestions have been offered, and to these I should like to add *"A College of the Medical Book."* I don't mean a course or two in medical bibliography but a 4-year college with all the courses devoted to the medical book. I mean buildings, campus, students, and faculty. I believe that our great universities are missing a golden opportunity. I believe that this college should be not only cultural but also practical. In this unique way, I think, desirable future librarians can be attracted. To be sure, we have library schools; but their courses aren't headed in this direction. Today, for example, their interest is focusing on mathematical solutions of library problems. They don't look at the complete problem. This can best be solved, I believe, by having a network of colleges of the medical book connected with university and commercial publishing houses.

Since I have devoted most of my career to medical librarianship I have changed Osler's title by adding the word "medical" to it. But such colleges would be equally applicable to all fields of knowledge. In fact, if he has not already attempted it, probably Doctor Lawrence Clark Powell, Dean of the University of California's Library School at Los Angeles, has ideas of a similar nature for the general book. I am always being drawn to the publications of Doctor Powell. Since my time at the Graduate Library School at the University of Chicago, when I was interested in Robinson Jeffers, Powell's *"Introduction to Robinson Jeffers"* and his *"Robinson Jeffers, The Man and His Work"* have intrigued me. In his most recent address before the American Library Association Powell[14] spoke of America as the "Great Land of Libraries." He stressed anew his perpetual belief that, above all, librarians should be bookmen: "Thus the good librarian is both doer and dreamer, producer and poet, statistician and story teller"; and again, "My interest in writing and writers was inevitable, for nothing in librarianship is more basic than writing and writers, the process and the people who produce information."

In another address Powell[15] stressed the importance of reading by librarians, with which I have always been in accord: "The two chief attributes of a good librarian are that he be a reader of books, and a servant of those in need of help . . . Given these two motivations in a young person, all the rest of the housekeeping jobs can be taught, in schools and on the job." Librarians, in other words, must be bookmen, quite distinct from administrators in general. To this I would only add that there is no reason why a successful bookman cannot be a successful administrator. Indeed, I believe I speak for Larry Powell[16] and many other librarians in saying that there are persons who combine both abilities. And, if I may paraphrase Powell, the following conventional characteristics make for a good librarian: energy, honesty, encyclopedic knowledge, selflessness, patience, orderliness, and tolerance. But the qualities he values most are curiosity, perception, courage, and dedication to the service of others. To me these elements combine in making librarians good administrators as well as good bookmen.

How, then, would I achieve this *"College of the Medical Book"?*

In the first place, I think that the West would be more receptive to such an idea than would the East or the Midwest. The first need is for a great university with an outstanding medical center to be made aware of and be receptive to this idea. The second would be to enlist the sympathy of one of our great philanthropic foundations, to make money available for such an enterprise. I am opposed to too much governmental intervention. And the third ingredient would be the necessary leadership to carry out such a project.

What, then, would be the curriculum and who would be the teachers?

On the basis of Osler's inspiration qualified by the word "medical," this college should include in its curriculum everything relating to the medical book. So, as early thoughts—not necessarily in their correct order and not necessarily final or complete, but merely as a trial effort—the following courses would be offered with the following distinguished persons in the professorial chairs.

I. Contents and Surrounding Cultures of Medical Writings
- A. Medical Writings in Ancient Cultures
  1. Babylonian Medical Clay Tablets—Doctor Martin Levei, Princeton Institute for Advanced Studies
  2. Egyptian Medical Papyri—Doctor Chauncy D. Leake, San Francisco
  3. Greek Medical Manuscripts—Doctor Owsei Temkin, Johns Hopkins Institute for the History of Medicine
  4. Japanese and Chinese Medical Manuscripts—Doctor Ilza Veith, University of California Medical Center (San Francisco).
  5. Ancient Indian and Persian Medical Manuscripts—Doctor Nand Keswani, All Indian Institute for Medical Science, New Delhi.
- B. Medical Writings in the Middle Ages—Doctor Dorothy M. Schullian, Cornell University
- C. Medical Incunabula—Doctor Max Fisch, University of Illinois
- D. Medical Writings in the Sixteenth Century—Doctor Maurice Walsh, Los Angeles
- E. Medical Writings in the Seventeenth Century—Doctor Lester King, Journal of the American Medical Association
- F. Medical Writings in the Eighteenth Century—Doctor Lloyd Stevenson, Yale University
- G. Medical Writings in the Nineteenth Century—Doctor F. Bradway Rogers, University of Colorado Medical School
- H. Medical Writings of the Twentieth Century—Mr. John Connor, Librarian, Los Angeles County Medical Association

II. Physical Makeup of the Medical Book
- A. Paper: Historical Development and Present-day Manufacture—Mr. Richard Wolfe, Rare Books Librarian, Harvard Medical School
- B. Printing Ink: Development and Present Concepts—Miss Brenda Crudge, University of California Medical Center, San Francisco
- C. Format and Binding: Historical Development From the Roll to the Codex to the Present Day—Mr. G.S.T. Cavanagh, Librarian, Duke University School of Medicine

III. Printing of the Medical Book
- A. Development ot the Medical Press From the 15th to the 20th Century—Miss Gertrude Annan, Librarian, New York Academy of Medicine
- B. The History of Medical Typography—Doctor James R. Eckman, Mayo Clinic
- C. Modern Typography—Mr. Adrian Wilson, University of California (Berkeley)

IV. Medical Illustration and the Book—Mrs. Lucille C. Innes, Loma Linda University

V. Medical Photography and the Book—Doctor Leonard Apt, University of

California Medical Center, Los Angeles, and Doctor Kenneth Arendt, Loma Linda University

VI. The Medical Manuscript

A. Problems of the Author—Doctor William Bean, Editor, *Archives of Internal Medicine.*
B. Problems of the Editor—Dr. Dwight Wilbur, Editor, *California Medicine*
C. Care of the Manuscript—Mrs. Mildred Langner, Librarian, University of Miami School of Medicine
D. Problems of the Publisher—Mr. Alexander M. Green, Year Book Publishers
E. Problems of the Medical Book Reviewer—Doctor Henry R. Viets, Boston Medical Library

VII. Administration of the Medical Book

A. Modern Medical Library Buildings—Mr. William Postell, Librarian, Tulane University School of Medicine
B. Acquisition of Medical Books and Periodicals—Miss Louise Darling, Librarian, University of California (Los Angeles)
C. Cataloging of the Medical Book—Mrs. Carmenina Tomassini, Librarian, University of California Medical Center Library (San Francisco)
D. Circulation of the Medical Book—Miss Sylvia Haabala, Circulation and Periodicals Librarian, Mayo Clinic
E. Interpretation of the Medical Book: Reference and Allied Services—Miss Clara S. Manson, Librarian, Stanford University School of Medicine
F. Storage of the Medical Book—Mr. Ralph Esterquest, Librarian, Harvard Medical School
G. The Use of the Computer in the Library—Mr. Scott Adams, National Library of Medicine

VIII. Reading, Including Audiovisual Aids

A. Reading: Speed and Comprehension—Doctor LeRoy Merritt, Assistant Dean, University of California School of Librarianship (Berkeley)
B. Reading: Selection of Books and Periodicals for the Physician—Miss Joan Titley, Librarian, University of Louisville Medical School
C. Reading: For the Patient—Miss Ruth M. Tews, Hospital Librarian, Mayo Clinic
D. Use and Design of Lantern Slides—Doctor Richard M. Hewitt, Clearwater Beach, Florida
E. Use of Phonograph Records and Tapes—Dean Merritt
F. Television for the Physician

IX. Selected Medical Masterworks—Doctor J.B. de C.M. Saunders, San Francisco

X. Auxiliary Medical Writings

A. The Great Medical Bibliographers—Doctor C. Donald O'Malley, University of California, Los Angeles
B. The Medical Novel—Doctor Wilder Penfield, Montreal, Canada
C. The Biography of Medicine—Doctor William C. Gibson, University of British Columbia
D. The Historiography of the Medical Book—Doctor Walton B. McDaniel, College of Physicians of Philadelphia

As mentioned earlier, this is only a rough outline of courses that could be taught in the College of the Medical Book. I can think of many things that have been overlooked or meagerly covered, such as the teaching of medical writing, the history of medicine, basic-science courses shaped for this new type of life-science librarian—and you can name many more.

As George R. Burns[17] wrote more than 15 years ago, "Dock's greatest work was in the training of other doctors; his great product was professors. . . .The group of teachers he helped to bring together made history. Members of the faculty of Washington University have won more Nobel prizes than those of all other U.S. medical schools combined."

I don't know whether the College of the Medical Book would produce any Nobel prize winners. But I should like to see what would happen if such a college were activated. I should hope for the improvement and growth of medical librarianship and also for a better interpretation of the resources of medical reading and consequently an improvement in the continuing education of the physician.

REFERENCES

1. FALLOT, SUZANNE C. Obituary. George Dock, MD. Bull M. Library A. 39: 382-383, Oct. 1951.
2. OSLER, WILLIAM: Quoted by HAWKINS, LELAND: Doctor George Dock. Ann. Int. Med. 35: 761-762, July-Dec., 1951.
3. KEYS, T.E., and WILLIUS, F.A. Cardiac Clinics. XCV. The Achievements of Karel Frederik Wenckebach. Proc. Staff Meet., Mayo Clin. 17: 332-336, May 27, 1942.
4. DOCK, GEORGE. Some Notes on the Coronary Arteries. M.&S. Rep. 75: 1-7, July 4, 1896.
5. HERRICK, J.B. Clinical Features of Sudden Obstruction of the Coronary Arteries. JAMA 59: 2015-2020, Dec. 7, 1912.
6. BLUMER, GEORGE. George Dock, 1860-1951. Tr. A. Am. Physicians 65: 16-17, 1952.
7. MACMICHAEL, WILLIAM. The Gold-Headed Cane. New York, Paul B. Hoeber, Inc., 1915, 261 pp.
8. KEYS, T.E. Sir William Osler and the Medical Library. Bull. M. Library A. 49: 24-41 (Jan.); 127-148 (Apr.) 1961.
9. CUSHING, HARVEY. The Life of Sir William Osler. Oxford, The Clarendon Press, 1925, vol. 2, pp. 81-82.
10. OSLER, WILLIAM. The Library School in the College. Library A. Rec. 19: 287-308, Aug.-Sept. 1917.
11. SHILLING, C.W. Special Training Program for Science Librarians. J. Education for Librarianship 5: 270-272, Spring 1965.
12. SHERA, JESSE. Little Girls Don't Play Librarian. Library J. 87: 4483-4487, Dec. 15, 1962.
13. STROUT, D.F. Personnel Shortages: The Library Profession's Number One Problem. Library J. 87: 38-42, Jan. 1, 1965.
14. Powell, L.C. Great Land of Libraries. ALA. Bull. 59: 643-648, July-Aug., 1965.
15. Powell, L.C. The Library Association Annual Lecture: Books Will Be Read. Library A. Conf. Proc. 47-52, 1957.
16. POWELL, L.C. The Elements of a Good Librarian. Wilson Library Bull. 34: 42-46, Sept. 1959.
17. BURNS, G.R. Men of Medicine: A Gifted and Inspiring Teacher. Postgrad. Med. 8: 325-330, 1950.

III
THE LIBRARIAN

Introduction

The medical librarian was born with a silver answer under his tongue. Verily, thou shalt not phaze him. He hath a liberal education and acquireth knowledge daily. He knoweth the names of the readers and greeteth them. Sometimes he remembereth their middle initials. If a woman, she recalleth also their neckties and the color of their eyes.

The medical librarian must have the agility of a robin, the eye of a hawk and the voice of a dove. When he refuseth it seemeth like conferring a favor. He loveth his books. He handleth a rare old volume like a newborn babe. The waste of time is unknown to him. He knoweth that while he listeneth to a tedious recital he can figure where the money is coming from to mend that leak in the roof.

He is not disturbed when a wild-eyed youth cometh up to demand, "What use are eyebrows anyway?" He beginneth with the antennae of insects and worketh up. He may not be certain at the moment whether cachexia is a troublesome cough or a skin disease, but tomorrow he will know ALL about it, and henceforth thou shalt not stick him on cachexia. Frequently he hath disciples to whom he sayeth not merely, "Thou shalt do thus and so," but, "Thou shalt do thus and so, and I will explain to thee WHY." He is always approachable, and usually available, for though he roameth afar thou canst get him by phone. He taketh notes and is able to read them. He treasureth old clippings and pasteth them in books for reference. Even a toothache doth not affect his invariable courtesy. He putteth himself out for people and LIKETH it. He is just. His fellow-workers speak kindly of him at other times than just before Christmas or pay-day. His library looketh like a library and not like an art exhibit, curiosity shop, or a club room. People come there to read, and he seeth that not one goeth away empty handed. Search, and thou shalt find him, maybe even in thine own home town[1].

Libraries are of three kinds. One has a quiet environment with an orderly collection of books and journals. Such libraries are run by custodians. A second type, besides being quiet and orderly, is efficient. These are in the charge of administrators. A few libraries are of the third class, orderly and efficient but also suffused with a spirit of scholarship, a reverence for knowledge, and a dedication to the concept that the people they serve are as important as the treasures on the shelves. These libraries are in the charge of unique individuals—those few librarians who have earned their "spurs" with consistent dedication, study, innovation, and contribution.

Selections for this chapter sample the literature dealing primarily with education and certification.

In 1925, Ballard[2] wrote a brief article stating his opinion that medical librarians should be specially trained. The idea that medical librarianship is a specialized field and as such deserved concomitant training grew. The culmination of these early considerations is embodied in the article by Mary Louise Marshall[3], who at that time was president of the Medical Library Association. She appointed a committee to consider the problems.

Janet Doe, in her 1949 presidential address, summarized the specialized education activities up to that year. By 1958, the need for another educational program for the practicing librarian was realized with the initiation of refresher courses (forerunners of the present Medical Library Association continuing education courses), provided at the annual meetings of the Association. These were well received. Continuing education programs, as can be noted today, have enjoyed healthy growth and expansion.

Louise Darling details the more sophisticated training programs involving internships and their value for communicating skills necessary to cope with the ever-growing complexities of a biomedical information world. Miriam Libbey reviews the Medical Library Association certification program. She also discusses some of the effects government monies, new techniques, and a certification program provoke in education requirements.

Dr. Martha Zachert describes educational programs necessary to prepare health sciences information personnel and notes the lack of evaluative criteria or studies in relation to these programs. Models depicting the range and relationships of the educational programs are used to present the concepts. She makes several basic recommendations pertinent to the role of the Medical Library Association in the educational process and concludes that vigorous involvement by the Association in its management/education role is essential if significant progress is to be made.

Dr. Arturo Castiglioni comments on the decisive influence that American medical libraries and librarians have had on both himself and the progress of medical science in this country. Dr. Merlin DuVal's theme is adaptation by libraries and librarians to changing needs, now that scientific information is being produced at an incredible rate. He makes a strong plea for the librarian to assume a more active role; to do research on how best to use the library in transmitting information; to take more responsibility for educating both providers and users in the management of scientific information; and, in general, to transform service philosophy so that the library is the key to effective use of biomedical information—an effective instrument in the delivery of quality health care.

If our health sciences library society successfully meets the challenges presented by a world of proliferating knowledge, it will continue to deserve the praise that Sir William Osler gave it many years ago when he said, "It is hard for me to speak of the value of libraries in terms which would not seem exaggerated[4]."

REFERENCES

1. Editorial: The medical librarian. Bull. Med. Libr. Assoc. 18: 26-27, 1929.
2. BALLARD, J.F. Training for medical librarianship. Bull. Med. Libr. Assoc. 15: 30-31, 1925.
3. Originally delivered as a presidential address to the Medical Library Association (New Haven, Connecticut, 1946). This article sparked the recognized need for special training of medical librarians, resulting in establishment of approved training in library schools and in a code for certification of graded qualification in 1950.
4. CAMAC, C.N.B. Counsels and Ideals: From the Writings of William Osler. Second edition. Boston, Houghton, Mifflin & Company, 1921, p. 159.

Training for Medical Librarianship

By MARY LOUISE MARSHALL, *President,*
Medical Library Association

THE FIELD of the medical library has grown in scope, in importance and in service beyond the fondest dreams of the group of far-seeing physicians and librarians who organized the Medical Library Association in 1898. The necessity for keeping abreast of the advance of medical thought, has made of the library a turn-stile on the broad highway over which must pass the march of medicine. Not only the faculties and students of medical schools, but practicing physicians, specialists and public health workers must travel the same way, for in a literal sense, completion of medical school training is only the first milestone on the road of medical education. The library offers the best opportunity for continued graduate study, desirable in other fields, but a necessity in medicine.

The medical library is distinguished from the general library by certain basic differences. First and most important is the subject specialization, with its extensive and individualistic vocabulary. Second is the type of clientele which the medical library serves. Most graduates of Class A medical schools have completed three to four years of college work before beginning the study of medicine. While this entrance requirement has been reduced to two years in the accelerated curriculum of the war years, prewar standards will doubtless be resumed as rapidly as possible. This background is evidenced in the research interest and study atmosphere in the medical library. The importance of at least a reading knowledge of several languages broadens the reference field proportionally. The fact that medical reference service is directed either immediately or ultimately toward the benefit of sick patients lends an urgency and importance to the contribution of the medical librarian which cannot be measured on a ledger sheet. There is an especial gratification if some new treatment thus suggested through the medium of print is later reported to have aided a patient to recovery. Medical reference work deals not

Originally published in *Bulletin of the Medical Library Association,* Volume 34 (October, 1946), pp. 247-252. Reprinted by permission.

with problems of industry or finance but with human life, and the trained scholarship and careful discrimination which the medical librarian brings to her task are in direct proportion to the contribution which the library may make to the alleviation of human suffering.

There are in addition certain variances in relative technical values in actual library administration as between medical libraries and those devoted to general subject fields: the essential importance of recent material in comparison to older publications; the greater use of periodicals rather than texts and monographs; the extensive development of gifts and exchanges as a source of acquisition; the fact that medical books and periodicals are usually more costly than those of other fields, necessitating careful study in budgeting, etc. These are matters concerning which little has been written and which are not always recognized by librarians engaged in general subject fields, although they are common knowledge to every experienced medical librarian.

If, then, the medical library and its services are distinctive, what of the medical librarian and her qualifications? What should be the educational background for service in our special field? What of her library school work? Is additional training necessary, and if so, of what should it consist? Those of us who have been faced with the problem of securing and maintaining an adequate staff during the past few years can but be interested in any program directed toward the betterment of the present situation as regards dearth of properly qualified personnel to staff the increasing number of medical libraries of all types. Perhaps the time has come for the Medical Library Association to establish standards of medical librarianship or even to sponsor a program of selective recruitment and training. Surely the subject merits careful study in the interests of medical library service in the years to come.

It has been said that "librarianship is a social activity—the establishment and maintenance of contact between men and books" (1). Certain it is that personal as well as acquired qualities make for success in library work. Carnovsky (2) names as the "qualities of librarianship, inherent or to be acquired in early life, ability to get along with people, bookish interest, imagination and a mind which prefers organization to confusion." Gapp (3) believes there should be in addition "a certain curiosity, an itellectual and emotional drive which gives some guarantee of future growth," as well as "an appreciation of the relation of routines to knowledge, the social structure and educational objectives." To these might be added adaptability, a pleasing personality, some nerve (rather than nerves), a sense of humor, and a strong constitution. All of these attributes apply equally well to medical librarianship.

Regarding the preprofessional training of the librarian, Wilson says (4) "Neither the scholar without library training, nor the librarian without scholarship of a high order can bring to the administration of . . . libraries all the abilities which are demanded if they are to be nicely adjusted to all the needs of organization, administration, scholarship and investigation." Jones (5) feels that "leadership in a librarian requires high intelligence, high scholarship, wide experience as well as linguistic ability" and that "Education and higher intelligence, when lacking in the staff members of the special libraries are qualities which are sadly missed, for here librarians have to condemn themselves to an intellectual level which is lower than that of their readers, if they are not well versed in the main subject of their collections." According to Hunt (6), the pre-library school training of the medical librarian should include a B.S. or B.A. with a major in the biological sciences and a reading acquaintance with German and French. Some training in several basic sciences is perhaps to be preferred to more profound knowledge of one subject, but study in one science should be sufficiently extensive to give the would-be librarian some knowledge of research method. Even a limited facility in Latin and Greek is a great aid in familiarizing one's self with medical nomenclature. Knowledge of other modern languages—Russian, Spanish, Italian, etc. approximately in the order named, represents a distinct advantage.

The second step in the training of the medical librarian is a year's course in professional librarianship, (a) "to give the student a broad overview of librarianship; (b) to acquaint her with the library's role in education; (c) to set forth for her in appropriate relationships the theories and principles underlying the major subjects in the field; (d) to acquaint her with the body of literature in the field; and (e) to give her command of library procedures fundamental for future professional performance." (7)

In the early library schools learning by doing was the basic plan. Modern curriculums tend to stress lectures on the theory of practical subjects such as Administration, Book selection, Cataloging, Reference and Bibliography, rather than actual practice work. Certain leaders seem to feel that the ideal might lie some place between these two methods. (8) Modern librarians have been branded technicians and it should be remembered that the merit of techniques is limited by the extent to which they serve a useful purpose. Librarians should be so familiar with means and devices that they may choose and employ them as need arises. "The mastery of skills, techniques and routines should not be permitted to eclipse the many other characteristics which in sum characterize the successful librarian" (2).

There still remains the need for specialized training in the medical library field. Until very recent years this problem has received little attention. The lack of planned training for medical work has in fact often resulted in the appointment of medical secretaries as librarians. Physicians have believed some knowledge of the subject field to be so important that in the absence of both medical and professional library training, the latter has been sacrificed for the former, and the technical organization of the library has suffered in consequence. The preferred method is assuredly library school training in addition to subject specialization.

Most of us in medical library work today entered this special field without other than library school training. We have learned other phases of our work by the system of trial and error, a process expensive both to the library and the librarian. We should thus be the first to advise planned and standardized training for those who follow us.

In attempting to fill this need, several short courses have been given, namely in Medical reference work, bibliography and administration, and in Hospital library work at the Columbia University School of Library Science and a course for Hospital librarians in the University of Minnesota. Instruction in the courses for hospital librarians includes not only the care and use of the hospital's medical library, but also the patients' library and lectures in bibliotherapy. These courses would seem to be inadequate to cover subject specialization in medical library work. Other than these, library schools have offered in their curriculums only two or three lectures on medical reference books.

It has been the belief of the author for some years, that training for subject specialization in library work might well follow the plan of training for specialization in medicine itself—that of the internship or residency. This method, as in medicine, superimposes a period of supervised experience on a foundation of theory.

In speaking of the internship as a method of training in library work, Metcalf and his collaborators say (8), "The introduction to library theory and practice comes from the first year of library school. Deeper insight into these matters can come from a period of internship and should lead, in the case of the student able to observe and reason for himself, to mastery of the subject. In such an internship there is the risk that the theoretical side may be limited to the principles illustrated and exemplified in the various parts of a particular library. The interne may not pursue any directed program of readings from library literature, but on the other hand, guidance from experienced and competent librarians may be more readily available and more significant than that obtainable in library schools. The program for a period of internship would in many ways be similar to a second-year library school program, since the interne would spend time in each of the various departments of a library with a major interest in some one of them.

"The important elements in the success of an internship are: first, that the student have the ability to observe and to reason for himself; and second, that one or more responsible people on the library staff have the time to discuss the administration and organization of the particular library, so that in this way the interne will not learn merely the practices of the one library, however good they may be. On the contrary, he is provided with opportunities to learn the principles and policies that are being applied, and thereby he is enabled to correlate the governing principles and the practical realities.

"What the interne gains that is different from the elementary library school program is, first, an intensive drilling in processes and routines under working conditions, and second, insight into underlying principles through directed thinking and through actual application of the principles. New areas of professional knowledge are not opened up to him, as he has already explored the general groundwork in the first year of library school where the studies were intended to give a view of the library in all its various general functions. What constitutes the advance is that deeper knowledge has come through an enlightened apprenticeship."

The internship is particularly advantageous in training for the special field of medicine in library work, since it furnishes opportunity for the student to learn the subject field, the nomenclature, the bibliography and the varying values of the different phases of medical library work and materials as previously mentioned. The value of a procedure may only be determined scientifically by experimentation and observation of results.

Some five years ago, therefore, it was decided to establish such a teaching unit in the Library of the Orleans Parish Medical Society, which is administered jointly with the Rudolph Matas Medical Library of Tulane University under the direction of the author. The period of training was set at twelve months, with a two weeks' vacation, corresponding to that of a medical internship. Since only one person could be accepted for training at a time, especial care has been used in the choice of each trainee. Scholarship records of college and library school have been examined and preliminary personal interviews required. Only persons evidencing a sincere interest in the medical field have been considered for appointment. A stipend to cover board and room only has been paid and it has been explained that the appointment is a training unit and in no sense a position.

The internes have worked as members of the staff under close personal direction, and have had a part in all phases of the libraries' work. Every effort has been made to explain not only methods used in our libraries, but in comparison those used in other medical libraries, with discussion as to reasons for selection of one method or another.

In providing opportunity for such supervised experience, services to different types of the medical library's patrons, is felt to be important, not only faculty, research workers and students, representing only the educational and research point of view, but also the general practitioner, the specialist, the medical interne, the nurse and the medical social worker. The joint administration of the libraries in question has offered service to this varied group.

It is felt that the experiment has been a success and that the internship is the method of choice for specialized training in medical library work. Four trainees have received certificates on completion of the course and a fifth will finish her work in another four months. Of the four who have completed the work, three hold responsible positions in medical libraries, the fourth has become a librarian of a Veterans' Hospital.

So much for the experiment, which will be continued as an accepted procedure, inasmuch as it has been proven worthwhile. A disadvantage has been that the training has been conducted independently and thus offers no library school advanced credit. One wonders why such a method of training for special library work might not be undertaken as a graduate project in some one library school. The argument that the regular library school faculty would not be qualified to supervise the work, is unsound, for to the special librarian directing the internship could be delegated temporary faculty status in each case, a medical librarian for a medical internship, a law librarian for a law internship—and the judgment of the specialist librarian could be accepted in grading the work of the intern. Location of the special libraries near the library school is likewise unnecessary, since the choice of the library and librarian is the important factor in the training, not adjacence to the undergraduate library school.

In summarizing, there are three factors of equal importance which lead to good medical librarianship—(1) Recruitment of carefully selected and properly qualified personnel; (2) Education both general and professional; and (3) Experience, preferably supervised experience as represented by internship in a medical library. Medical library service of the future will depend on the successful correlation of these three factors, and the problem of recruitment and standardized training of medical librarians is deserving of careful study by the Medical Library Association.

REFERENCES

1. KOLITSCH, MYRA: Toward a philosophy of librarianship. Library quarterly, 15: 25-31. 1945.
2. CARNOVSKY, LEON: Preparation for the librarian's profession. Library quarterly, 12:404-11. 1942.
3. GAPP, K. S.: Librarian's task in improving personnel. College and Research libraries, 1:132-37. 1940.
4. WILSON, L. R.: Aspects of librarianship in America. Library quarterly, 2:1-10. 1932.
5. JONES, H. W.: Editorial. Bull. Med. Lib. Assn., 30:183-84. 1942.
6. HUNT, J. W.: Medical librarian (in Doe, Janet, ed. Handbook of medical library practice. 1943. p. 28-32)
7. WILSON, L. R. and others: Essentials in the training of University librarians. College and Research libraries, 1:13-38. 1939.
8. METCALF, K. D. and others: Program of instruction in library schools. Urbana, Univ. of Ill. pr. 1943. 140p.
9. BRODMAN, ESTHER: Education of medical librarians. To be published.

Libraries and Librarians

By ARTURO CASTIGLIONI, *M.D., Research Associate*
Historical Library, Yale Medical Library

I AM VERY honored to be with you today, having the opportunity of saying some words to you in this place, which is enhanced by the memory of Harvey Cushing the scientist, the artist, the passionate book-lover. I believe that there is only one fact that may justify my addressing you on this occasion, and that is my age. Sixty years have passed since I for the first time attempted as a young boy to make a catalogue of my small library. The love for books has accompanied me and often comforted me during my wandering life. A book-collector myself, I had the privilege of knowing Cushing and his admirable work, of meeting him several times in Italy, discussing with him many things in which we had a common interest. I hoped to be able at last to leave my books, very modestly and inconspicuously, to this same library, where his treasured collection has found a resting place. But unfortunately in the course of the Nazi invasion of Italy my books and the precious volumes which I possessed were looted. When I first came to Yale seven years ago, too late to find Cushing alive, I was very sorry to have no longer the opportunity of meeting him, holding discussions with him and enjoying the privilege of his invaluable help. But later, working in this room in which his treasures are kept, I felt that just the same I was working under his auspices, in this library where his spirit is always present. This library seems to me to have a peculiar characteristic which distinguishes it among others, because he has impressed on it, and I may say, on any one of his books, the indelible mark of his personality. He was the bibliophile who had the mental preparation of a humanist and the qualities of a great scientist and of an outstanding librarian, and in many books of this library you find notes written or dictated by him which are the personal introduction of the reader to the book and the author, by Harvey Cushing, who seems to take you by the hand, showing

Originally published in *Bulletin of the Medical Library Association,* Volume 34 (July, 1946), pp. 180-183. Reprinted by permission.

you the way. You are encouraged and inspired by his expert guidance. Here I met the living presence of two great professors of Padua, my alma mater: Andreas Vesalius, who was introduced to a large American public by Harvey Cushing, and Girolamo Fracastoro, the epidemiologist, poet, astronomer, whose masterly bibliography we owe to my illustrious friend, John Fulton. This library offered me the first opportunity of knowing more than superficially the great American medical libraries and to come in contact with American librarians. But I would like to tell you that even though this is the first time that I have had the pleasure of attending a meeting of your Association I have appreciated your work for a long time. I have had the opportunity of being in contact with many of you and to be acquainted with the fine work which is accomplished by the American librarians. Like all people who are accustomed to working in public libraries, I went through the shyness of the newcomer, when as a young boy, at Vienna, I had to face for the first time the imposing librarian of the University Library, and it was perhaps this psychic trauma which left in my mind for many years a feeling of frustration and a desire of escape as the first reaction when facing the librarian's desk. I have had the experience of working in small libraries of provincial towns, where the visitor appeared to the librarian as a very disagreeable surprise, which could but disturb his quiet, regular life—and I have had many contacts with the big bosses of the librarians' world, scientists and scholars, who did not conceal their slight contempt for the inadequate knowledge of editions, of printers, of dates. One I remember, a very respectable old man, whom I never had met before, and who greeted me, as he heard my name, with the words: "I know you, I have read your paper on medical history a couple of years ago." And as I bowed, very flattered, he added: "There is a bad mistake concerning the date of the first Greek edition of Dioscorides."

That explains the psychology of a book-lover, who had begun as a boy to search for old editions in the small book-shops of his native Italian city, and considered books as a treasure, but was always scared by the custodians of the treasure, who appeared in his eyes as the mythical dragons. Maybe this is one of the symptoms of an incipient bibliomania. Later, when I worked in the great and famous libraries all over the world my psychological relation with the librarians became easier and better but something of the first impressions remained, something that gave me a certain shyness when I approached the desk of the librarian, asking for a book or for information. My sojourn and my work in this country, ladies and gentlemen, have brought about my recovery. I have had the privilege of working and studying in this and some other wonderful medical libraries, surrounded by a congenial atmosphere, becoming acquainted with librarians whom I considered, as they always have been, colleagues and friends, and from whom I have learned a lot of things—unfortunately not (but that is my fault) the classification of the Library of Congress. Here I noted not only the riches and the admirable order of the medical libraries, but first and most important of all, the expert knowledge, the excellent preparation, the vast culture of the people whom I met. The American librarian, in the judgment of an impartial observer who had at the beginning to fight the difficulties of the language, of the classification and of many different customs, is not only a specialist who is perfectly at ease in his difficult job, able to find with wonderful comprehension the most recondite book, print, manuscript or periodical: he is also a man who has an unusual background of humanistic and of medical education. He is no less versed in the editions of old books than in the names of modern magazines, no less acquainted with the printers of the Renaissance than with the modern eponyms. He is no longer, as librarians have been for a long time, the man, or the girl, on the other side of the fence, whose job was accomplished with the finding of a date, with providing a superficial information, given with more or less evident annoyance. He is a valuable collaborator who takes a lively interest in one's work and is eager to help. He is, I may say, the modern American, realistic and practically efficient, in the mental attitude and the garb of the humanist. Very often, as I know by my personal experience, the interest he shows, the advice he gives are encouraging and inspiring to further researches, to a deeper study in a subject, and it happens in this way that many subtle bonds of understanding, of cooperation, of friendship, are formed. And to your outstanding credit are the great kindness, the smiling attitude, the extreme patience—your national characteristics—with which you are able to listen to the most strange requests, to face problems, to solve some often difficult riddle, to answer questions posed by the readers to whom you appear as an oracle. I am accustomed to call my librarian-friends wandering encyclopedias.

I think that it is possible and obvious to discuss and disagree on different ways of education in different schools and countries, on various tendencies and various degrees of humanistic or historical trends in medical studies. But there is one subject on which, I am quite sure, all those who are able to pass judgment on the evolution of medical thought must agree, that is the remarkable, decisive influence that the splendid organization of the American medical libraries and the work of their librarians has had in the progress of medical science in this country. The possibility of finding in a short time, thanks to the *Catalogue of the Surgeon General's Library,* of the *Index Medicus* and of many other excellent sources and reference works, any possible literary information, of locating any book and any journal, and of obtaining it; the splendid service of the microfilms; and in the first line, the gracious help of the expert librarian in the most difficult emergencies, have made the task of research an agreeable and easy one. All of us whose work is founded and depends on this kind of research, are now accustomed to consider the hours spent in the libraries, having the privilege of your presence and your kind help, as the agreeable and useful introduction to a scientific work. And only somebody who has had the experience of working in libraries for half a century and has often the feeling of being himself an old and therefore rare, but surely not precious edition, is able to appreciate what has been done in America in this field, and the great credit that belongs to people who are working in silence, never boasting nor telling what they have done and are doing, often seeing their name and their work ignored.

That is what I wanted to say today, as a deferent and cordial collective homage. There are here some among you today, whom I consider as the prototype, not only of the good librarian but also of the excellent companion and the reliable friend. I wanted to thank you, all of you, for the help you give to the medical historian, to the physician, to the writer, to the foreigner among you, who is in need of a friendly word and of a kind smile. I wanted to tell you that your intelligent and cordial cooperation is and will remain in my recollection among the most charming souvenirs of my American experience. You have accomplished in the American libraries and in your Association and your journal, which I am reading wth great pleasure and profit, a great deal of remarkable work and I am sure that this work forms one of the pillars of scientific and of historical research in America and in the world. There is no place in which the scientist and the historian feel so perfectly at home as in an American library and that is due not only nor chiefly to the treasure of their collections, but in the first instance to your knowledge, to your kindness, to the charming way in which you have been able to introduce the profane to the acquaintance and the use of these treasures. With these feelings I present you my best wishes for the success of this meeting and the progress of your Association, with the classic motto: *Vivat, crescat, floreat!*

The Development of Education For Medical Librarianship[1]

By JANET DOE, *Librarian,*
New York Academy of Medicine

A description of the development of education for medical librarianship can be brief indeed. Such education has been almost wholly the old apprenticeship method of learning on the job, until within a very few years. Medical libraries seem to have existed apart from ordinary library currents almost up to the present time, and are only just beginning to be drawn into the main stream. The cause lies probably in the difference in the evolution of medical librarians and of general librarians.

In medicine, the books existed first, producing eventually the need for a librarian. General librarians undoubtedly began in this way, too, but they have for a long time now attained a point in development where the librarian comes first and is often engaged to produce and organize a book-collection into a library. This latter stage is now being reached in the medical library world, but it is just barely starting. It is still seldom that one hears of a medical librarian in search of a library: it is nearly always the medical books that are in search of a librarian!

In medicine, collections of books for the use of students and practitioners were a necessity from the earliest times. Until the late nineteenth century, they formed the comparatively small working collections cared for by some responsible soul among the users who valued his literary tools enough to try to keep them in order. Some of these workers became the great bibliographers of science, scholars like Gesner and Haller. The rank and file, however, were the physicians who used the books in their daily practice, in their teaching, or for their recreation. Their care was either a labor of necessity or of love.

Most such collections were comparatively small private ones until the freshet of medical periodical publishing started gushing in the middle of

[1]Presidential address, 48th Annual Meeting, Medical Library Association, Galveston, Texas, April 13, 1949.

Originally published in *Bulletin of the Medical Library Association,* Volume 37 (July, 1949), pp. 213-220. Reprinted by permission.

the nineteenth century. The gathering volume resulted in the pooling of literary wealth by groups of individuals, and thus the medical society libraries and some of the older hospital medical libraries came into being. These collections were still small by present standards, and in only occasional instances acquired the full-time attention of a caretaker. Most of them doubtless maintained the same sort of precarious existence which an unattended departmental library still does, new books being supplied by the authorities fairly regularly and being just as regularly drained off by nonchalant borrowers who neglected to return them.

In spite of these adverse circumstances, collections began to become sizable, and took more time than even a book-loving medical man could spare; by the last quarter of the century, the physician-librarian had become only the titular head of the library while to the physician's secretary had been turned over the technical and physical chores of the now firmly established library. Small collections in hospitals, especially, would be cared for by a secretary in her spare time, or by the record-room assistant—a condition still obtaining frequently today. And as the collections grew larger and more staff was required, it was normally drawn from sources with which the medical authorities, who were the owners, were familiar: their secretarial or technical assistants—though there were, of course, occasional exceptions in librarians coming from among the physician-users themselves, like John Shaw Billings and Fielding H. Garrison.

By the end of the century, then, we find that the medical profession had developed its individual book collections into more or less formal libraries supported by groups or institutions, whose moving-spirits were the medical men themselves and whose technical workers were recruited from the clerical services auxiliary to medicine. This was the situation at the time of the founding, in 1898, of the Medical Library Association. Its charter members numbered four physicians, Dr. George M. Gould, Dr. John L. Rothrock, Dr. E. H. Brigham, and Dr. William Browning, and four librarians, Miss Margaret R. Charlton, Miss Marcia C. Noyes, Mrs. Elizabeth Thies-Meyer, and Mr. Charles Perry Fisher. Of these librarians—who may be assumed, from their taking part in such an association, to have been among the outstanding members of their profession—as far as I could learn, only one had had any library school education, a short summer course, while three had previously had brief library experience. They learned their work by doing it—and they learned and did it well!

As libraries began to grow apaçe after the beginning of the twentieth century and new collections to start up, the demand for librarians increased. These continued to be recruited in part from the secretarial and record-room staffs, but some came, too, from the outside world who had been to library school. It was found that the methods learned there could be applied, sometimes with adjustment, to medical libraries. With the continued rapid increase in the need for medical librarians in the last two decades, more and more of them have come from the general field. And yet the apprentice-system of instruction has continued to a large extent in effect: the only way to know medical library methods was to work in a medical library. And this is still true! Except for the handful of students who took the medical library course at the Columbia University School of Library Service in the last few years, every medical librarian has had to learn through apprenticeship most of what he knows, by working under someone who could teach him the tools and methods of his special field.

Apparently through preoccupation with their affairs in their own world, medical librarians remained for years little affected by advances made in general library education. In 1898, as we have seen, only one of the four librarians who helped to found our Association had had a short course in library work, although there were then four schools functioning, one of them for over ten years. Few of their graduates seemed to go into medical libraries, however; perhaps because few of the medical librarians ever vacated their posts till retirement removed them. It would surprise us, I think, to find how small was the number of library school graduates in medical libraries even as late as the 1920's. In 1926, for instance, the staff of one of our larger libraries, numbering ten in all, included just one library school graduate—and that one was not the librarian in charge. It must make us very proud of our colleagues to contemplate what they accomplished through native intelligence, common sense, industry, and unsurpassed devotion to their profession. While the infiltration of trained librarians into the medical field has been remarkably slow, it has been increasing, and library school graduates in medical libraries are now becoming the rule instead of the exception.

A few figures from the personnel survey conducted last year by a committee of the Medical Library Association under the chairmanship of Mrs. Breed Robinson* show the advances in this direction. A comparison was made between the percentage of library school graduates among those who entered the field some twenty-five years ago and those entering now. Of the ninety-two of our librarians now over fifty years of age, fifty-one, or 55 percent, have had no library school training; whereas, of the sixteen librarians listed in the survey files who have joined the Association in the

*My warm thanks are due her for gathering the statistics given here.

past two years, only five, or 31 percent, are without library training. While it is possible for an individual to become an excellent medical librarian without formal library training, there can be little question that on the whole it is an advantage for our librarians to have it. When physicians inquire if we know of someone to take charge of their hospital library, they are now apt to say, "I suppose we should get a *trained* librarian?" Other things being equal, they should!

But the other things must be equal. The medical background which the older secretary-librarian or record-room assistant brought to his task, the familiarity with medical literature and medical bibliographical methods and the peculiarities of medical library administration which the apprenticed worker in a medical library acquired as he went along, must somehow be learned by the fresh-water library student, if he is to be immediately and fully useful to his prospective employer. Basic library training should be supplemented by a course in medical terminology, in the extensive bibliography of medicine, its specialties and the allied sciences, and in the varying methods of administration, and in values in medical libraries. A course was formulated for hospital and medical librarians during the session of 1923-24 by Dr. Richard O. Beard, secretary of the medical faculty at the University of Minnesota. A special bulletin was issued which outlined a sequence of three years of collegiate study with special emphasis on biology and social service, a year of general library training, and a fifth year devoted to the theory and practice of hospital library service. But there was at that time no organized course of library training offered at the University, and this Special Bulletin evidently did not produce enough enthusiasm, for though the course was included in the University's Bulletin for several years, no applicants materialized and it was cancelled.* The earliest course pointing in this direction actually given was that instituted in the spring of 1937 by the University of Minnesota Division of Library Instruction. Lectures on medical library work were delivered for this course by Miss Isabelle T. Anderson and Miss Helen H. Norris. As a course for hospital librarians, however, most of its emphasis was on patients' libraries, so that comparatively small attention fell to the hospital medical library. It remained for the Columbia University School of Library Service to offer in its summer session of 1939 the first course devoted entirely to medical library matters. Taught by Mr. Thomas P. Fleming, Librarian of the College of Physicians and Surgeons of Columbia University, this course

*Mr. Thomas P. Fleming kindly brought this interesting item to my attention. It will be found in: Frank K. Walter, *Training for Librarianship at the University of Minnesota; a Historical Summary,* Minneapolis, The University, 1942. 32 p. (p.10-11)

covered only medical bibliography and reference. In this, however, it began with the most important point of difference between medical and general libraries: the subject matter and the keys to it.

Meanwhile, new ideas were fermenting in general library education. Library administrators were dissatisfied with the product turned out by the library schools, while the school directors were sure they knew better than the librarians themselves what was wanted in the trained assistant. Conferences between representatives of both camps were held in which each side continued to assert it was right. In this impasse, the Council of National Library Associations stepped in, convinced that a frank and thorough searching of the general situation was called for. Its conference held at Princeton in December 1948 cleared the air to the extent of a plain statement that library administrators want differently trained assistants from those the schools have been turning out. The Council of National Library Associations is forming a Joint Committee on Education for Librarianship, and further discussions conducted under this same aegis of honest and searching inquiry are in prospect.

While this investigation of general library education has been in progress, medical librarians have also been gradually becoming aware that the preparation of candidates for their field needed more attention than it had had so far. Eileen R. Cunningham in an article in *Special Libraries* in January 1940, called attention to the inadequacy of the library school undergraduate curriculum as a preparation for special librarianship, and discussed the difficulties the library schools faced in attempting to provide courses to meet all sorts of special fields' requirements. She also drew up tentative courses for special librarianship in the natural and applied sciences, outlining the work which should be emphasized during the four years of college and the one year of library school.

Active investigation of the possibilities for education directed towards preparing library school students for work in medical libraries was not started, however, until Miss Mary Louise Marshall at the Annual Meeting of Medical Library Association in 1946 gave a report showing what she had been able to accomplish in the Orleans Parish Medical Society Library through supervised instructional internships one student a year. The Medical Library Association voted then to establish a committee to consider the possibilities of adoption of a training program and standards for medical librarianship. This Committee, under the chairmanship of Miss Marshall, began a study of the problem through questionnaires to medical librarians, and recommended in 1947 that the Association sponsor a program of training and the establishment of a plan for certification. In addition, a recruitment campaign was urged. By the end of the second year of investigation, the first course attempting to cover medical library work with any completeness had been started in the spring of 1948 at the Columbia University School of Library Service, being taught by Miss Estelle Brodman, for which twelve students received credit; and, further, the Association had voted to establish certification. A by-law enabling it to undertake this is about to be presented at this meeting.

Education for medical librarianship is at present in a healthy state of flux. A candidate taking the full library schedule of three semesters at the Columbia school, with the medical course included, will receive an M.S. degree. When there are enough applicants to justify additional facilities, we hope that one or two other library schools in different sections of the country will inaugurate a medical course. In time, with the development of more advanced courses, a Ph D. may perhaps be earned. All such courses need periods of internship in medical libraries, and all would benefit by some practical means of acquiring subject knowledge along with library techniques and principles. This might be done either by affiliation with schools of nursing, physical education, public health, or medical welfare work. The new combined three-year curriculum of the Graduate Library School at the University of Chicago has in it the seeds of such a possible combination of subject specialization and technical library instruction, a system which might be followed with particularly happy results for medical librarianship.

Such specialization cannot be asked of the library schools, however, until it is made economically possible through sufficient demand, and demand is not likely until there is sufficient remuneration. We believe that the increase in the number of medical libraries, the great shortage of librarians — and particularly librarians with medical backgrounds — and the improving salary situation are already making convincing proof of its possibility. We believe that no kind of library work is more rewarding than that for medicine. If advances are to be made by the profession, however, it must train its newcomers to make them — otherwise we are trying the old and impossible trick of raising ourselves by our own bootstraps. We who learned and have spent our working-years with the old apprentice-method are eager to see new and better methods instituted. Candidates with the best training in library techniques should be able to add to this the special methods of their chosen field, a good general grounding in their subject-matter of medicine, and a chance to apply their new knowledge under supervision through a reasonable period of internship. When this is true, medical librarianship will have emerged from the apprentice stage into that of a full-fledged profession.

In closing, I should like to recall to your minds one of the great physicians of modern times who was among the outstanding knowers and lovers of libraries, Sir William Osler. He was constantly giving choice volumes to the libraries of his acquaintance — which was wide, not confined just to the institutions with which he had been connected. The Boston Medical Library and the Library of the New York Academy of Medicine each possess a first edition of Vesalius, gifts from him, and they are merely examples of the many recipients of his bounty and his encompassing eagerness to see the treasures of his profession's literature made accessible to every member of it. Innumerable libraries in this country, as well as some in England and France, can show rarities in their exhibition cases labeled, "Gift of Dr. Osler". His own marvelous collection of some 7,600 books significant in the development of medicine went back to his medical school at McGill. The monumental annotated catalogue of this collection was outlined by him and begun under his direction, then completed after his death by four of his close friends: two of them were our physician-librarians, Dr. W. W. Francis and Dr. Archibald Malloch, while the others were Mr. R. H. Hill of the Bodleian Library and the late Mr. Leonard Mackall, the eminent bookman. It is an immensely valuable contribution to medical bibliography.

But what I wanted to speak about especially was the keen first-hand knowledge which Osler had of library practices and pitfalls. I wonder how many of you are familiar with his address at the opening of the Summer School of Library Service, Aberystwyth, Wales, in 1917. It demonstrates an amazing understanding of the ways of libraries. He mentions, for instance, the use of "printed cards, free from slips in copying." Only one who had made such slips and caught them would be aware of the bane of their existence. Because he did know what went on in libraries, Osler knew also the educational equipment which their librarians ought to have. He called attention, with sorrow, to the scarcity of college-bred individuals on library staffs: out of 650 library school graduates in the previous 20 years, not 6 were college graduates (this was in Wales, and is happily not true in America). I might mention parenthetically that the lack of a college education is not an insuperable handicap to either librarians or prime-ministers: Churchill has just remarked that in spite of his not having college training, he seemed to have picked up a few things as he went along! But to go back to Osler, he made comparison with the apprentice-method so long in vogue in medical education (and still in effect, as we have seen, in medical library education). The lack of adequate preparation for the tasks of a librarian was very disturbing to him.

I wish I could quote at length from his entertaining and instructive discourse, but time allows me to repeat only a few phrases showing his acute awareness of the position the librarian fills in the world's economy. He calls them "the purveyors of knowledge," "the universal providers of the mental food of the public . . . often called upon to do the work of cooks and doctors." Of them he says, "No man in the community requires a more comprehensive and thorough education. All knowledge is his province. A common tap for the waters of wisdom, he should not perhaps know everything, but he should know where everything may be found . . . He is the badly salaried intellect of the community, and if fortunate enough to be able to suffer fools gladly, he leads a life of surprising usefulness. And let us not forget other qualifications — an ability to manage a business as complicated as a department shop, and a knowledge of men and a gift of manners that will enable him to drive his Committee or Council without strain on bit or rein." I wish I could go on quoting from Osler's incisive, humorous, and human examination of librarians, but you will have to read it for yourselves in the *Library Association Record* for August and September 1917. I cannot refrain from one last bit, however, his injunction to the young librarians he was addressing, which is quite as applicable to ourselves today: "Strive for mental accuracy and independence, cultivate the critical investigating faculty, keeping at the same time your mouth shut. In a profession demanding an amazing measure of equanimity, you cannot afford either to fight or to fret."

ABSTRACTS OF REFRESHER COURSES TO BE GIVEN MAY 31, 1958

Medical Library Association Annual Meeting, Rochester, Minnesota

1. Acquisition

Instructor—Louise Darling

Because of the instructor's personal experience, the course unavoidably will be slanted somewhat to the point of view of a larger medical library in a medical center setting, but every effort will be made to adapt material to what preliminary registration indicates will be the needs of the students.

There will be time only to mention a good number of the topics listed in the outline. As far as possible, details and references covered in Isabelle Anderson's chapter on acquisitions in the 2d edition of the *Handbook of Medical Library Practice* will be omitted and students referred to the *Handbook*. If time permits, a certain amount of class discussion will be included where it seems profitable to do so, particularly if the group is very small.

I. *Selection*

1. *Types of materials* in medical libraries: serials, monographs, texts, historical materials, ephemera, and special collections; basic science materials vs. clinical materials.
2. *Criteria*
    a. Needs of various types of clientele; participation of readers in the acquisitions program.
    b. Relative importance of types of material in relation to budgetary limitations: e.g. evaluation of new journal titles, balance between serials on the one hand, text and monographs on the other.
    c. Standard lists and bibliographies: types and examples.
    d. Book reviews
    e. Publisher and dealer catalogs and announcements; announcements of societies, institutions and congresses.
    f. Evaluation of material in light of staff time required to obtain it.
3. *Special Problems*
    a. Government documents and reports
    b. Reprints
    c. Gifts: collections, etc.

Originally published in *Bulletin of the Medical Library Association,* Volume 46 (January, 1958), pp. 122-132. Reprinted by permission.

II. *Techniques for Securing What Is Selected*
   1. *Purchases*
      a. Current materials, domestic and foreign.
         (1) Serials: agents, publishers.
         (2) Texts and monographs: agents, publishers, local bookstores.
      b. Out of print materials
         (1) Wants lists: bids and quotations, responsibility toward dealer, etc.
         (2) Dealers catalogs: reservations, special handling arrangements etc.
         (3) Auctions
   2. *Gifts and Exchanges*
   3. *Problems*
      a. Order information: bibliographic tools, letters of request for prices, publishers, series etc.
      b. Legal or administrative requirements for annual bidding on orders.

III. *Organization of Work*
   Emphasis on avoiding duplication of files and information and othei kinds of waste motion.
   1. Bibliographical checking: how far to go with verification of information.
   2. Records of order, claim, receipt, and payment.
   3. Serials record: receipt, claims, payment.
   4. Accessioning: to do or not to do.

2. Administration

Instructor—Mildred Jordan

As nearly everyone knows, an executive has practically nothing to do, except to decide what is to be done; to tell somebody to do it; to listen to reasons why it should not be done, why it should be done by someone else, or why it should be done in a different way; to follow up to see if the thing has been done; to discover that it has been done incorrectly; to point out how it should have been done; to conclude that as long as it has been done, it may as well be left where it is; to wonder if it is not time to get rid of a person who cannot do a thing right; to reflect that he probably has a wife and a large family, and that certainly any successor would be just as bad, and maybe worse; to consider how much simpler and better the thing would have been done if one had done it oneself in the first place; to reflect sadly that one could have done it in 20 minutes, and, as things turned out, one has to

> spend two days to find out why it has taken three weeks for someone else to do it wrong.*

So Dr. Harry Levinson of the Menninger Foundation is reasonably funny but what's that got to do with us? We are librarians, not executives. But please remember that administrative work must be performed through people. And that the minute there is one other human being involved in the accomplishment of the library's objectives you are in the business—usually without an Executive Suite, whether you like it or not. This business and/or art of getting things done through people as well as yourself—as everyone knows—demands planning, organizing, staffing, directing, co-ordinating, reporting, and budgeting. But how many librarians, male or female, don their gray flannel suits with ease and wear them comfortably? Currently the styles are being designed and reported by the American Management Association, Harvard's Graduate School of Business Administration, Fortune Magazine, etc., etc., etc. With the assist from such sources and with the cooperation of the enrolled students (if any) the instructor will attempt in the brief time to direct and restrict the concentration of the group to the basic job of the supervisor or administrator: The selection, development, and effective utilization of people.

3. Architecture

Instructor—William D. Postell

Medical institutions have undergone a tremendous expansion program since the end of World War II. Libraries serving those institutions have been a part of this expansion program. With the emphasis on the use of current literature as a teaching aid, the research programs, and the tremendous advances made in the health sciences in recent years, there have necessarily been significant changes in medical library planning. This discussion of library planning will be directed towards the small or medium size libraries serving hospitals, societies, institutions and schools. The principles of organization of the library in relation to the objectives of the institution which it must serve, the organization and size of the collection, readers' and technical needs, and space allotted as exemplified by the plans of recently constructed libraries will be discussed. With these principles in mind, individual case studies will be made of libraries to determine how they solved their problems. Final discussion will be directed to how well the plans have worked out, and any changes that could be made as a result of experience. Not only will different types of libraries be studied, but different types of building problems such as libraries housed in a separate building, and

* Quoted by Ralph T. Collins in The Man in the Gray Flannel Suit—As a Psychiatrist Sees Him, New York, American Management Association, Personnel Series no. 167, [c1956], p. 47–48.

those occupying one of several floors as part of a hospital, medical school or other institution will be brought up for discussion.

4. Binding

Instructor—Paul Berrisford

Binding problems of the library are reflected in the words preservation, use, and money. These words and their interrelationships should be the basis of any decision concerning funds for the care of the library collection.

Aesthetics is a criteria for making binding decisions but preservation makes a greater appeal to those concerned with the library budget. Preservation, therefore, will be the central theme of the discussion.

Can the library afford preservation costs? Yes, it can and must, to save its collection and protect its investment. Without this expenditure costly materials will have to be replaced at prices often higher than those of the binder. There will be instances where replacement, regardless of cost, will be impossible. Without a well preserved collection, the patron will seek other sources of greater convenience and the function of the collection will decline.

Must all material be bound? No, this would be a financial impossibility and beyond adequate defense in the majority of cases. However, all material of anything more than the most casual and fleeting interest should be preserved in some manner. In all cases, the individual material in question, the patrons use of it, and the objectives of the library, in terms of money available, should be reflected in any decision made.

Class "A" binding, as prescribed by the American Library Association and the Library Binding Institute, is usually the first method of preservation considered but not always the best in terms of the individual item to be preserved. Librarians should also consider other alternatives in a preservation program. Prebinding, purchase of working and storage copies of inexpensive materials, storage boxes, pamphlet binders, some type of organized mending program, and variations of class "A" binding should be part of a preservation program. A variation of class "A" binding, of recent interest, is "lumbinding" approved at the 1957 American Library Association Convention. This is a uniform method of binding library materials less often used than those requiring class "A", and yet used often enough to rule out boxing or tying.

The greater percentage of binding cost may be found in labor. It is, therefore, necessary for any library to establish an over all binding policy which will give adequate protection to the collection, convenience to the patron, and allows for the maximum standardization for binding specifications. The use of standardized lettering in periodical binding, for example, is one possible labor saving device. This reduces and simplifies routines requiring extra time saving on binding charges. Other forms of standardization should also be considered.

The binding or preservation program is an individual problem from library to library. It is, therefore, important that each librarian in any system be aware of the library policy and various methods recommended, so that he or she can facilitate its effectiveness.

5. Cataloging and Classification

Instructor—Mary Louise Marshall

The criteria for choice of a classification scheme for use in a medical library will be outlined, with brief descriptions of the salient features of the principal general library classification schemes and their use in a medical library and of the several medical classification schemes.

Sources from which subject headings may be chosen will be enumerated with comment on criteria for choice of heading and forms of subheadings. Suggestions will be given for the establishment of a subject authority list for the individual medical library. The advantages and possible problems arising from the use of printed cards will be presented.

The final thirty minutes of the period will be reserved for the open discussion of questions raised by members of the group. Those planning to register for this course are requested to send the questions they wish to have discussed, to Miss Mary Louise Marshall, 1430 Tulane Ave., New Orleans 12, La.

6. Equipment

Instructor—Scott Adams

This course will consider equipment in the sense of tools for the accomplishment of the basic library functions of organization, storage, and use. The useful instruments and devices of utility in small and medium size libraries will be considered under seven headings as follows:

1. Things to shelve with
2. Things to write with
3. Things to communicate with
4. Things to move with
5. Things to copy with
6. Things to have around (furniture)
7. Things to play with (gadgets)

Emphasis will be placed on the practical and inexpensive.

7. Medical Nomenclature

Instructor—Frank B. Rogers

Language and meaning; the symbolic character of language; the difference between things and processes; problems and possibilities in the stabilization of scientific terminology; language roots and new term formation; abstractions from context and the problem of foreshortening and stereotyping for special purposes; foreign terms; methods and aids for individual study and familiarization.

8. Medical Writing

Instructor—George G. Stilwell

Perhaps no other professional group, with the exception of those persons who write for a living, do as much writing as physicians. The amazing total of approximately 1,500 medical journals in the United States alone attests to the prolificacy of physicians as scriveners. However, the sheer bulk of this "medical literature" is in somewhat of an inverse relationship to its scholarly quality, succinctness, clarity and readability.

Physicians have many reasons, some good and some bad, for writing articles. Most medical papers are written with an honest desire to impart information to other physicians and scientists and to advance the practice of medicine. Yet many medical writers fall far short of producing a short, clear-cut, simple and unambiguous exposition of their ideas.

This presentation will consider some of the reasons for the cloudy character of much medical writing. Emphasis will be placed on many of the common errors and faults in medical papers, and suggestions will be made for their correction and avoidance. Lantern slides will be employed to illustrate many examples of poor usage and how such faulty constructions can be improved. An exercise will be performed in which copies of a typical case report before and after editing will be distributed to the participants; detailed analysis of the changes incorporated in the edited version of this manuscript will be made.

9. Periodicals

Instructor—Eleanor Steinke

Introduction. The periodical, indispensable from the standpoint of research and information, presents serious and complex problems of selection, cataloging, indexing, preservation, cost, and maintenance. Medical librarians are aware that the true value of their collections is found in the periodical files. It has become increasingly necessary for a highly competent and well-trained staff member to be in charge of periodicals; and the trend is toward centralization of the handling of periodicals. This is as important for a small library as it is for the large library.

In this discussion, the broadest interpretation of the term"periodical" will be used, that which Grenfell stated "as a publication in a continuous series with consecutive number and no predetermined end, as distinct from a single work in separate parts."[1] It includes any title which lends itself to listing in visible indexes and other specialized periodical records. This includes independent journals, and the publications of professional organizations, institutions, and societies, such as their bulletins, memoirs, proceedings, and transactions, and presupposes their treatment as magazines.

No attempt is being made to cover all aspects of the subject, which is far-reaching in content and nature, but shall be limited to Evaluation and Selection; Cataloging; Records; and Circulation.

Evaluation and Selection. Current periodical titles will be stressed, concentration being placed on the principles and methods of selection. Brief discussion will pertain to back files, multiple copies, treatment of ephemeral material such as reprints, and the importance of regional cooperation.

Cataloging. Since the policy of filing periodicals alphabetically, rather than by subject arrangement, is advocated, this section of the course will deal with arrangement and listing of titles, form of entry, references, the catalog, and shelf list.

Records. The visible index will be discussed, as well as the accession record, special files, claims for non-receipt, and payment of subscriptions. It is planned to illustrate with examples of new developments as well as established methods.

Circulation. The principles and methods of circulation of periodicals will be described. Interlibrary loans and the advantages of union lists will be included.

Since indications are that periodical activity will continue to increase in the future, librarians will be wise to review their policies of collection, of processing, and of making the maximum use of this important form of publication. Methods must be adopted which will prove most suitable to the individual medical library, methods which are based on sound principles, but with sufficient flexibility to fulfill present requirements and at the same time provide for future growth.

10. Photoduplication

Instructor—Mildred E. Walter

The Photoduplication talk will give practical information on photostats, lantern slides, photographs, microfilms, microcards and motion pictures, including location or source of supply, price where obtainable, care and storage. Any new equipment necessary to the reading or projection of lantern slides, microfilms, microcards and motion pictures will be considered as will be copying devices such as Verifax, Contura, Copease, Cormac and Thermo-Fax.

[1] Grenfell, David. Periodicals and Serials; Their Treatment in Special Libraries. London, Aslib, 1953. p. 1.

11. Rare Books

Instructor—Gertrude Annan

In this brief time some aspects must be eliminated. Reference and cataloging will not be considered. Instead there will be an attempt to answer those questions most frequently raised and a few which should be frequently asked and are not.

1. What makes a book rare? A book is rare when it is desirable for some reason or reasons: importance, age, scarcity, illustrations, beauty, printer or place of publication, particulary copy (condition, binding, provenance, etc.)

2. How can the price of a particular item be determined? There is no easy way. For books under $50. the time spent searching through auction records and catalogs of secondhand dealers make the book cost far more than its worth. The prices found may be erroneous. For very expensive volumes consult a knowledgeable librarian or dealer. The main consideration is *not* its price in money but its value to the library as part of its collection.

3. How should such a collection be started and developed? All depends upon the funds available for both the present and the future. Are they sufficient to buy valuable material, or should purchases be restricted to reference books, histories, biographies, facsimiles, modern editions? If funds are not ample enough to provide for a continuing program of purchasing early and expensive material should any be collected at all? In a library which has money for building a collection of original material, selection depends upon the resources of the library and the resources of the community. The contents of the library should point the way to grow in specific subject strength and interests. The collections in the community should point the way to a sensible policy of cooperation instead of duplication. In all a most important factor is the relationship of the librarian with the dealers.

4. What special care is needed? Medical books like any other early material should receive reasonable protection. They should be kept in an atmosphere not too moist or too dry. Marking should be avoided. Binding and repairs should be done *only* by expert craftsmen. Inexpert staff members should be *warned*! Use should be restricted as little as possible without courting damage.

5. How can the purchase of defective copies be avoided? Only by carefully collating an early book by signature and checking to see if other copies have plates can the librarian make sure money is not being wasted on imperfect books. The purchase policy should be to buy *only* perfect copies. Some staff member in every library containing books before 1800 should be able to collate books by signature—for ensuring that a copy is perfect and for describing books for scholars too distant to come to examine them. Some knowledge is needed of the history of the book—paper, printing, binding, illustrating processes.

6. What materials and information should be saved for future historians? Large books, important items are usually treasured. The historian seeks small bits of information, odd bits of material. Librarians should be particularly alert for: archives of the organization; archives of the community; ephemera.

12. Reference

Instructor—Bertha B. Hallam

Development of the course on Reference is planned on the following basic outline.

The concept of reference service in libraries has been the subject of study by a number of individuals. Rothstein (1) has pointed out that such service did not develop as an entity in the United States until about 1875. Since then, however, it has shown a steady pattern of growth corresponding to the ascendancy of research and scholarship as professions and of the research library as "a service agency for scholarship." It has become a distinct and important function and responsibility of libraries for the librarians to give personal assistance to aid readers in the pursuit of information. Herein lies the spark which makes the library a vital and vibrant adjunct in the quest for the extension of knowledge.

In accordance with this philosophy, health science libraries at the present time offer reference service and in many libraries this service occupies a large proportion of the time of the staff. The clientele of these libraries varies with the aims of the parent institution or organization. As has been ably pointed out by Eileen R. Cunningham and Mary Grinnell (2), the library may be used by people who may be categorized as Professional, Semi and Preprofessional, Professional Laity, Non-professional Laity. For any or all of these people, as circumstances dictate, the librarians stand ready to give guidance through the mass of past and present scientific literature which may aid in solving study problems. This guidance carries with it the connotation of teaching. In many instances, instruction in the use of library materials is indicated while the aid is being given, or, as in the case of students, prior to their entering upon the work on a problem.

The librarian giving reference service in a health science library, therefore, needs to be a person vitally interested in the pursuit of research and in people. The greater the librarian's fund of general information, especially on the subject fields in the library and on library techniques and resources, plus skill in reading various languages, the greater is the efficiency of the reference service given. Withal, the reference librarian needs a flair for sleuthing so that each new topic presents a welcome challenge.

Reference service procedures vary in different health science libraries depending on local conditions of time, space, book stock, skills, clientele, research problems and other factors. One person may have to sandwich in this vital service between multidinuous other duties. Various staff members may have to aid in the work of reference. What serves well as a routine request form in one library may be totally inadequate in another. Clearness of the stated question, coverage desired and purpose the inquirer has in mind are essentials. A routine to suggest to students who are learning to make reference use of the library is helpful.

In the field of the health sciences, there is a vast array of source material which serves a reference purpose. Witness the 1965 items in this area listed by Eileen R. Cunningham, Gertrude L. Annan and Mary E. Grinnell (3), and the summary by Frances B. Jenkins on medical reference sources added during the past decade (4). However, time and health science literature do not stand still. Almost daily it seems additional publications appear which may serve as reference guides to health science subject material. Some of these sources and their coverage will be listed for the Refresher Course.

Discussion of the background, philosophy, purposes, procedures, materials, needs and other aspects of library reference service in the health sciences may redound to the advantage of librarians and of clientele. At this refresher course, it is hoped there will be much discussion, even debate.

REFERENCES

1. ROTHSTEIN, SAMUEL. The Development of Reference Services through Academic Traditions, Public Library Practice and Special Librarianship. ACRL Monograph #14. Chicago, Association of College and Reference Libraries, June 1955.
2. CUNNINGHAM, EILEEN R. AND GRINNELL, MARY E. Reference and Bibliographic Service. Medical Library Association Handbook of Medical Library Practice. 2nd ed. rev. and enl. Janet Doe and Mary Louise Marshall, Editors. Chicago, American Library Association, 1956, p. 265.
3. CUNNINGHAM, EILEEN R., ANNAN, GERTRUDE L., AND GRINNELL, MARY E. A Bibliography of the Reference Works and Histories in Medicine and the Allied Sciences. Medical Library Association Handbook of Medical Library Practice. 2nd ed. rev. and enl. Janet Doe and Mary Louise Marshall, Editors. Chicago, American Library Association, 1956, pp. 337–537.
4. JENKINS, FRANCES B. Medical Reference Sources—A Backward Glance. BULLETIN. 45: 361–370, July 1957.

Development of Training Programs in American Medical Libraries

By Louise Darling, *Librarian*

Biomedical Library
University of California Center for the Health Sciences
Los Angeles, California

Training for personnel to man science libraries has reached a cross-roads in its development, with new directional signs posted in growing profusion, though all read to the same final destination.* The cause behind this confusing situation is obviously the ever more critical need for ordered and intelligent handling of the vast stores of information produced by the expansion of research the world over, coupled with the shortage of personnel equipped to deal with any phase of the problem. Conferences, articles, and reports are devoted to recommendations for education and training for a new profession of information specialists. Librarians claim that they are already in this business, and with a good deal of justice, too, for, as pointed out in a recent paper by Dr. Jesse Shera, "special librarians may be found abstracting, indexing, searching, editing, translating, and performing a variety of other miscellaneous duties associated with the organization, retrieval, dissemination, and communication of recorded information" (1). But regardless of where the training is to be offered, or how, or by whom, there is agreement that subject background and foreign language facility are prime requisites, if not absolute essentials, for anyone working on a professional level in either a science library or information center. There are, to be sure, numerous examples of people who have entered this field very successfully without such a background. Indeed, at present such a background is more the exception than the rule, but it would be foolish to deny the advantages of knowledge and training for even the most able or the shortcuts they provide to the expertness so greatly needed today. The question is whether it will be any easier to recruit

* A number are described in *Proceedings of the Conferences on Training Science Information Specialists*, Georgia Institute of Technology, Atlanta, Georgia, October 12–13, 1961, April 12–13, 1962.

Originally published in *Bulletin of the Medical Library Association*, Volume 51 (July, 1963), pp. 339-353. Reprinted by permission.

science students for a new information profession than it has been in the past to recruit them for the library field. Would more and better opportunities for special training be an inducement? Would such opportunities stimulate superior students with nonscience backgrounds to acquire at least a modicum of proficiency for work in science libraries? Could not such opportunities be used to equal advantage by the library profession if equal financial support were made available?

The answers to these questions are still largely in the realm of speculation, but librarians have experimented on a small scale with two kinds of specialized training programs. The purpose of this paper is to examine their development and effectiveness in the medical library field. Consideration will be limited primarily to the internship, though the work-study program will also be taken into account. Many medical libraries, of course, give in-service training, chiefly of an orientation nature, but such training is designed to facilitate work in a specific institution rather than to educate for general professional competence.

Internship is commonly accepted as a period of around a year's duration in which the novice works intensively at the graduate level under expert supervision to gain broad professional experience by applying theory to practice. Associated since the nineteenth century with medicine, this type of training has been widely adopted in other fields during the twentieth century. It began to be seriously and hopefully talked of for librarianship in the mid-thirties, although the idea of a practicum was basic in all the early library schools (2). The practicum, however, frequently took the form of apprenticeship-type field work, which interfered with acquiring the broad basis of professional education which even in the early twenties was recognized as essential by leading library educators.

A significant study made at this time was Charles C. Williamson's report on *Training for Library Service*. In this he concluded that "the place for the field practice as a means of imparting skill in professional grades of library work is not in the one-year general course, but in a second year devoted to advanced study in some special field" (3). Medical library interest in Williamson's plan is evidenced in a keynote paper given by Margaret Brinton at the Medical Library Association's annual meeting in Chicago in 1924 (4). Then some months later in an editorial in the Association's BULLETIN the late James Ballard proposed a year of postgraduate work in a large, modern, medical library following library school (5). Almost without exception, however, no training of this kind was developed in either the general or the medical library area until after publication in 1938 of the feasibility study made by Francis St. John for the American Library Association Board of Education for Librarianship

(6). As a result of this study the Tennessee Valley Authority internship program of the early forties was inaugurated. A curious aspect of the development during this period was the stimulus produced by the great depression, which made jobs hard to come by and additional training for subsistence pay quite acceptable. The manpower shortages of World War II brought an end to this situation. Significantly, when the Library of Congress established its program in the following decade, it offered full salary at the beginning level to its trainees plus the prospect of permanent employment if desired and the likelihood of rapid advancement (7).

Simultaneously with the TVA plan, a medical library internship was independently initiated at Tulane's Rudolph Matas–Orleans Parish Medical Society Library by Miss Mary Louise Marshall. The announcement appearing in the BULLETIN for March 1941 stated that an appointment for a residency in medical library work was available for a twelve-months term, that it carried a salary supported by the Orleans Parish Medical Society, and that "the course proposes to cover a study of the various phases of medical library administration as used in these libraries and a comparison with varying methods used elsewhere" (8). Also included was the opportunity to attend daily medical school lectures, see surgical operations, visit other libraries, and attend library meetings. This pioneer program sparked a development that has continued without interruption to the present time. It was followed in 1944 with a similar program at Vanderbilt University School of Medicine Library under the direction of Mrs. Eileen Cunningham.

In 1946, at the first postwar meeting of the Medical Library Association, Miss Marshall's presidential address concerned training for medical librarianship. Discussions which followed resulted in the appointment of a Committee on Training for Medical Librarianship, whose work in turn brought about the Association's well-known plan for certification of medical librarians at Grades I, II, and III, Grade II requiring an internship period of at least six months plus meeting requirements at Grade I.† Requirements for a teaching library and qualifications for interns were published in 1949 (9), and in 1952 the programs at Vanderbilt and Tulane were approved on a retroactive basis. The way was clear for widespread development of the internship plan, but, instead, when with the retirement of Mrs. Cunningham in 1956 and Miss Marshall in 1959 the Vanderbilt and Tulane internships closed, only one new training center had been

† Requirements are graduation from an American Library Association–approved library school and successful completion of an approved course of approximately forty hours on medical librarianship.

established and that not until 1957. The problems behind this lag and the resulting changes in present-day programs will be discussed below.

The early programs are still too close to be assessed adequately or with complete objectivity, but in a first attempt to do so the writer has talked with or written to all those interns who are still active in the field as well as to the two program directors and has checked on manuscript records at Tulane, at Vanderbilt, and in the files of the MLA Subcommittee on Internships. Detailed thesis reports on two of the Tulane internships have also been consulted (10, 11). Even this superficial survey shows that a high order of professional achievement resulted from the sixteen-year span of training supported by these two libraries. Statistically, perhaps, the group will be thought too small to be of significance, yet it is the largest on record except for the much more recent Library of Congress group and is thus a unique source for studying the library internship concept.

Nineteen librarians in all were trained—thirteen at Tulane and six at Vanderbilt. Additionally, at Vanderbilt there were two informal work-study arrangements which in several respects paralleled internships and which therefore are included in the following statistics to bring the total to twenty-one. Of these, fifteen are still actively engaged in medical library work and a sixteenth was active up to the time of her death. In the active group, five are head librarians, two are assistant librarians, and three are department heads in medical school or medical center libraries, and one is head of a major medical society library. Two others hold responsible posts in important medical research information centers. One was Editor of the BULLETIN for several years, four have served as elected officers of the Association, most have held important committee assignments in professional organizations, and several have contributed to the literature of the field. All but two of the total used their internship experience in at least one medical library position before retiring into marriage or turning to other library fields.

Written replies from thirteen of this group indicate that for twelve of them the internship was a factor of primary importance in shaping their subsequent careers; five state that it was *the* deciding element, for the opportunity brought them into the medical library field and the experience determined their remaining there.

Most frequently cited as enduring values gained during the training period were a philosophy of medical librarianship, self-confidence in work, dedication to service, development of professional attitudes, a feeling for professional ethics, and practice in thinking through problems in terms of real situations, which infused meaningfulness into theories learned in library school. More specific gains reported include a knowledge of methodology in reference work and of professional approaches to problem solving, experience in comparative cataloging and classifying, a new respect for foreign medical literature, a better understanding of the relationships between the basic and clinical sciences, and an appreciation of the interdependency of various library functions. Another advantage was the time saved in breaking into positions held later because of the basic training received in routines in the various phases of the teaching library's work. Nonlibrary aspects of the programs were praised too; for example, the stimulus of attending medical lectures and clinics, of living in a different part of the country, and of making new friends with different social outlooks.

Many specific skills and techniques were mentioned also—learning to search for historical items, to run a circulation department, to be on the alert for the idiosyncracies of serials publishing, to handle exchanges, to prepare materials for binding, etc.—but it was generally felt that, profitable though experience in these areas had been, the less tangible values were what really carried over into later professional life.

Criticism turned up four or five times regarding individual training schedules not being as well rounded as they should have been. There were also a few comments on undue emphasis on clerical tasks as compared with time allotted for professional work. In these instances the difficulties seemed to be caused by unexpected pressure on the small staff of the teaching library, which was temporarily unable to manage the training period to the best advantage of the interns.

A frequent and interesting comment was that in retrospect it was impossible to separate appraisal of the value of an internship as such from the personality of the director. The early plans were indeed reflections of the professional competence, drive, and enthusiasm of the women who conceived them and were possible only because of their willingness to sacrifice other interests to these ventures in training for medical librarianship.

Before we pass on to the new group of programs, a few words should be said about the plan sponsored by the University of Texas Graduate School of Library Science. At Texas the thesis required for the master's degree may take one of three forms: a research paper, a group project, or a report on an internship served in a library approved by the school after all degree requirements have been met. The internship must be for at least six months, with the teaching library responsible for providing a stipend sufficient to cover the cost of living (12). A review of this interesting and unique plan has recently been prepared by Dr. Esther Stallman (13). Among the students who elected the internship, four to date have gone to medical libraries—three to Tulane and one to the Squibb Institute for Medical Research in New Jersey. The latter had no regular program of its own, but accepted the student under the University's plan for an eleven-months period; at the end of this time, incidentally, the student joined the Squibb staff. The other students have been included in the statistics given for the Tulane and Vanderbilt courses, since they became eligible for Medical Library Association certification when their library school degrees were awarded them.

". . . to offer an internship a library must devote much time to advance planning, must have varied kinds of experience to present to its interns, and must have enough other staff to be able to spend the necessary time to guide and teach the newcomer. Moreover, this staff must be aware of what is being thought and done throughout the profession and be capable of transmitting the information to the student" (14). Dr. Estelle Brodman used these words in her defense of internships in a symposium on continuing education held in 1960. Mr. William Postell, on the opposite side in the same symposium, pointed out that in this statement is the crux of the problem of developing internships into an integral part of medical library education (15). There must be a seasoned staff with time to devote to teaching, and that in turn means extra financial support. There must also, of course, be funds for adequate stipends for trainees and for an active recruitment campaign, for recruitment is a basic problem in this type of training.

Staff time, support for adequate stipends, and recruitment problems all played a part in the termination of the early programs. The stipends were set at subsistence level, but fell below as living costs rose. Simultaneously, as job opportunities began rapidly to exceed the supply of librarians, it became unrealistic to expect top-notch graduates to be attracted to subsistence wages even for an additional year of training, unless to meet a requirement, as in the case of the University of Texas students. Staff time, too, had ever greater drains upon it as the explosion of biomedical literature and the rise of interdisciplinary research brought new complexities to all areas of the teaching library. These changes, in turn, meant that a well-rounded internship plan must cover more ground than heretofore. Other libraries could not respond to the Medical Library Association's call for additional teaching libraries because the budget choice was always between full-time staff salaries and training stipends. This was a choice in name only, if one considers that the first requisite of a teaching library is that it be equipped to give above-average service, and that without dependence on its interns.

It was against this background that the National Library of Medicine announced its training plan in 1957. As at the Library of Congress, recruiting needs were the wellspring of the program, but again there was the further hope that individuals who went through the year's training would make contributions to the field as a whole. This broader goal is underscored by the fact that application for MLA approval of the program for Grade II certification was sought at the outset and received at the end of the first six months trial period.‡

Three training positions at the minimum professional salary were set up as a regular part of NLM's budget. A full-scale recruiting plan preceded selection of the first group of interns. A leaflet describing the Library and the advantages of Washington living was prepared for distribution. Information was sent to all the accredited library schools of the country and requests made to interview interested students and, if possible, to talk to classes as a whole about the National Library of Medicine and its training positions. Recruiting trips have preceded selection every year since, though the number of schools visited varies. Recruiting is geared to library school students, but this does not mean that recent graduates are not considered.

The program is planned and administered by a Training Committee composed of the NLM division chiefs and the Executive Officer, with the Assistant to the Director as Chairman. In addition, there is an Intern Advisor, a post filled at one time by the Executive Officer, then by the Assistant to the Director, and now by the Personnel Officer. The original twelve-month program consisted of rotating assignments in the various divisions, with the interns assigned as a group. Last year they were assigned individually so that they might be more closely involved in the administrative demands of the work, become better acquainted with the staff, have fewer special assignments, and not feel that they were competing with one another as in a class. The Training Committee has divided the program into two parts this year, the first nine months for the established rotating assignments, the last three for assignment to regular library positions.

An account of the content of the rotating assignments is given in a paper by Maxine Kennedy Hanke, 1958/59 intern (16). Of one she writes, "The period spent in the Catalog Division was arranged to permit study of methods of classification and subject heading, and to engage in the cataloging of monographs and serials, recataloging of the old collection, catalog maintenance routines, and card editorial processes." Special projects are also assigned from time to time; for example, a survey of book dealers

‡ Information on current internship programs is based on correspondence with program directors at the National Library of Medicine and the A. W. Calhoun Medical Library, Emory University, on experience at the UCLA Biomedical Library, and on conversation with interns from all three programs.

based on percentage of orders received was done for the Acquisitions Division. The program also includes visits to related libraries in the Washington area, attendance at professional meetings, seminars given by the Director and division chiefs for the professional staff, assigned readings on medical and library subjects, individual conferences with division chiefs, and provision for study in pertinent subject or language areas in local institutions. Included in the latter provision is the MLA-approved course on medical libraries at Catholic University.

Since 1957 sixteen internships have been awarded, with eleven completed, two now in process of completion, and three resigned. In the graduated group eight now hold responsible posts at the National Library of Medicine and two are in medical school or center libraries. It is too soon to trace the influence of the internship on career development in so young a group, but the percentage remaining in the medical field has been exceptionally high. Without the internship opportunity, it is unlikely that more than a fraction would even have thought of working in medical libraries.

Internships at the National Library of Medicine have been criticized as not offering a learning experience that can be transferred to other situations because of the Library's great size and special mission. Dr. Brodman answered this criticism with the proposition that only in very large libraries is the intern likely in a single year to run into most of the kinds of problems he may meet in the course of work in later posts (14). If internships are designed as lessons in applying theory to practice, the knowledge gained should be transferable to any similar situation, regardless of its size. However, the very large institution does not offer the best opportunity for the intern to feel an intimate part of the overall operation or to become well acquainted on either a professional or personal basis with all the regular staff. The informality of smaller institutions is a very important condition for learning for some people. Intern training cannot become a part of the general pattern for medical library education unless the number and kinds of teaching libraries are large enough to allow students a choice of type, size, and location best suited to their needs.

The two new internship programs which opened in 1961 offer, combined with NLM, a varied and nicely graduated first series. On the Atlantic coast is the A. W. Calhoun Medical Library, which not only serves the Schools of Medicine and Nursing and related programs at Emory University in Atlanta but also has long functioned as the regional medical library for the area. It has a medium-sized staff and book collection with a high reputation for excellent service. On the Pacific coast is the University of California Biomedical Library, which serves the Schools of Medicine, Public

Health, Dentistry, and Nursing and the Life Sciences Division on the Los Angeles campus. This is one of the largest of the academic medical libraries with an unusually broad subject scope. The settings of the two new teaching libraries are thus rather different in several respects but alike in that both are centered on university campuses and are in close proximity to library schools which offer approved medical library courses. Though plans began independently in each library, they were coordinated at an early date, with the Emory plan submitted in February and the UCLA plan in July 1959 to the U. S. Public Health Service for support as part of the broad training program funded by the National Institutes of Health in the interest of medical research. The National Library of Medicine participated in the review procedure and gave warm endorsement to the plans. All three programs cooperate on an informal basis and look forward to further coordination when NLM's Extramural Program is able to implement its training proposals. It should be emphasized that only outside support has made the Emory and UCLA programs possible or feasible, even though the administration of each institution was extremely sympathetic with its library's goal. The grants include not only stipends, tuition, and student fees, but funds for recruiting purposes, salary for a training officer, and all incidental expenses to the libraries.

The UCLA program will be described in some detail because the writer is most familiar with it. Here the intern is enrolled as a post-master's degree student in the School of Library Service and must meet all requirements of both the Graduate Division and the School. Stipends are set a step below the beginning professional salary, with two weeks vacation granted during the course of the twelve-month period. During each full-length semester the intern takes from six to ten units of formal course work selected from the biomedical sciences, history of science, computer science, languages, and science librarianship. Additionally, he attends the lecture courses on the history of the basic medical sciences and the history of the clinical sciences and takes the eight-hour beginning Fortran course to gain an idea of the elements in machine programming. The advanced Fortran course is optional. The interns, also, soon after arrival receive the general type of orientation given all new professional staff on the structure of the University, the University Library system, personnel policies, and the organization of the Medical Center. Tours of the Medical Center and of campus libraries are included.

Opportunities are given for visits to other institutions and to campus laboratories. Typical of the latter are attendance at a demonstration of an electron microscope in action and trips to the Laboratory of Nuclear Medicine, the prosthetics research project, the University Herbarium, the Brain

Research Institute, the Heart Laboratory, the X-ray Department, and the ophthalmic pathology collections, where in every instance research staff explain work in progress. The possibilities are legion, but only a small number can be included from year to year. Visits to other institutions are generally only to their libraries, though they may include tours of hospitals and selected laboratories. The interns are encouraged to attend as many special lectures in the Library School, the Medical Center, and the Life Sciences Division as they are able to work into their schedules. They attend local professional meetings as well as the annual meeting of the Medical Library Association, with expenses covered for the latter.

The work in the library is divided into four quarters, one intern at a time scheduled for the three divisions of acquisitions, cataloging, and public services on a rotating basis, with the choice open to return to any one of the three during the summer when generally no formal classes are taken. All three interns also collaborate during the summer on assembling a major exhibit, which requires much outside reading as well as exercise of bibliographical and reference skills. A staff member and/or a faculty member serve as exhibit consultants. Within each division the intern is scheduled to observe and participate in all operations, both clerical and professional; the major time goes to the latter, but an understanding of the former, with emphasis on areas where supervision is most needed, is expected. Special projects are sometimes included; e.g., last year the interns were asked to study the arrangement of the Catalog-Bindery Division and to draw up a plan to improve the work flow. The plan was then discussed with the division staff, modified, and carried through.

Assignments within divisions are scheduled by the division head, who holds frequent informal conferences with the trainees. Arrangement of order of rotation is the responsibility of the Training Officer, but teaching and supervision are handled by the division heads and appropriate staff members, except that the Training Officer handles the basic instruction in cataloging and classification, where teaching requires more concentrated daily time than in any other area (the Training Officer must, it goes without saying, have special competence in this field). Originally, seminars were given every two weeks in each division. This schedule proved unworkable because the zest of the division staff was quite diluted by the time the third intern came round. Now seminars are scheduled once a month in one division or another for all three interns at once. Readings are assigned as preparation for participation in the seminar.

The Training Officer is the key to smooth and full functioning of the program in a larger library, where liaison is necessary between the divisions, between the library and the library school, and between the library and a host of offices such as the Registrar's, Housing, University Library departments, etc. The Program Director also must be kept informed of details and have someone to rely on to execute plans. In addition to the duties already enumerated, the Training Officer handles the grant forms and reports, advises on courses and problems of all kinds, writes and sends publicity notices, assists with the Library School's biomedical libraries course, works with division heads on seminars, and arranges for all outside demonstrations and visits. This position at present is filled on only a half-time basis, so it is a very busy one.

The Emory and UCLA programs have much in common, yet differ in several respects, the most important of which are as follows: (1) On the score of course work, at Emory the interns all take the same classes, with primary emphasis on acquiring subject background in medicine. They audit the lectures designed as an introduction to the clinical sciences for third year medical students. Beginning language courses are not approved, but a course such as medical German would be. The courses taken for credit—History of the Basic Sciences, Mechanized Systems of Information Retrieval, Science Literature, and Medical Librarianship—are similar to courses included in the group from which selection may be made at UCLA. (2) Emory interns have full standing as students in the Graduate School, but are not required by University regulations to be attached to a particular school or department. (3) The greatest difference in the two programs is the way in which provision is made for supervised experience in the library. At Emory this is done through imaginatively planned special projects which are organically related to the regular work of the library. One project, for example, was the organizing of the Nursing School collection. The basic problems here were understanding and application of the National Library of Medicine Classification and Subject Headings. Administrative experience was gained from planning how to do the job and how to integrate it with the work of the regular staff. A current project of some magnitude is concerned with weeding and book selection at the Library's hospital branch. As preparation for this, the interns have worked on foreign and domestic periodicals for two specific situations and in doing so have handled all steps of serials work from selection through bindery preparation. Selection was done individually for joint discussion and justification of choices with the Program Director and supervisors.

Last year Emory awarded four fellowships, with one dropout, and UCLA three, with one dropout. The five who completed their internships had interesting positions waiting for them, with salaries well above the beginning professional average. At present both programs carry a complement of three each with no fatalities in view.

Teaching libraries receive high interest on the time they invest in training. They are in a favored position to recruit from a carefully selected group whose abilities have been tested and observed under a wide variety of circumstances. They have the satisfaction of making a contribution to the profession as a whole, a stimulus to keep well abreast of current trends in the field, and, most important, a difficult-to-escape need for critical and continuous examination of the philosophy and procedures they seek to teach. Even in the more tangible terms of work hours, the consensus of the UCLA staff is that now that the general pattern of the program has been set up, even though much experimenting and improving are needed, there is a fair overall balance between staff time and contributions made by the interns. Time spent in familiarizing the interns with nonprofessional routines is more or less a dead loss to the library. The same is largely true for cataloging and classification. In acquisitions work, on the other hand, the library almost breaks even, and in public services it is definitely well ahead. This ratio varies with the background and ability of the individual intern, as would be expected, but by and large holds true insofar as can be judged by so limited a sampling.

The major obstacle to the wider development of internship training, in our view at least, is the difficulty of recruiting. The National Library of Medicine reports for 1962/63, the sixth year of its training program, fourteen applicants and for the previous year, a record eighteen. Applicants for the two new programs are, of course, fewer. Complete records are not available, but, since some candidates investigate more than one program, it is probably accurate to estimate the total of qualified candidates for 1962/63 at from twenty to twenty-five. "Qualified" is, of course, an important element in the estimate, for only those meeting the standards of the programs can be properly counted as candidates. All three require above-average scholarship, with preference given to those with good backgrounds in science and languages, and stress desirable personal attributes as shown in careful personal interviews as well as in written recommendations from library schools, college instructors, and former employers. In general, selection is made from young library school students or recent graduates.

Training programs are thus competing for those to whom many job possibilities are open in a variety of locations and frequently at higher salaries than training stipends. Moreover, internships tend to be more demanding than most beginning-level positions. By the time students have finished college and library school, they are often reluctant to take on still another year of study before settling into their careers, especially since the extra year is in no way mandatory. Sometimes family ties make it impossible or impractical to take an internship in a distant part of the country—and certainly the three geographical choices now open are distant for many. It therefore seems urgent to establish three or four additional training centers in other parts of the country for a trial period to determine once and for all whether the values of this type of training will prove to have strong enough attraction to give it an accepted place in the general scheme of professional education for medical and science libraries. A matching program such as that now employed for medical internships in hospitals would very likely be required to assure enough good recruits to fill an increased number of training centers. Much more data needs to be accumulated and studied to prove that the internship is indeed a prime preparation for handling the problems bursting all over the library horizon. Evidence to date is good, but there is not enough of it, and what there is needs refinement so that factors such as the academic background of the intern can be correlated with career success.

Additionally, the present job market, the overcrowding and understaffing of many potential teaching libraries, and the lack of enthusiasm for an intermediate level of training as demonstrated in the demise of the two-year master's degree suggest that alternate plans should be developed within the prevalent library school framework. The most feasible alternate would seem to be an extension of the work-study program that has been developed with such success in a number of public library systems, notably in the New York–New Jersey area. "Work-study" in its proper sense has been well defined by Lowell Martin as "a *balanced* program, which brings financial, personnel, and educational considerations into a working relationship. Further, it is a *cooperative* program between libraries and a library school, that takes into account the interests of both institutions" (17). Recruiting is done jointly by library schools and libraries, a time plan for completing the library school degree is established (generally two years), and a scheme for salary and work assignments is set up, beginning at the clerical level and progressing to the professional as the trainee gains in experience and moves ahead with his library courses. Obligation to remain in the library's employ in a professional position for a given period of time following completion of the degree requirements may or may not be a condition of the program.

The first program of this type in the medical library field was instituted in April 1959 by the Veteran's Administration for its hospital library service (18). It offers experience in both patients' and medical libraries, with salary set at one step below or at the minimum professional level, depending on qualifications. Half a dozen or so VA installations now have flourishing programs and have been able to recruit graduating trainees as permanent staff.

The New York Academy of Medicine Library has also in the past few years supported two part-time training positions in reference work. Students in library schools in the New York area are eligible as candidates for the two available posts.

The new Columbia University Libraries program, at present in its first year of operation, includes one trainee in the Medical Center Library and one assigned to the Natural Sciences Libraries out of a total of fourteen. Prospective trainees must, among other things, "be qualified for admission to the Columbia School of Library Service (preferably exceeding minimum requirements by a wide margin), be judged as possessing aptitude for handling supervisory responsibilities and as qualified in terms of education, language skill, and aptitude to fill any one of several positions on the library staff (initially in pre-professional status and following completion of the Master of Library Science degree, as a member of the professional staff)."§ The degree must be completed within a three-year period, during which the salary increases from $3,600 to $5,000 in terms of the full-time rate. General orientation meetings are planned for the group as well as individual and small-group sessions to acquaint trainees with operations of departments directly related to their own assignments. Special effort is made to coordinate job experience with formal course work.

Some other university libraries have arrangements with the library schools of their institutions akin to those at Columbia, but, for the most part, work-study programs as yet play no great part in any kind of special librarianship. This would seem a training area which could be expanded more easily than internship programs, because a part of it is at the pre-professional level and all of it involves assignments which are part of the library's regular workload. Most important, it is a means of financing required basic professional education. As a result, there is a much larger group of potential candidates than is ever likely to exist for the internship plan, which in contrast is designed for advanced training for those with well-defined career goals.

A limiting factor in the work-study scheme is the need for sponsoring libraries to be within commuting distance of the cooperating library schools, though arrangements are sometimes made for students to alternate periods of full-time work and full-time school attendance. Another aspect of this same factor is that libraries are in turn limited to selecting trainees from nearby schools and may not always find candidates qualified for work in science libraries. Internships, too, are advantageously situated near library schools, but are not dependent upon them, nor is the library confined to any particular school in selecting its interns. In any case, there

§ Based on January 1963 correspondence and a copy of a 1962 memorandum from the Office of the Director, Columbia University Libraries.

is ample room for expansion of both types of training; the two plans are not mutually exclusive. Moreover, there is no reason why a student in a work-study program should not go on to an internship, where he could be given experiences tailored to his needs, especially if he chose teaching libraries of different types.

Well-publicized training opportunities requiring a high level of performance and ability and with reasonable compensation provided should be a major means of leading students with the needed qualifications to consider a career in medical librarianship. Once recruited, the practical experience combined with his library school education should give the intern the confidence and the interest to adapt to changing patterns on his own initiative and to become expert in handling some of them. It will take many measures, including some basic changes in professional education, to solve all the problems of personnel shortages, but a step by step expansion in training opportunities would check the worsening situation with which we are faced at present. It could, moreover, be begun almost immediately and with relatively small support and would be permanently useful. The history of medical library training programs attests to this.

ACKNOWLEDGMENTS

Grateful acknowledgment is made to Miss Mary Louise Marshall, Mrs. Eileen Cunningham, the interns of their programs at Tulane and Vanderbilt Universities, Miss Ruth MacDonald of the National Library of Medicine, and Miss Mildred Jordan of Emory University School of Medicine for their kindness and help in furnishing information for this paper.

REFERENCES

1. Shera, Jesse H. An educational program for special librarians. J. Educ. Librarianship 1: 121–128, Winter 1961.
2. Stallman, Esther L. Library internships: History, purpose and a proposal. Univ. of Ill. Libr. Sch. Occasional Pap. 37: 1–23, Jan. 1954.
3. Williamson, Charles C. Training for Library Service; a Report Prepared for the Carnegie Corporation of New York. New York, 1925. 165 p.
4. Brinton, Margaret. Medical librarianship: Some of its present day problems. Bulletin 14: 28–38, Oct. 1924.
5. Ballard, James. Training for medical librarianship. Bulletin 15: 30–31, Oct. 1925.
6. St. John, Francis R. Internship in the Library Profession. Chicago, American Library Association, 1938. 40 p.
7. Goodrum, Charles A. L.C. trains recruits. Libr. J. 77: 393–395, March 1, 1952.
8. Marshall, Mary Louise. A training program in medical librarianship. Bulletin 29: 178–179, March 1941.
9. Medical Library Association. Report of the Subcommittee on Internship. Bulletin 37: 333–336, Oct. 1949.

10. RUDD, JOEL WILLIAM. Report of an Internship Served in the Rudolph Matas Medical Library of Tulane University School of Medicine and the Orleans Parish Medical Society Library, July 1954–January 1955. University of Texas, 1957. 76 p. Unpublished M.L.S. thesis.
11. SYKES, CHRISTA MARIE. Report of an Internship Served at the Rudolph Matas Medical Library, New Orleans, January 1–June 30, 1956. University of Texas, 1956. 67 p. Unpublished M.L.S. thesis.
12. A Proposal for Library Internships for Students from the University of Texas Graduate School of Library Science. Austin, Texas, University of Texas, 1956. 13 p. Mimeographed.
13. STALLMAN, ESTHER L. Review and Evaluation of the Internship Program Conducted by the Graduate School of Library Science of the University of Texas, February 1954 to June 1962. Austin, Texas, University of Texas, 1962. 7 p. Mimeographed.
14. BRODMAN, ESTELLE. Continuing education for medical librarianship; a symposium: Internships as continuing education. BULLETIN 48: 408–412, Oct. 1960.
15. POSTELL, WILLIAM D. Continuing education for medical librarianship; a symposium: Some practical thoughts on an internship program. BULLETIN 48: 413–414, Oct. 1960.
16. KENNEDY, MAXINE. An internship. BULLETIN 49: 423–425, July 1961.
17. MARTIN, LOWELL. Work-study programs—recruiting breakthrough? Libr. J. 82: 2743–2749, Nov. 1, 1957.
18. U. S. VETERANS ADMINISTRATION. DEPT. OF MEDICINE AND SURGERY. Circular 10–72: Librarian Work-Study Programs. Washington, D. C., April 28, 1959. 3 p. Mimeographed.

MLA Certification: The Certification Program And Education For Medical Librarianship*

By Miriam Hawkins Libbey, *Librarian*

A. W. Calhoun Medical Library
Emory University
Atlanta, Georgia

ABSTRACT

The certification program was formally adopted by the Medical Library Association in 1948 in an attempt to establish standards for medical librarians. The program is reviewed, and some of its effects on education for medical librarians are discussed. At the time of its adoption the program defined the kind of education librarians in the field thought necessary for work in medical libraries. New techniques and a shortage of personnel demand consideration of new educational programs, and the Medical Library Assistance Act will provide the means for their establishment. The Association should assume leadership in determining what and where these programs should be and should evaluate its certification and standards programs as often as current needs require.

THE standards program, of which the certification program is a part, had its beginning at the 1946 annual meeting in New Haven, Connecticut. At that meeting Mary Louise Marshall's presidential address was on training for medical librarians and the prevailing lack of standards. She named three factors as equally important in bringing qualified persons to the profession: (1) recruitment, (2) education, both general and professional, and (3) experience, preferably supervised, as represented by an internship. She further pointed out that as long as the Association had no training program or recognized standards it had no basis for concerted action[1]. After a long and spirited discussion, a Committee on a Training

*Presented as part of a general session on "Issues of 1966" at the Sixty-fifth Annual Meeting of the Medical Library Association, Boston, Massachusetts, June 8, 1966.

Originally published in *Bulletin of the Medical Library Association,* Volume 55 (January, 1967), pp. 5-8. Reprinted by permission.

Program for Medical Librarians was appointed to make recommendations at the next annual meeting.

During the year the Committee formulated a questionnaire which was mailed to the administrators of each library belonging to the Association and, in addition, to each professional member who would not be reached as the head of a library[2]. Overwhelmingly, these medical librarians expressed the need for special instruction in medical bibliography subsequent to some technical library training and stated that this should be followed by a period of supervised experience in a medical library. Results of the questionnaire also indicated almost unanimous approval of the adoption of a certification program; 91 of the 128 persons who replied favored it, 14 did not favor it, and the remainder expressed no opinion.

At the 1947 annual meeting the Committee presented its recommendations based upon the opinions expressed in the questionnaire. It recommended training at three levels[3]:

Grade I. Library school training with work in library administration, medical bibliography, etc. (It was hoped that the cooperation of three library schools could be secured in offering courses in medical bibliography—one school in the East, one in the Middle West, and one in the Far West—and it was suggested that about twenty persons could be absorbed in the field annually).

Grade II. Requirements for Grade I plus six months' experience under an approved librarian.

Grade III. Training leading to an advanced degree or its equivalent.

As an adjunct, the Committee recommended a plan of certification at the three grades.

Again, the discussion was long and heated. The arguments of proponents of certification were later summarized in an articleby Mildred Jordan as follows: (1) it would serve as a method of establishing minimum standards and training for the group, thus assuring a higher level of service to the medical public; (2) it would assist in marking the boundaries between professional and nonprofessional personnel working in libraries; (3) it might induce new workers in the field to meet the educational standards established by the Association, while serving as a means of recognizing older members of the profession who met the standards; (4) it would establish standards useful to administrators and accrediting bodies concerned with medical libraries; and (5) it would lend prestige to the profession and improve working conditions[4].

The views of opponents to certification were voiced in a minority report by Sanford V. Larkey: (1) medical libraries vary greatly as to function and size, and, as a corollary, the qualifications necessary for workers in various types of libraries differ; (2) the disparity between Charter and Grade Certification would be too great; and (3) the role of the Medical Library Association as an accrediting body was open to question[5].

The Committee's recommendations for training were finally adopted unanimously, but, because no agreement could be reached on the proposed certification program, the matter was tabled and a committee was appointed to study it further.

At the 1948 annual meeting the Committee on Training for Medical Librarianship again recommended that a certification program be adopted which would include Charter Certification for those who had had five years of experience by April 1, 1954, when Charter Certification was to be closed; Certification at Grades I, II, and III, corresponding to the levels of medical library training approved by the Association the previous year; and Special Certification, in exceptional cases, of those presenting credentials other than the ones specified[6]. This program was adopted, and the name of the Committee on Training was changed to Committee on Standards for Medical Librarianship, with Subcommittees on Recruitment, Curriculum, Internship, and Certification.

The Committee and the Association were then faced with the problem of implementing the program. They had to encourage the establishment of courses in medical librarianship, decide what these courses should cover, persuade medical libraries to offer internships, and seek to provide scholarships and subsidies.

In the first year of its existence, the Subcommittee on Curriculum defined its scope as investigation into the education of medical librarians along formal lines, including the goals such education should have and the method of attaining these goals. As an initial step a questionnaire was distributed to selected librarians[7]. Information from the questionnaire and collection and analysis of data on library education from other sources formed the basis for the Subcommittee's "Minimum Standards for the Training of Medical Librarians," which has been revised a number of times to meet changing conditions. "Minimum Standards" is designed as a guide in the organization and administration of courses and is used as a measuring stick in approving or disapproving courses offered.

When the certification program was adopted, a course in medical librarianship was being offered at Columbia University. In addition, in 1949 and 1950 the Veterans Administration arranged for intensive short-term courses in medicine and medical bibliography for its medical librarians at four universities. These Veterans Administration courses were not offered again after 1950, possibly because the number of courses in medical librarianship regularly scheduled in library schools began to increase rapidly. Between 1951 and the present time, nine courses have been established in library schools throughout the country, bringing the total number of courses now offered to ten. Each is taught by a medical librarian, and each has been reviewed every five years by the Subcommittee on Curriculum. In addition to providing guidance in establishing these courses, the Medical Library Association has offered a number of scholarships each year.

Like the Subcommittee on Curriculum, the Subcommittee on Internships set as its first goal the establishment of standards. In 1949 it drew up requirements for a library which might give intern training, requirements for librarians applying for internships, and a general outline of the training that should be offered[8], [9]. The Subcommittee also sent out questionnaires to selected libraries in an effort to determine how many libraries were qualified to offer internships.

There were two internship programs in existence at the time, one at Tulane and one at Vanderbilt. In 1952 both programs were approved retroactively. In its statement of approval the Subcommittee noted:

> The establishment and carrying through of an internship program requires much time and effort on the part of the librarian and the other staff members of the teaching library. Indeed, it cannot be done without their willingness to sacrifice many of their own desires in order to further this program of training for medical librarianship. . . . These two libraries, with one intern apiece each year, can provide a most limited amount of training, not sufficient to meet the demand[10].

Both Vanderbilt and Tulane discontinued their programs, and from 1957 until 1961 the only program available was offered by the National Library of Medicine. In 1961 the U.S. Public Health Service awarded five-year grants for graduate training to the A.W. Calhoun Medical Library, Emory University School of Medicine, and to the Biomedical Library, University of California, Los Angeles. In 1964 the Library of the National Institutes of Health established a training program for library interns, but in the same year the National Library of Medicine discontinued its program. Since only three traineeships have been available yearly at any one library, there have never been more than nine offered in any one year.

The lack of success in increasing the number of internship programs has been a matter of concern, not only to the Subcommittee on Internships, but also to many other members of the Association, some of whom have stated that it is unrealistic or unwise to include internships as a part of the standards program when so few opportunities for training are available. Now that money is available for training through the Medical Library Assistance Act, a greater number and a greater variety of internships may certainly be expected to develop.

Although minor changes were made in the Certification Code in 1956, no major revisions occurred until 1964[11], when the Standards Committee presented recommendations which the membership at large voted to accept. Under the revised Code, a passing grade on an examination covering the materials usually included in an approved course in medical librarianship or an internship may be substituted for completion of a formal course. Prior to this change, interns who had not attended a course could not be certified at any level. Convinced that graduate work in subject fields related to the life sciences or librarianship should be recognized, the Standards Committee revised Grade II to permit a master's degree in an appropriate subject field as an alternate to an internship. Since only two persons had ever received Special Certification, this provision of the Code was dropped; the credentials of persons holding foreign degrees or with unusual backgrounds are now evaluated in terms of Grade equivalencies.

By the end of the reporting year 1964/65, 671 persons had been certified: 309 with Charter Certification, 332 at Grade I, 26 at Grade II, 2 at Grade III, and 2 with Special Certification.

Not all of the early hopes for the Certification Program have been realized. It has served, however, to define the kind of education that medical librarians working in the field thought necessary, and it has stimulated the establishment of courses and internships to provide that education. Medical libraries are now faced with a world of new techniques and a shortage of personnel. Not only are more librarians needed, but librarians already in the field must learn new techniques, and the introduction of new techniques requires a growing number of non-librarian specialists, e.g. programmers and other machine experts. A variety of new educational programs is required to meet these needs.

One program which has been under discussion is the training of medical library technicians. Last year in a survey of institutions offering library courses at the subprofessional level, the Institute for Advancement of Medical Communication made the surprising discovery that twenty-four such programs were already in existence and two institutions planned to start programs in the fall of 1965[12]. Although none of these courses is designed for medical library technicians, members of the Medical Library Association have supported technician training. In a paper presented at the Second International Congress on Medical Librarianship, Gertrude Annan said:

> Just as the training and accreditation of practical nurses have elevated standards of the registered nurses and freed them from routine duties, so could the training and accreditation of library technicians favorably affect programs of libraries[13].

A grant application recently was made to establish a course for medical library technicians at the Upstate Medical Center in Syracuse, New York. Interested librarians have suggested that the Medical Library Association should set up standards for such courses, encourage their development, and provide certification to persons who complete the courses.

The recent passage of the Medical Library Assistance Act will provide the means for new educational programs which could not have been financed before. It remains for the Association to determine what and where these programs should be and to evaluate and revise its standards program as often as current needs require.

REFERENCES

1. MARSHALL, M.L. Training for medical librarianship. BULLETIN 34: 247-252, 1946.
2. Results of the questionnaire as submitted by the Committee on the Training for Medical Librarianship. BULLETIN 35: 94-96, 1947.
3. Report of the Committee on Training for Medical Librarianship. BULLETIN 35: 201-105, 1947.
4. JORDAN, M. Certification; a stage of professionalism. BULLETIN 36: 108-116, 1948.
5. Statement on proposed certification; minority report. BULLETIN 35: 206-208, 1947.
6. Report of the Subcommittee on Training. BULLETIN 36: 292-293, 1948.
7. Report of the Subcommittee on Curriculum. BULLETIN 37: 327-333, 1949.
8. Report of the Sub-Committee on Internship. BULLETIN 37: 333-336, 1949.
9. Report of the Subcommittee on Internship. BULLETIN 38: 348-349, 1950.
10. Report of the Subcommittee on Internship. BULLETIN 40: 441-442, 1952.
11. Code for the training and certification of medical librarians. BULLETIN 52: 784-788, 1964.
12. MARTINSON, JOHN. Vocational training for library technicians: A survey of experience to date. Philadelphia. Institute for Advancement of Medical Communication, 1965.
13. ANNAN, G. Library technicians: Need, training, potential. BULLETIN 52: 72-80, 1964.

The Changing Role of the Library*

By Merlin K. DuVal, M.D., *Dean*

College of Medicine
The University of Arizona
Tucson, Arizona

ABSTRACT

This article reviews the extraordinary growth in the scientific literature that has resulted from increased federal expenditures in the past decade or two. The article further notes that the impact of the knowledge explosion has impinged on the Health Sciences Library as well as on the individual scientist who needs access to the information. A strong plea is made for the librarian to assume a more active role in: (1) doing internal research with respect to how best to use the library as a tool in the dissemination of new information; (2) educating newcomers to the field of library science with respect to the management of scientific information; and (3) converting the library from a passive to an active instrument in disseminating the scholarly record to and among those who require access to it. Medical center administrators are reminded that if the librarian succeeds in these ventures then he will fulfill all of the research, teaching, and service requirements ordinarily made of other academic departments and, in turn, should be rewarded with departmental status for the library.

SINCE the Second World War the health service industry has become one of the largest employers in the United States. It is said to be exceeded only by agriculture, manufacturing, and the construction industry. A very wide spectrum of activity is encompassed by those who toil in these vineyards and, as the "team" concept of health care becomes increasingly prevalent, it is only reasonable to expect that more people will become involved, and their spectrum of interests will become even broader. Already these changes have stimulated the development of many new programs in education for the health sciences and, for those of us who are deeply involved in the general field of medical education, it has forced us to

*Presented as part of a general session on "The Emerging Role of Medical Libraries" at the Sixty-sixth Annual Meeting of the Medical Library Association, Miami, Florida, June 14, 1967.

Originally published in *Bulletin of the Medical Library Association,* Volume 56 (January, 1968), pp. 32-35. Reprinted by permission.

reexamine the resources that are available to support those educational programs.

One of the reexaminations that has occupied a great deal of our attention during the past year and one-half has been a survey of a large number of health science libraries across the United States. This survey had as its objective the preparation of a report for the National Library of Medicine and the definition of the changing role of the medical library as an instrument in education for health sciences. The contents of this report are available to you elsewhere[1].

There can be little disagreement that the principal influence on the health industry has been the federal government. In the twenty years that have gone by since the end of World War II our government has invested over 100 billion dollars for health and medical services. This is greater than the total expenditures our government has encumbered throughout all the years of its history. If I were to single out one prototype of this investment, I would pick the National Institutes of Health, which is only one of several agencies within the structure of the U. S. Public Health Service. The Institutes are currently supporting over 16,000 individual research grants each year, nearly 500 research contracts, and over 8,000 training grants and fellowships. Health scientists have responded to this nourishment by increasing the number of personnel who are actively engaged in research from 19,000 in 1954 to over 50,000 ten years later. As a result, it has been estimated that almost 90 percent of all scientists who have ever dedicated their lives to research are alive and working in their laboratories today.

The impact which this investment has had on the scholarly record can only be described as staggering. There are currently over 75,000 scientific and technological journals available in sixty-five different languages, and there are over 3,500 journals which have as their only concern the publication of abstracts of material which has already been published somewhere else. In a nutshell—new knowledge is being generated at a rate which is straining our capacity to synthesize it, index it, store it, and retrieve it.

Ultimately, this knowledge explosion has its greatest impact at the level of the individual scientist who needs access to it. For the scientist who is currently working in the health field, there are over 800 medical journals now being published in the United States alone. Of course, the scientist is spared the assignment of reading all of these journals because the great majority of information they contain has already been screened and selected, for both interest and pertinence, by editorial boards and peer groups. Theoretically, this should permit our scientist to limit his own current awareness tools to areas of his personal concern. Unfortunately, it doesn't work this way because much of the research currently being done is so complex, and has become so interdisciplinary, that it may be reported in any of several journals. This has the effect of bypassing the scientist. What we are learning from all of this is that most of the old tools and devices on which the scientist formerly relied are rapidly losing their effectiveness.

In the specific area of patient care, there has been an honest fear expressed that the knowledge explosion has produced a "knowledge gap." The essence of the argument is that the rate at which new information is accumulating in the laboratory, and as a result of clinical experience, is so rapid that the individual physician cannot possibly be current in his awareness of it. Thus, some have concluded that a gap of this kind may have the effect of delaying, or even denying, the benefit of new discoveries to the patient who may be in need.

Others have taken quite a different position. They suggest that if any such gap does exist it would be dangerous to have it closed completely since it is not only preferable, but safer, for the patient if an appropriate interval of time is allowed to pass between the announcement of something new and its application in the field. Either way, there seems to be an agreement that much of the new information is not immediately relevant nor useful in the majority of clinical situations. In other words, if a "knowledge gap" does exist between the laboratory and the bedside, it is probably less harmful than one might suspect.

The extraordinary rate at which progress has been made in recent years has added a substantial burden to those like yourselves who are charged with responsibility for maintaining the scholarly record; and, although academic institutions, industry, and government are rapidly becoming partners in an effort to assist you in the management of this information explosion, a great deal of progress has still to be made. In this context, it is reasonable to predict that the role of the library as an instrument in education in the health sciences will undergo some revision, inasmuch as the library of the future is destined to undergo a very substantial change itself.

In our society we have always looked to the university as the instrument of primary responsibility for knowledge; its creation through research, its dissemination through teaching, and its application through service. With respect to the health professions, educational centers have developed as subdivisions of the universities so that this same role can be carried out with respect to knowledge in health-related matters. In this setting, it is the health sciences library that is the focal point for housing and storing the resources which serve the many educational programs involved. However, changes in the techniques of information storage and retrieval are occurring so very rapidly that the somewhat more passive role of the traditional health sciences library will not long withstand the light of the future. Instead, the health sciences library is slated for a new role.

This is not to say that some of the aspects of a traditional library will not continue to serve as an instrument in the educational process. Certain documents are classic or original in their presentation, and the traditional library makes the best housing for such documents. In spite of the information which is now accumulating in media other than the printed word, there is going to be a continuing place for the presentation of printed material for a very long time. When there is a strong local emphasis on research, the participating scientists will need access to a broad portion of the scholarly record, and there is little likelihood that it will become either economical or feasible to transfer many of the older portions of this record into the newer media—especially in view of the fact that it is already available in an acceptable form. Later, when the student has left the educational institution, his primary exposure to new information will continue to be the printed word for quite some time. His very best introduction into the usefulness of this medium is in the traditional library.

But even though we may concede that the traditional aspects of the library will remain on the scene for a substantial number of years, there is a new dimension that the contemporary health sciences library should be claiming. Specifically, it has already been noted that there is a gap between the discovery of information and its use, even though the magnitude and relevance of this gap may vary substantially for scientists in different endeavors. Nothing has happened to suggest that this gap will disappear by itself and, although the use of new devices such as automated literature searches, cathode-ray display tubes, light pens, and individual terminals may increase the efficiency with which one can confront the scholarly record, by and large it has remained up to the individual scientist to keep himself as up to date as possible. Now, however, there are reasons to believe that the health sciences library may be developing much of the capability, and all of the potential, to solve this specific problem for the individual scientist. Furthermore, I am personally confident that this capability can be achieved if the librarian and the medical center administrator will accept certain responsibilities which, until recently, have generally been accorded little more than lip service. Let's consider these responsibilities for a few moments.

First, the librarian is going to have to begin a very active period of research into the most feasible and realistic modalities for disseminating the scholarly record to the scientist and the student. The answers he obtains to such research will not always be the same from campus to campus, because they will necessarily reflect the characteristics of the specific market served by the individual health sciences library. For example, where the emphasis on research is heavy, the requirements will be different than when there is a heavy emphasis on service. Briefly, the librarian must accept the obligation for doing whatever research is necessary to give him an insight into the best possible ways for him to disseminate the information that his collection harbors. The opportunity for research of this type has never been greater—the Medical Library Assistance Act will support it; other health sciences librarians want and need the answers to some of the questions that are involved, and the scientist who is working in the health field is hungry to cooperate since he knows he will be the ultimate beneficiary of the results.

Second, the librarian is going to have to accept a role as an educator much beyond anything he has been requested to accept up to this time. Generally, the educational programs in which he will engage will have two objectives: to educate and familiarize the student in health sciences with the form in which the scholarly record is contained—and the means through which one may gain access to it; and the identification, attraction, and education of new talent in the increasingly specialized field of information management. The first of these objectives will probably require that the librarian participate in the curriculum itself, along with the other academic departments. From the viewpoint of the student, the librarian's contribution to learning can be every bit as important an educational experience as any other he may undergo while in a student capacity. Furthermore, it is very likely that the success with which the student remains current in his thinking, after he has left the educational institution, will in all likelihood bear a direct relationship to the familiarity and ease with which he utilizes the library.

In anticipating educational programs for new talent in the field of information management, it is reasonable to assume that many of the librarians of the future will continue to emerge via the traditional route of the library school. On the other hand, there is new evidence that some candidates for careers in this very interesting field will be coming from mathematics, biology, engineering, chemistry, and perhaps even merchandising. As he assumes the role of "information specialist," the librarian can look forward to becoming a manager of a team of experts, each of whom may have particular competence in managing only one or two of the several media and carriers of information that are coming into the fore.

Third, the health sciences library will probably have to adopt an entirely new philosophy in the area of service, if the information gap is to be meaningfully narrowed. It seems likely that such service will become increasingly active in character and less passive. Indeed, I think we can look forward to an era in which health sciences information is actually disseminated in much the same manner that information is disseminated in the nonacademic sectors of society. Specifically, the range of services which the library of the future might offer could include the provision of linkages between people with information, as well as between people and documents. It could provide up-to-date directories of persons who are known to be doing certain types of research and where their latest results are published. It could maintain a continuous display of materials which relate to national meetings, either by organization or by subject. It could expand and develop current awareness tools, introduce selective dissemination of information, publish regular announcements or bulletins containing brief reviews of "what's new," telecast graphic images of the tables of contents of newly arrived journals, and so forth. The possibilities seem unlimited.

If the librarian can be persuaded to accept these responsibilities, then so also must the central administration of the medical center be willing to accept certain commitments. Since the library will be assuming responsibility for research, education, and service, it will have fulfilled all of the customary requirements that one makes of any other instructional department. Therefore, the library should be accorded full academic partnership in the educational endeavor, as a department. Second, if the library is to meet the requirements that will be imposed upon it as an educational instrument, it will have to be granted all of the rights and privileges that other academic departments enjoy, including a voice in the structure and makeup of the curriculum. Last, the library should be allowed to compete, on equal terms with other academic departments, for its proper share of the instructional budget. In the past, the library has generally occupied a position which, at best, can only be described as anomalous with respect to the sources and munificence of its budgeted support.

Now you may be saying that this is heady stuff—of which these dreams are made. And frankly, I wish that it was possible for me to speak on behalf of all my administrative colleagues and tell you that we will do our absolute best to meet our half of these responsibilities as we move toward this future goal together. But even though that is not my privilege, I can state with some confidence that the administrators have become increasingly sensitive both to your needs and to your capabilities, and I believe they will be receptive to your aspirations. But, if the time is right for a favorable response from them, so also is it time for you to reach beyond those precepts which you have accepted for so long and come into your own as professional managers of the scholarly record so that its usefulness as an instrument in education for the health sciences can be enhanced

REFERENCE

1. The health sciences library; its role in education for the health professions. J. Med. Educ. 42: No. 8, Pt. 2, Aug. 1967.

Preparation for Medical Librarianship: Status and Potential*

BY MARTHA JANE K. ZACHERT, *Associate Professor*

School of Library Science
Florida State University
Tallahassee, Florida

ABSTRACT

The educational programs for the preparation of health sciences information personnel are described and the lack of evaluative criteria or studies in relation to these programs is noted. The author recommends an extension of MLA's role in four areas of the educational process: curriculum design, teacher development, development of learning materials, and evaluation of the educational effort. Preconditions for the fulfillment of the projected MLA role are identified as unity of purpose, leadership by the headquarters staff, and money.

THE assignment for this paper was that I "present the various programs for medical librarianship, evaluating each type of program and indicating results and recommendations." I shall proceed in a rather straightforward way to cover two elements of this assignment; the third I shall bypass.

The educational programs are presented by means of a model (see Fig. 1) designed to show both the range and the relationships of these programs. The components at the top of the figure represent five categories of formal educational programs, identified by their degrees. Each component (i.e., 1-5) includes the title of the position appropriate to that degree on the basis of the ALA policy[1]. Each of these educational programs is time-bound just as each of them, with one minor exception, is degree-bound. The component at the bottom of the figure (i.e., 7) represents the informal educational program (which is shown as a unit, though actually it should not be so considered). Each of the formal programs potentially leads into the informal program, which is neither time-bound nor degree-bound.

*Presented June 1, 1971, at the Seventieth Annual Meeting of the Medical Library Association, New York, New York, as a part of a panel on manpower for medical libraries.

Originally published in *Bulletin of the Medical Library Association,* Volume 60 (April, 1972), pp. 301-309. Reprinted by permission.

The big advantage of a model, or picture, is that it describes a complex phenomenon better than a thousand words, so I shall add very few words. I included component 2, the bachelor's level programs in library science, which, ALA states, provide an appropriate educational base for the position of library associate, because these programs do exist and in them people are being trained for positions at a paraprofessional level in all libraries[2]. By using dotted lines, I have tried to indicate the rather tenuous inclusion of this component, at the moment, in the overall picture for health sciences information personnel.

Component 4 is more complex than the others. It includes both the sixth-year or postgraduate programs that are degree-granting and those that are not. It includes programs that are primarily classroom experiences and those that emphasize work experience in the formalized pattern of internship.

Among the problems of modeling the multifaceted situation in education for health sciences librarianship, none is more complex than that presented by the Association's certification courses. The same course serves as part of three components in the model, because individuals may choose to take it (or have it thrust upon them) at the fifth-year degree level, the sixth-year level—either degree or nondegree—or at the continuing education level, which is nondegree.

I hasten to point out that this is a hypothetical model based on the observations of one person and that, at best, it is a generalization of the situation only in the United States. I hope many others will study and criticize it, for its usefulness as a description depends on logical testing. Even if it turns out to be completely valid, this model merely describes. What we desperately need is *evaluation* of each of these components and, thus, of our educational base.

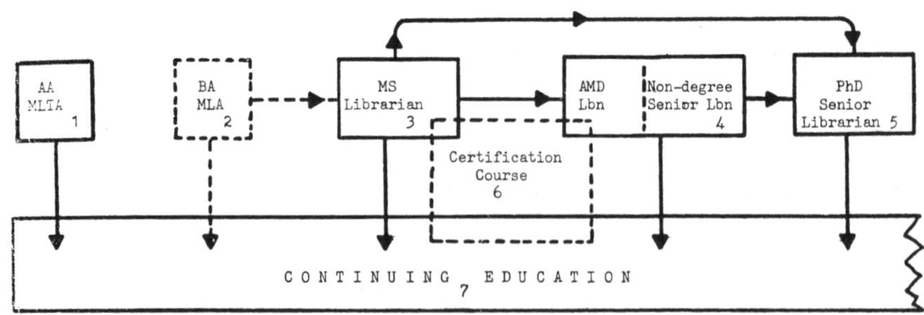

FIG. 1. Range and relationships of educational programs for health sciences information personnel.

One looks in vain for evaluation criteria, procedures, results. True, the Committee on Curriculum has provided standards for the certification courses[3], and it does accredit those individual courses meeting the standards[4]. Accreditation, however, is a means of describing the quality of the offering. It does not tell us anything about the results in terms of people with regard to quality or anything else. The Committee on Certification has similarly provided standards. By definition, certification is granted to those who satisfactorily complete an accredited course, among other qualifications, and who request certification. Conversely, the certification examination is, by definition, for those who have not taken an accredited course. So whatever facts about certification may be available, they do not help us *evaluate* the certification course component in the picture.

MLA has also adopted standards for training programs for medical library technicians. These standards, however, are too recent for implementation or evaluation[5].

To look at another component—the postmaster's internships—the only published study evaluated these programs primarily in terms of recruitment and endorsement by the participants[6]. No other evaluation of the educational components was found in the literature. Judging by the length of time MLA has expressed interest in education for medical librarianship and the paucity of data, it seems obvious that no emphasis has been placed on the evaluation of the educational programs.

In postulating the research design for their manpower study, Kronick, Rees, and Rothenberg included as their final step "evaluation of present educational programs in relation to present and projected needs and requirements[7]." I am afraid they are just going to have to carry out their study because, given the limitations of available information and resources, I can make no objective evaluative statements on the complex subject of education for health sciences information service.

Recommendations

The major part of my assignment is to provide recommendations for the future. In attempting to do this, I have not felt restricted by tradition. Rather, I have sought—and received—considerable input from a variety of sources, both printed and personal. For all of this I am appreciative. Let me remind you, however, that these recommendations are a personal opinion, their weaknesses not to be accounted to any source other than myself. Their strength, if they have any, will come from the validity they hold in the face of testing and from the conviction with which you, the Association members, feel compelled to accept them.

The recommendations I am about to make envision a new and more vigorous role for MLA in relation to education for health sciences information service. The implication of this statement may come as a surprise to some. MLA has been an innovator among library associations in relation to professional education, and it enjoys a healthy and deserved respect for its accomplishments in certification and continuing education. Why rock the boat?

Margaret Mead encapsulated the need to "rock the boat" when she said:

> To the multiple (existing) functions of an educational system we must add a quite new function: education for rapid and self-conscious adaptation to a changing world. No one will live all his life in the world into which he was born, and no one will die in the world in which he worked in his maturity[8].

Whether you began your career in 1925 or 1965, 1971 is a different world. Change has become an everyday phenomenon in medical libraries, scarcely even commented upon except when the pace accelerates. Precisely because MLA has been an innovator in this climate of change, an enhanced role in innovation is appropriate. The time is right to build on past successes.

This future role for MLA I call the role of management of education for health sciences information service, because it focuses on two prime management responsibilities, planning and evaluation. Examination of this concept suggests four immediate tasks that are incumbent on the Association:

1. Curriculum design
2. Teacher development
3. Materials preparation
4. Evaluation.

Each of these tasks must be implemented for all levels of personnel from MLTAs to senior librarians, thus at all levels of education, from junior college certificate programs through doctoral degree programs and continuing education, both institutional and noninstitutional. My recommendations relate to these four tasks.

First, curriculum design. I recommend that MLA initiate a systems study to redesign the gamut of educational experiences for all levels of health sciences library personnel.

This is not a new idea except, perhaps, in placing the responsibility on MLA and in including all personnel levels. What I want to emphasize is the systems approach to the objective of curriculum design. It was suggested, with an appropriate model, by Richard Orr in 1967[9]. The systems concept is just as valuable now as then, and much more urgent. I would make two major modifications in Orr's statement. His process model (see Fig. 2) appears to be linear, with a modification loop[10]. I prefer to visualize a spiral model (see Fig. 3). Those who prepare the design and those who live with it as students and practitioners must conceptualize a system in continuous change in the operational mode. This is implied by Orr; I simply say that the concept will probably be better understood by all concerned if the working model is more specific.

The second modification I would make stems from Orr's statement that "unless separate schools, or separate curricula, are established specifically for training medical library personnel, any really major improvement in the education of medical librarians depends upon *general* changes in library education[11]." Orr was looking only at the fifth-year programs aimed at producing master's degree level librarians—the journeymen of ALA policy. Needs of the master's curriculum notwithstanding, the major curriculum inadequacies at the moment appear to me to be in education for medical library technical assistants and in continuing education. I feel we must design curricula for all positions and that we need not—in fact, cannot—wait for changes in the general master's degree curriculum.

I see the Association as having the major responsibility for the process of design, bringing into its orbit the accredited library schools with medical librarianship courses, the junior colleges with LTA courses, the four-year colleges which train library associates (if there is a role for them in health sciences information service), and the National Library of Medicine. Further, I see the Association as having major responsibility for curriculum content. Let me hasten to emphasize that curriculum content is not the same as course design, which is, and must remain, the province of the institution which offers the courses. Though curriculum design is a complex task, expert help is available, and the responsibility is clearly ours.

Let me restate, then, that the recommendation is for an Association-initiated systems design for the gamut of educational experiences for health sciences information service personnel.

The second task is teacher development. I recommend that MLA develop a cadre of teachers with both substantive knowledge and instructional expertise, teachers specifically prepared to respond to the varied needs of individuals at whatever point in their own education these individuals may be vis-à-vis health sciences information service.

Again, we would be building on strength. The medical library expertise of experienced administrators in our master's level and continuing education classrooms is a priceless asset. But I know that very few administrators have the time—and some lack the inclination—to keep up to date on current trends in educational psychology and methodology. Yet students, who benefit from teaching expertise in other classrooms, have little patience with lack of skill in the library science classroom even when it is coupled with depth of substantive knowledge. Further, much current research has addressed itself to the effectiveness of classroom methodologies, linking these with learning theory. Students and the profession deserve to benefit from this research with less time lag than at present. As we think about the education of MLTAs and MLAs, we must face the possibility that persons in these categories will be trained in classrooms with nonmedical LTAs and nonmedical LAs and that they will be taught by teachers who are not experienced in the spcifics of medical information service[12]. It appears to me that among teachers we have, and will continue

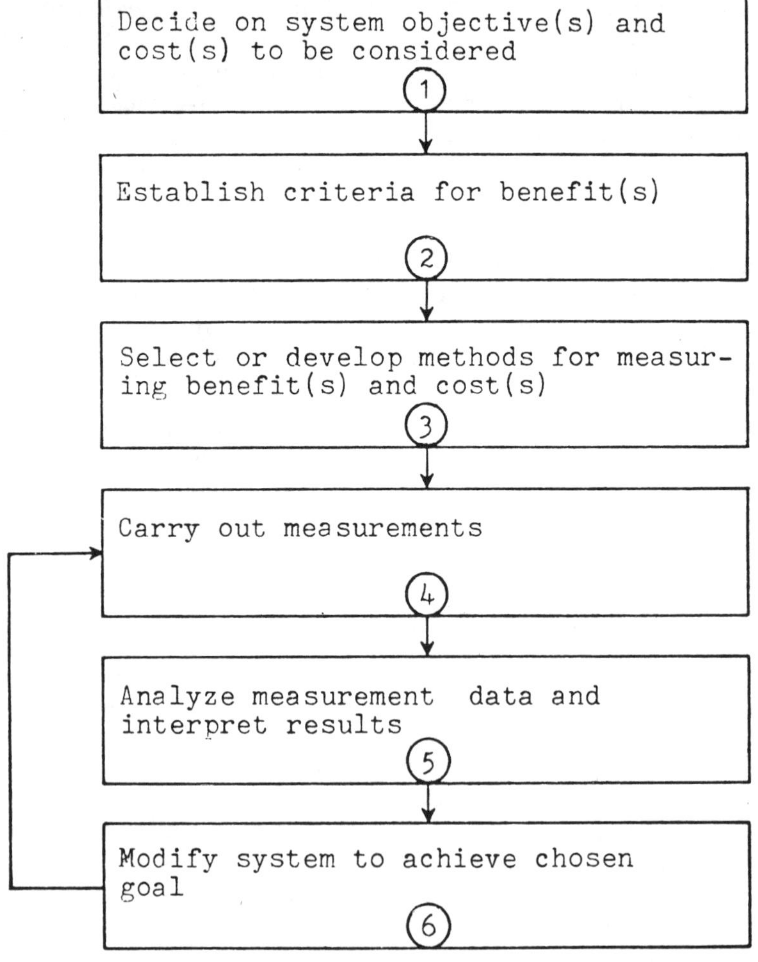

FIG. 2. Systems approach to redesign of education for medical librarianship (Orr).

to have in the future, two separate and quite distinct groups: (1) experienced medical librarians who need to be introduced to, or kept abreast of, developments in instructional methodologies and (2) experienced instructors in general librarianship who need to be introduced to or kept abreast of developments in medical librarianship. (Occasionally there is even a third group, the inexperienced in both librarianship and teaching. Its members present special problems.)

The teaching corps is an important subsystem in the total educational system. If MLA has a commitment to that total system, the responsibility is clear. Two highly significant aspects of this responsibility are (1) preparation of those who wish to, or find they have to, teach health sciences library personnel, and (2) assistance in the preparation of materials for use by both inexperienced and experienced teachers.

Since I am going to concentrate on the preparation of materials in just a moment, let me here expand only on the matter of initial preparation and updating in classroom methodologies and related pedagogical areas (see Fig. 4). MLA is in a position to facilitate the provision of a variety of learning activities for both groups of teachers (e.g., observation in medical libraries or in innovative classrooms—even personal experience if this is needed; formal learning experiences such as short courses, up-to-date seminars, and workshops; and direct communication for interchange of ideas among teachers at various educational levels).

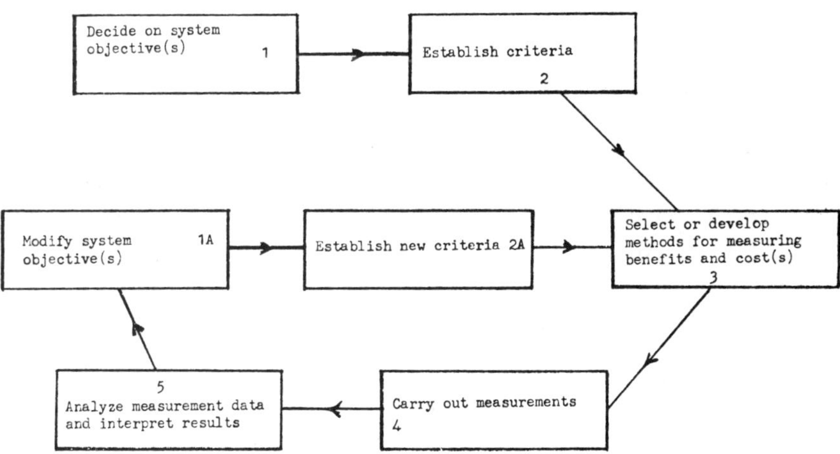

FIG. 3. Modified systems approach to redesign of education for medical librarianship (Zachert).

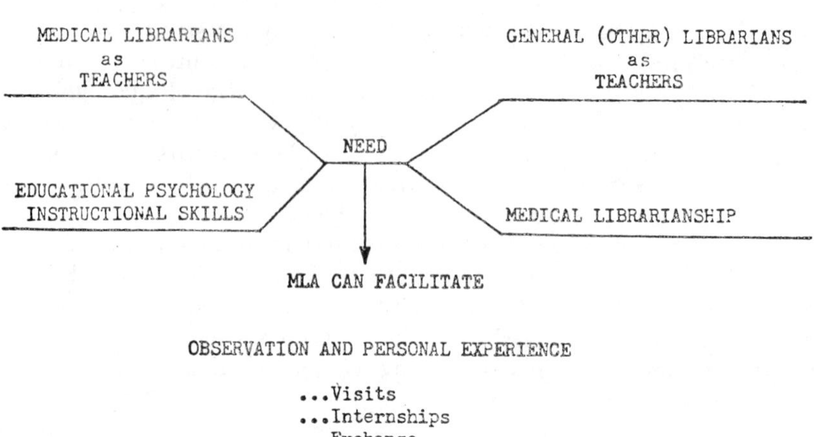

FORMAL LEARNING EXPERIENCES

...Short Courses
...Seminars
...Workshops

COMMUNICATION PATHWAYS

...Meetings
...An "Invisible College"
...Publications

FIG. 4. MLA's role in teacher development.

MLA has been exceptionally lucky in its volunteer teachers and their willingness to educate themselves for teaching and to undertake the preparation of all of their teaching materials, even the most duplicative. But when we are talking about planning a system, we can no longer depend on luck. Therefore, the recommendation is for Association development of a cadre of teachers meeting the specifications of our educational design.

The third task in this new role I am projecting for the Association is that or all levels of instruction, we postulate a situation in which numbers of teachers are presenting the same content and therefore face the prospect of duplicating necessary basic teaching materials. I am suggesting that the Association should take the responsibility for providing a wide range of such materials—making more alternatives available to each teacher than he could possibly produce himself; saving him the time of preparing duplicative materials; and providing the examples and a base line from which he can develop his own materials. I do not view the responsibility for the production of materials as related to any specific compulsion to use these materials. They should be available to teachers, not forced upon them. A teacher's time is best used in interaction with students. I am suggesting that, in order to leave the teacher sufficient time for preparation for that interaction, we should delegate a large part of the job of producing basic materials. The best materials will result if their production is delegated to experts who can devise, test, reshape them, and bring them to a level of effectiveness currently unavailable. The Association's responsibility, as I see it, is to initiate, facilitate, and disseminate.

I believe the greatest need at the moment is for the individualization of instruction at all educational levels. This suggestion is an acknowledgment in medical librarianship of what the educator in more general fields of study is finding out. Groups of students—whether in the classroom or out of it—are made up of individuals, and individuals are different in their educational interests, needs, motivations, and learning modes. In practical terms, individualized instruction means, among other things, that we must prepare units of learning materials in small packages and that these units must be essentially replicated in a variety of learning modes in order that the student may learn what he needs to learn when he feels the need for learning it and in the mode that suits him best. In short, the student should be free either to choose a single learning experience or to "freight train" by coupling units meaningful to himself.

For example, let us choose a task from the list of those identified as appropriate for MLTAs: "verifying references[13]." This is a well-defined task (see Fig. 5). A student can learn this technique from a short personal demonstration by a teacher or a supervisor; from a cassette-recorded explanation accompanied by illustrative material; from a learning program; or perhaps in still other ways. The choice depends on the answer to the question: How does this student learn best?

"Verifying references" is a unit task in the sense that it is an element in several procedures used in library work; for example, it is a unit in the order process, in checking the card catalog for a circulation desk request, in preparing a bibliography in response to a reference request, and so on. Sometimes verification of a reference is the complete and sole response to a request; at other times it is part of a complex procedure. Thus, sometimes a learning unit on the verification of references would be used as a solitary unit; at other times it might be coupled into its appropriate place in a series of learning experiences. In learning a different task, for example, preparing an interlibrary loan request, a different freight train would be assembled, but the unit, "verifying references," would be included.

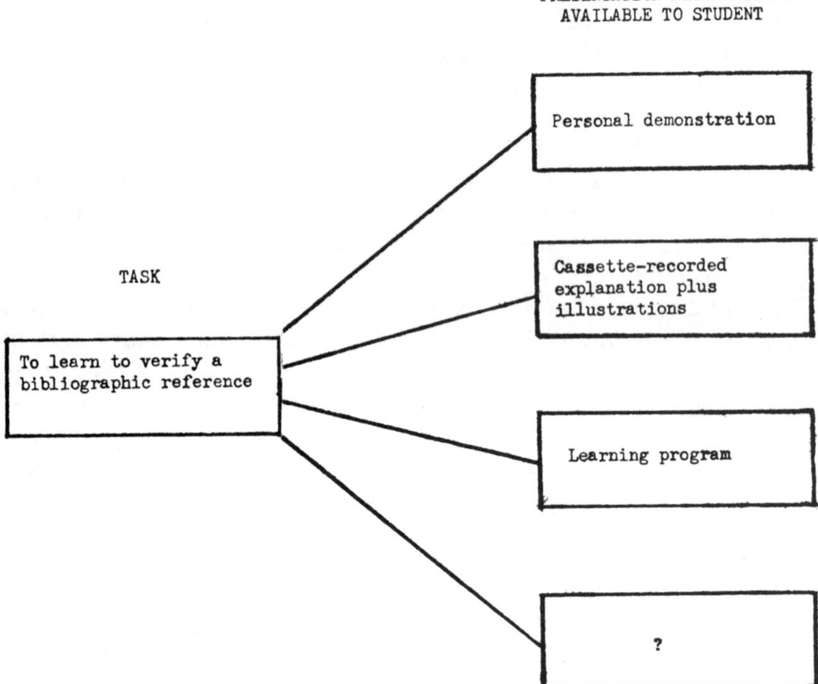

FIG. 5. Example of individualized instructional alternatives.

I have deliberately chosen a very simple example, but the principle of individualized learning materials for individualized needs can be applied to many more complex and more provocative learning situations. I am saying that we need to turn our attention, as a group, to individualized instruction and, consequently, to the preparation of materials.

It will be obvious to many of you that the kind of individualized instruction I am describing has particular relevancy to training of MLTAs (whether this is formal classroom training or one-by-one on-the-job training) because of the routine nature of the tasks and the need to teach standardized procedures to this level of personnel. Advantages in continuing education situations are, perhaps, also obvious. Continuing education in medical librarianship is now available only to those who can attend the courses offered at the national and regional meetings. Individualized packaged materials can provide continuing education anywhere, on demand. The major technological devices used in individualized instruction (projectors, recorders, teletype terminals, touch-tone telephones) are present in large medical libraries and in many medium sized and small ones. Pilot projects are under way which demonstrate their feasibility. Only our corporate commitment is necessary to implement this strategy in a significant way.

In considering the potential for individualized instruction in the training of paraprofessionals and in continuing education, do not overlook the possibilities for this mode of education in the certification course. The students in every certification course that I have observed have reflected a wide range of experience and/or prior training. Neophytes who have never worked a day in any library, and who may actually be enrolled in master's degree programs, are locked into the same courses, use the same syllabi, and undergo the same learning experiences as students whose formal education was completed five, ten, or more years ago, and who have spent some or all of the intervening years in a variety of library positions, medical and otherwise. Every teacher of an MLA accredited course with whom I have talked has described this problem as the most perplexing with which he has to contend. Conversations with students have convinced me that they are frustrated and often feel they are required to waste time or to do "Mickey Mouse" busy work. Only in the internships, and to a lesser extent in the advanced and doctoral programs, does individualization appear to play a significant role. We cannot afford the wasted time and effort implicit in lockstep certification courses.

Perhaps the most compelling reason of all for placing so much emphasis on individualized instruction derives from what I said earlier about the rapidity of change in our world and in our profession. It has been estimated that the half-life of library school education is five years. That is to say, in five years after graduation, half of your library school education is obsolete. In medical library education, the margin may be even narrower. A healthy professional career depends on an individual's ability to develop insight into his own functioning as a learner and to sustain motivation and self-direction in relation to continuous learning. Individualized instruction emphasizes learner autonomy. What Virgil M. Howes said with reference to individualized instruction of children applies also to that of adults. Howes said that "goals stress the development of individuals who are self-directive, self-disciplined, self-responsible, and capable of making intelligent choices[14]" in relation to the society in which they function. Can medical librarianship afford less at any personnel level? It is because I believe medical librarianship cannot even survive unless we increase our total potential by increasing each individual's personal learning effectiveness that I recommend the Association's immediate attention to the implementation of individualized instruction for medical library personnel at all levels.

The fourth task in MLA's role as manager of education is the design and implementation of a means of evaluating our total educational effort. Our curriculum designers need to know whether or not their plans are effective in meeting goals. Employers need to know what to expect from personnel at stated levels of accomplishment, what they need to supplement as in-house training, and how best to do that job. Teachers need to know which methods are most effective. Budget makers want to know how much has been learned, in relation to what objectives, and at what cost. Further, they want to know whether the same financing could have produced greater benefits. It behooves us to provide curriculum designers, teachers, employers, and budget makers with precise input for making wise decisions, decisions we can live with. The field of educational testing is developing more sophisticated techniques than ever before, and experts to assist in this task can be drawn from its ranks. The best agency available to initiate action, to monitor the entire scene, and to disseminate information salient enough to influence all parties concerned seems to me to be a strong professional association. This is the role I see for MLA.

To summarize, there are four recommendations:

1. that MLA initiate a systems study to redesign the gamut of educational experiences for all levels of health sciences information service personnel;
2. that MLA develop a cadre of teachers meeting the specifications of its educational design;
3. that MLA provide a wide range of teaching materials for use in the implementation of its educational design, with particular attention to the urgency of the need for materials for individualized instruction;
4. that MLA evaluate continuously the total educational effort for health sciences information service personnel and provide its evaluation as feedback to the system.

I would be remiss if, before closing, I did not point out certain preconditions to the successful implementation of these recommendations. Very briefly, first, there must be a unity of purpose in this regard within the Association. I have deliberately not specified details, because it cannot be assumed that we can or should agree initially on details. Indeed, the first order of business for each recommendation should be the identification of alternatives, so that the best *modus operandi* will eventually be chosen. Unity of purpose, however, is essential.

Second, the implementation will require more man-hours than even the sizable number now expended in pursuit of the Association's educational activities. There will continue to be a role for committees and volunteers. There is also, now, an obligatory role for specialized consultants from related fields such as educational psychology, educational testing, curriculum design, educational technology, and biomedical education. Additionally, there is more than a hint of need for a full-time health sciences library education officer on the staff of the Association. Acceptance and realization of this precondition might well be the single act most determinative in bringing forth a new generation in medical library education.

The third precondition is, simply, money. It's obvious and doesn't need to be elaborated.

It is my belief that we can move on these recommendations immediately; furthermore, I believe it is essential that we do so. The time is now. MLA, right on!

REFERENCES

1. Library Education and Manpower: a Statement of Policy Adopted by the Council of the American Library Association, June 30, 1970. Chicago, American Library Association, 1970. Offprint.
2. ZACHERT, MARTHA JANE K. Objectives and Patterns in Undergraduate Library Science Education. Columbia University, 1967. (Unpublished doctoral dissertation.)
3. MEDICAL LIBRARY ASSOCIATION. Minimum Standards for the Training of Medical Librarians. Adopted June 6, 1958; revised 1959, 1962. Mimeographed.
4. MLA NEWS, No. 37: 4, Feb. 1971.
5. MEDICAL LIBRARY ASSOCIATION. Ad Hoc Committee on Standards for Medical Library Technicians Training. Definition of medical library technician and analysis of duties. Bull. Med. Libr. Assoc. 58: 266-268, 1970.
6. MARTIN, JESS A. What happens to medical library interns? Bull. Med. Libr. Assoc. 55: 416-417, 1967.
7. KRONICK, DAVID A.; REES, ALAN M.; AND ROTHENBERG, LESLIEBETH. An investigation of the educational needs of health sciences library manpower. Bull. Med. Libr. Assoc. 58: 7-17, Jan. 1970.
8. MEAD, MARGARET. Quoted in : UMANS, SHELLY. The Management of Education. New York, Doubleday, 1970. p. 40.
9. ORR, RICHARD H. Systems Concepts and Library Education. In: Proceedings of an Invitational Conference, September 10-12, 1967, ed. by IRVING LIEBERMAN. Seattle, School of Librarianship, University of Washington, 1968. p. 107-121.
10. *Ibid.*, p. 119.
11. *Ibid.*, p. 107.
12. Library Education and Manpower. Chicago, American Library Association 1970. p. 7.
13. MEDICAL LIBRARY ASSOCIATION. Ad Hoc Committee on Standards for Medical Library Technicians Training. Definition of medical library technician. Bull. Med. Libr. Assoc. 58: 266-268, 1970.
14. HOWES, VIRGIL M. Individualization of Instruction: A Teaching Strategy. New York, Macmillan, 1970. p. 76.

IV
THE ECOLOGY OF MEDICAL LIBRARIES

Introduction

The library is not a shrine for the worship of books. It is not a temple where literary incense must be burned. A library, to modify the famous metaphor of Socrates, is the delivery room for the birth of ideas—a place where history comes to life[1].

A medical editor once wrote that, as an ideal, "Whenever a doctor meets a new patient or a new problem, he ought to have at his disposal every known fact that may help him[2]." In this regard, the biomedical literature, the medical library, and modern retrieval methods are essential for rapid dissemination of needed information. Particularly in medicine, information is of value only if it is accurate and can be made available at the right place and time.

The medical library is the major access point to health sciences information. It is a storehouse for the knowledge of the past. It provides the avenues for connecting the past with the present and for presaging the future. Perhaps the most practical value of the medical library is that it acquires, organizes, houses, and provides to users whatever information is required—for example, the latest developments in medicine or surgery. Of course, the space, resources, and services offered by the library depend, to a large extent, on the size of the institution it serves and the financial support available. Generally, most medical libraries, regardless of size, have a similar mission, which is to acquire, classify, catalog, house, and circulate needed materials and to perform a myriad of other services, such as reference and interlibrary loans. The main emphasis is on efficient retrieval and transfer of information to support education, research, and clinical practice goals of their institutions. *Service* is the basic commodity.

The title of this chapter implies that medical libraries have essential properties similar to an organism. Medical libraries are as dynamic as living, breathing things. They are growing in physical size, in numbers, in numbers of persons, in the variety of their activities, and, one hopes, in the quality of services. Like organisms, medical libraries are changing in response to changing environments. There are changes in the admixtures of basic functions, in organization, in specific means for achieving goals, and in relationships with host bodies, other libraries, and governmental agencies. The organism even seems to reproduce, as evidenced by increasing numbers and specialized extensions. The most important elements of our organism, of course, are its people, who are its gray-matter cells and its nourishing lifeblood, and the principles of the profession, which provide its spirit.

Change has been a constant factor in the development of medical libraries and services. Indeed, the rate of change appears to be increasing. Planning has become more complex, requiring more time, energy, and skill to ensure that future changes in response to the changing environment meet the tests of desirable improvement. Information needs are great and management problems difficult, but the organism is improving.

Selections for this chapter are a potpourri of interesting and important contributions to the literature of medical librarianship. Dr. Oliver Wendell Holmes shares his thoughts on medical libraries, librarians, books, journals, and services.

Dr. John Shaw Billings addresses problems associated with both the worthless and the valuable literature of medicine; gives statistics on the number of medical publications and the number of persons producing them throughout the world; emphasizes the importance of bibliographic methodology; comments on the utility of catalogs, indexes, and bibliographies; and appeals to authors and editors to pay more attention to the problems of defective or misleading titles.

The name Sir William Osler is frequently encountered by medical librarians. Osler enriched the lives of many librarians and made numerous contributions to libraries of each community in which he lived. The Osler selections are comments on what he sees as necessities central to the collections of a good medical library and on the importance of the medical library in postgraduate work.

Dr. William Mayo recounts personal experiences, valuable to his intellectual and professional growth, of encounters with books and libraries.

The heart of the teaching effort of a medical or health center, as depicted by Chauncey Leake, is the library. He discusses at length the role and scope of the library in the medical school teaching program.

Jacqueline Felter presents a progress report, with evaluations describing functions of the Medical Library Center of New York after 4 years of experience. This library for other libraries was initially set up as a joint housing facility of less-used library materials in medicine and its related disciplines and to render needed services for the participating member libraries.

Dr. Martin Cummings and Mary Corning present an excellent overview of the impact of the Medical Library Assistance Act through the National Library of Medicine's extramural programs and conclude that it has done much to upgrade medical library services to the nation's health community. The centralized operation of the Pacific Northwest Regional Health Sciences Library, one of the 11 Regional Medical Library programs supported by the National Library of Medicine, is the subject described by Gerald Oppenheimer. One of his grateful users enthusiastically claimed *that* enterprise the "single most effective piece of health legislation yet."

This chapter is rounded out with a longitudinal study, by Dr. Susan Crawford, describing the development of medical school libraries in the stimulating and expansive period 1960 through 1975, "an era of great social and technological change."

The first library was a small chest containing a few tablets of baked clay. Today a great library may house millions of volumes on—literally—miles of shelves. There is one work, however, found neither in the chest nor on the shelves, and that is the library's final book.

No library is ever completed. It cannot be until people stop thinking, for ideas beget ideas, and no one has yet devised a better place for preserving them than the pages of a book. Since no library is ever perfected, no good library is ever static. It expands with human learning, and its collections shift with human interests. Its needs are continuous, as is the good it yields[3].

REFERENCES

1. Cousins N: Editor's Odyssey: gleanings from articles and editorials by N.C. Saturday Review, vol 5, no. 14, April 15, 1978, p. 11.
2. Fox T: Crisis In Communication: The Functions and Future of Medical Journals. London, University of London Athlone Press, 1965, p. 1.
3. Fairfax M. Cone (1903-1977), Former Chairman of the Board of Trustees, The University of Chicago.

DEDICATORY ADDRESS.

BY OLIVER WENDELL HOLMES, M. D.,
President of the Association.

It is my appointed task, my honorable privilege, this evening, to speak of what has been done by others. No one can bring his tribute of words into the presence of great deeds, or try with them to embellish the memory of any inspiring achievement, without feeling and leaving with others a sense of their insufficiency. So felt Alexander when he compared even his adored Homer with the hero the poet had sung. So felt Webster when he contrasted the phrases of rhetoric with the eloquence of patriotism and of self-devotion. So felt Lincoln when on the field of Gettysburg he spoke those immortal words which Pericles could not have bettered, which Aristotle could not have criticised. So felt he who wrote the epitaph of the builder of the dome which looks down on the crosses and weathercocks that glitter over London.

We are not met upon a battle-field, except so far as every laborious achievement means a victory over opposition, indifference, selfishness, faintheartedness, and that great property of mind as well as matter, — inertia. We are not met in a cathedral, except so far as every building whose walls are lined with the products of useful and ennobling thought is a temple of the Almighty, whose inspiration has given us understanding. But we have gathered within walls which bear testimony to the self-sacrificing, persevering efforts of a few young men, to whom we owe the origin and development of all that excites our admiration in this completed enterprise; and I might consider my task as finished if I contented myself with borrowing the last word of the architect's epitaph and only saying, Look around you!

The reports of the librarian have told or will tell you, in some detail, what has been accomplished since the 21st of December, 1874, when six gentlemen met at the house of Dr. Henry Ingersoll Bowditch to discuss different projects for a medical library. In less than four years from that time, by the liberality of associations and of individuals, this collection of nearly ten thousand volumes, of five thousand pamphlets, and of one hundred and twenty-five journals, regularly received, — all

Originally published in *Dedication of the New Building and Hall of the Boston Medical Library Association,* (1881), Cambridge: Riverside Press, pp. 1-21.

worthily sheltered beneath this lofty roof, — has come into being under our eyes. It has sprung up, as it were, in the night, like a mushroom; it stands before us in full daylight as lusty as an oak, and promising to grow and flourish in the perennial freshness of an evergreen.

To whom does our profession owe this already large collection of books, exceeded in numbers only by four or five of the most extensive medical libraries in the country, and lodged in a building so well adapted to its present needs? We will not point out individually all those younger members of the profession who have accomplished what their fathers and elder brethren had attempted and partially achieved. We need not write their names on these walls, after the fashion of those civic dignitaries who immortalize themselves on tablets of marble and gates of iron. But their contemporaries know them well, and their descendants will not forget them, — the men who first met together, the men who have given their time and their money, the faithful workers, worthy associates of the strenuous agitator who gave no sleep to his eyes, no slumber to his eyelids, until he had gained his ends; the untiring, imperturbable, tenacious, irrepressible, all-subduing agitator who neither rested nor let others rest until the success of the project was assured. If, against his injunctions, I name Dr. James Read Chadwick, it is only my revenge for his having kept me awake so often and so long while he was urging on the undertaking in which he has been preëminently active and triumphantly successful.

We must not forget the various medical libraries which preceded this: that of an earlier period, when Boston contained about seventy regular practitioners, the collection afterwards transferred to the Boston Athenæum; the two collections belonging to the University; the Treadwell Library at the Massachusetts General Hospital; the collections of the two societies, that for Medical Improvement and that for Medical Observation; and more especially the ten thousand volumes relating to medicine belonging to our noble public city library, — too many blossoms on the tree of knowledge, perhaps, for the best fruit to ripen. But the Massachusetts Medical Society now numbers nearly four hundred members in the city of Boston. The time had arrived for a new and larger movement. There was needed a place to which every respectable member of the medical profession could obtain easy access; where, under one roof, all might find the special information they were seeking; where the latest medical intelligence should be spread out daily as the shipping news is posted on the bulletins of the exchange; where men engaged in a common pursuit could meet, surrounded by the mute oracles of science and art; where the whole atmosphere should be as full of professional knowledge as the apothecary's shop is of the odor of his medicaments. This was what the old men longed for, — the prophets and kings of the profession, who

> "desired it long,
> But died without the sight."

This is what the young men and those who worked under their guidance undertook to give us. And now such a library, such a reading room, such an exchange, such an intellectual and social meeting-place, we behold a fact, plain before us. The medical profession of our city, and, let us add, of all those neighboring places which it can reach with its iron arms, is united as never before by the *commune vinculum*, the common bond of a large, enduring, ennobling, unselfish interest. It breathes a new air of awakened intelligence. It marches abreast of the other learned professions, which have long had their extensive and valuable centralized libraries; abreast of them, but not promising to be content with that position. What glorifies a town like a cathedral? What dignifies a province like a university? What illuminates a country like its scholarship, and what is the nest that hatches scholars but a library?

The physician, some may say, is a practical man and has little use for all this book-learning. Every student has heard Sydenham's reply to Sir Richard Blackmore's question as to what books he should read, — meaning medical books. "Read Don Quixote," was his famous answer. But Sydenham himself made medical books and may be presumed to have thought *those* at least worth reading. Descartes was asked where was his library, and in reply held up the dissected body of an animal. But Descartes made books, great books, and a great many of them. A physician of common sense without erudition is better than a learned one without common sense, but the thorough master of his profession must have learning added to his natural gifts.

It is not necessary to maintain the direct practical utility of all kinds of learning. Our shelves contain many books which only a certain class of medical scholars will be likely to consult. There is a dead medical literature, and there is a live one. The dead is not all ancient, the live is not all modern. There is none, modern or ancient, which, if it has no living value for the student, will not teach him something by its autopsy. But it is with the live literature of his profession that the medical practitioner is first of all concerned.

Now there has come a great change in our time over the form in which living thought presents itself. The first printed books — the *incunabula* — were enclosed in boards of solid oak, with brazen clasps and corners; the boards by and by were replaced by pasteboard covered with calf or sheepskin; then cloth came in and took the place of leather; then the pasteboard was covered with paper instead of cloth; and at this day the quarterly, the monthly, the weekly periodical in its flimsy unsupported dress of paper, and the daily journal, naked as it came from the womb of the press, hold the larger part of the fresh reading we live upon. We must have the latest thought in its latest expression; the page must be newly turned like the morning bannock; the pamphlet must be newly opened like the ante-prandial oyster.

Thus a library, to meet the need of our time, must take, and must spread out in a convenient form, a great array of periodicals. Our active practitioners read these by preference over almost everything else. Our specialists, more particularly, depend on the month's product, on the yearly crop of new facts, new suggestions, new contrivances, as much as the farmer on the annual yield of his acres. One of the first wants, then, of the profession is supplied by our library in its great array of periodicals from many lands in many languages. Such a number of medical periodicals no private library would have room for, no private person would pay for, or flood his library with if they were sent him for nothing. These, I think, with the reports of medical societies and the papers contributed to them, will form the most attractive part of our accumulated medical treasures. They will be also one of our chief expenses, for these journals must be bound in volumes and they require a great amount of shelf-room; all this, in addition to the cost of subscription for those which are not furnished us gratuitously.

It is true that the value of old scientific periodicals is, other things being equal, in the inverse ratio of their age, for the obvious reason that what is most valuable in the earlier volumes of a series is drained off into the standard works with which the intelligent practitioner is supposed to be familiar. But no extended record of facts grows too old to be useful provided only that we have a ready and sure way of getting at the particular fact or facts we are in search of.

And this leads me to speak of what I conceive to be one of the principal tasks to be performed by the present and the coming generation of scholars, not only in the medical, but in every department of knowledge. I mean the formation of *indexes*, and more especially of indexes to periodical literature.

This idea has long been working in the minds of scholars, and all who have had occasion to follow out any special subject. I have a right to speak of it, for I long ago attempted to supply the want of indexes in some small measure, for my own need. I had a very complete set of the *American Journal of the Medical Sciences;* an entire set of the *North American Review*, and many volumes of the reprints of the three leading British quarterlies. Of what use were they to me without general indexes? I looked them all through carefully and made classified lists of all the articles I thought I should most care to read. But they soon outgrew my lists. The *North American Review* kept filling up shelf after shelf, rich in articles which I often wanted to consult, but what a labor to find them, until the index of Mr. Cushing, published a few months since, made the contents of these hundred and twenty volumes as easily accessible as the words in a dictionary! I had a copy of good Dr. Abraham Rees's Cyclopædia, a treasure-house to my boyhood which has not lost its value for me in later years. But where to look for what I wanted? I wished to know, for instance, what Dr. Burney had to say about singing. Who would have looked for it under the Italian word *cantare?* I was curious to learn something of the etchings of Rembrandt, and where should I find it but under the head "Low Countries, Engravers of the," — an elaborate and most valuable article of a hundred double-columned close-printed quarto pages, to which no reference, even, is made under the title Rembrandt. There was nothing to be done, if I wanted to know where that which I specially cared for was to be found in my Rees's Cyclopædia, but to look over every page of its forty-one quarto volumes and make out a brief list of matters of interest which I could not find by their titles, and this I did, at no small expense of time and trouble.

Nothing, therefore, could be more pleasing to me than to see the attention which has been given of late years to the great work of indexing. It is a quarter of a century since Mr. Poole published his Index to Periodical Literature, which it is much to be hoped is soon to appear in a new edition, grown as it must be to formidable dimensions by the additions of so long a period. The *British and Foreign Medical Review*, edited by the late Sir John Forbes, contributed to by Huxley, Carpenter, Laycock, and others of the most distinguished scientific men of Great Britain, has an index to its twenty-four volumes, and by its aid I find this valuable series as manageable as a lexicon. The last edition of the Encyclopædia Britannica had a complete index in a separate volume, and the publishers of Appleton's American Cyclopædia have recently issued an index to their useful work, which must greatly add to its value. I have already referred to the index to the *North American Review*, which to an American, and especially to a New Englander, is the most interesting and most valuable addition of its kind to our literary apparatus since the publication of Mr. Allibone's Dictionary of Authors. I might almost dare to parody Mr. Webster's words in speaking of Hamilton, to describe what Mr. Cushing did for the solemn rows of back volumes of our honored old *Review* which had been long fossilizing on our shelves: "He touched the dead corpse of the" *North American*, "and it sprang to its feet." A library of the best thought of the best American scholars during the greater portion of the century was brought to light by the work of the index-maker as truly as were the Assyrian tablets by the labors of Layard.

A great portion of the best writing and reading—literary, scientific, professional, miscellaneous—comes to us now, at stated intervals, in paper covers. The writer appears, as it were, in his shirt-sleeves. As soon as he has delivered his message the book-binder puts a coat on his back, and he joins the forlorn brotherhood of "back volumes," than which, so long as they are unindexed, nothing can be more exasperating. Who wants a lock without a key, a ship without a rudder, a binnacle without a compass, a check without a signature, a greenback without a goldback behind it?

I have referred chiefly to the medical journals, but I would include with these the reports of medical associations, and those separate publications which, coming in the form of pamphlets, heap themselves into chaotic piles and bundles which are worse than useless, taking up a great deal of room, and frightening everything away but mice and mousing antiquarians, or possibly at long intervals some terebrating specialist.

Arranged, bound, indexed, all these at once become accessible and valuable. I will take the first instance which happens to suggest itself. How many who know all about osteoblasts and the experiments of Ollier, and all that has grown out of them, know where to go for a paper by the late Dr. A. L. Peirson, of Salem, published in the year 1840, under the modest title, Remarks on Fractures? And if any practitioner who has to deal with broken bones does *not* know that most excellent and practical essay, it is a great pity, for it answers very numerous questions which will be sure to suggest themselves to the surgeon and the patient as no one of the recent treatises, on my own shelves, at least, can do.

But if indexing is the special need of our time in medical literature, as in every department of knowledge, it must be remembered that it is not only an immense labor, but one that never ends. It requires therefore the coöperation of a large number of individuals to do the work, and a large amount of money to pay for making its results public through the press. When it is remembered that the catalogue of the library of the British Museum is contained in nearly three thousand large folios of manuscript, and not all its books are yet included, the task of indexing any considerable branch of science or literature looks as if it were well nigh impossible. But many hands make light work. An "Index Society" has been formed in England, already numbering about one hundred and seventy members. It aims at "supplying thorough indexes to valuable works and collections which have hitherto lacked them; at issuing indexes to the literature of special subjects; and at gathering materials for a general reference index." This society has published a little treatise setting forth the history and the art of indexing, which I trust is in the hands of some of our members, if not upon our shelves.

Something has been done in the same direction by individuals in our own country, as we have already seen. The need of it in the department of medicine is beginning to be clearly felt. Our library has already an admirable catalogue with cross references, the work of a number of its younger members coöperating in the task. A very intelligent medical student, Mr. William D. Chapin, whose excellent project is endorsed by well-known New York physicians and professors, proposes to publish a yearly index to original communications in the medical journals of the United States, classified by authors and subjects. But it is from the National Medical Library at Washington that we have the best promise and the largest expectations. That great and growing collection of fifty thousand volumes is under the eye and hand of a librarian who knows books and how to manage them. For libraries are the standing armies of civilization, and an army is but a mob without a general who can organize and marshal it so as to make it effective. The "Specimen Fasciculus of a Catalogue of the National Medical Library," prepared under the direction of Dr. Billings, the librarian, would have excited the admiration of Haller, the master scholar in medical science of the last century, or rather of the profession in all centuries, and if carried out as it is begun will be to the nineteenth all and more than all that the three Bibliothecæ — Anatomica, Chirurgica, and Medicinæ-Practicæ — were to the eighteenth century. I cannot forget the story that Agassiz was so fond of telling of the king of Prussia and Fichte. It was after the humiliation and spoliation of the kingdom by Napoleon that the monarch asked the philosopher what could be done to regain the lost position of the nation. "Found a great university, Sire," was the answer, and so it was that in the year 1810 the world-renowned University of Berlin came into being. I believe that *we* in this country can do better than found a national university, whose professors shall be nominated in caucuses, go in and out, perhaps, like postmasters, with every change of administration, and deal with science in the face of their constituency as the courtier did with time when his sovereign asked him what o'clock it was: "Whatever hour your majesty pleases." But when we have a noble library like that at Washington, and a librarian of exceptional qualifications like the gentleman who now holds that office, I believe that a liberal appropriation by Congress to carry out a conscientious work for the advancement of sound knowledge and the bettering of human conditions, like this which Dr. Billings has so well begun, would redound greatly to the honor of the nation. It ought to be willing to be at some charge to make its treasures useful to its citizens, and, for its own sake, especially to that class which has charge of health public and private. This country abounds in what are called "self-made men," and is justly proud of many whom it thus designates. In one sense no man is self-made who breathes the air of a civilized community. In another sense every man who is anything other than a phonograph on legs is self-made. But if we award his just praise to the man who has attained any kind of excellence without having had the same advantages as others whom, nevertheless, he has equalled or surpassed, let us not be betrayed into undervaluing the mechanic's careful training to his business, — the thorough and laborious education of the scholar and the professional man.

Our American atmosphere is vocal with the flippant loquacity of half knowledge. We must accept whatever good can be got out of it, and keep it under as we do sorrel and mullein and witchgrass, by enriching the soil, and sowing good seed in plenty; by good teaching and good books, rather than by wasting our time in talking against it. Half knowledge dreads nothing but whole knowledge.

I have spoken of the importance and the predominance of periodical literature, and have attempted to do justice to its value. But the almost exclusive reading of it is not without its dangers. The journals contain much that is crude and unsound; the presumption, it might be maintained, is against their novelties, unless they come from observers of established credit. Yet I have known a practitioner — perhaps more than one — who was as much under the dominant influence of the last article he had read in his favorite medical journal as a milliner under the sway of the last fashion-plate. The difference between green and seasoned knowledge is very great, and such practitioners never hold long enough to any of their knowledge to have it get seasoned.

It is needless to say, then, that all the substantial and permanent literature of the profession should be represented upon our shelves. Much of it is there already, and as one private library after another falls into this by the natural law of gravitation, it will gradually acquire all that is most valuable almost without effort. A scholar should not be in a hurry to part with his books. They are probably more valuable to him than they can be to any other individual. What Swedenborg called "correspondence" has established itself between his intelligence and the volumes which wall him within their sacred enclosure. Napoleon said that his mind was as if furnished with drawers, — he drew out each as he wanted its contents, and closed it at will when done with them. The scholar's mind, to use a similar comparison, is furnished with shelves, like his library. Each book knows its place in the brain as well as against the wall or in the alcove. His consciousness is doubled by the books which encircle him, as the trees that surround a lake repeat themselves in its unruffled waters. Men talk of the nerve that runs to the pocket, but one who loves his books, and has lived long with them, has a nervous filament which runs from his sensorium to every one of them. Or, if I may still let my fancy draw its pictures, a scholar's library is to him what a temple is to the worshipper who frequents it. There is the altar sacred to his holiest experiences. There is the font where his new-born thought was baptized and first had a name in his consciousness. There is the monumental tablet of a dead belief, sacred still in the memory of what it was while yet alive. No visitor can read all this on the lettered backs of the books that have gathered around the scholar, but for him, from the Aldus on the lowest shelf to the Elzevir on the highest, every volume has a language which none but he can interpret. Be patient with the book-collector who loves his companions too well to let them go. Books are not buried with their owners, and the veriest book-miser that ever lived was probably doing far more for his successors than his more liberal neighbor who despised his learned or unlearned avarice. Let the fruit fall with the leaves still clinging round it. Who would have stripped Southey's walls of the books that filled them, when, his mind no longer capable of taking in their meaning, he would still pat and fondle them with the vague loving sense of what they had once been to him — to him, the great scholar, now like a little child among his playthings?

We need in this country not only the scholar, but the *virtuoso*, who hoards the treasures which he loves, it may be chiefly for their rarity and because others who know more than he does of their value set a high price upon them. As the wine of old vintages is gently decanted out of its cobwebbed bottles with their rotten corks into clean new receptacles, so the wealth of the New World is quietly emptying many of the libraries and galleries of the Old World into its newly formed collections and newly raised edifices. And this process must go on in an accelerating ratio. No Englishman will be offended if I say that before the New Zealander takes his stand on a broken arch of London bridge to sketch the ruins of Saint Paul's in the midst of a vast solitude, the treasures of the British Museum will have found a new shelter in the halls of New York or Boston. No Catholic will think hardly of my saying that before the Coliseum falls, and with it the imperial city, whose doom prophecy has linked with that of the almost eternal amphitheatre, the marbles, the bronzes, the paintings, the manuscripts of the Vatican will have left the shores of the Tiber for those of the Potomac, the Hudson, the Mississippi, or the Sacramento. And what a delight in the pursuit of the rarities which the eager book-hunter follows with the scent of a beagle! Shall I ever forget that rainy day in Lyons, that dingy bookshop, where I found the Aëtius, long missing from my Artis Medicæ Principes, and where I bought for a small pecuniary consideration, though it was marked *rare*, and was really *très rare*, the Aphorisms of Hippocrates, edited by and with a preface from the hand of Francis Rabelais? And the vellum-bound Tulpius, which I came upon in Venice, afterwards my only reading when imprisoned in quarantine at Marseilles, so that the two hundred and twenty-eight cases he has recorded are, many of them, to this day still fresh in my memory. And the Schenckius, — the folio filled with *casus rariores*, which had strayed in among the rubbish of the bookstall on the boulevard, — and the noble old Vesalius with its grand frontispiece not unworthy of Titian, and the fine old Ambroise Paré, long waited for even in Paris and long ago, and the colossal Spigelius with his eviscerated beauties, and Dutch Bidloo with its miracles of fine engraving and bad dissection, and Italian Mascagni, the despair of all would-be imitators, and pre-Adamite John de Ketam, and antediluvian Berengarius Carpensis — but why multiply names, every one of which brings back the accession of a book which was an event almost like the birth of an infant?

A library like ours must exercise the largest hospitality. A great many books may be found in every large collection which remind us of those apostolic looking old men who figure on the platform at our political and other assemblages. Some of them have spoken words of wisdom in their day, but they have ceased to be oracles; some of them never had any particularly important message for humanity, but they add dignity to the meeting by their presence; they look wise, whether they are so or not, and no one grudges them their places of honor. Venerable figure-heads, what would our platforms be without you?

Just so with our libraries. Without their rows of folios in creamy vellum or showing their black backs with antique lettering of tarnished gold our shelves would look as insufficient and unbalanced as a column without its base, as a statue without its pedestal. And do not think they are kept only to be spanked and dusted during that dreadful period when their owner is but too thankful to become an exile and a wanderer from the scene of single combats between dead authors and living housemaids. Men were not all cowards before Agamemnon or all fools before the days of Virchow and Billroth. And apart from any practical use to be derived from the older medical authors, is there not a true pleasure in reading the accounts of great discoverers in their own words? I do not pretend to hoist up the Bibliotheca Anatomica of Mangetus and spread it on my table every day. I do not get out my great Albinus before every lecture on the muscles, nor disturb the majestic repose of Vesalius every time I speak of the bones he has so admirably described and figured. But it does please me to read the first descriptions of parts to which the names of their discoverers or those who have first described them have become so joined that not even modern science can part them; to listen to the talk of my old volume as Willis describes his circle and Fallopius his aqueduct and Varolius his bridge and Eustachius his tube and Monro his foramen — all so well known to us in the human body; it does please me to know the very words in which Winslow described the opening which bears his name, and Glisson his capsule and De Graaf his vesicle; I am not content until I know in what language Harvey announced his discovery of the circulation, and how Spigelius made the liver his perpetual memorial, and Malpighi found a monument more enduring than brass in the corpuscles of the spleen and the kidney.

But after all, the readers who care most for the early records of medical science and art are the specialists who are dividing up the practice of medicine and surgery as they were parcelled out, according to Herodotus, by the Egyptians. For them nothing is too old, nothing is too new, for to their books of all others is applicable the saying of D'Alembert that the author kills himself in lengthening out what the reader kills himself in trying to shorten.

There are practical books among these ancient volumes which can never grow old. Would you know how to recognize "male hysteria" and to treat it, take down your Sydenham; would you read the experience of a physician who was himself the subject of asthma and who, notwithstanding that, in the words of Dr. Johnson, "panted on till ninety," you will find it in the venerable treatise of Sir John Floyer; would you listen to the story of the King's Evil cured by the royal touch, as told by a famous chirurgeon who fully believed in it, go to Wiseman; would you get at first hand the description of the spinal disease which long bore his name, do not be startled if I tell you to go to Pott — to Percival Pott, the great surgeon of the last century.

There comes a time for every book in a library when it is wanted by somebody. It is but a few weeks since one of the most celebrated physicians in the country wrote to me from a great centre of medical education to know if I had the works of Sanctorius, which he had tried in vain to find. I could have lent him the "Medicina Statica," with its frontispiece showing Sanctorius with his dinner on the table before him, in his balanced chair which sunk with him below the level of his banquet-board when he had swallowed a certain number of ounces, — an early foreshadowing of Pettenkofer's chamber and quantitative physiology, — but the "Opera Omnia" of Sanctorius I had never met with, and I fear he had to do without it.

I would extend the hospitality of these shelves to a class of works which we are in the habit of considering as being outside of the pale of medical science, properly so called, and sometimes of coupling with a disrespectful name. Such has always been my own practice. I have welcomed Culpeper and Salmon to my bookcase as willingly as Dioscorides or Quincy, or Paris or Wood and Bache. I have found a place for St. John Long, and read the story of his trial for manslaughter with as much interest as the laurel-water case in which John Hunter figured as a witness. I would give Samuel Hahnemann a place by the side of Samuel Thomson. Am I not afraid that some student of imaginative turn and not provided with the needful cerebral strainers without which all the refuse of gimcrack intelligences gets into the mental drains and chokes them up, — am I not afraid that some such student will get hold of the "Organon" or the "Maladies Chroniques" and be won over by their delusions, and so be lost to those that love him as a man of common sense and a brother in their high calling? Not in the least. If he showed any symptoms of infection I would for once have recourse to the principle of *similia similibus.* To cure him of Hahnemann I would prescribe my favorite homœopathic antidote, Okie's Bonninghausen. If that failed, I would order Grauvogl as a heroic remedy, and if he survived that uncured, I would give him my blessing, if I thought him honest, and bid him depart in peace. For me he is no longer an individual. He belongs to a class of minds which we are bound to be patient with if their Maker sees fit to indulge them with existence. We must accept the conjuring ultra-ritualist, the dreamy second adventist, the erratic spiritualist, the fantastic homœopathist, as not unworthy of philosophic study; not more unworthy of it than the squarers of the circle and the inventors of perpetual motion, and the other whimsical visionaries to whom De Morgan has devoted his most instructive and entertaining "Budget of Paradoxes." I hope, therefore, that our library will admit the works of the so-called Eclectics, of the Thomsonians, if any are in existence, of the Clairvoyants, if they have a literature, and especially of the Homœopathists. This country seems to be the place for such a collection, which will by and by be curious and of more value than at present, for Homœopathy seems to be following the pathological law of erysipelas, fading out where it originated as it spreads to new regions. At least I judge so by the following translated extract from a criticism of an American work in the *Homœopatische Rundschau* of Leipzig for October, 1878, which I find in the *Homœopathic Bulletin* for the month of November just passed: —

"While we feel proud of the spread and rise of Homœopathy across the ocean, and while the Homœopathic works reaching us from there, and published in a style such as is unknown in Germany, bear eloquent testimony to the eminent activity of our transatlantic colleagues, we are overcome by sorrowful regrets at the position Homœopathy occupies in Germany. Such a work [as the American one referred to] with us would be impossible; it would lack the necessary support."

By all means let our library secure a good representation of the literature of Homœopathy before it leaves us its "sorrowful regrets" and migrates with its sugar of milk pellets, which have taken the place of the old *pilulæ micæ panis*, to Alaska, to "Nova Zembla, or the Lord knows where."

What shall I say in this presence of the duties of a Librarian? Where have they ever been better performed than in our own public city library, where the late Mr. Jewett and the living Mr. Winsor have shown us what a librarian ought to be — the organizing head, the vigilant guardian, the seeker's index, the scholar's counsellor? His work is not merely that of administration, manifold and laborious as its duties are. He must have a quick intelligence and a retentive memory. He is a public carrier of knowledge in its germs. His office is like that which naturalists attribute to the bumble-bee, — he lays up little honey for himself, but he conveys the fertilizing pollen from flower to flower.

Our undertaking, just completed — and just begun — has come at the right time, not a day too soon. Our practitioners need a library like this, for with all their skill and devotion there is too little genuine erudition, such as a liberal profession ought to be able to claim for many of its members. In reading the recent obituary notices of the late Dr. Geddings of South Carolina, I recalled what our lamented friend Dr. Coale used to tell me of his learning and accomplishments, and I could not help reflecting how few such medical scholars we had to show in Boston or New England. We must clear up this unilluminated atmosphere, and here, — here is the true electric light which will irradiate its darkness.

The public will catch the rays reflected from the same source of light, and it needs instruction on the great subjects of health and disease, — needs it sadly. It is preyed upon by every kind of imposition almost without hindrance. Its ignorance and prejudices react upon the profession to the great injury of both. The jealous feeling, for instance, with regard to such provisions for the study of anatomy as are sanctioned by the laws in this State and carried out with strict regard to those laws, threatens the welfare, if not the existence of institutions for medical instruction wherever it is not held in check by enlightened intelligence. And on the other hand the profession has just been startled by a verdict against a physician, ruinous in its amount, — enough to drive many a hard-working young practitioner out of house and home, — a verdict which leads to the fear that suits for malpractice may take the place of the panel game and child-stealing as a means of extorting money. If the profession in this State, which claims a high standard of civilization, is to be crushed and ground beneath the upper millstone of the dearth of educational advantages, and the lower millstone of ruinous penalties for what the ignorant ignorantly shall decide to be ignorance, all I can say is

God save the Common*h*ealth of Massachusetts!

Once more, we cannot fail to see that just as astrology has given place to astronomy, so theology, the science of Him whom by searching no man can find out, is fast being replaced by what we may not improperly call theonomy, or the science of the laws according to which the Creator acts. And since these laws find their fullest manifestations for us, at least, in rational human natures, the study of anthropology is largely replacing that of scholastic divinity. We must contemplate our Maker indirectly in human attributes as we talk of Him in human parts of speech. And this gives a sacredness to the study of man in his physical, mental, moral, social, and religious nature which elevates the faithful students of anthropology to the dignity of a priesthood, and sheds a holy light on the recorded results of their labors, brought together as they are in such a collection as this which is now spread out before us.

Thus, then, our library is a temple as truly as the dome-crowned cathedral hallowed by the breath of prayer and praise, where the dead repose and the living worship. May it, with all its treasures, be consecrated like that to the glory of God, through the contributions it shall make to the advancement of sound knowledge, to the relief of human suffering, to the promotion of harmonious relations between the members of the two noble professions which deal with the diseases of the soul and with those of the body, and to the common cause in which all good men are working, the furtherance of the well-being of their fellow creatures!

NOTE. — As an illustration of the statement in the last paragraph but one, I take the following notice from the *Boston Daily Advertiser* of December 4th, the day after the delivery of the address: —

"Prince Lucien Bonaparte is now living in London, and is devoting himself to the work of collecting the creeds of all religions and sects, with a view to their classification, — his object being simply scientific or anthropological."

Since delivering the address, also, I find a leading article in the *Cincinnati Lancet and Clinic* of November 30th, headed "The Decadence of Homœopathy," abundantly illustrated by extracts from the *Homœopathic Times*, the leading American organ of that sect.

In the New York *Medical Record* of the same date, which I had not seen before the delivery of my address, is an account of the action of the Homœopathic Medical Society of Northern New York, in which Hahnemann's theory of "dynamization" is characterized in a formal resolve as "unworthy the confidence of the Homœopathic profession."

It will be a disappointment to the German Homœopathists to read in the *Homœopathic Times* such a statement as the following: —

"Whatever the influences have been which have checked the outward development of Homœopathy, it is plainly evident that the Homœopathic school, as regards the number of its openly avowed representatives, has attained its majority, and has begun to decline both in this country and in England."

All which is an additional reason for making a collection of the incredibly curious literature of Homœopathy before that pseudological inanity has faded out like so many other delusions.

Our Medical Literature

By John Shaw Billings, M.D.

When I was surprised by the honour of an invitation to address this Congress, my first thought was that it must be declined, for the simple, but sufficient reason that I had nothing to say that would be worth occupying the time of such an assemblage as it was evident this would be. But while thinking over the matter, and looking absent-mindedly at a shelf of catalogues and a pile of new books and journals awaiting examination, it occurred to me that perhaps some facts connected with our medical literature, past and present, from the point of view of the reader, librarian, and bibliographer, rather than from that of the writer or practitioner, might be of sufficient interest to you to warrant an attempt to present them; and, the wish being probably father to the thought, I decided to make the trial.

When I say "Our Medical Literature," it is not with reference to that of any particular country or nation, but to that which is the common property of the educated physicians of the world as represented here to-day—the literature which forms the intra- and international bond of the medical profession of all civilized countries; and by virtue of which we, who have come here from the far West and the farther East, do not now meet, for the first time, as strangers, but as friends, having common interests, and though of many nations, a common language, and whose thoughts are perhaps better known to each other than to some of our nearest neighbours.

It is usual to estimate that about one-thirtieth part of the whole mass of the world's literature belongs to medicine and its allied sciences. This corresponds very well to the results obtained from an examination of bibliographies, and catalogues of the principal medical libraries. It appears from this that our medical literature now forms a little over 120,000 volumes properly so called, and about twice that number of pamphlets, and that this accumulation is now increasing at the rate of about 1,500 volumes and 2,500 pamphlets yearly.

Let us consider the character of this annual growth somewhat in detail, first giving some figures as to the numbers of those who are producing it.

There are at the present time scattered over the earth about 180,000 medical men, who, by a liberal construction of the phrase, may be said to be educated; that is, who have some kind of a diploma; and for whose edification this current medical literature is produced. Of this number about 11,600 are producers of, or contributors to, this literature, being divided as follows: United States, 2,800; France and her Colonies, 2,600; the German Empire and Austro-Hungary, 2,300; Great Britain and her Colonies, 2,000; Italy, 600; Spain, 300: all others, 1,000.

Originally published in *Transactions of the International Medical Congress* (7th, London), Volume I (1881), pp. 54-70.

These figures should be considered in connection with the number of physicians in each country; but this I can only give approximately, as follows: United States 65,000; Great Britain and her Colonies, 35,000: Germany and Austro-Hungary, 32,000; France and her Colonies, 26,000; Italy, 10,000; Spain, 5,000; all others, 17,000.

It will be seen from these figures that the number of Physicians who are writers, is proportionately greatest in France and least in the United States. As regards France, this is largely due to the requirement of a printed thesis for graduation, which of itself adds between six and seven hundred annually to the number of writers.

Excluding popular medicine, pathies, pharmacy and dentistry, all of which were included in the figures for the annual product just given, we find that the contributions to medicine, properly so called, form a little over 1,000 volumes and 1,600 pamphlets yearly.

For 1879, Rupprecht's *Bibliotheca* gives as the total number of new medical books, excluding pamphlets, periodicals and transactions, 419; divided as follows, viz.: France, 187; Germany, 110; England, 43; Italy, 32; United States, 21; all others, 26. These figures are, however, too small, and especially so as regards Great Britain and the United States. The Index Medicus for the same year shows by analysis that the total number of medical books and pamphlets, excluding periodicals and transactions was 1,643; divided as follows: France, 541; Germany, 364; United States, 310; Great Britain, 182; all others, 246. This does not include the inaugural theses, of which 693 were published in France alone.

The special characteristics of the literature of the present day are largely due to Journals and Transactions, and this is particularly true in medicine. Our periodicals contain the most recent observations, the most original matter, and are the truest representations of the living thought of the day, and of the tastes and wants of the great mass of the medical profession, a large part of whom, in fact, read very little else. They form about one-half of the current medical literature, and in the year 1879 amounted to 655 volumes, of which the United States produced 156; Germany, 129; France, 122; Great Britain, 54; Italy, 65; and Spain, 24. This is exclusive of journals of pharmacy, dentistry, &c., and of journals devoted to medical sects and isms. These are given in an appended table from which it appears that the total number of volumes of medical journals and transactions of all kinds was for the year 1879,—850 and for 1880,—864. The figures for 1880 are too small, but the real increase is slight. During the year 1879, the total number of original articles in medical journals and transactions which were thought worth noting for the *Index Medicus* was a little over 20,000. Of these there appeared in American periodicals 4781, in French, 4608; in German, 4027; in English, 3592; in Italian, 1210; in Spanish, 703; in all others, 1248. The figures for 1880 are about the same. It will be seen that at present more of this class of literature appears in the English language than in any other, and that the number of journal contributions is greatest in the United States. The actual bulk of periodical literature is, however, greatest in Germany, owing to the greater average length of the articles. With regard to the mode of publication, I will only say that in all countries except Spain, the greater number of medical periodicals are monthly, while in Spain they are semi-monthly. It is this periodical literature which, more than anything else, makes medicine cosmopolitan, and although as regards new discoveries or methods of treatment, it is still somewhat farther from London or Berlin or Paris to New York, than it is from New York to either of these places, the discrepancy is gradually becoming less.

Many of the medical journals are very short lived, but the total number is increasing. In 1879, 23 such journals ceased, but 60 new ones appeared, and in 1880 there were 24 deaths and 78 births in this department of literature. Over one-third of this fluctuation occurs in the United States alone, France being next in the scale, Spain third and Italy fourth, while Great Britain is the most stable of all.

This merely quantitative classification gives of course no idea as to the character, and very little as to the value of the product. Let us now consider it by subjects. During 1879 there were published 167 books and pamphlets and 1,543 articles relating to anatomy, physiology and pathology—that is, to the biological or scientific side of medicine. Dividing this again by nations, we find that Germany produced a majority of the whole, France being second. The proportionate production by nations of this class of literature is perhaps better shown by an analysis of the bibliography of physiological literature for the year 1879, as published by the *Journal of Physiology*. This shows 59 treatises and 500 articles in German, 17 treatises and 227 articles in French, 5 treatises and 77 articles from Great Britain, 8 treatises and 41 articles from Italy, and 2 treatises and 24 articles from the United States. The number of authors for this product was, German, 393, French, 119, English, 59, Italian, 39, United States, 19, all others, 41. For the year 1880 the same journal reports 62 treatises and 452 articles from Germany, 23 treatises and 216 articles from France, 12 treatises and 76 articles from Great Britain, 4 treatises and 51 articles from Italy, 6 treatises and 25 articles from the United States, and 10 treatises and 31 articles from all other countries.*

When we turn to the literature of the art, or practical side of the profession the figures are decidedly different. We find over 1200 treatises and 18,000 journal articles which come under this head, and the order of precedence of countries as to quantity is: France, United States, Germany, Great Britain, Italy and Spain. The appended tables give still further subdivisions, showing by nations the number of works and journal articles upon the practice of medicine, surgery, obstetrics, hygiene, etc., for the years 1879 and 1880, and some of the figures will be found interesting. A marked increase has occurred in the literature of hygiene during the last two years, and this especially in England, France, Germany and the United States. The literature of diseases of the nervous system of ophthalmology, otology, dermatology, and gynæcology, is also increasing more rapidly than that of the more general branches.

It would of course be extremely unscientific to use these figures as if they

* The difference between these figures and those of the *Index Medicus*, is due, on the one hand, to the fact that the *Journal of Physiology* includes articles which are placed under other headings in the *Index Medicus*, and on the other hand, to the fact that the Journal has a different standard of excellence from that of the Index, rejecting many articles which the latter must accept as original.

represented positively ascertained and comparable facts, the accuracy of which, as well as of the classification, could be verified. They represent merely the opinions of an individual—first as to whether each treatise or pamphlet included in these statistics was worth noting, and second as how it should be classed. Had everything been indexed the figures, for journal articles at least, might have been nearly doubled ; while if the selection had been made by a more severe critic they might have been reduced one-half.

If I had to do the work again I should not obtain the same results. The prevailing error is that, as regards journal articles, the figures are too large, for some of those included are of so little value or interest that they are, I fear, never read by more than two persons.

Be that as it may, I think we can take them as indicating certain differences in the direction of work of the medical authors of the great civilized nations of the earth ; but they must be considered as approximations only; and the statistical axiom must be remembered that the results obtained from a large number of facts are applicable to an aggregate of similar facts but not to single cases. There will be a certain number of medical books and papers printed next year, just as there will be a certain number of children born ;—and as we can within certain limits predict the number of these births and the proportion of the sexes, or even of monsters ;—so we can within certain limits predict the amount and character of literature that is yet to come, the ideas that are yet unborn. The differences are due to race, political organization, and density of population. As Dr. Chadwick has pointed out, in speaking of the statistics of obstetric literature, one of the chief causes of the multiplication of medical societies is geographical. "In England it is possible for those who are specially interested in gynæcology and obstetrics to attend the meetings of the Obstetrical Society of London, whereas in America the distances are so great that this is impossible." Speaking broadly we may say that at present Germany leads in scientific medicine both in quantity and quality of product, and that the rising generation of physicians are learning German physiology. But the seed has gone abroad and scientific work is receiving more and more appreciation everywhere.

Seven years ago Professor Huxley declared that if a student in his own branch showed power and originality he dared not advise him to adopt a scientific career, for he could not give him the assurance that any amount of proficiency in the biological sciences would be convertible into the most modest bread and cheese. To-day I think he might be bolder, for such a fear would hardly be justifiable ; at all events, in America; where such a man as is referred to could almost certainly find a place, bearing in mind the Professor's remark that it is no impediment to an original investigator to have to devote a moderate portion of his time to giving instruction either in the laboratory or in the lecture room.

Within the last ten years the literature of France, Germany, Great Britain, and the United States has contained much with regard to medical education and the means for its improvement. In all these countries there is more or less dissatisfaction with the existing condition of things, although there is no general agreement as to the remedy. Solomon's question, "Wherefore is there a price in the hands of a fool to get wisdom, seeing he hath no heart to it?" is now easily answered, for even a fool knows that he must have the semblance of wisdom, and a diploma to imply it, if he is to succeed in the practice of medicine; but to ensure the value of a diploma as a proof of education is the difficulty.

This evidence of discontent and tendency to change is a good sign. In these matters stillness means sleep or death—and the fact that a stream is continually changing its bed shows that its course lies through fertile alluvium and not through sterile lava or granite.

I have said that as regards scientific medicine we are at present going to school to Germany. This, however, is not the case with regard to therapeutics either external or internal,—in regard to which I presume that the physicians of each nation are satisfied as to their own pre-eminence. At all events it is true that, for the treatment of the common diseases, a physician can obtain his most valuable instruction in his own country; among those whom he is to treat. Just as each individual is in some respects peculiar and unique, so that even the arrangement of the minute ridges and furrows at the end of his forefinger differs from that of all other forefingers, and is sufficient to identify him; and as the members of certain families require special care to guard against hæmorrhage, or insanity, or phthisis; so it is with nations and races. The experienced military surgeon knows this well, and in the United States, which is now the great mixing ground, illustrations of race peculiarities are familiar to every practitioner.

Neither the tendency nor the true value of this current medical literature can be properly estimated by attending to it alone. It is a part of the thought of the age—of that wonderful kaleidoscopic pattern which is unrolling before us, and must be judged in connection with it. From several sources of high authority there have come of late years warnings and laments that science is becoming too utilitarian. For example, Prof. Du Bois-Reymond in his address upon civilization and science, says that that side of science which is connected with the useful arts is steadily becoming more prominent, each generation being more and more bent on material interests. "Amid the unrest which possesses the civilized world men's minds live as it were from hand to mouth. . . . . And if industry receives its impulse from science it also has a tendency to destroy science. In short, idealism is succumbing in the struggle with realism and the kingdom of material interests is coming." Having laid down this rather pessimistic platform, he goes on to state that this is especially the case in America which is the principal home of utilitarianism, and that it has become the custom to characterize as "Americanization" the dreaded permeation of European civilization by realism. If this characterization be correct it would seem that Europe is pretty thoroughly Americanized as regards attention to material interests and appreciation of practical results. But the truth of the picture seems to me doubtful. Science is becoming popular, even fashionable, and some of its would-be votaries rival the devotees of modern Æstheticism in their dislike and fear of the sunlight of comprehensibility and common sense. The languid scientific swell who thinks it bad style to be practical, who takes no interest in any thing but pure science, and makes it a point to refrain from any investigations which might lead to useful results lest he might be confounded with mere "practical men" or "inventors," exists and has his admirers. We have such in medicine, and their number will increase.

The separation of biological study from practical medicine, which has of late years become quite marked in the literature of the subject, has its advantages and disadvantages. Thus far the former have far outweighed the latter, and both the science and the art of medicine have been promoted thereby. But are not the physiologists, or as I believe they prefer to be called, the biologists, separating themselves too completely from medicine for the best interests of their own science, in that they are neglecting human pathology? In our hospital wards and among our patients, nature is continually performing experiments which the most dexterous operator cannot copy in the laboratory—she is, as Professor Foster says, "a relentless and untrammelled vivisector, and there is no secret of the living frame which she has not laid, or will not at some time or place lay, bare in misery and pain."

Now while it is true that Professor Foster, in his address before the British Medical Association last year (which address is the clearest exposition of the aims of the physiology of the present day that I have seen), insists upon the fact that all distinctions between physiology and pathology are fictitious, and declares that attempts to divide them are like attempts to divide meteorology into a science of good and a science of bad weather, his conclusion that the pathologist should be trained in methods of physiological investigation seems to me to be only a part of the truth. The tacit assumption is that all, or at least the most important, phenomena of human disease may be reproduced in the physiological laboratory. If this were only true, what a tremendous stride would have been taken towards making medicine a science. Unfortunately it is not so. Many of the most interesting of these phenomena—the most interesting because as yet the most unexplainable—can only be observed in the sick man himself. Nor have the physiologists as yet made much use of that field which ought to be specially inviting to them—namely: comparative pathology; although the literature of the present time already indicates that a change has begun in this respect.

While it is true that to the graduate of thirty years ago much of the physiological literature of the present day is in an unknown tongue, it is also true that the physiologist of the present, who confines himself to laboratory work, will find himself distanced by the man who keeps his clinical and pathological studies and his experimental work well abreast.

The increase in both the amount and value of the literature of the several specialities in medicine is readily seen by a comparison of recent catalogues and bibliographies with those of twenty or thirty years ago, and this increase still continues at a greater rate than prevails in the more general branches. There are great differences of opinion as to the relative value of this increase and as to its future effect upon the profession, but there can be no doubt as to the fact. There must be specialities and specialists in medicine, and the results will be both good and evil; but the evils fall largely upon those specialists who have an insufficient general education,—who attempt to construct the pyramid of their knowledge with the small end as a foundation. It has been said by Dr. Hodgen that "in medicine a specialist should be a skilled physician and something more, but that he is often something else—and something less." There is truth in this: truth which the young man will do well to consider with care before he begins to specialize his studies; but on the other hand it is also true that the great majority of men must limit their field of work very much and very clearly if they hope to achieve success. The tool must have an edge if it is to cut. It is by the labour of specialists that many of the new channels for thought and research have been opened, and if the flood has sometimes seemed to spread too far, and to lose itself in shallow and sandy places, it has nevertheless tended to fertilize them in the end.

The specialists are not only making the principal advances in science but they are furnishing both strong incentives and valuable assistance towards the collection and preservation of medical literature and the formation of large public libraries.

Burton declares that a great library cannot be improvised, not even if one had the national debt to do it with—thinks that 20,000 volumes is about the limit of what a miscellaneous collection can bring together, and refers especially to the difficulty in creating large public libraries in America. My experience would show that these statements do not apply to medical books. Of these the folios and quartos of three and four hundred years ago seem to have had great capacity for resistance to ordinary destructive forces. Perhaps much of this is due to the fact that they are not usually injured by too much handling or perusal. True, they are gradually becoming rarer, but at the same time by means of properly organized libraries they are becoming more accessible to all who wish to really use them, and not merely to collect and hide them away. They drift about like the sea weed, but the survivors are gradually finding secure aud permanent resting-places in the score of great collections of such literature which the world now possesses. At present the currents of trade are carrying them in relatively large numbers to the United States, where medical collectors and specialists are among the best customers of the antiquarian booksellers of Europe. I could name a dozen American physicians who have given to European agents almost unlimited orders for books relating to their several specialities, and upon their shelves may be found books of the fifteenth and sixteenth centuries, which may be properly marked as "rarissime."

Not that the rarest books are by any means the oldest. The collector who seeks to ornament his shelves with the "Rose of John of Gaddesden," or the "Lily of Bernard de Gordon," the first folios of "Avicenna" or "Celsus," or almost any of the eight hundred medical incunabulæ described by Hain, will probably succeed in his quest quite as soon as the one who has set his heart on the first editions of Harvey or Jenner, the American tracts on inoculation for small-pox, or complete sets of many of the Journals and Transactions of the present century.

Whatever may be the chosen line of the book collector, he is the special helper of the public library, and this whether he intend it or not. In most cases his treasures pass through the auction room, and sooner or later the librarian, who can afford to wait, will secure them from further travel. Thanks to the labours of such collectors, I think it is safe to say,—what certainly would not have been true twenty years ago,—that if the entire medical literature of the world with the exception of that which is collected in the United States, were to be now destroyed, nearly all of it that is valuable could be reproduced without difficulty.

What is to be the result of this steadily increasing production of books? What will the libraries and catalogues and bibliographies of a thousand, or even of a hundred years hence be like, if we are thus to go on in the ratio of geometric progression, which has governed the press for the last few decades? The mathematical formula which would express this, based on the data of the past century, gives an absurd and impossible conclusion, for it shows that if we go on as we have been going there is coming a time when our libraries will become large cities, and when it will require the services of every one in the world, not engaged in writing, to catalogue and care for the annual product. The truth is, however, that the ratio has changed, and that the rate of increase is becoming smaller. In western Europe, which is now the great centre of literary production, it does not seem probable that the number of writers or readers will materially increase in the future, and it is in America, Russia, and southern Asia, that the greatest difference will be found between the present amount of annual literary product and that of a century hence.

The analogies between the mental and physical development of an individual and of a nation or society, have been often set forth and commented on, but there is one point where the analogy fails as regards the products of mental activity,—and that is that as yet we have devised no process for getting rid of the exuviæ. Growth and development in the physical world imply the changes of death as well as of life—that with the increase of the living tissues there shall also be the excretion and destruction of dead, outgrown, and useless matters which have had their day and served their purpose. But *litera scripta manet.* There is a vast amount of this effete and worthless material in the literature of medicine, and it is increasing rapidly. Our literature is in fact something like the inheritance of the golden dustman, but with this important difference—viz., that when the children raked a few shells or bits of bone from the dustman's heap—and, after stringing them together and playing with them a little while, threw them back—they did not thereby add to the bulk of the pile; whereas our preparers of compilations and compendiums, big and little, acknowledged or not, are continually increasing the collection, and for the most part with material which has been characterized as "superlatively middling, the quintessential extract of mediocrity." A large medical library is in itself discouraging to many inquirers, and I have become quite familiar with the peculiar expression of mingled surprise, awe, and despair which is apt to steal over the face of one not accustomed to such work when he first finds himself fairly in the presence of the mass of material which he wishes to examine for the purpose of completing his ideal bibliography of—let us say epilepsy, or excisions, or the functions of the liver.

Let such inquirers, as well as those who regret that they have no access to large libraries, and must therefore rely on the common text books and current periodicals for bibliography, console themselves with the reflection that much the larger part of all of our literature which has any practical value belongs to the present century, and indeed will be found in the publications of the last 20 years.

There are a few books written prior to 1800 which every well educated medical man should—I will not say read but—dip into, such as some of the works of Hippocrates and Galen, of Harvey and Hunter, of Morgagni and Sydenham—but this is to be done to learn their methods and style rather than their facts or theories, and by the great majority of physicians it can be done with much more profit in modern translations than in the originals. The really valuable part of the observations of these old masters has long ago become a part of the common stock, and the results are to be found in every text book.

If, perchance, among the dusty folios there are stray golden grains yet ungleaned, remember that just in front are whole fields waiting the reaper. There is not, and has not been any lack of men who have the taste and time to search the records of the past, and the man who has opportunities to make experiments or observations for himself wastes his time, to a certain extent, if he tries to do bibliographical work so long as he can get it done for him. He wishes to know whether this problem has been attacked before, and with what result—whether there are accounts of any other cases like the one he has in hand. In ninety-nine instances out of a hundred if the answer to these questions is not given in the current text books or monographs it is not worth prolonged search by the original investigator. Yet he should know how to make this search, if only to enable him to direct others, and it is for this reason that a little acquaintance with bibliographical methods of work ought to be obtained by the student.

When a physician has observed (or thinks he has observed) a fact, or has evolved from his inner consciousness a theory which he wishes to examine by the light of medical literature, he is often very much at a loss to know how to begin, even when he has a large library accessible for the purpose.

The information he desires may be in the volume next his hand, but how is he to know that? And even when the usual subject-catalogue is placed before him he finds it very difficult to use it, especially when, as is often the case, he has by no means a well defined idea as to what it is he wishes to look for. Upon the title page of the Washington City Directory is printed the following aphorism, "To find a name you must know how to spell it." This has a very extensive application in medical bibliography. To find accounts of cases similar to your own rare case you must know what your own case is.

To return to the Subject-Catalogue. If it is a classed catalogue, a catalogue raisonnée—it will often seem to be a very blind guide to one who is not familiar with the classification and nomenclature adopted by the compiler. And certainly some of these classifications are very curious—reminding one of Heine's division of ideas into reasonable ideas, unreasonable ideas, and ideas covered with green leather. But if the inquirer has mastered the arrangement of the catalogue it is two to one that it will not help him. It is a catalogue of the titles of books, but very often the title of a book gives very little information as to its contents, if indeed it is not actually misleading. Now suppose the particular case he has in hand is one of a new-born infant having one leg much larger and longer than the other. He will find no book title relating to this. There may be a book in the library on diseases of the lymphatics which contains just what he wants, but unless he knows that his case is one affecting the lymphatics he will hardly get the clue. There may also be in the library twenty papers, in as many different volumes of journals and transactions, the titles of which show that they probably relate to similar cases, but the titles of such papers do not appear in the catalogue.

It should also be observed that Subject-Catalogues may easily be put to improper uses, or thought to give more information than they really do. They are not bibliographies, but mechanical aids in bibliographical work.

You will, perhaps, pardon me for taking as an illustration the Index Catalogue of the library of the Surgeon-General's office in Washington, as being one with which I am familiar, and which I can venture to comment on without risk of its being thought that I wish to depreciate its value. Taking any given subject in medicine, it is possible for a fairly educated physician to obtain from this catalogue a large proportion of all the references which have any special value, and by so doing to save a vast amount of time and labour. On the other hand, he will find when he comes to examine the books and articles referred to, that at least one-half of them are of no value so long as the other half are accessible, seeing that they are dilutions and dilatations, re-hashes and summaries of the really original papers. If the seeker is in the library itself, this does not cause a great waste of time, as he can rapidly examine and lay aside those that do not serve his purpose But if he is using this catalogue in another library—say here in London, the case is different. It is highly improbable that he will find in any other collection all the books referred to, and then comes the annoyance of the doubt as to whether he may not be missing some very valuable paper. How is he to know whether or not Smith, in his pamphlet on the functions of the pneumogastric, has anticipated his own theory of its relations to enlarged tonsils? And in all such cases "omne ignotum est pro magnifico." In a bibliography of the subject, prepared from the same material as the catalogue, he would either find no mention of Smith's paper, or, better still, a note that his paper is merely an abstract, or compilation. The fact that he does not find Smith's book in the London library, nor any allusion to it in the best works on the subject, ought to induce him to ignore it altogether.

In proportion to the energy of the young writer, and his determination to not only note everything that has been written about his subject, but to carry out the golden rule of verifying all his references, he is apt to be led off from his direct research into the many attractive by-paths of quaint and curious speculation which he will find branching off on every side, and this danger must be guarded against, or he will find that he is wasting his time and energy in turning over chaff which has long ago been pretty thoroughly threshed and winnowed.

It is, however, no part of my present purpose to set forth the methods and principles of bibliography; it is sufficient to point out their importance, and to call attention to the point that a knowledge of how and where to find the record of a fact is often of more practical use than a knowledge of the fact itself, just as we value an encyclopædia for occasional reference, and not for the purpose of reading through from cover to cover.

Instruction in the history and literature of medicine forms no part of the course of medical education in English and American schools; nor should I be disposed to recommend its introduction into the curriculum if it were to be based on French and German models, but it does seem possible to take a step in this direction which would be of great value, not only as a means of general culture, as teaching students how to think, but from a purely practical point of view, in teaching them how to use the implements of their profession to the best advantage—for books are properly compared to tools of which the index is the handle. Such instruction should be given in a library, just as chemistry should be taught in a laboratory. The way to learn history and bibliography is to make them—the best work of the instructor is to show his students how to make them.

In the absence of some instruction of this kind the student is liable to waste much time in bibliographical research. There has been much more done in this direction than many writers seem to suppose, and there are not many subjects in medicine which have not been treated from this point of view. Of course all is not bibliography which pretends to be such. Very many of the exhaustive and exhausting lists of references which are now so common in medical journal articles have been taken largely at second-hand, and thereby originate or perpetuate errors. It is well to avoid false pride in this matter. To overlook a reference is by no means discreditable,—but a wrong reference, or an unwitting reference to the same thing twice, gives a strong presumption of carelessness and second-hand work. Journal articles, however, and especially reports of cases, undergo strange transmogrifications sometimes, and I have watched this with interest in the case of a French or German paper, translated and condensed in the *London Record*, then appearing in abstract under the name of the translator in a leading journal, then translated again, with a few new circumstances, in a continental periodical, and finally perhaps reversed and appearing as an original contribution in the pages of the *Little Peddlington Medical Universe*.

In this connection it is well to remember that a mere accumulation of observations, no matter how great the number, does not constitute science, especially if these observations have been recorded under the influence of the same theories and in essentially similar conditions.

Science seeks the law which governs or explains the phenomena, and when this is found the records of isolated instances of its action usually become of small importance so far as that law is concerned. We care little now for the records of the chemical experiments of a century ago, and the many detailed accounts of the earlier cases of the use of ether or chloroform are of so little interest at the present time that it is not worth while to refer to them in a bibliography of the subject. And although much has been done towards classifying and indexing our medical records, more in fact than most physicians suppose, still, as Helmholtz points out, such knowledge as this hardly deserves the name of science, since it neither enables us to see the complete connection nor to predict the result under new conditions yet untried.

Do I seem to depreciate the value of the thoughts which our masters have left us, and which have furnished the foundations on which we build—or to undervalue the importance of the great medical libraries in which are stored these thoughts—or to speak slightly of the utility of the catalogues, and indexes, and bibliographies, without which such libraries are trackless and howling wildernesses? If so, I have said what I did not mean to say. The subject has been considered from the point of view of what used to be called the division of labour, but which now I suppose should be called evolution and differentiation, and this has been done because life is short and the art is long,—with fair prospect of becoming longer. It is surely unnecessary for me to enter upon any panegyric of books or libraries. As Dr. Holmes says: "It is not necessary to maintain the direct practical utility of all kinds of learning. Our shelves contain many books which only a certain class of medical scholars will be likely to consult. There is a dead medical literature, and there is a live one. The dead is not all ancient, the live is not all modern. There is none, modern or ancient, which, if it has no living value for the student, will not teach him something by its autopsy. But it is with the live literature of his profession that the medical practitioner is first of all concerned."

In medicine, as in social science, we must depend for many facts upon the observation of conditions which occur very rarely, and which cannot be repeated at pleasure. I have already alluded to the importance of Nature's vivisections to the physiologist, and a record of a case written a century ago may be just the link that is needed to correlate the results of his experiments of yesterday with existing theories. The case, which at first seems unique and inexplicable, both receives and furnishes light when compared with ancient records.

A science of medicine, like other sciences, must depend upon the classification of facts, upon the comparison of cases alike in many respects, but differing somewhat either in their phenomena or in the environment. The great obstacle to the development of a science of medicine is the difficulty in ascertaining what cases are sufficiently similar to be comparable—which difficulty is in its turn largely due to insufficient and erroneous records of the phenomena observed. This defect in the records is largely due—first, to ignorance on the part of observers; second, to the want of proper means for precisely recording the phenomena; and third, to the confused and faulty condition of our nomenclature and nosological classification.

Let us consider each of these points briefly. Very, very few are the men who can, by and for themselves, see and describe the things that are before them. Just as it took thousands of years to produce a man who could see what now any one can see when shown him, that the star Alpha in Capricorn is really two separate stars, so we had to wait long before the man came who could see the difference between measles and scarlatina, and still longer for the one who could distinguish between typhus and typhoid. Said Plato, "He shall be as a god to me, who can rightly divide and define." Men who have this faculty—the *Blick* of the Germans—we cannot produce directly by any system of education; they come we know not when or why, "forming a small band, a mere understanding of whose thoughts and works is a test of our highest powers. A single English dramatist, and a single English mathematician have probably equalled in scope and excellence of original work in their several fields all the like labours of their countrymen put together."*

But cannot we do something to increase the number of observers by telling them what to observe? It is probable that much may be accomplished in this direction provided that care be taken to limit the field. Manuals of "what to observe at the bedside and in the post-mortem room" are very well in their way, but can never be made to reach the great majority of the profession, nor would they be of much use if they did. If a few, a very few, distinct specific questions are brought to the attention of the general practitioner, he will often be on the alert for their answer. And it should be remembered that chance may present to the most obscure practitioner an opportunity for observation which the greatest master may never meet.

The great difficulty is to get such questions prepared. They must relate to matters that are just in the nebulous region between the known and unknown—to

* Iles, Mathematics in Evolution. *Pop. Sci. Monthly*, 1876, ix. p. 207.

points not yet clear, but of which we know enough to make it probable that by observing in a definite direction they can be made clear; and to prepare them requires not only knowledge, but a certain reaching out beyond knowledge. It usually happens that the man who has this faculty strives to answer his questions himself; and no doubt he can usually do it better than another. But much can be done towards defining and marking out what we do not know, and this has been a powerful aid to the progress of physiology in recent years.

I have had occasion to refer to this in speaking of Professor Foster's work on physiology, in each section of which an attempt is made to separate that which may be considered as proved from that which is merely probable; and thus almost every page becomes suggestive of work to be done.

Another example of what I mean will be found in a paper on the collection of data at autopsies by Professor H. P. Bowditch of Boston (*Trans. Mass. Med.-Legal Soc.* i., 1880, p. 139). Taking the results of an investigation into the absolute and relative size of organs at different periods of life, and in connection with different morbid tendencies, recently published by Professor Beneke of Warburg, Dr. Bowditch urges the securing as large a number as possible of such data, and selects certain of Professor Beneke's results for special inquiry; as, for instance, that "the cancerous diathesis is associated with a large and powerful heart, capacious arteries, but a relatively small pulmonary artery, small lungs well developed bones and muscles, and tolerably abundant adipose tissue." It can hardly be doubted that those who read the papers of Professors Bowditch and Beneke will be induced to examine things which before would have had for them no interest, and therefore to make and record observations in pathological anatomy which otherwise would have been lost.

The second difficulty referred to—viz.: the want of means for making accurate records, is one that is yearly growing less. It behoves us to be modest in our predictions as to what may be accomplished in the future towards the solution of our Sphinx's riddle. We see as through a glass darkly, and except through the glass, in no wise; but at least we have made such progress that what we do see we can to a great extent so record that our successors yet unborn can also see—and it is owing to this fact that a part of the medical literature of the last quarter of the nineteenth century will be more valuable than all that has preceded it.

The word-pictures of disease traced by Hippocrates and Sydenham, or even those of Graves and Trousseau, interesting and valuable as they are, are not comparable with the records upon which the skilled clinical teacher of the present day relies. Yet how imperfect in many cases are even the best of these records as compared with what might be given with the resources which we have at our command. The temperature chart has done away with the errors which necessarily follow attempts to compare the memory of sensations perceived last week with the sensations of to-day—and the balance and the burette enable us to estimate with some approach to precision the tissue changes of our patients by the records of change in the excretions which they furnish; but we must still trust to our memory, or to the imperfect descriptions of what others remember, when we attempt to compare the results obtained on successive days by auscultation or percussion, although the phonograph and microphone strongly hint to us the possibility of either accurately reproducing the sounds of yesterday, or of translating them into visible signs, perhaps something like the dot and dash record of the telegraph code, which could then be given to the press, and so compared with each other by readers at the Antipodes.

We are beginning to count the blood corpuscles, and to use photomicrography, but we do not yet apply the latter process to the former so as to enable every reader to count for himself.

The connections of medicine with the physical sciences are yearly becoming closer, and the methods by which these sciences have been brought to their present condition are those by which progress has been, and is to be, made in therapeutics as well as in diagnosis or in physiological research. These methods turn mainly upon increasing the delicacy and accuracy of measurements: of expressing manifestations of force in terms of another force, or of dimension in space or time. The balance and the galvanometer, the microscope and the pendulum, the camera, the sphygmograph and the thermometer are some of the means by which investigators, at the bedside and in the laboratory, are seeking to obtain records which shall be independent of their own sensations or personal equations; which shall be taken and used as expressing not opinions but facts; and with every addition to or improvement in these means of measurement and record, the field of observation widens, and new and more reliable materials are furnished for the application of logical and mathematical methods.

Upon the third difficulty which has been referred to,—viz: our confused and defective terminology I need not dwell. "Science," said Condillac, "is a language well made," and though this is far from being the whole truth, it is an important part of it. In examining medical reports and statistics, it is necessary to bear constantly in mind that to understand many terms you must know what the individual writer means by them. When, for example, we find in such statistics a certain number of deaths attributed to gastro-enteritis, or croup, or scrofula, we have to take into account the country, the period and the individual author in order to get even a fair presumption as to what is meant.

The three difficulties which have been referred to, although the most important, are by no means the only causes of the confusion and imperfection of our records.

Prominent among the minor troubles of the investigator are defective or misleading titles; and in behalf of the readers and bibliographers of the future I would appeal to authors, and more especially to editors, to pay more attention than many of them do to the matter of titles and indexes. The men to whom your papers are most important, and who will make the best use of them provided they knew of their existence, are for the most part hard workers, busy men, who have a right to demand that their literary table shall be provided with properly prepared materials and not with shapeless lumps.

The editors of transactions of societies, whether these are sent to journals, or published in separate form, often commit numerous sins of omission in the matter of titles. The rule should be that every article which is worth printing is worth a distinct title, which should be as concise as a telegram, and be printed in a special type. If the author does not furnish such a title it is the editor's business to make it, and he should not be satisfied with such headings as "Clinical Cases," "Difficult Labour," "A Remarkable Tumour," "Case of Wound, with Remarks." The four rules for the preparation of an article for a journal will then be: 1. Have something to say; 2. Say it; 3. Stop as soon as you have said it; 4. Give the paper a proper title.

Some societies and editors do not seem to appreciate fully their responsibility for the articles which they accept for publication, a responsibility which cannot be altogether avoided by any formal declaration disclaiming it. This is due to the fact that while the merits of a paper can usually be determined by examination, this is by no means always the case. In every country there are writers and speakers whose statements are received with very great distrust by those best acquainted with them. Supposing these statements to be true, the papers would be of much interest and importance; but the editor should remember that a certain number of readers, and especially those in foreign countries, have no clue to the character of the author, beyond the fact that they find his works in good company. In medical literature, as in other departments, we find books and papers from men who are either constitutionally incapable of telling the simple literal truth as to their observations and experiments, although they may not write with fixed intention to deceive, or from men who seek to advertise themselves by deliberate falsehoods as to the results of their practice. Such men are usually appreciated at their true value in their immediate neighbourhood, and find it necessary to send their communications to distant journals and societies in order to secure publication.

I presume that you are all familiar with the peculiar feeling of distrust which is roused by too complete an explanation. The report of a case in which every symptom observed, and the effect of every remedy given, is fully accounted for, and in which no residual unexplained phenomena appear, is usually suspicious, for it implies either superficial observation, or suppression, or distortion of some of the facts. A diagrammatic representation is usually much plainer than a good photograph, but also of much less value as a basis for further work.

No fact is more familiar to this audience than the vast extent of the field of the science of to-day—so vast that few may hope to master more than a small part of it, and yet so closely connected that even the small part cannot be fully grasped without some acquaintance with a much wider field.

But little over a hundred years ago, Haller in Göttingen was professor of anatomy, botany, physiology, surgery, and obstetrics, and lecturer on medical jurisprudence. At the same time he was writing one review a week, and summing up existing medical science in his bibliothecæ. To-day any one of these branches requires all the time of the most energetic and learned of our contemporaries; but, on the other hand, the well-educated medical graduate of to-day could give Haller valuable instruction in each of the branches of which he was professor. It is also true, as I have pointed out, that our actual progress is by no means in proportion to the work done, nor as great as these merely quantitative statements would seem to make it.

Science has been termed "the topography of ignorance." "From a few elevated points we triangulate vast spaces, enclosing infinite unknown details. We cast the lead and draw up a little sand from abysses we shall never reach with our dredges. If it is true that we understand ourselves but imperfectly in health, it is more signally manifest in disease, where natural actions imperfectly understood, disturbed in an obscure way by half seen causes, are creeping and winding along in the dark toward their destined issue, sometimes using our remedies as safe stepping stones, occasionally, it may be, stumbling over them as obstacles."*

In days of old, when the profession of medicine, or of a single medical specialty, was an inheritance in certain families, a large part of their knowledge, and the efficiency of their remedies was thought to depend upon these being kept a profound mystery. Among the precepts of magic there was no more significant one than that which declared that the communication of the formula destroyed its power, and that hence attempts to reveal the secret must always fail. We have changed all that. Every physician hastens to publish his discoveries and special knowledge, and a good many do the same by that which is not special, or which is not knowledge. For the individual, in a degree—for the nation or the race in a much greater degree—the literature produced is the most enduring memorial. The whole result of civilization has been cynically defined as being roughly, "Three hundred million Chinese, two hundred million natives of India, two hundred million Europeans and North Americans, and a miscellaneous hundred million or two of Central Asians, Malays, South Sea Islanders, &c., and over and above all the rest the Library of the British Museum. This is the net result of an indefinitely long struggle between the forces of men and the weights of various kinds in the attempt to move which these forces display themselves."†

And thus in our great medical libraries each of the folios or quaint little black letter pamphlets which mark the first two centuries of printing, or of the cheap and dirty volumes of more modern days with their scrofulous paper and abominable typography, represents to a great extent the life of one of our profession and the fruit of his labours, and it is by the fruit that we know him.

After stating that modern physicists have concluded that the sun is going out, that the earth is falling into the sun, and therefore that it and all things in it will be either fried or frozen, Professor Clifford concludes that "our interest lies so much with the past as may serve to guide our actions in the present, and with so much of the future as we may hope will be affected by our actions now. Beyond that we do not know and ought not to care. Does this seem to say let us eat and drink for to-morrow we die? Not so, but rather let us take hands and help for this day we are alive together." To this I join a verse from the Talmud which will remind you of the first aphorism of Hippocrates, and is none the worse for that. "The day is short, and work is great,—the reward is also great, and the master presses. It is not incumbent on thee to complete the work, but thou must not therefore cease from it.

* "Border Lines of Knowledge," &c., by O. W. Holmes, Boston, 1862, pp. 7-8.
† "Liberty, Equality, and Fraternity," by James Fitz James Stephen, N.Y., 1873, p. 18.

TABLE I.

The Number of Volumes of Medical Journals and Transactions Published in the Years 1879 and 1880.

Subjects.	Journals and Transactions.	United States.		Gt. Brit. and Colonies.		France & Colonies.		Germany		Spain.		Italy.		All Others.		Total.	
		1879	1880	1879	1880	1879	1880	1879	1880	1879	1880	1879	1880	1879	1880	1879	1880
General and Miscellaneous, Practical Medicine, &c.	Journals	75	83	26	26	60	63	41	43	22	26	42	42	70	72	336	355
	Transactions ...	56	54	11	12	30	19	31	31	1	1	9	7	31	27	169	151
Anatomy, Physiology, Morphology, Biology.	Journals			4	4	5	5	15	17	1		1			1	26	27
	Transactions ...	1	1			4	2									5	3
Diseases of Nervous System and Insanity.	Journals	3	5	4	4	2	3	5	5			3	4			17	21
	Transactions ...					1										1	
Surgery.	Journals		1					3	3							3	4
	Transactions ...					1	1	1	1							2	2
Ophthalmology.	Journals	1	1	1	2	4	4	5	5	3	3	3	3	2	2	19	20
	Transactions ...							1	1			1				2	1
Skin Diseases.	Journals	1	1	1	1	1	1	1	1			1	1			5	5
	Transactions ...	1	1													1	1
Otology.	Journals	2	2			1	1	3	3							6	6
	Transactions ...	1														1	
Gynæcology and Obstetrics.	Journals	2	2	1	1	5	7	6	6	1		2	2	1	2	18	20
	Transactions ...	3	1	2	1											5	2
Hygiene and Medical Jurisprudence.	Journals	6	6	2	3	5	5	13	13	1	3	3	4	6	6	36	40
	Transactions ...	3	3	2	4	3	2	4	3					1	1	13	13
Pharmacy and Medical Chemistry.	Journals	7	9	7	6	5	5	15	15	5	5	5	5	9	9	53	54
	Transactions ...	4	3			3	1	1								8	4
Dentistry.	Journals	6	10			2	2	2	3							10	15
	Transactions ...																
Homœopathy.	Journals	12	16	4	4	3	3	7	7	1	1	3	2	3	3	33	36
	Transactions ...	3	3			2	1									5	4
Eclectic, Botanic, Physio-Medical, &c.	Journals	11	13													11	13
	Transactions ...	2	2													2	2
Popular, Advertising, Mineral Waters, &c.	Journals	8	10	4	4	12	8	5	5	2	2	2	2	2	2	35	33
	Transactions ...					1	1									1	1
Veterinary.	Journals	1	3	3	3	4	4	11	10			4	5	4	4	27	29
	Transactions ...																
Laryngology .	Journals		1				1										2
	Transactions ...		1														1
Total	Journals	135	163	57	58	109	112	132	136	36	40	69	70	97	101	635	680
	Transactions ...	74	69	15	17	45	27	38	36	1	1	10	7	32	28	215	184

TABLE II.

The Medical Literature of 1879 *and* 1880.

Subjects.	No. of	United States.		England.		France.		Germany.		Italy.		Spain.		Others.		Total.	
		1879	1880	1879	1880	1879	1880	1879	1880	1879	1880	1879	1880	1879	1880	1879	1880
Anatomy and Physiology.	Books	7	17	19	18	60	32	54	31	5	2	1	1	26	8	172	106
	Theses					25	24	4							6	29	30
	Jour. Articles ...	162	177	157	176	385	351	458	420	109	105	26	32	74	68	1371	1329
Pathology	Books	2	3		2	13	5	7	6							22	16
	Theses					11	7	3	1					2	1	16	9
	Jour. Articles ...	32	32	25	27	36	51	35	56	13	12	5	5	12	19	158	202
Practice of Medicine.	Books	52	27	39	51	132	104	78	56	7	12	9	2	55	12	372	264
	Theses					248	216	7	12					2	7	257	235
	Jour. Articles ...	1454	1154	1085	918	1340	1056	1001	812	316	257	198	171	405	348	5799	4716
Diseases of Nervous System.	Books	38	32	19	30	33	48	32	23	1	4	1		11	7	135	144
	Theses					56	51	3	4					4	4	63	59
	Jour. Articles ...	406	410	342	303	380	355	372	332	112	124	50	43	99	100	1761	1607
Surgery.	Books	18	27	5	23	62	63	36	29	2	4	1		16	15	135	150
	Theses					144	144	15	6	1				5	11	165	161
	Jour. Articles ...	894	823	844	706	706	597	539	513	198	180	136	23	160	145	3477	3087
Opthalmology.	Books	10	15	7	7	13	18	20	17		1	5	1	5	5	60	64
	Theses					41	32	1	1					2	1	44	34
	Jour. Articles ...	187	228	81	101	310	252	254	271	59	58	52	52	49	45	992	1007
Otology.	Books	3	9	3	1	2	7	2	6					2		12	23
	Theses					7	9	1								8	9
	Jour. Articles ...	114	185	38	74	31	73	102	158	11	9	5	16	12	20	313	535
Skin Diseases.	Books	3	9	2	8	11	12	15	10	1	2		2	1	1	33	44
	Theses					21	24	1								22	24
	Jour. Articles ...	63	95	115	101	62	138	99	109	51	53	20	27	31	24	441	547
Venereal.	Books	1	2	4	4	19	13	5	6		3			6	1	35	29
	Theses					19	19									19	19
	Jour. Articles ...	76	72	45	31	106	96	94	56	42	31	17	22	19	32	399	348
Gynæcology.	Books	12	16	2	6	12	13	13	12	3	2	1		4	1	47	50
	Theses					40	25	3	2					1		44	27
	Jour. Articles ...	364	416	239	189	200	200	192	186	60	66	27	27	48	48	1130	1132
Obstetrics.	Books	6	7	6	8	17	16	8	13		5	1	1	7	1	45	52
	Theses					33	47	2	1					1	1	37	49
	Jour. Articles ...	435	430	216	195	293	211	173	142	80	55	22	30	51	57	1270	1114
Hygiene.	Books	62	80	29	48	39	80	29	28	3	5		2	16	4	178	247
	Theses					2	13								3	2	16
	Jour. Articles ...	173	239	161	237	186	271	235	202	27	26	33	30	76	56	891	1061
Jurisprudence.	Books	2	2	1	1	9	18	2	4		4			1	1	15	30
	Theses					8	9		2							8	11
	Jour. Articles ...	72	167	44	103	85	173	80	160	33	46	18	28	36	49	368	726
General and Miscellaneous.	Books	94	96	46	52	119	144	61	64	6	6	2	2	52	13	382	377
	Theses					22	50	2	7					5	6	29	63
	Jour. Articles ...	349	476	200	274	488	556	393	411	99	142	94	79	176	178	1799	2116
Total by Countries.	Books	310	339	182	259	541	573	364	306	28	50	21	11	197	58	1643	1596
	Theses					677	670	42	36	1				23	40	743	746
	Jour. Articles ...	4781	4904	3592	3443	4608	4380	4027	3828	1210	1164	703	685	1248	1183	20,169	19,587

On the Library of a Medical School*

By William Osler, M.D.

One day last spring a London bookseller called and said he had a library of seventeenth and eighteenth century medical books for sale, which had been gathered by the physicians connected with the Warrington Dispensary. Looking over the catalogue I saw at once that it was a collection of value, and knowing that it would supplement very nicely the special libraries which have gradually grown up in connection with the Johns Hopkins Medical School, I wrote to Mr. W. A. Marburg and he authorized me to purchase it and to have it put in good order, and this has been done, and to complete his generous gift, Mr. Marburg has furnished bookcases as well. Dr. Welch will speak of some of the special works. I may mention in passing that the library is very rich in English medical pamphlets of the seventeenth and eighteenth centuries, and contains a large number of the works of classical medical authors which we had not in the library.

A word or two on Warrington and the men who collected these books: This old town on the banks of the Mersey, partly in Chester, partly in Lancashire, had in the middle and latter part of the eighteenth century a notable group of scientific and professional men. The Aiken family made the place celebrated as a literary center, as it was largely through the Rev. John Aiken that the Warrington Academy became so famous. His son John became well known through his "Biographical Memoirs of Medicine in Great Britain," and the large work on "General Biography." A sister of the elder Aiken was the distinguished authoress, Mrs. Barbauld, and Lucy Aiken, a daughter of Dr. John, became a well-known figure in English literature. But by far the most important of the scientific men who lived here in the eighteenth century was Joseph Priestly, who was tutored in "classics and polite literature" at the academy for six years, from 1761. He must have had a very stimulating effect on his colleagues. A very notable character who also has a strong interest for us on this side of the water is Thomas Percival, who was born at Warrington and practiced there before going to Manchester. Upon his work, "Medical Ethics, 1803," was founded

Originally published by Osler W: On the Library of a Medical School in *Bulletin of the Johns Hopkins Hospital,* Volume 18 (April, 1907), pp. 109-111. u 1907 by The Johns Hopkins University Press. Reprinted by permission.

the code of ethics of the American Medical Association. I see it stated that a brother of this Percival was also a well-known physician at Warrington, and at his death left a very large library; some of the books may possibly be those before us this evening. James Kendrick was a physician and naturalist of the same type. It was by the exertions of these men and their colleagues that this library was formed. The influence of the Warrington Academy, the educational college of the Unitarians of England, made the town a literary and scientific center, and the medical profession must have benefited largely from the intellectual environment of the place. So prominent indeed did it become that a Press was organized, and in looking over Miss Nutting's interesting collection of books on "Nursing," to which I shall refer later, I noticed that from it the works of the celebrated philanthropist, John Howard, were issued. Altogether, the collection has an affiliation with a remarkable group of men, and its value is not a little enhanced to know that it has been used by such men as Priestly, and John Aiken, and Thomas Percival.

The occasion offers an opportunity to make a few remarks upon the future of the libraries connected with this school.

Books are the tools of the mind, and in a community of progressive scholars the literature of the world in the different departments of knowledge must be represented. With the existing arrangements we have gradually built up two libraries, one connected with the hospital and the other with the university. In the former are to be found the modern works and journals relating to medicine, surgery, obstetrics, and the various specialties. Under Dr. Hurd's fostering care this side of the library has grown rapidly, and we have had several valuable donations from the libraries of the late Dr. Donaldson and the late Dr. Chatard. Files of all the more important medical journals are there to be found, and we can all testify to the very stimulating influence which this library had had upon the hospital staff and upon the senior medical students.

After the medical school had opened and the laboratories of anatomy, physiology and pharmacology been erected, the University began the collection which is in this building and which represents the modern works and journals in those scientific subjects upon which medicine is based. There are now very complete files of the scientific journals of anatomy, embryology, physiology, pharmacology, and physiological chemistry. While, in some ways, the ideal plan is to have a special library of each subject in each laboratory, the buildings here are so close together that it was thought best to concentrate all of the collections in this building.

Now it is along these two lines that a library of a medical school should progress, but there are one or two other sides of the question which may be considered. In a large city with another active medical library supported by the profession, the two should work in harmony, as great economies could be effected, particularly in the purchase of the more expensive works and journals. I am glad to know that the library of the Medical and Chirurgical Society is prepared to co-operate with the other medical libraries in this city in some such plan. It is not worth while for the library of the medical school to deal extensively with local literature or with the transactions of the State societies, or to attempt to keep files of all the smaller American journals. There are two other directions in which the library of a medical school should grow, and they are well represented by the collections presented to-night. When a man devotes his life to some particular branch of study and accumulates, year by year, a more or less complete literature, it is very sad after his death to have such a library come under the hammer—almost the inevitable fate. Fortunately, such libraries are very often offered for sale *en bloc*, and this was the case with the large collection of works on teratology and embryology formed by the late Professor Ahlfeld, of Germany. Through the liberality of Mr. W. F. Jencks this very valuable library has been secured for us and will be presented to-night by Dr. Williams. These special groups of books are of the greatest value to the student. It is interesting to know that in connection with the training school of the hospital Miss Nutting has gradually formed a library of all the works relating to nursing and to the care of the sick in peace and war, and I may remind you that we are already the fortunate possessors of another remarkable collection, that of the late Dr. Fisher, who gathered together the set of portraits which was presented to the hospital a few years ago by Dr. Kelly.

This Warrington collection represents a fourth side of the library work. I think you will all agree with me that the interest which has been taken here in the history of medicine and in the biography of the great men of our profession has had a very stimulating influence on the younger men, in giving to them that historical outlook so important in scientific research. The library of a great medical school should contain the original works of all the great masters of medicine. No book should be added to a library simply on account of its age. As in modern literature so in that of the sixteenth, seventeenth, and eighteenth centuries, there is an enormous quantity of trash which is hardly worth shelf room. I would have *all* of the original works of *all* of the great men; and one special value of this Marburg gift is that it is so rich in original editions of many of our masters. For example, I would have in such a library a carefully selected group of the works of Hippocrates, not everything, of course, but the standard editions, such as the Aldine folio, and the editions Frobenius and the more important translations; the editio princeps of Celsus, 1479; the more important of the works of Galen, including the fine Aldine edition, 1525;

good editions of Dioscorides, Aretaeus, and of Pliny, and of the other great medical writers of the Greco-Roman school. On the same principle should be collected the chief works of the Arabian physicians, and a shelf or two should be devoted to the school of Salernum. The great medical Humanists should be well represented—Linacre, Caius, and others. Every scrap of the writing of such a man as Vesalius should be collected. A good beginning has been made with the 1543 edition of the "Fabrica," but of such a man all the editions of all his works should be here. The same may be said of such great anatomists as Fabricius, Malpighi, Eustachius, Sylvius, and many others of the sixteenth century. The original works of the great physiologists should be sought for. Every scrap of the writings of Harvey (and they are not numerous) and every edition should be here. In practical illustration of my remarks I beg to present to the Marburg collection an original edition of the "De Motu Cordis," 1628, perhaps the greatest single contribution to medicine ever made, and which did as much for physiology as the "Fabrica" of Vesalius did for anatomy. The "De Motu Cordis" has become an excessively rare book. I had been on the outlook for a copy for nearly ten years. It had not appeared in an auction catalogue since 1895. Then in August of last year a very much cut, stained and unbound copy was offered to me at a very high figure. It had come from the library of Dr. Pettigrew, the author of a work on "Medical Biography." I had been waiting a long time for a copy, but this looked so shabby and dirty that I decided not to take it. Some months later the booksellers sent the copy back nicely cleansed and beautifully bound, and this time I succumbed. Within forty-eight hours the same dealers sent me another copy from the library of the late Professor Milne Edwards, of Paris, uncut and very nicely bound, which they offered at the same price. Naturally, I took the larger copy and the other one went to a friend in this country. The copy I here present to the library has been a little too energetically cleansed, so that the leaves are very tender and in places have had to be repaired. It came from the library of a physician in London and the bibliographical data are found attached.

I would have the complete works of the Hunters, every fragment available of John Hunter's; everything of Haller—and that means a great deal—of Majendie, and a complete collection of the monographs of great modern physiologists, such as Claude Bernard. The original works of the great clinicians, of Boerhaave, Morgagni, Bichat, Laennec, Louis, Corvisart, Bright, and Addison should be on our shelves; and lastly the great works relating to the history of medicine and to medical bibliography should be collected. Books in the special historical and bibliographical department of the library could very well be added to this Warrington collection, in which way the university could express its appreciation and gratitude for the very generous gift received from Mr. Marburg.

And one word in conclusion—when the plans for the medical school were under discussion, I drew in outline what I should have liked to see on this plot of land. Very much idealized it would have taken many millions for its realization. Surrounding the entire square ran beautiful stone cloisters (ornamented with busts and statues of the great men of the profession), and uniting the four chief buildings which stood in the middle of the sides of the square. On the Monument Street front was a beautiful structure in stone devoted to the library and museum. This part of my plan could yet be realized. As the museum collections grow, and as year by year the books increase in number such a building will become a necessity, and in it these special libraries will find their appropriate home.

*Remarks made on the occasion of the presentation of the Marburg Collection of books to the Johns Hopkins Medical School, January 2, 1907.

Remarks on the Medical Library in Post-Graduate Work*

By William Osler, M.D., F.R.S.,
President of the Medical Library Association

WITH collectivism the order of the day it is very natural that those interested should associate themselves in an organization which has for its object the welfare of the Medical Library. As stated in the circular, the Provisional Committee has given the new society a wide basis. The objects are:

(a) To bring together those engaged in or interested in medical libraries and medical literature, and for the discussion of matters associated with their fostering and care;
(b) To maintain an exchange for the distribution of duplicate books and periodicals;
(c) To increase the facilities for reference work;
(d) To encourage the study of the history of medicine;
(e) To issue publications dealing with medical library work;
(f) To form a library union amongst those of the medical libraries between which the exchange of books can be arranged—

all unexceptionable objects, and with the additional merit of being within reach of accomplishment.

Let me say at the outset that this is not to be simply a society for those whose work is more or less officially concerned with libraries, but it is for all interested in the book as a living factor in the education of the members of a learned and consequently of a very bookish profession. Whether the British doctor has been a better book-lover or book-maker is an open question, but from the first Oxford movements in the thirteenth and in the early fifteenth centuries we find him ever in the ranks of the keenest bibliophiles. He has never been a great student of the book as such, and it is strange not to find in the long line of splendid bibliographers, from the

*Delivered at the inaugural meeting of the Medical Library Association, held at Belfast, July 28th, 1909.

Originally published in *British Medical Journal*, Volume 2 (October 2, 1909), pp. 925-928 and reprinted as a separate by the Medical Library Association. Reprinted by permission.

lovable Conrad Gesner to the encyclopaedic Billings, an Englishman of the first rank. I do not forget the useful books of Douglas, of Young, and of Forbes, nor the Rabelaisian (in the mirth-loving sense) two-letter bibliography of Atkinson†; but they are feeble efforts in comparison with the works of our foreign and American brethren. But the Englishman has made up by being a great book-lover. Some of the best known of collections have been made in this country by physicians. It would be impossible to parallel elsewhere the libraries of Mead, Askew, and William Hunter. The sale catalogues of the former tell of treasures (and of prices) that send a thrill of regret through the book-lover that his lot was not cast in those happy days. The William Hunter Library met a better fate, and in the University of Glasgow is an enduring and worthy monument to the elder of the two great brothers, so unlike in mind and manners, so like in the capacity to see the true value of collections. It is to be hoped that a complete catalogue of this library may be issued before long, in companion volumes to the splendid catalogue of the manuscripts recently edited as a memorial to the late Professor Young.

It is safe to say that in proportion to population there are more medical libraries in these islands than in any other country in the world. We hope before long to have a proper census of them, and meanwhile I base the statement on casual observation. One of the first questions I ask on visiting a new town is, "Where is your medical library?" and I have been astonished at their extent and value. Usually in connexion with the county hospital or the medical society, or both, many of them go back to the middle or later part of the eighteenth century, and bear witness to the culture and intelligence of the provincial physicians of those days.

There are three groups:

First, in the national libraries of the capitals and of the universities, such as the British Museum and the Bodleian, are large collections of medical books—that of the British Museum the largest in the country. Upon these public storehouses of bibliographical knowledge we all draw freely. In many of the small libraries there are special collections of great intrinsic or historical value. The college libraries of Oxford and Cambridge contain manuscripts and old books of exceptional interest. Diel's topographical catalogue shows how rich some of the colleges are in the Greek medical manuscripts, particularly Balliol, New, Merton, All Souls, and Caius. Stowed away on their shelves are many fine folios, the gift of old members. Gulston's books are at Merton; New College has a very choice collection, including some of Walter Bayley; Floyer's books are at Queen's, Paddy's at St. John's, Coggan's at Oriel—indeed there is scarcely a college library without interesting medical associations.

Secondly, the medical libraries proper, among which those of the Royal

†The only man, so far as I know, who has had the courage to write a diverting bibliography, but unfortunately he only got through A and B.

Colleges of the three capitals are the most important. Easily first in extent and in the wide sphere of its influence is that of the Royal College of Surgeons of England, which is a model of good management. The library of the Royal Society of Medicine is the largest, I believe, connected with any medical society, and with the new organization is rapidly growing. The libraries of the Faculty of Physicians and Surgeons of Glasgow, of the Medical Institution of Liverpool, of the Birmingham Institute, of University College, Bristol, the Worth Library of the Steevens Hospital, and the Manchester Medical Society, form collections of the first rank. One of the most valuable of professional libraries is that of the British Medical Association, under whose auspices, so to speak, we meet to-day. Founded in 1889, it now possesses more than 20,000 volumes, with a card catalogue. The books are chiefly modern, with a large proportion of monographs and valuable sets of foreign periodicals. It receives also, and this is a very important point for borrowers, the theses of the French universities. Through it the Association has already done good work by aiding in the formation of local libraries, and between 6,000 and 7,000 duplicates have already been distributed. An important step has recently been taken to make this a lending library for members of the Association, who will be able to borrow expensive works and periodicals such as are only occasionally required for consultation. Having frequently visited the library in the old building, I very gladly bear testimony to its usefulness and to the admirable way in which it is managed by the librarian, Mr. Honeyman. I am not surprised to hear that the annual number of readers is very large, more than 6,000 in 1906. In the new building the arrangements are excellent, and I have no doubt that provincial members visiting London will more and more resort to this library. In all matters of management and detail these large libraries will be able to guide and assist us with their experience. Certainly we shall get much more from them than they from us, but theirs will be the richer blessing of the giver. With a well-managed exchange we may be able to help them fill the lacunae on their shelves, and it should be our aim to make these national collections more and more complete.

By far the best work we can do is in the organization, preservation and extension of the smaller libraries already existing in the provincial cities and towns. Many of these are already well housed and well arranged, as for example the Reading, York and Norwich libraries, to speak of those which I know personally. There are scores of hospitals with good collections, some of the greatest value, as those of Exeter and Bath and the Brackenbury Library, Preston. Some of them have associations of exceptional interest. I have always been an admirer of Caleb Hillier Parry of Bath, type of the old naturalist-physician, more common a few generations ago than now. His library in the Royal Hospital remains a fitting monument to a scholarly man of wide sympathies, and who left a deep impression on that part of the West Country which has given us such men as Jenner, Pritchard and Symonds. In those days life was not so full, and competition was less keen, so that men had more time to read and to think. Many of the best of these smaller libraries date from the latter part of the eighteenth century and the beginning of the nineteenth century. Some of them have died into cupboards and barrels, and sadly need the kind care of a Philip de Bury, one of the founders of Oxford libraries, who, in the fourteenth century, complained bitterly that he found precious volumes defiled and injured by mice, worms and moths. A collection of this sort, offered me a few years ago, I was able to buy through a friend, for the Johns Hopkins Medical School. It had associations with Joseph Priestley, with John Aikin, Thomas Percival and James Kendrick, well-known names in the North. As illustrating how valuable may be some of these out-of-the-way collections, there were in this one scores of seventeenth and eighteenth century pamphlets which were not in the London libraries.

Our best work will be in stimulating an interest in these smaller libraries, either in connexion with the medical society or with the hospital, and in helping to organize them; and from every one of them we hope to have in our society a representative.

And, lastly, there is the private library of the practitioner, the scope of which will depend on his training, his tastes, and his purse; and this brings me to the subject of my remarks, "the value of the library in post-graduate study."

Some of the best of men have used books the least, and there is good authority for the statement that shallowness of mind may go with much book-learning. Descartes, one of the most brilliant of thinkers and observers, had no library. At Egmond, asked by a friend the books he most read and valued, he took him into his dissecting room and showed him a calf—"There is my library." An identical anecdote is told of John Hunter. But these were exceptional men; and few will be found to doubt the importance of books as a means to what the same author called the end of all study—the capacity to make a good judgement.

It cannot be denied that many men practise, and do so successfully, with few journals and still fewer books. Radcliffe, whose memory is enshrined in two of the finest library buildings in the kingdom, and whose travelling Fellows are supposed to have at least a triennial thirst for new knowledge, neither read nor wrote books; and he is credited with the famous *mot* that he could set down the whole art of medicine on a sheet of paper. But conditions have changed, and medicine is now a rapidly progressive science, as well as an exceedingly complicated art, of which, at qualification, a man has only laid the foundation; and if he is to develop his intelligence—that is, get an education—it must be by systematic post-graduate study. Out of leading-strings he must himself be at once teacher and pupil, and make and keep certain self-made laws. Whether he will get this education, whether, indeed, he will be able to keep what he has, will depend in part upon the sort of training he has received, and in part upon the type of mind with which he has been endowed. Unless as a student he has got that "relish of knowledge" of which Locke speaks; unless he has got far enough to have his senses well trained to make accurate observations; unless he has been taught how to use his intelligence so as to form a good judgement, the teacher will have more or less of a fool for a pupil, and between them make a sad mess of an education. After a few years such a man gives up in despair, and without mental exercise grows stale and is fit to do only the ordinary reflex practice, in which cough means an expectorant mixture, and heart disease digitalis, just as surely as a tap on the patellar tendon brings out the knee-jerk. A glance at the consulting-room suffices for the diagnosis of this type: the BRITISH MEDICAL JOURNAL or *Lancet* lies uncut in heaps on the table, and not a book is in sight! Some of the men of this type play a good game of tennis, others shoot and ride well, more play a good game of bridge, but they are lost souls, usually very dissatisfied with the profession—the kickers, the knockers, the grumblers, without a glimmer of consciousness that the fault is in themselves.

Post-graduate study is a habit of mind only to be acquired, as are other habits, in the slow repetition of the practice of looking at everything with an inquiring spirit. A patient with pneumonia has grass green sputum. "Have I ever seen it before? Have I a note of it? Where can I get a good description of it? What does it signify?" These are questions preliminary to getting a bit of clinical education, trifling in itself apparently, but when stored up and correlated with other facts may become the basis for an intelligent judgment on an important case.

There are many factors in this training—note-taking, reading, the medical society, and the quinquennial brain-dusting at a hospital or a post-graduate school. But I am only here concerned with one—books. I would like to speak of the value of notes, however brief, collected through long years as the sole means whereby a man gets his experience codified and really helpful; but I cannot wander to-day from the book, in which I include the JOURNAL.

But how can a busy man read, driven early and late, tired out and worried? He cannot. It is useless to try, unless he has got into the habit when he was not so busy; then it comes easy enough, and the hardest-worked man in the land may read his journals every week, even if he has to do it in his carriage. My old teacher and colleague at McGill, Palmer

Howard, was the busiest practitioner in Montreal, but the weeklies and the monthlies, English and French, the good old Quarterly, the hospital reports, the new monographs—nothing escaped him, and I have often heard him say that he did his best reading as he drove from patient to patient.

It is not so much a question of *when* but of *what* and of *how*. What sort of reading will best help a man in his education, will help him to keep up with the times and to develop into a thinking, reasoning practitioner? Let him get rid of the notion that much has to be read; one or two journals, a good weekly—the *Lancet* or the BRITISH MEDICAL JOURNAL—a good monthly—the *Practitioner* or the *American Journal of the Medical Sciences*—suffice; but let them be read thoroughly. Then each week strip the husk of advertising sheets, and keep on the desk a file of reasonable proportions, and to the articles which have been of interest refer again and again. At the end of the half-year bind your journals and insert slips where you have found articles bearing directly on your cases.

Carefully studied, a couple of journals are the very basis of post-graduate work, and year by year the files on the shelves become not simply the nucleus of, but actually a good working library, and, well marked in his mind, he has in them volumes on every special disease and a complete summary of the progress of medicine.

Let him follow the same practice with books. Buy with discrimination, and not too many, as here again it is a question of reading. If, as is said, the man of one book is dangerous, the man of a few books is more useful and more apt to keep the open, plastic mind. A good "System" of medicine and of surgery, an occasional monograph or work on special diseases, a new edition of a favourite textbook (when you can trust that it is really an editor's, not a publisher's, edition!), should suffice, and do not mean a large annual expenditure.

It is much simpler to buy books than to read them, and easier to read them than to absorb their contents. Too many men slip early out of the habit of studious reading, and yet this is essential to a man if he is to get an education. To be worth anything it must be associated with concentration—with that mental application which means real effort. Of the new Allbutt and Rolleston "System" I can read comfortably about twenty pages in an hour—sometimes of a tough author not more than fifteen. Half an hour a day would finish the six volumes already published within a year.

More than once I have referred to the three essentials in the house of the general practitioner—the library, the laboratory, and the nursery—and of these the first is much the easiest to get, as he starts with a nucleus in his students' textbooks. Effort and system gradually train a man's capacity to read intelligently and profitably, but only while the green years are on his head is the habit to be acquired, and in a desultory life, without fixed hours, and with his time at the beck and call of everybody, a man needs a good deal of reserve and determination to maintain it. Once the machinery is started, the effort is not felt in the keen interest in a subject. As Aristotle remarks, "In the case of our habits we are only masters of the beginning, their growth by gradual stages being imperceptible, like the growth of a disease"; and so it is with this habit of reading, of which you are only master at the beginning—once acquired, you are its slave.

So far as the library is a factor, the greater part of a man's post-graduate education must be at home. In this country no man practises very far from a county town in which there is a medical society or a general hospital with a library attached. A notebook for special points to look up, or for certain books of reference, will get him into the habit of frequenting it, and he should become a subscriber, as in this way not only does the library widen its influence, but finds means for its support. The county library, wherever situated, should be the much-esteemed consultant of the general practitioner.

But it is in the towns of 20,000 in population and upwards that the library is of the greatest value, and where it becomes a factor of the first importance in the development of the progressive man. These are days of great opportunities, when we have discovered other ways to the top, toilsome all the same, than up the old rungs of the academic ladder, or the weary climb of the stairs of a London hospital. We are waking up to the fact that the man may make his own environment, and may make it just what and where he pleases; he may even perform a miracle—the mountain may come to Mahomet. Let me give you a notable illustration.

A few years ago when two young Irish-Americans called Mayo began to frequent the surgical clinics of Europe, no one knew where they came from; no one had ever heard of Rochester, Minnesota, and when informed that it was on the "Prairies," about 1,000 miles north-west of Chicago, there was a shrug of the shoulders and "Oh!" Self education, post-graduate study, books, journals, laboratory work, have enabled these remarkable men to build up one of the largest and in some respects the most important surgical clinic in the world, and a town of less than 20,000 inhabitants has become the Mecca of all surgeons.

To the man who is ambitious to use his opportunities in a town or city, a well selected library is essential, and whether he be surgeon, physician, or specialist, he needs as a rule more than his own shelves supply, often indeed a good deal more than the library can offer. As I have already stated, the library of the British Medical Association is offering great facilities to its members. In England, too, he can and should join the Royal Medical

Society, from which monographs and special journals may be had, but he cannot always wait, and there is no reason why in the larger towns there should not be a library which ministers to the ordinary wants of all ranks. The journals at once become a serious consideration—French, German, and American—but a few of the best suffice when supplemented by the admirable German *Centralblätte*. By means of an exchange this association can render great assistance, while in the thickly populated districts a system of exchanges between libraries would cut in half the cost of the more expensive journals. In this matter, too, a central library like that of the British Medical Association may be most helpful.

In large cities the profession should have its own home in connexion with the leading medical society, and of such an organization the library forms an important part. Belfast has set a good example, and through the munificence of Sir William Whitla you have a splendid building for the Medical Institute. About such rooms or buildings should centre the life of the profession, present and past. Portraits of the old worthies, memorials of friends, and to our heroes (such as the beautiful stained-glass window in the Institute here to Dr. William Smyth), show-cases full of the interesting relics of the profession, with manuscripts and books illustrative of local history—all these memorials make the past live again. At York you may see in the medical library the actual foceps with which Dr. Slop broke the bridge of Tristram Shandy's nose, and in every county there are relics of the profession well worth preserving.

It should be the ambition of the men in each county to have well-equipped rooms, such as those I have visited with much pleasure at York and Norwich. If, as at Reading, Exeter, Preston, and Dublin (Steevens' Hospital), rooms have been furnished in the hospital, see that the equipment is attractive; many libraries have deservedly fallen into disuse because men will not seek books or journals in dull, dark, cold, dusty, uninviting rooms.

Like everything else that is worth having, a library costs money. Do not try to do too much, strive to have a large membership, which enables the fees to be low; and when the library is in connexion with a hospital, the current English journals should be furnished by the governors to the staff. In towns with a tax for the upkeep of a public library, a grant should be made for the medical library. But the financial and other questions of organization and support will be discussed, I hope, at an early meeting.

Were there time I should like to say a few words on the subject of *how* to read, but the essence of the whole matter I found the other day in the Bibliotheca Lancisiana, Rome (founded in 1711, and containing the books of the famous Lancisi). In the opening address, 1714, *De recto usu Bibliothecae*, the Abbé[6] Carsughi discusses the subject in three sections, and gives some good rules. The first section, *Librorum scilicet delectum,* need not detain us, but in the second, *Legendi methodum,* he urges two important points—to read in a certain order and with a definite object, and *lente festinans,* "unhasting but unresting." In the third section, *Adnotandi modum,* he urges the necessity of careful note-taking, quoting the praise of Clement of Alexandria, "Oblivionis medicamentum, monumentum senectutis et adjumentum memoriae." He dwells upon the importance of study in the morning, which was all very well in those days, but is not one hour after six in the evening worth now two before eight in the morning? (I am sure it is to me!) With half an hour's reading in bed every night as a steady practice, the busiest man can get a fair education before the plasma sets in the periganglionic spaces of his grey cortex.

But there is another side of the question of books and libraries—man does not live by bread alone, and while getting his medical education and making his calling and election sure by hard work, the young doctor should look about early for an avocation, a pastime, that will take him away from patients, pills and potions. One of the best features I find in my "old country" colleagues is the frequency with which they have hobbies. No man is really happy or safe without one, and it makes precious little difference what the outside interest may be—botany, beetles or butterflies, roses, tulips or irises, fishing, mountaineering or antiquities—anything will do so long as he straddles a hobby and rides it hard. I would like to make a plea for the book, for the pleasant paths of bibliography, in which many of us stray to our great delight. Upon this how charming is old Burton (really one of us, "by profession a divine, by inclination a physician," he says), whose *Anatomy of Melancholy* is the only great medical work ever written by a layman. "For what a world of books offers itself, in all subjects, arts, and sciences, to the sweet content and capacity of the reader! In arithmetic, geometry, perspective, optics, astronomy, architecture, sculpture, painting, of which so many and such elaborate treatises are written; in mechanics and their mysteries, military matters, navigation, riding of horses, fencing, swimming, gardening, planting, great tomes of husbandry, cookery, falconry, hunting, fishing, fowling, etc., with exquisite pictures of all sports, games, and what not! In music, metaphysics, natural and moral philosophy, philology, in policy, heraldry, genealogy, chronology, etc., they afford great tomes, or those studies of antiquity, etc., *et quid subtilius Arithmeticis inventionibus, quid jucundius Musicis rationibus, quid divinius Astronomicis, quid rectius Geometricis demonstrationibus!* What so sure, what so pleasant?"

Our society will, I am sure, be very helpful to men who take up this study. We hope to have two groups, mutually helpful—the professional bibliographers, the men in charge of our libraries, who have to do with the book, as such, and who care little or nothing about its contents; and amateurs, like myself. As Professor Ferguson says in his charming essay[1]:

> He (the bibliographer) has to do with editions and their peculiarities, with places, printers, and dates, with types and illustrations, with sizes and collation, with binding and owners, with classifications, collections and catalogues.

There are scores of book collectors whose hobby also takes them in this direction, but we should have a large amateur group who will be happier in following other lines. Personally, I collect on two principles—first, interest in an author, which is a good guide, as the book illustrates the biography, a principle which has the advantage of helping at least to keep you within the limits of purse and shelves, more the latter than the former. Take, for example, the two small groups of books I have placed in our exhibition, the one illustrating Servetus, the other Ulrich von Hutten. Valuable as they are from the standpoint of the professional bibliographer, this is nothing to the interest awakened in the men themselves, in their aspirations, their labour, and their tragic fates. For the amateur this personal note clothes the dry bones of bibliography and makes them live. And my other principle is this: a student of the history of medicine, I look out for books which have left their impress on it in some special way. If one is particular to examine carefully into the claims of a book before admitting it to the select company on your shelves, you here again cultivate a due regard for purse and space. For example, five or six books illustrate the whole subject of auscultation and percussion, only the masterpieces are chosen. I confess there may be a certain satisfaction in tracing out the biography of a book, but it is cold work unless you love the author.

Judiciously cultivated, bibliography has many advantages as a pastime for the doctor; a little patient care, a very small expenditure of money, and a constant look-out for the books wanted are the essential requisites. Nor is there ever any difficulty in the choice of a subject—anything he may be interested in has its bibliographical side. One friend (Dr. Turrell), a very busy man, is a keen fisherman, and has found the time to collect a library on this subject, and has written the article on it for the *County History of Oxfordshire*. Another man has kept up his classics, and collected everything relating to Horace. Another has a library relating to the order of St. John. Another friend in large general practice has found time to make a collection of the masterpieces of English literature, which has not only been a diversion and an edcation, as it has brought him into the best company of the past four centuries, but he tells us there is another side—it has been a better investment than life insurance. A member of our profession, the late Professor Corfield, made one of the best modern collections of bindings, the sale of which at Sotheby's in 1904 was one of the bibliographical features of the year. Once in a subject it is extraordinary how it grows and develops. As Atkinson says, "It is an art of itself, which is not easily sought into or acquired, but which, if so acquired, may stand both his pleasure and profit in very great stead in a very long or a short life." And the busiest general practitioner may find the time for first-class work. Many of you may have seen a book issued two years ago from the Oxford Press on Greek and Roman medical and surgical instruments, the only separate treatise on the subject which has appeared in English. It illustrates the hobby of a very hard-worked practitioner in the town of Hartlepool—John Milne, whose spare time and whose vacation have been spent in studying this aspect of Greek and Roman archaeology.

We shall hope to have in our society both the professional and the amateur—the man whose life-work is in libraries, and those of us who are fond of books, either from a biographical or a bibliographical standpoint. We should be able to encourage library organization, and once established as a common meeting ground for all interested, the society should be of great value to the profession. We look for a large membership, and many will join who do not belong to either of the above-mentioned groups, the men who feel that, as a matter of policy, such a society should be supported. *Non sibi sed toti*—let us work in the spirit of this motto, and our future is assured.

In starting an organization of this sort the work always falls on one or two men. We have to thank Dr. Stanley Hall, of Bristol, and Mr. C. E. A. Clayton, of the Manchester Medical Library, to whom is due entirely the success of this preliminary meeting. We have also to thank the university authorities for allowing us to meet here, and furnishing us with rooms for the exhibit.

REFERENCE

1. Some Aspects of Bibliography, Edinburgh.

LIBRARIES USEFUL IN THEIR DAY *

WILLIAM J. MAYO, M.D.

Rochester, Minnesota

LADIES and Gentlemen: We are very glad to have as our guests in the Clinic the members of the Medical Library Association.

To be brought up in an atmosphere of books is a rare privilege for which one should be grateful for life. There is a friendliness about books, an appeal to the emotions perhaps as much as to the intelligence. Books become friends that never fail; and as we advance in years, until we find that we belong to the vanishing generation, and see our friends among men and women passing away one by one, we find increasing comfort in our libraries, in taking down books with gentle hands, visiting again and again our friends in their pages. Even to stand in a loved library and look at the books, so well known that we are at once aware if a volume has been misplaced, gives a sense of rest and sustainment.

My brother, Dr. Charles H. Mayo, and I had the good fortune to grow up in the atmosphere of books. Our father, Dr. W. W. Mayo, had, for his day, an excellent medical library at his office, with all the medical journals then available, a fine microscope, and a human skeleton, that of Cut-Nose, an Indian chief, who had been executed after the Indian massacres in southern Minnesota in 1862. Father had prepared the skeleton with his own hands, and from it my brother and I learned osteology. In our home was an unusually large general library, not in a separate room, but in the living-room, on open shelves which reached to the ceiling and occupied all the wall space in the room. I can see Father now, standing on a wooden chair, reaching up to take books down, or, with one book under his arm, another held between his knees, looking into the pages of a third. And our mother, with her keen, inquiring, and studious mind, was a source of inspiration to us. An excellent amateur astronomer, she had a four-foot telescope which she herself had assembled, and she was a well-versed botanist, finding interest and recreation in her garden. Mother always encouraged us in our preparation for our profession, and after we had entered medicine, she spurred us on to travel and to scientific reading and writing.

In that early day we were encouraged to read Sir Walter Scott, because Scott's books, instead of giving series of dates and indigestible historical facts, picture the customs and habits of peoples and historic events in such fashion that much clings to the mind because it appeals to the emotions as well as to the intelligence. Dickens served as a basis for our reading in

*** Read at the Annual Meeting of the Medical Library Association, Rochester, Minnesota, June 24, 1936.**

Originally published in *Bulletin of the Medical Library Association,* Volume 25 (September, 1936), pp. 70-72. Reprinted by permission.

sociology. His arguments for social welfare, as presented in his books, did much to bring about reforms in England in the manner of dealing with the poor, the ignorant, and the unfortunate.

When I was about sixteen, at Father's suggestion I read Darwin, and soon after that Haeckel, the German biologist who followed Darwin. Then I dipped into a variety of subjects and authors, always with the idea that I was to be a doctor, and to this day I remember distinctly many of the things I read at that period. In the reign of Queen Elizabeth (1558–1603), as a result of the spirit of investigation which rose from the great mental and moral disturbances of the time, intellect was freed from dogma. There were, for instance, during this period, and in the decades immediately following, Shakespeare (1564–1616), supreme dramatist; Sir Francis Drake (1545–1595), great navigator; Francis Bacon (1561–1626), logician and statesman; John Mayow (1643–1679), one of the first to investigate medical physicochemistry; and the great clinicians, of whom Sydenham (1624–1689) was a fine example.

Those early clinicians were clear thinkers and critical observers, as shown in many instances. They were men who studied man in relation to disease and reasoned directly from cause to effect, in a manner which made a lasting impression, as contrasted with much of the writing of the present day. They pointed out the difference in what might be called insulation against heat and cold in women and men. Women, because of a particular panniculus, are less affected by heat and cold than are men, who even when clothed in heavy dress suits are often chilly, whereas women in light dress or decolletage are comfortable. They observed that the kidneys in women are more active than in men, maintaining circulatory equilibrium, perhaps one reason why high blood-pressure in women may not carry with it so great a cardiac danger as in men. They called attention, too, to the fact that swollen ankles in men are a sign of grave import, whereas swollen ankles in women are often of less significance.

And there was the clinical pathologist, Sir James Paget (1814–1899). I have not read anything in Paget for nearly sixty years, but certain comments of his have remained with me since boyhood. He wrote of atheromatous conditions, that man as he grew older became earthy in his blood-vessels, and other structures of his body, as though he were preparing for the grave; that organs which are becoming obsolete in the species, wisdom teeth and the little toes, for instance, are frequently found to be undergoing changes of obsolescence; that steady pressure on the body would lead to local ulceration, such as bed sores, whereas intermittent pressure would lead to callus and corns.

There is something about the very atmosphere of books which stirs certain emotions within us, even though the contents of the books may not of themselves be of great value. To books we turn to learn of the past, opinions of the present, and prognostications of the future. To quote Patrick Henry's never to be forgotten aphorism, " I have but one lamp by which my feet are guided, and that is the lamp of experience. I know no way to judge the future but by the past."

In 1825, when Thomas Jefferson dedicated the University of Virginia, he made one statement which epitomized an educational viewpoint which it has taken the people of this country more than 100 years to appreciate. He said, in substance, "This institution is for the purpose of diffusion of knowledge useful in its day."—Useful in its day.—At the present time it seems as though many libraries consist too largely of any kind of printed matter that has covers, much of it material not necessarily of real value, occupying space which more precious volumes ought to have, interfering sometimes with the essential purpose of the library.

I do not mean by this that libraries should not contain miscellaneous books of unequal value, because all books have some value, if only to increase the impressive size and learned appearance of the library, but size should not be overrated in building up a library. If we could but have those books which are useful in their day, even if that day is one long past, which are of value in prognosticating the future, on Patrick Henry's summation, the great quantities of mediocre books could still be held as secondary and tertiary reserves.

During the two years that my brother and I spent in Washington during the War, in the office of the Surgeon-General, we went often to the Army Medical Library, the library of the Surgeon-General, of which Col. John Shaw Billings was the founder. We wandered through those great stacks of books, impressed by the tremendous collection of material, and when we wanted to find anything, with the assistance of the library force it eventually could be found. I read recently that Major Edgar Erskine Hume, the latest of a long line of successors of Colonel Billings, has finally brought out the first volume of the fourth series of the *Index-catalogue* of this vast library of 394,003 medical volumes and 558,616 pamphlets.

In many cities in this country there are great collections of medical literature. The University of Minnesota has a superb library; there is the John Crerar Medical Library in Chicago, the Library of the Surgeon-General, already mentioned, and others. Because of their beneficent custom of lending books, medical institutions and individual workers can obtain from them those rare and unusual books which sometimes may be needed to complete certain investigations. Because of this inestimable aid, the average medical library is left free to spend its funds for books useful in their day, and of course may accept gifts of old books, which have come through the generosity of friends, usually from the private libraries of members of the medical profession who have passed on.

We have increasing satisfaction in our own reference medical library in the Clinic, which receives constant use by the staff of The Mayo Clinic and the Fellows of The Mayo Foundation.

The Role of the Medical School Library in the Medical School Teaching Program*

By Chauncey D. Leake, Ph.D., *Executive Director*
University of Texas Medical Branch
Galveston, Texas

One of the most important current developments in medical education is the increasing use of the medical school library as an essential instrument in the medical school teaching program. This is an inevitable feature of the overwhelming mass of detailed material we are accumulating through research regarding health and disease. While the prime function of any scientific library is the accumulation and preservation of knowledge about ourselves and our environment, it is increasingly apparent that this vast information must be used if it is to have any significance at all in our culture.

The accumulation of knowledge in regard to medicine has had enormous effects on the character of the professional medical effort. One may note four phases in man's approach to disease: (1) the primitive fear of disease, with resulting superstitious attempts to handle it, which unfortunately persists even to the present; (2) the gradual accumulation of knowledge about disease through the centuries of experience gained by a professional group particularly interested in managing disease; (3) the gradual accumulation of precise knowledge about the cause of disease, resulting in a shift of emphasis at the beginning of this century toward the prevention of disease; and (4) the current appreciation that we know enough about disease and have devised skilled enough methods of handling it, so that we can turn our attention toward the promotion of optimum health.

These four phases are of great importance. While the primitive fear of disease still persists with us, and while the traditional methods of handling disease result in physicians sitting back to wait for disease to come along, the accumulation of knowledge about disease has resulted in a much more aggressive attitude now in trying to prevent disease. The difficulty is that our eco-

* Read at the 52nd Annual Meeting, Medical Library Association, Salt Lake City, June 16, 1953.

Originally published in *Bulletin of the Medical Library Association,* Volume 41 (October, 1953), pp. 369-378. Reprinted by permission.

nomic imagination has not kept up with our accumulation of knowledge, so that doctors still cannot make a living by practicing on the basis of preventing disease. Maybe this can develop as doctors learn that people are willing to pay to keep healthy. The success of the Armed Forces in maintaining optimum health in our fighters shows the way by which civilian practice may satisfactorily be turned toward the promotion of optimum health. Certainly people would be willing to pay well for such service.

In these significant changes in approach to the practice of medicine, medical libraries have played a leading part. From remotest antiquity doctors found that the empirical knowledge about disease and its management was too much for memory. Records and texts began to be kept even as early as the fourth millennium B.C. The early Egyptian physicians had exceptionally well organized surgical texts, as the existing Edwin Smith Surgical Papyrus clearly shows. This document is a series of typical case histories organized for injuries from the top of the head running down through the body, with each case developed upon the basis of examination, diagnosis, prognosis, and treatment. This text, now in the New York Academy of Medicine, was copied by a scribe about 1800 B.C., from a much older original. The copying scribe had to explain terms already archaic, which indicate that the original document must have been written about 3500 B.C. Similarly, the great Ebers Papyrus, which was destroyed in World War II in Leipzig, was a medical text with some 800 prescriptions and a few monographic discussions of diseases and anatomical conditions; it too was written about 1800 B.C. Even the general practitioners of old Egypt had their formularies copied for them by scribes from the scrolls kept in the centers of teaching. The Hearst Medical Papyrus at the University of California and the Berlin Medical Papyrus are of this sort. Similar texts from old Egypt have been preserved for gynecology (the Petrie Papyrus in London), and for proctology (the Chester Beatty Papyrus in London). There must have been collections of texts in the major teaching centers of old Egypt, and there is similar evidence that collections of recipes and procedures were made by the ancient Sumerians.

In ancient Greek times it is apparent that the great teaching schools of medicine at Cos, Cnidus, Pergamon, and Epidaurus must have had libraries of reference. The teachers at these schools were encouraged to make records of their observations. The great Hippocratic collection represents the accumulated wisdom of the school at Cos. This remarkable library of medical material indeed became one of the most important sources for the development of rational medicine in western culture. Its philosophical impact is powerful even now, in connection with the high ethical standards of practice which were encouraged, and in the naturalistic approach to disease. The high value always placed on this great collection is clear from the care with which it has been preserved through two and a half millennia.

Similarly, great collections of medical works were made in the ancient Chinese and Hindu cultures, and were used as the basis for medical teaching for centuries. Unfortunately, in the case of Chinese and Hindu medicine, the ancient texts became stereotyped, were followed blindly, and few additions were made as a result of original observations. The result was an unfortunate static condition for medicine, reflecting the stagnation of all scientific or exact knowledge in these lands.

When the Romans inherited Greek culture, they developed libraries of great size and importance. Individual physicians, such as Galen, must have had relatively large collections of manuscripts, to judge from the many references to previous writers which occur in their own records. The great library at Alexandria, known throughout all antiquity, unfortunately was burned and later pillaged in religious riots.

During the Dark Ages in Europe, the ancient glories of Greco-Roman medicine were carefully preserved in the rapidly expanding Arabian culture. The significant contributions from antiquity were translated into Arabic and Hebrew, and studied and hoarded in libraries throughout the Mohammedan empire, and later were translated back into Latin for the benefit of the teaching centers which gradually developed in Italy and western Europe.

The Medical School of Salerno, which was the center for medical training through the 13th century, must have had a considerable library. In the manuscript collections preserved there were translations into Latin from Arabic sources, and there were also gradually accumulated manuscripts in original Greek from the old Greek tradition in medicine. This material was commented upon and expanded by the Salerno teachers, and set the example for the later university studies in medicine as reflected at Bologna, Padua, Paris, Oxford, Cambridge, Montpellier, Basle, and Prague.

With the development of printing in the 15th century and the mass production of books, libraries became an essential part of the working equipment not only of individual physicians, but of all medical training centers. The books were precious. They were kept carefully, and often were chained to the reading desks in the libraries. They were sumptuously bound, with the leaves pressed by clasps, so that they would not buckle or warp, and were considered to be the prize possessions of the teaching institutious. Since the books in the library were so precious, they were kept locked up. The librarian was personally responsible for them. The library could only be opened for use to fully accredited people. It apparently was open only for a limited period of time. Unfortunately, these medieval traditions shackle too many of our own modern medical libraries, but the tradition of the precious value of medical books is well worth maintaining.

As the great medical organizations and academies developed in Europe in the 17th century, libraries became their special interest. The library of the

Royal College of Physicians in London was outstanding. Similarly the library of the Royal College of Surgeons was a center for postgraduate teaching and learning. Unfortunately, these libraries maintained medieval traditions with respect to the care with which they were used. Only individuals with the most critically screened qualifications were allowed to use the books, and otherwise they remained locked in their cases. This unhappily is still the case in many of these fine institutions.

Thus, the great medical teaching centers in Europe became relatively static with respect to libraries. During the 19th century most of the medical schools in the Germanic sphere of influence developed on the basis of separate institutes for each discipline, and each institute had its library. As a result there was much duplication. The head of the institute usually contributed most of the books himself, and they were, in effect, his personal property. Accordingly, they could be used only by the special pupils working under his direction for graduate degrees in the disciplines involved. The average medical student could do little more than buy the books he needed for his own studies; in addition, he had little access to medical libraries for reference use or reading.

Nevertheless, the example of the brilliant clinical teachers in Paris, London, Edinburgh, and in the German centers of Vienna, Berlin, Leipzig, and Munich stimulated the more eager students, among them many Americans, to accumulate helpful personal libraries. In the 19th century it was still possible for an energetic physician to have a personal library reasonably satisfactory for the knowledge available at the time. Certainly three to five thousand volumes would cover the entire range of important medical contributions, even including the rapidly growing special periodicals, for personal use.

Only recently have European medical training centers followed the example developed at American medical schools in having a central library for student use. The many new medical schools established in India, China, Japan, South Africa, and Latin America have attempted to develop student-use libraries. The most important example set here was by the Peking Union Medical College, under Rockefeller Foundation influence. What has happened to this important library, following Japanese and Communist China domination, is unknown.

Meanwhile, there was rapid mushrooming of medical schools in the United States during the 19th century. This was necessary under the speedy expansion of the country, with frontier conditions and relatively poor communication. The early American medical schools had poor library facilities; however, attempts were made to develop student-use libraries at Harvard, at the College of Physicians and Surgeons in New York City, at Pennsylvania, at the University of Virginia, at Tulane, and even at the frontier school at Transylvania.

As medical education in the United States was stabilized at the beginning of this century, with the elimination of proprietary and ill-equipped schools, medical libraries became a standard part of the medical school program. Special libraries were developed at some schools, such as the great Lane Library at Stanford Medical School in San Francisco. Outstanding has been the splendid student-use library at the Johns Hopkins Medical School, and at Yale Medical School. Very helpful has been the influence of the New York Academy of Medicine, the Philadelphia College of Physicians, the Boston Medical Library, the John Crerar Library in Chicago, and the Mayo Clinic Library in setting examples for helpfully organized medical library development in connection with medical teaching, research, and professional service.

The Scope of Modern Teaching Medical Libraries

Modern medicine has expanded enormously. We are entering the fourth phase of medical service, directed toward the promotion of optimum health. Under these circumstances many auxiliaries play a role in the medical team. Indeed, some universities, such as Ohio State, are wise enough to designate such a combination of activities as "The Health Center." These various auxiliaries to the health team use the library as much as medical students. Accordingly, provision must be made in the modern teaching medical library for full reference service in all fields of medicine and also in dentistry, public health, nursing, veterinary medicine, pharmacy, clinical psychology, clinical laboratory technology, radiation technology, physical therapy, occupational therapy, sociology and social service, dietetics, and hospital administration. Indeed, the alert medical librarian must now be prepared to anticipate the needs of intelligent laymen in health affairs, and have material which may bear upon all sorts of aspects of the current health effort, including economics, philosophy, esthetics, and general literature.

The modern teaching medical library is in fact a general reference center, with special collections expanded in the fields of the various health disciplines. The general reference sources in the humanities, in literature, in esthetics, in philosophy, and in mathematics, chemistry, physics, and biology remain the firm foundation of the first-class medical library, as of any other general library. If the health center is part of a general university campus, these general library sources will be available in the general university library. Even under such circumstances, however, there is much to be gained in developing a special health center library, where there may be much duplication of material in the main university library, but where the morale of the growing health team can be well nurtured by close association in a conveniently arranged and working health library.

The arrangement of a health library is extremely important. Primarily it should be designed for convenience of use. All students in the health fields can be assumed to be mature and responsible individuals, who are working in the health fields for serious ends. Under these circumstances the health library can well be developed on an open shelf basis, so that the users may find the material they want themselves. There should of course be full indices and a relatively large area for general reference works, near the entrance, so that the library users can get essential general information readily. Here may also be the bibliographical and abstract tools for systematic study. Let pencils and note-paper be handy!

It matters little what classification is used in a modern health library. The point is to get the books out where they can be seen, where people can take them down and look at them, and where the library is arranged openly and conveniently for such a purpose. An apron shelf along widely spaced stacks, arranged in cubicles, makes for convenience. A table with chairs in the center of the cubicle makes it easy to sit down and make such notes or do such reading as may be pertinent to the books at hand.

Even if the health center library is part of a great university library, arrangements can be made for its individuality, and for promoting the team work of the health group. Would that all great university libraries could be as conveniently and comfortably arranged as the new Princeton Library! Here in addition to large general reading rooms and special rooms for special collections, are vast open shelves throughout the building in close proximity to seminar rooms, individual cubicles, lounging areas, and rooms pleasantly devised for group discussion and study. With the stacks in the center, and the lounge and seminar rooms arranged peripherally, the library works smoothly and efficiently. With open shelves students are encouraged to find for themselves the material they wish. The check out desk is efficient, and the library is open from 7:00 in the morning until midnight every day, including Sundays and holidays.

This is really the way to run a large modern library. Such a place is, of course, the intellectual center for an intellectual institution. In any health center the library should be the intellectual heart of the effort. To function in this manner, every effort must be made to have the material in the library reasonably comprehensive, as conveniently arranged as possible, and always in fairly good order. Convenience, comfort, and cleanliness may well be the slogan for a medical library prepared for teaching use.

If the health library can be developed as an independent unit, it should still preserve the general features of ready accessibility of all material, ease in using the books directly where they may be stacked, and with full provision for many seminar rooms, lounging rooms where tea may be served, special study rooms, and individual cubicles.

There is little purpose in a modern health center library acquiring and keeping textbooks. The students get these on their own. A small file of current textbooks might be maintained for reference purposes, and the first editions of important texts might be kept for historical interest, but the main type of material for a first-class modern health library is comprehensive periodical files and well-selected monograph publications.

If the health library is properly arranged with cubicle shelving, seminar and study rooms, and with full conveniences for readers throughout the stacks, the bound periodicals and monographs may be run together. This helps frequently when the library is not too large. On the other hand when a health library exceeds 50,000 or 60,000 volumes, it seems preferable to keep the monographs in cubicle arrangements for ease in reference and use, and to keep the periodical files in stacks. Sometimes it helps to have the last five years of a periodical in the monograph cubicles, in order to provide ready reference. However, this may result in a lot of unnecessary movement, if much reference work is undertaken in the library.

Current periodicals can be conveniently located in a special cubicle or area. Upon arrival periodicals might be placed on tables in the main reading room for a day or so to give those sturdy regular readers of every good medical library a chance to check them over day by day as they come. The major periodical sets, such as the *Journal of the American Medical Association*, *The British Medical Journal*, *Lancet*, and *Science* may be conveniently shelved in the general reading room. Here also should be kept the general reference works, and of course the major indices and the abstract journals.

Whatever promotes the ease of use of a health library will contribute significantly to the teaching effort in the health center. Students can readily learn where the books in which they may be interested are located, and they may be stimulated and encouraged to browse frequently and often throughout the library if it is open for their convenience. With comfortable chairs and lounges, with desks and tables frequently placed, with easy arm chairs, and with paper and pencils liberally supplied, the library can indeed become the real center of the entire teaching effort.

The difficulty is that many teachers in medical schools and most medical students do not know how to use a medical library. The librarian can help. An orientation in the use of the library to first year students is a real aid. This should include orientation for the students in all of the health auxiliaries. It is wise for the librarian to speak frequently at faculty meetings regarding the activities of the library, so that all members of the teaching staff will know what is available, and what is planned in connection with the development of the health library. An imaginative library committee can really assist.

While funds may be a limiting factor in the character of the health center library and in the books arranged in it, wise care in the selection of books and periodicals is paramount. The exercise of such wisdom will inevitably bring its own rewards in increased funds, as the usefulness of the library becomes increasingly apparent.

If the central health library in a teaching health center is not large enough or cannot be satisfactorily designed to provide seminar and conference rooms or lounges, the health library may be decentralized in part by placing appropriate periodical files and monographs in departmental seminar rooms and libraries. This might require some duplication of material, but it would certainly greatly assist the teaching effort. An alert health library staff could keep the departmental libraries coordinated with the main health center library, see to it that the books in the departmental seminar rooms are kept in order, and promote some competitive morale by seeking gifts for departmental libraries from departmental staff members. Pooling of departmental resources might assist in developing strong departmental libraries to supplement the main health center library. Such a program has worked successfully for many years at Western Reserve Medical Center in Cleveland. In the clinical departments, especially, many of the departmental staff members would be willing to donate to their own departmental libraries some of the periodicals to which they personally subscribe. Such departmental libraries, conveniently arranged in the departmental seminar rooms, are helpful in course study work on the part of the students. Ready accessibility and informality of the small book collection in the seminar room promotes use.

One of the most important features of a departmental teaching library for use in the departmental seminar room, or in the main health center library, is a carefully organized reprint collection. Reprints of significant articles can readily be obtained on request. Such articles may be treated as special items and may be bound in pamphlet binders and cataloged. Reprints of review articles are particularly useful in the health teaching effort. The accumulation of detailed knowledge in special health fields is so great that it is impossible even for experts to digest it adequately, and the original articles and abstracts are very confusing, particularly to students. Critical reviews summarizing and analyzing significant contributions in a field are extremely helpful to students. Each article in *Medicine*, *Physiological Reviews*, *Pharmacological Reviews*, and *Biological Reviews* is worth treating as a separate article in binding and cataloging. The topical character of *Annual Reviews* render them less satisfactory for teaching than for research. We need more critical review journals to aid our health teaching program.

It is pertinent for the health center librarian to know fully what the teaching curriculum may be in each of the health fields. Careful selection of periodicals and books to supplement the curriculum, and to add interest to the students taking the various courses, will result in increased use of the library, and thus in an increased efficiency in the teaching effort. Book and periodical reference lists may be posted daily or weekly to correlate with the subject matter of the different courses.

Fortunate is the health center where there is a good book store. This can well supplement the library of the institution, particularly in making available appropriate texts for the students, and by encouraging the purchase of special professional items in which the individual student may be interested. Such a store can also encourage the development of a small personal library containing some of the well-known classics related to medicine, and thus help promote the general cultural effort of the health teaching program.

The health center library itself would add greatly to the curriculum effort by having special collections relating to general cultural publications with a medical flavor, including poetry, novels, medicated essays of various sorts, and a wide collection of the major literary classics. These can frequently be obtained by gifts, especially from older physicians on the staff.

Of major importance is the historical collection in a health center library. This should serve as the archives for the institution, where all the important records of activities may be preserved for future study and use. Here, also, may be arranged exhibits from time to time to give the cultural background for the institution, and of course of the various health fields. As far as possible, this historical collection should foster study and quiet readings. If possible one copy of an early edition of an outstanding work of every great medical contributor should be obtained for the historical collection. This will add to the interest of orientation in the health disciplines; we all know best what we learn from its beginning. And it adds greatly to the interest of the complex fields related to medicine to see something of the ancient volumes which have contributed to the growth of the professional effort.

An interesting feature of a teaching health center library would be a collection of reprints and publications of staff members. Not only would this provide an important record of achievement in the institution, but it would help in the teaching effort by aiding the students in knowing at first hand what their teachers actually contribute. Such a collection is a considerable morale builder and may help maintain a wholesome competition among the staff members.

A recent development in American health teaching centers is the establishment of a "house organ." Some of these periodicals are maintained by alumni interest; most of them are quarterlies, some with considerable dignity and distinction. The *Yale Journal of Biology and Medicine* has had over 25 years of outstanding leadership, while the *Bulletin of the Johns Hopkins Hospital* has long been widely recognized as one of the most important monthly journals in medicine.

There are many interesting aspects to these local publishing efforts. Primarily, they provide an opportunity for the local teaching staff and student body to publish significant contributions. With the increasing centralization of editorial activity in the northeast part of this country, where the editors see each other frequently and talk things over, thus learning each other's whims and biases, there is often difficulty in obtaining publication from a provincial area which is unknown to the editorial staff. It is very easy for the editors on a great national journal, who may never have travelled much, to think of a health training area in some outlying part of the country as being a small and inconsequential affair from which nothing very worthwhile could ever come. The provincial health centers should, therefore, support their own publishing endeavor. Such a publication can be in the best democratic tradition. To obtain reasonable policy agreements, we must all, as John Locke long ago showed, have access to the same body of verifiable knowledge. Science has a great part to play in the democratic process. It was on this principle that Thomas Jefferson and his followers in this country advocated the establishment of the free public school. This was for the purpose of providing an opportunity for all of the citizens of a democracy to have available to them verifiable information about themselves and their environment. It was on this same basis also that the free public library has developed in this country. Now it would seem appropriate that on the same general principle all institutions supported at public expense should make freely available the results of their independent investigations and research. Hence the local journal in the health fields can really be a most significant factor in the general teaching program, particularly if it is distributed without cost to the libraries of medical institutions all over the world. The practical response in exchange is more than worth the effort!

Summary

Medical and health libraries can well be the heart of the teaching effort of a medical or health center. Books and periodicals may be obtained, arranged, and listed in accordance with the teaching program of the institution, with material organized especially for ease of reference and use, as correlated with the content of courses. Physical accessibility to monographs and periodicals, plenty of space for note-taking and reading, lounges, conference and seminar rooms, and individual study cubicles, contribute greatly to the teaching use of a medical library. Most important, however, in the success of correlating a medical library with a modern medical or health center curriculum is the skill, adaptability, good sense, and good humor of the health center library staff. That they are succeeding so well in promoting the teaching use of medical libraries throughout this country is testimony to their judgment and ability.

The Medical Library Center of New York: A Progress Report

By Jacqueline W. Felter, *Acting Director*

Medical Library Center of New York
New York, New York

ABSTRACT

An article published in the BULLETIN in 1963 outlined the proposed program of the Medical Library Center of New York. This progress report describes actual functions of the Center and attempts to evaluate them after four years of experience. Details of adapting a building intended for other use, financing this cooperative enterprise, applying standard library techniques and equipment to an atypical library, and acquiring materials that complement, rather than duplicate, the collections of member libraries are given. New services, not envisioned in detail in the initial program, but initiated during this period of operation, are mentioned. The report ends with a tentative look into the future.

AT the Medical Library Center we have a saying that, if one were to cross the Center for Research Libraries in Chicago with the Philadelphia Union Catalog, the Medical Library Center of New York would be the result. Certainly the objectives of MLC are similar to both of these prototypes, but the narrowly defined area MLC serves and the needs of the community make implementation of the objectives unique. In 1962 Erich Meyerhoff wrote an article which tells the history of the Medical Library Center and outlines its proposed program[1]. This paper was an architect's rendering, so to speak; now it is possible to view the actual structure. After four years of successful operation it can no longer be called an "experiment."

The Building

Even though the Medical Library Center purchased its building toward the end of 1961, the staff was not able to occupy its permanent quarters until January 1964. It is obvious that actual operation did not start with lightning speed. The building, designed as a garage, but with two floors suitable also for light industry, was not suited to library use without

Originally published in *Bulletin of the Medical Library Association,* Volume 56 (January, 1968), pp. 15-20. Reprinted by permission.

extensive renovation. Financial help was needed to make the alterations possible. Caution urged that final architectural plans should be drawn and remodeling begun only after funds for the purpose were assured. Matching grants from the Alfred P. Sloan Foundation and the Rockefeller Foundation, together with a grant received previously from the Department of Health of the City of New York through its Health Research Council, finally made it possible to start construction. Even then the increase in building costs over the earlier estimate made it necessary to defer renovation of the sixth floor and convert only the seventh floor to offices for the staff and book stacks capable of housing approximately 200,000 items.

A building designed for another purpose offers both disadvantages and advantages to its new occupant. Contrary to expectation the floor load capacity—120 pounds per square foot—prevented us from using book stacks especially constructed for compact storage. Therefore, to make storage as compact as possible with standard library book stacks, textbooks and monographs are shelved by size in fixed locations. This arrangement is possible because MLC is not open to the reader, except by special arrangement; it circulates its material as interlibrary loans. It is not a browsing library. Journals and other materials, however, are shelved in the conventional ways. On the other hand, the unusually high ceilings made it possible to accommodate ventilator ducts and electrical conduits and, in the office area, conceal them with hung ceilings. The resulting quarters are well-lighted, air-conditioned, and, except for the stack area which is more functional than decorative, brightly painted.

The seven floors not occupied by the Medical Library Center are rented to other organizations. Half of the space is occupied by a garage, sorely needed in a neighborhood characterized by expanding medical institutions with large numbers of personnel and visitors. The remaining space was formerly occupied by other commercial enterprises, but, as the leases have expired, the space has been taken by the New York Medical College and Mount Sinai School of Medicine. Thus, the building has become, in part, an educational and professional center; the property and neighborhood have been improved, and the taxes have been reduced by the tenancy of our tax-free neighbors.

Membership

Though the original Sponsoring Institutions have some of the largest and strongest libraries, it was not intended that the Center should serve only to relieve their growing pains. It was conceivable that a center which could house the overflow of large libraries could also serve as a back-up facility for institutions that might well maintain the smaller working literature collections. We welcome and have acquired a number of hospital libraries as participating members. Serving both large and small libraries does not result in a dichotomy, because both are doing the same work on a difficult scale, but the different types of libraries do make different demands on the Center.

To the nine original Sponsoring Institutions have been added two medical schools: New Jersey College of Medicine and Dentistry, and the newly incorporated Mount Sinai School of Medicine. There are now also twelve Participating Institutions, of which eleven are hospitals, making a total of twenty-three member institutions.

The annual membership fees are: Sponsoring Institutions, $10,000, Participating Institutions, $2,000, and Commercial Firms, $5,000. As yet, no commercial firms have become members. Nonmembers in the New York Area may borrow items, but thy must pay a unit transaction fee.

Administration

Operation of The Medical Library Center is guided by the Director. Professional librarians head the Technical Services Division and the Union Catalog of Medical Periodicals. Building maintenance and services are supervised by a part-time engineer. The Assistant Treasurer, or business manager, is also a part-time employee.

In the normal operating staff, excluding the part-time engineer and business manager, the ratio of professional to nonprofessional employees is 1:4. During the period of compilation of the Union Catalog, however, while there is need for considerable cataloging expertise and grant funds provide an augmented budget, the UCMP staff includes three additional librarians. Similarly, the Technical Services Division had as an additional cataloger for six months, Mrs. Elfrida Ureta of the Biblioteca Escuela de Medicina Universidad de Chile, Santiago, Chile, who was in New York while her husband was on a medical fellowship here. During this time the ratio of professional to nonprofessional employees was 1:2.

The Board of Trustees consists of one administrator from each Sponsoring Institution and is concerned mainly with financial affairs. The Board meets three times a year to vote on the budget and consider any facets of fiscal policy that are brought to its attention by the Director and Business Manager.

The librarians of the member institutions form the Advisory Committee of Librarians. This committee meets several times a year, usually at the request of the Director. Its function is to give the Director the members' views on the existing services, suggest changes or additional services, and act on those the Director proposes. The chairman is one of the librarians, elected by the membership; the Director of the Center serves as secretary. *Ad hoc* committees wrestle with special problems and procedures. Because the membership in the Center has increased, the Advisory Committee has become too large to function efficiently as a steering committee, and recently a Planning Committee was appointed to study current conditions and recommend future programs of service and acquisitions.

FINANCES

The Medical Library Center is a nonprofit organization. It was anticipated at first that surplus income from rentals would pay more than half of the operating expenses of the Medical Library Center, thereby enabling us to reduce the amount of the members' fees. In practice, thus far, this hope has not been realized. The building had not been well maintained by the previous owner, and most of the rental income has been reinvested in expensive repairs and replacement of equipment. The operating expenses of MLC, therefore, are still paid by the members' fees. In time,however, the original plan should become fact.

The income was augmented by an extension of the John A. Hartford Foundation grant which supported the Union Catalog of Medical Periodicals entirely through October 31, 1965. From November 1, 1965 through May 31, 1968, grant funds, first from the Department of Health of the City of New York (Grant No. U—1653 of the Health Research Council) and then from the National Library of Medicine (Grant No. LM00042—01 and 02), have partially spported the Union Catalog. The grant funds are applied to the expense of completing the conversion of the original records to machine-readable form. Operating expenses of the Union Catalog are included in the MLC budget.

SERVICES

The first service to be initiated was the delivery service; it continues to be the most popular of the various services. Driving a Hertz rented truck, our driver makes daily trips to the member libraries in Manhattan, the Bronx, and Brooklyn; on three days a week he includes New Jersey in his rounds, and on the remaining two days he stops at libraries in Nassau County on Long Island. The speedometer clocks 450 miles a week. The messenger not only delivers and picks up for return the items borrowed from MLC, but also delivêrs the interlibrary loans the member libraries exchange with each other. One librarian of a Sponsoring Institution has said that the delivery service saves her library the salaries of two messengers. The truck service is possible, of course, because MLC serves a compact geographic area. Such an arrangement would not be possible for an organization such as the Center for Research Libraries, whose service area includes many states.

A Xerox copy reimbursement service, begun in 1966, is also generally satisfactory. This service was designed to speed interlibrary loan transactions and reduce paper work. It speeds loans by eliminating the negotiations necessary for advance payment when the borrowing library requests an article in a journal that is restricted from circulation by the lending library. The lending library simply fills the request with a photocopy and sends to MLC a statement of the amount due at ten cents per page. The Center does the paper work, reimbursing each library once a month for the Xerox copies it has made for other members. Actually the Center is paying the members with their own money because it comes out of their dues, but it saves them nuisance and labor.

A TWX network was inaugurated on May 1, 1967. While it may be argued that TWX is not necessary in a restricted geographic area where telephone service is as fast and possibly cheaper, it was the consensus of the librarians of the member institutions that the written record TWX provides would improve the accuracy of interlibrary loan requests. A written record is made, of course, if the ALA interlibrary loan form is used; but, sent by mail or even picked up and delivered by the MLC messenger, the ALA form cannot be transmitted as rapidly as the TWX message. The Medical Library Center pays the cost of installation and monthly rental of the equipment; the member libraries pay for their messages. Thus far, TWX has been installed only in the libraries of Sponsoring Institutions. This policy does not reflect discrimination against the smaller Participating Institutions, for there certainly is as much justification for facilitating the interlibrary loan transaction in the library that is mainly a borrower as in the one that is mainly a lender. It is not discrimination; it is simply a matter of money. Here again, when MLC pays the equipment rental charge, it is only spending the member library's dues, and it cannot include TWX in the services to a Participating Institution that pays $2,000 a year and still make ends meet. If the participating libraries can manage an increase in membership fees, MLC can manage to include TWX.

The Depository Collection

The depository collection, which initially seemed to hold great promise, has perhaps, not completely fulfilled our expectations. There are two basic categories of deposit: deposit without expectation of return, and rental storage. Rental storage was intended to be of limited duration, an expedient for a library in the process of moving, temporarily in need of extra space, or awaiting completion of a larger stack area. For this, the member library pays a small fee to cover service, for books to and from rental storage are charged out and delivered by messenger, as are items from the permanent depository collection. Some rental storage collections do fit the initial specifications. Other collections, however, consist of long runs of common journals that might well be on permanent deposit (and often duplicate permanent deposits). They come from libraries where, as much as can be judged, there is little hope of larger book stacks to house them or little evidence of need, so long as the volumes are available for loan from MLC's permanent collection. Rarely would a volume be unavailable, because generally Xerox copies of the articles requested are supplied. This use of rental storage implies a lack of commitment to the idea of the central depository collection. It also reflects an outmoded belief on the part of institution administrators rather than librarians that the size of a library is a status symbol, even though a large proportion of the volumes are too old or unsuitable to earn their keep. Reluctance of large libraries to commit to the Center back files of common journals also does not enable MLC to fulfill as readily as we wish the objective of using the resources of the large libraries to back up the working collections of small ones.

Nevertheless, a considerable depository collection has been acquired. MLC has accepted what the member libraries have chosen to separate from their collections. In other words, the term "less-used" in the original policy statement has, in reality, meant that the donor library determines what is less-used and expendable in its collection. Thus, from one library we may have received a collection of institutional annual reports, while from another we have a large number of runs of journals including quite recent volumes. The term "less-used" is, of course, subject to different interpretations. Take state medical journals, for instance; they lend themselves to deposit because, though less-used in a research library, they may be much used in a library serving mostly clinicians.

Textbooks and monographs are noncurrent editions, less-used by everyone. The Center is the one place in the area where one copy of each edition of long-lived, frequently revised publications should be retained for historical reference and comparison. It is the logical resting place for the aforementioned administrative annual reports of medical institutions, organizations, and government agencies. The medical and paramedical dissertations from foreign universities, formerly held by the New York libraries, have been collected in MLC.

At the end of 1966 the holdings of the Medical Library Center included:

Journals	108,744
Textbooks and monographs	20,830
Government documents and institutional reports	20,665
Medical dissertations	209,000

The journals are a mixed lot of bound and unbound pieces; the figure 108,744 is items, not volumes.

Acquisitions

While it is evident that the periodical holdings of the Medical Library Center duplicate those of some of its members, and the duplication is justified by the aforementioned use to fill requests of small libraries, in general the policy of MLC is to complement, rather than duplicate, the libraries of its members. For this reason, MLC does not acquire current textbooks and monographs. In a region as richly endowed with medical libraries as New York, complementary materials are likely to be the less-used types that fit comfortably into the MLC acquisitions policy. Current journals is an example. At present, subscriptions are maintained only for medical journals indexed in *Index Medicus* that are not received currently by any library in the New York area. The Center has entered subscriptions also for thirty-six uncommon veterinary journals, a scarce commodity in this urban area. Current journals in other subject areas, such as nursing and dentistry, should be added to the subscription list in the future. The Center not only houses the dissertations of foreign medical faculties but has assumed responsibility for keeping the collection up to date. Gaps in journal holdings are filled from exchange lists, and there is a long-range plan to assemble from member libraries their fragments of foreign journals to make stronger sets in MLC, using the Union Catalog as a guide.

A modest reference collection is maintained. Back volumes of indexing services are usually gifts, but current issues are obtained by subscription. An extensive collection of union lists has been acquired for reference by the staff of the Union Catalog of Medical Periodicals.

The cooperative acquisition of expensive and/or infrequently used reference works, outlined in the original policy statement, has only just begun. The first such purchase was a subscription to the costly periodical, *Adverse Reactions Titles*, with the multiple copies distributed to the member libraries that wish to have them.

Cataloging and Physical Care

Cataloging procedures are simple. Journals, as is customary, are shelflisted by title, with holdings given in detail. They are, of course, included in the Union Catalog of Medical Periodicals. Inasmuch as MLC is not a browsing library, subject control of monographs and textbooks is unnecessary. Being shelved by size in fixed location, the books are identified by a location mark rather than a classification number. An author catalog only is maintained because all loans are interlibrary loans, and the items are requested by main entry, presumably verified in advance. Nevertheless the reference collection is useful for the checking of occasional puzzling requests.

Dissertations published during the last five years are shelved alphabetically by author. As they are retired from the current shelves, the older dissertations are arranged by university and year. To make author cards for over 200,000 dissertations would be a considerable undertaking and will be done only if experience shows that the present system is unworkable or if a bonanza and sufficient demand should justify publication of a dissertations catalog.

Annual reports are shelved in the conventional way, grouped by corporate body. A catalog of these is also a project for the distant future if the need is apparent.

Even though many of the periodicals are unbound, MLC has no binding program. Xerox copies are supplied in lieu of hard copy whenever it is possible. Therefore, we can preserve unbound issues, and it is often easier to copy pages in them. The Center owns a microfilm camera and will eventually film deteriorating journals, especially medical newspapers.

Union Catalog of Medical Periodicals

The computer-based Union Catalog of Medical Periodicals has been described elsewhere[2,3]. The articles referred to, however, do not describe its service policy.

The Union Catalog publishes volumes of selected periodical titles with library holdings and provides by telephone holdings information for the journals not included in these works. The policy, at present, is not to publish lists of journals that ceased publication before 1929, because such older material will not be sought frequently. The Union Catalog is, therefore, a service rather than a product.

The service and published volumes are included in membership in the Medical Library Center. Within MLC's service area—the New York Metropolitan Area—the service and publications are available also to nonmembers for a graduated annual subscription fee that is determined by the subscribing library's budget. In addition, libraries outside the New York Metropolitan Area may purchase the published volumes at cost and, presumably, they would not be interested in the telephone service at long distance rates. The installation of TWX, however, might result in a contradiction of this supposition.

Now that the conversion of the retrospective records to machine-readable form is nearly finished, it is possible to contemplate the addition of more contributing libraries. The first additions are about twenty libraries in Nassau County that had formerly compiled their own local union list. In the spring of 1966, when this list was in need of revision, the Medical Librarians of Long Island entered into an agreement with the Union Catalog for the preparation of a new Long Island Union List. The Union Catalog is absorbing the Long Island Union List but, at the same time, preserving its integrity on a separate computer tape so that a separate printout can be produced. The Union Catalog has assumed responsibility for updating its own and the Long Island lists as the librarians send in current information. The Medical Librarians of Long Island reimburse the Union Catalog for computer time and pay the cost of making multiple copies of the printout for local distribution. The Long Island Union List is not in competition with the Union Catalog; it enables the Long Island libraries to help one another with a compact local union list that is easy to use.

The new and revised computer programs of the Union Catalog of Medical Periodicals and the role that the Union Catalog is playing in helping other regional union lists develop should be the subjects of a separate article.

The Future

After only four years of operation, the present stack area of MLC is filled to capacity, and shelving has been installed on another floor. The additional stack area has 10,000 square feet and should hold another 100,000 items.

In the future, the strength of the Medical Library Center may be in rendering services rather than in warehousing books. That is the reason why, with the aid of a Resource Grant from the National Library of Medicine, a study of the feasibility of centralized and automated record keeping for circulation and serials control for our member libraries is in progress. The study is being made by Nelson Associates in collaboration with the Theodore Stein Company. They have been commissioned to determine how much each library should benefit by centralized record keeping; whether each library should delegate to MLC both functions, or one, or none; to recommend equipment to be used if the routines are automated; and to estimate the costs of the service. At the Jacobi Library,

Mount Sinai School of Medicine, a current periodicals control system is being designed that makes use of data prepared for the Union Catalog of Medical Periodicals and may well be a prototype for serials control systems for other members.

The progress that has been reported is the result of the foresight, imagination, and energy of Erich Meyerhoff, the first Director of the Medical Library Center; the support of the member institutions; and the cooperation of the librarians of the member institutions. While new projects will undoubtedly pass through trial periods, the Medical Library Center as a whole appears to have survived the era of experimentation.

REFERENCES

1. MEYERHOFF, E. The Medical Library Center of New York: An experiment in cooperative acquisition and storage of medical library materials. BULLETIN 51: 501-506, Oct. 1963.
2. FELTER, J. W., AND TJOENG, D. S. A computer system for a union catalog: Theme and variations. BULLETIN 53: 163-177, Apr. 1965.
3. FELTER, J. W. The Union Catalog of Medical Periodicals of New York. In: Information Retrieval with Special Reference to the Biological Sciences. Minneapolis, University of Minnesota, Nolte Center for Continuing Education, 1966, p. 117-131.

The Medical Library Assistance Act: An Analysis of the NLM Extramural Programs, 1965-1970*

BY MARTIN M. CUMMINGS, M.D., *Director*

MARY E. CORNING, *Special Assistant to the Director*

National Library of Medicine
Bethesda, Maryland

ABSTRACT

The imbalance between medical library resources and information needs of the health professional led to a reexamination of the mandate for the National Library of Medicine. Legislation known as the Medical Library Assistance Act (MLAA) was passed in 1965 which enabled the NLM to (1) initiate programs to assist the nation's medical libraries and (2) develop a medical library network with the establishment of regional medical libraries to link the NLM with local institutions.

The National Library of Medicine, through the MLAA, has made available $40.8 million to the medical library community under a competitive grant and contract mechanism for the period July 1965—June 1970. A total of 604 projects has been executed in resources, research and development, training, construction, regional medical libraries, publications, and special scientific projects. An assessment is given of each of these programs and their impact on both the National Library of Medicine and individual medical libraries. In the aggregate, these programs have significantly improved library and information services to the professional health user. The principal limitation has been inadequate funding to accomplish the level of originally stated objectives.

INTRODUCTION

THE Medical Library Assistance Act, PL 89-291, (MLAA), was enacted by the U.S. Congress in October 1965. In the five fiscal years (FY 1966-1970) which have elapsed, 40.8 million dollars have been made available to the medical library community from the National Library of Medicine under a competitive grant and contract mechanism. The length of time and the amount of money expended justify an assessment of

*Presented at the Seventieth Annual Meeting of the Medical Library Association, New York, New York, June 3, 1971, as part of the General Session.

Originally published in *Bulletin of the Medical Library Association,* Volume 59 (July, 1971), pp. 375-391. Reprinted by permission.

1. The fundamental concepts embodied in the Act
2. The allocation of resources to fulfill the expectations of the Act
3. The impact on the National Library of Medicine
4. The performance and level of accomplishment by the medical library community which received these funds, and
5. The impact on users.

Status of the Medical Library Community Prior to the MLAA

The concepts developed and embodied in the MLAA reflected both the strengths and weaknesses of the U.S. medical library community.

In 1964, the National Library of Medicine (NLM) was serving as a national resource; it had a budget of $4 million, a staff of 350 provided services nationwide, and was an innovator in the use of technology to develop a computer-based information storage and retrieval system (MEDLARS) which had just become operational.

The weak status of the medical libraries in this country had been described by Deitrick and Berson[1] and Bloomquist[2]. In 1962, the Surgeon General held a Conference on Health Communications[3]. The recommendations related to the need for improved communications research, training, and the use of libraries as communications centers and resources.

The National Academy of Sciences—National Research Council (NAS-NRC) studied "Communication Problems in Biomedical Research"[4] in 1963. The NAS-NRC conclusions and recommendations emphasized the responsibilities of the biomedical community for facilities and services, research and development, training and coordination of the biomedical information complex. The U.S. President's Commission on Heart Disease, Cancer and Stroke[5] assessed communications problems within the context of three specific diseases; and its communications recommendations were specifically addressed to the need for better facilities, resources, and legislation. Thus, significant studies and evaluations from professional user groups highlighted the need for improved biomedical communication.

Activity in the medical library world was reflected in the substantive articles of the 1964 issues of the *Bulletin of the Medical Library Association*[6] which reviewed the National Library of Medicine's new computer-based system, MEDLARS, *Medical Subject Headings (MeSH)*, and the NLM bibliographic services. The relative service roles of both the NLM and individual libraries in interlibrary lending and photocopying, and the establishment of an MLA Committee on the NLM were treated in Editorials and News Notes[7].

Other articles in the *Bulletin* described an International Congress on Medical Librarianship; operating aspects of individual medical libraries; mechanization; library statistics; the growth of the literature in specialized areas of health. A special section was devoted to "Regional Plans for Medical Library Service" with representatives from six states assessing independently their current and potential scope of services. There was a recurring theme: librarians were interested in responding to more than their immediate local clientele; but they were hampered by lack of facilities, equipment, staff, and money.

This can be expressed as the imbalance between library resources and users' demands for services. This imbalance can be traced to the greatly increased funding of medical research and education with no attendant disparity between the present and potential roles of a medical library. Problems existed in meeting the needs of the professional user, whether he worked in health research, education or practice. These problems were traceable to the fundamental issues of the nature, availability and utilization of resources—both human and material. Some physicians and scientists, geographically distant from modern library facilities, were found to be isolated from current information sources. Some libraries could be characterized not only by inadequate funding but by a low level of performance. The NLM commissioned studies to be done by the Association of American Medical Colleges[8], [9], [10] on needs of medical school libraries, and requested assistance from the Medical Library Association to crystalize data and statistics on problems facing medical libraries[11].

NLM also reexamined the NLM mandate from the U.S. Congress to serve as a national resource and "to assist the advancement of medical and related sciences and to aid the dissemination and exchange of scientific and other information important to the progress of medicine and to the public health." As a result of these examinations, Cummings recommended that the future role of the National Library of Medicine should include programs to upgrade the nation's medical libraries and recommended regional and local interrelationships in which the constituent elements would have clearly defined roles and responsibilities. The totality would then be a strong entity which would encompass a sharing of talent and resources to achieve the primary objective of responding more effectively to the information needs of the health professional.

Specifications were then developed for legislation which would create new programs directed at both the individual and the institution, and at local, regional and national levels. Cummings[12] described NLM's proposed supporting functions and activities at the dedication of the Countway Library in 1965. He presented the philosophy underlying the pending legislation, which was subsequently enacted by the U.S. Congress in October 1965, as the Medical Library Assistance Act (PL 89—291):

It is my view that the time has come for rapid expansion of library resources locally. Continued dependency of the more than 6,000 medical libraries upon the services of the National Library of Medicine would lead ultimately to the evolution of a monolithic medical library resource in this nation. For the convenience of the user, for the inspiration which the presence of the local library gives to its own community, for the serendipity which accompanies browsing and search, strong medical libraries must exist wherever there are strong biomedical interests.

In my view, our country requires the development of a complex of regional medical libraries with adequate facilities, resources, and personnel to serve those sections of the nation with underdeveloped library facilities. NLM has submitted legislative specifications to Congress and the Administration requesting authority and funds to provide assistance to local and regional libraries for (1) library construction, (2) training of librarians, (3) research in the field of information sciences, (4) library resources, (5) development of regional libraries, (6) publications and translations support. I am encouraged by the favorable reaction of librarians, physicians, and scientists to these proposals.

During this same year (1965), articles published in the *Bulletin* showed a continued preoccupation with MEDLARS activities; and the Medical Library Assistance Act occupied the Editorial and News Notes Sections.

By contrast, in 1970, 25 percent of the papers published in the MLA *Bulletin* described activities funded by the Medical Library Assistance Act. Subjects included educational needs of health sciences library manpower; information needs of specialty groups; mechanization of library procedures; automated serials accession systems; library management data; and regional medical libraries—their services and functions.

Interrelationship of NLM and the Medical Library Community (FY 1966-1970)

During the period of the MLAA (July 1965-June 1970), the total five-year cumulative budget of the NLM was approximately $87.6 million. Of this, NLM provided 49 percent or $43 million to the U.S. medical library community: 40.8 million under the MLAA and 2.2 million through contracts for MEDLARS Centers and other library-based activities. This sum is relatively large when viewed against a prior base of no federal support for medical libraries. It is small in comparison with the total national expenditures for health care, medical research, and communications. The total (extramural and intramural) efforts of the National Library of Medicine in 1969 represented only 0.03 percent of the overall national funding for health activities (Fig. 1). However, the very existence of these funds is significant because they are unique and are the principal existing mechanism for the exclusive improvement of the resources and services of U.S. medical libraries.

In any federal grant program, the funding institution cannot dictate the usage of these funds. It can only present the philosophy, the objectives, the criteria, and then respond to the submitted proposals which are evaluated by an external review group for technical merit and priority. Accordingly, the usage of the NLM funds essentially reflects the perspective and priorities of the medical library community.

Programs Executed Under the MLAA

The underlying purpose of the MLAA is to improve biomedical information services. This assumes a conversion from traditional attitudes and mechanisms to emphasize that (1) the modern medical library is part of the communication process, and (2) improved communication is necessary for advances in medical research, education and practice.

The MLAA (1965) authorized the following programs:

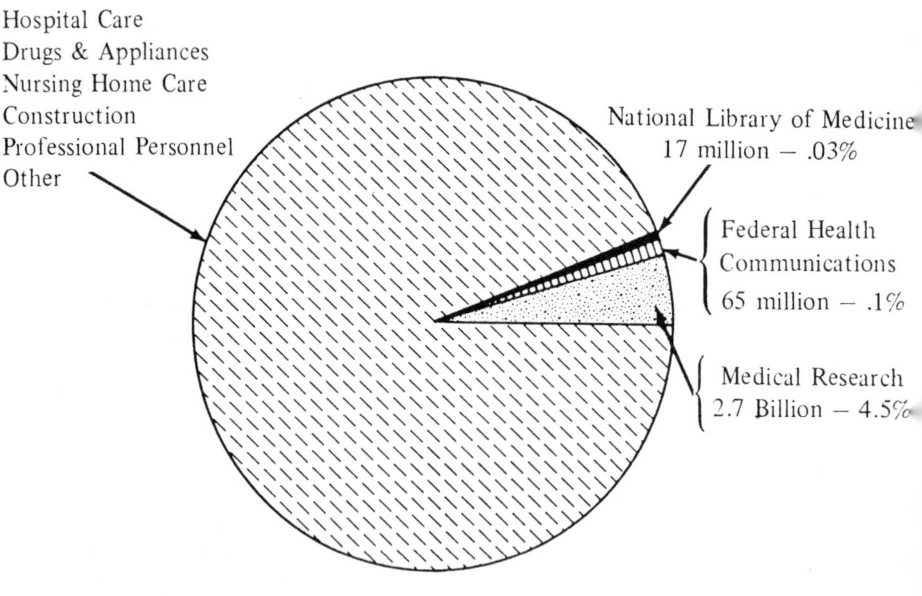

FIG. 1. National health expenditures in 1969 for health care, medical research and communications.

1. Construction of facilities
2. Training in medical library sciences
3. Special scientific projects
4. Research and development in medical library science and related fields
5. Improvement and expansion of the basic resources of medical libraries and related instrumentalities
6. Establishment of regional medical libraries
7. Biomedical publications, and
8. Regional branches of the National Library of Medicine.

TABLE 1

COMPARISON OF NLM AUTHORIZATION, APPROPRIATIONS, AND UNFUNDED PROJECTS UNDER THE MEDICAL LIBRARY ASSISTANCE ACT OF 1965 FOR FY 1966–1970 (JULY 1, 1965—JUNE 30, 1970)

(Million $)

(A)

Program	Funds Authorized	Funds Appropriated and Awarded	Percentage of Authorized Funds Appropriated	Number of Projects
Resources	$15	$11.8	79%	402
Construction	40	11.3	28	11
Research and Development	15	6.0	40	103
Regional Medical Libraries	12.5	4.7	38	10
Training	5	4.5	90	28
Publications	5	2.3	46	43
Special Scientific Projects	2.5	.2	8	7
NLM Regional Branches	10	0	0	0
Totals	$105	$40.8	39%	604

(B)

Program	Difference Between Authorized and Appropriated Funds	Project Funds Requested but Unavailable
Resources	$ 3.2	$ .9
Construction	28.7	34.8
Research and Development	9.0	.5
Regional Medical Libraries	7.8	.9
Training	.5	.3
Publications	2.7	.2
Special Scientific Projects	2.3	0
NLM Regional Branches	10	0
Totals	$64.2	$37.6

The NLM has acted to implement all of these programs with the exception of establishing our own Regional Branches. We decided, instead, to try to improve existing resources rather than to create competitive federal entities.

Comparison of the level of funding authorized by Congress under the MLAA and the funds actually appropriated (Table 1A) indicates that only 39 percent of the total authorization was made available to the NLM. The distribution of authorized and appropriated funds by program illustrates two program areas received 50 percent or more of funds authorized; Training Grants and Resource Grants.

The NLM has maintained records of those projects which have been approved but could not be supported due to inadequate funding. The amount of monies represented by these unfunded projects (Table 1B) are identified by program areas. Only in the construction program does the sum of the funded and unfunded projects total more than the original estimate of needs as reflected in the basic Congressional authorization. In all other program areas, the level of unfunded projects does not equal, and

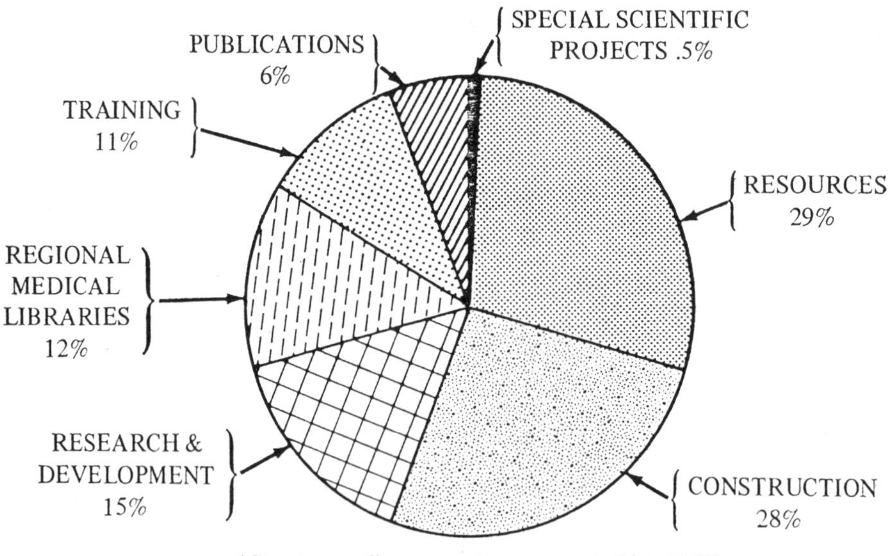

FIG. 2. Percentage distribution of funds by program for the period July 1, 1965 through June 30, 1970.

oftentimes is a small percentage of what had been originally estimated as needed by the medical library community. There are three interpretations for this: (1) the original estimate in the Act was not realistic, (2) the scarcity of funding tempered the number of requests received by the NLM, or (3) the medical library community was unable to convince those who authorized appropriations of its needs. We believe the interpretations (2) and (3) are the primary reasons for the failure to achieve more adequate funding.

The total number of grants awarded through the MLAA was 604, and the distribution by programs and funds is shown in Table 1A. Figure 2 gives the percentage distribution of MLAA funds by program areas. Resource Grants utilized 29 percent; Construction 28 percent; Research and Development 15 percent; Regional Medical Libraries 12 percent; Training/Fellowships 11 percent; Publications 6 percent; and Special Scientific Projects 0.5 percent.

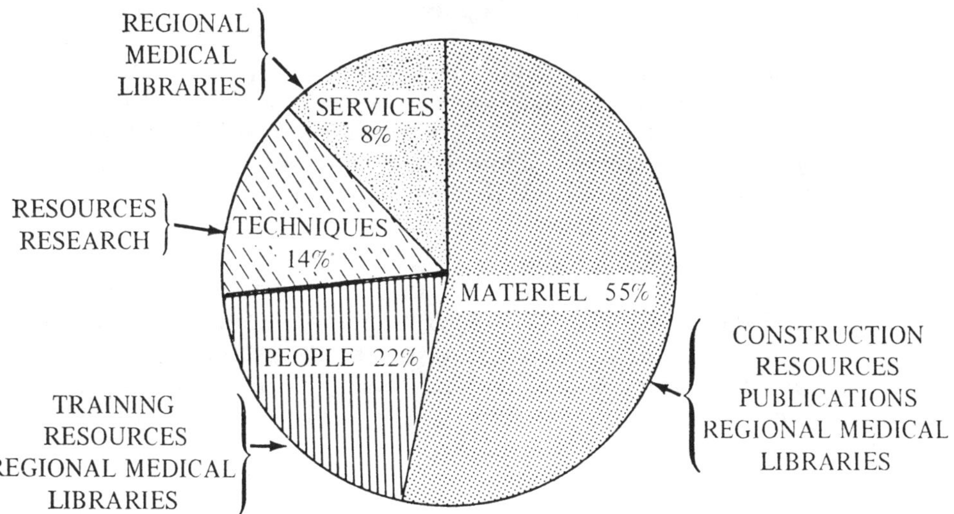

FIG. 3. Percentage distribution of program funds by personnel, materiel, techniques and services for the period July 1, 1965 through June 30, 1970.

We have tried to estimate how the MLAA funds have been utilized in terms of personnel, material, services and techniques. These figures are shown in Figure 3. Although there needs to be some refinement of the data, the gross picture is clear. Assistance for material has been provided within the Construction, Resource, Publications, and Regional Medical Library (RML) Grants. The Training Program emphasis has been on people, and salaries have been provided for medical library staff through both the Resource and Regional Medical Library Programs. Techniques (development and utilization of technologies) are made possible through both the Resource and the Research and Development Programs. The service function is primarily reflected within the RML program. Overall, it is clear that emphasis has been overwhelmingly on material (55 percent), with relatively little emphasis on new services (8 percent).

Some specific details on the individual programs follow.

Research and Development

The Research and Development Program was intended to encourage research in medical library science and the development of new techniques, systems and equipment for information storage and retrieval. The projects have been grouped in three categories.

1. Library Services, Operations and Manpower—projects concerning development and evaluation of information activities in libraries, and studies of manpower needs and training to provide these services
2. Biomedical Communications Usage and Tools—projects, studies, publications in the broad field of biomedical communications
3. History of Medicine and the Life Sciences—historical studies of matters related to health and medicine

The distribution of the number of grants and contracts and funds among the three program categories is given in Table 2. Library services accounted for 13 percent of the projects and 35 percent of the funds; biomedical communications 42 percent of the projects and 49 percent of the funds; and history of medicine 45 percent of the projects and 16 percent of the funds.

Projects supported have included surveys on health library manpower, an on-line computer serials control system, studies of communication patterns among medical researchers, development of standard nomenclatures, evaluation of self-instruction materials, and language analysis for information retrieval. There has been heavy emphasis within the program on history of medicine projects. New research methodology was not a prominent feature of grant applications by librarians and information specialists. Thus, few research projects to date have led to the application and implementation of new modes of biomedical communications.

Training

The Training Program included both training grants and fellowships as follows:

(1) Traineeships and fellowships for advanced academic degrees in library or information science
(2) Retaining or special training for health science librarians or information specialists
(3) Institutional programs for training in library science and communication
(4) Establishment of internship programs in medical libraries.

A summary of the training grants and fellowships is shown in Table 3. The training funds made available by the NLM for FY 1966—70 will have provided for the training of approximately 350 individuals. The average cost per trainee is $8,100, of which 57 percent covers stipend and trainee expenses, and 43 percent is nontrainee expenditures. Insufficient emphasis was placed on retraining existing librarians in modern information-handling methods, and there were no grants to train library assistants.

Publications

Forty-three scientific health publications, critical reviews, atlases, compendia, and abstracting and indexing tools were supported, with an expenditure of $2.3 million under this program. Many secondary literature services and specialized subjects series have resulted and these would not have been supported by commercial ventures (Table 4).

Special Scientific Projects

This program provided ten special fellowships for preparing scholarly studies on topics such as discovery, regulation and use of drugs, and interorganizational aspects of urban community health. Approximately $200,000 was expended for this program. Although the quality of work seems uniformly good, the small number of participants who applied has been disappointing.

TABLE 2

NLM RESEARCH AND DEVELOPMENT PROGRAM GRANTS AND CONTRACTS AWARDED, FY 1966–70 (JULY 1, 1965—JUNE 30, 1970)

Category	Number of Projects	Amount (Million $)
Library Services, Operations and Manpower	14	2.1
Biomedical Communications Usage and Tools	43	3.0
History of Medicine	46	1.0
Total	103	6.1

TABLE 3

NLM TRAINING PROGRAMS, FY 1966–70 (JULY 1, 1965—JUNE 30, 1970)

	Projects Funded	Individuals Supported[1]
A. Training Grants:		
Non-Degree Programs	6	77
Degree Programs		
Masters	9	143
Ph.D.	5	33
Total	20	253*
B. Fellowships:		
Postdoctoral Research		
History	6	6
Biomedical Communications	2	2
Total	8	8

*Training programs funded during 1966-70 will have provided training for approximately 350 individuals, some of whom will actually receive this training in FY 1971. Funds awarded totaled $4.46 million.

[1]During 1966-70; some for more than one year.

TABLE 4
NLM PUBLICATION PROGRAM GRANTS AND CONTRACTS, FY 1966-70
(JULY 1, 1965—JUNE 30, 1970)

Category	No. of Projects
Abstracts	8
Atlases	6
Bibliographies	6
Critical Reviews	1
Handbooks and Catalogs	8
Monographs	3
Translation Projects	6
Other Media	5
Total	43
Total $ Awarded	2.3 Million

It is evident that few scholars accepted this opportunity to do creative writing and study. The deficiency rests with the U.S. medical community and not with librarians.

CONSTRUCTION

Construction grants were made to eleven institutions: nine Medical Schools; one School of Optometry; and one School of Veterinary Medicine. The specifics are given in Table 5. It is clear that this program will have a profound impact on improving library resources in those areas where they are being constructed. There is a great need to expand this program to other needy institutions (approximately twenty-five to forty).

RESOURCES

Under the Resource Grant Program 401 grants have been made, totaling 11.8 million dollars. The distribution and utilization of these grants provides us with an interesting commentary on medical library operations. Approximately 50 percent of the number of resource grants went to hospital libraries, whereas 63 percent of the funds went to medical libraries within academic institutions (Figures 4 and 5). Over 50 percent of the funds expended under the resource grants were used to acquire journals, books, and informational materials. Approximately 24 percent of the monies enabled the medical libraries to increase the number of their staff, and 16 percent was for the purchase of equipment.

Thus, this program has had a major impact on the enlargement of collections. More than 400 local libraries have been assisted, but most did not use the funds to improve the nature and scope of service through increased manpower or by the application of new technology.

Regional Medical Libraries

As noted earlier, the NLM decided not to establish its own Regional Branches but chose to support regional services through existing libraries of excellence or those with potential. We tried to develop a "network" to achieve the goal of responding more effectively to the needs of the health professionals. We did not define the "network" as a rigid unchanging snare of interconnections; we visualized a planned sharing of resources systematically so that improved services could be provided with maximum efficient utilization of available resources—manpower, fiscal, and technological. Thus, the underlying principle was "cooperative service."

In order to assist the local institutions in a systematic and constructive manner, we established a regional link to interrelate the national and local institutional levels. This link was the Regional Medical Library. Regional Medical Libraries were principally university-based, were selected competitively from libraries with strong collections, well-trained staffs,

TABLE 5

List of Institutions Receiving NLM Construction Grants (Fiscal Years 1967—1970)*

	RML Region	Type of Institution	Award	Net S.F. Area	Volume Capacity
Boston University Boston, Massachusetts	I	Medical School	$ 1,017,891	29,900	100,000
Brown University Providence, Rhode Island	I	Medical School	536,331	14,119	100,000
Rutgers, The State University New Brunswick, New Jersey	II	Medical School	541,293	12,498	100,000
Jefferson University Philadelphia, Pennsylvania	III	Medical School	1,765,636	44,465	145,000
George Washington University Washington, D. C.	IV	Medical School	1,295,595	29,271	80,000
Wayne State University Detroit, Michigan	V	Medical School	1,459,567	50,107	130,000
Auburn University Auburn, Alabama	VI	Vet. Med. School	101,229	4,000	17,000
Southern College of Optometry Memphis, Tennessee	VI	Optometry School	176,525	5,924	20,000
University of Nebraska Omaha, Nebraska	VIII	Medical School	1,636,077	59,629	273,000
University of Utah Salt Lake City, Utah	VIII	Medical School	1,121,450	35,425	190,000
University of Texas (Medical Branch) Galveston, Texas	IX	Medical School	1,598,406	48,783	150,000
Totals			$11,250,000	334,121	1,305,000

* Congressional appropriations were not made for Construction until FY 1967.

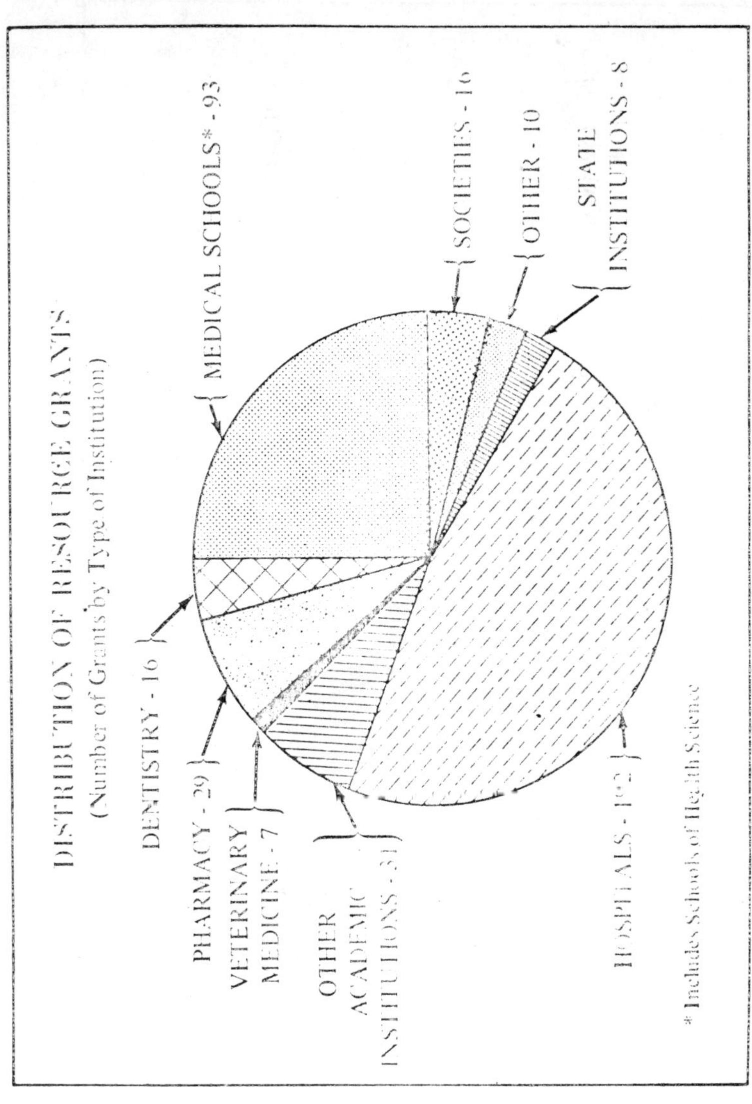

FIG. 4. The number of resource grants distributed by type of institution.

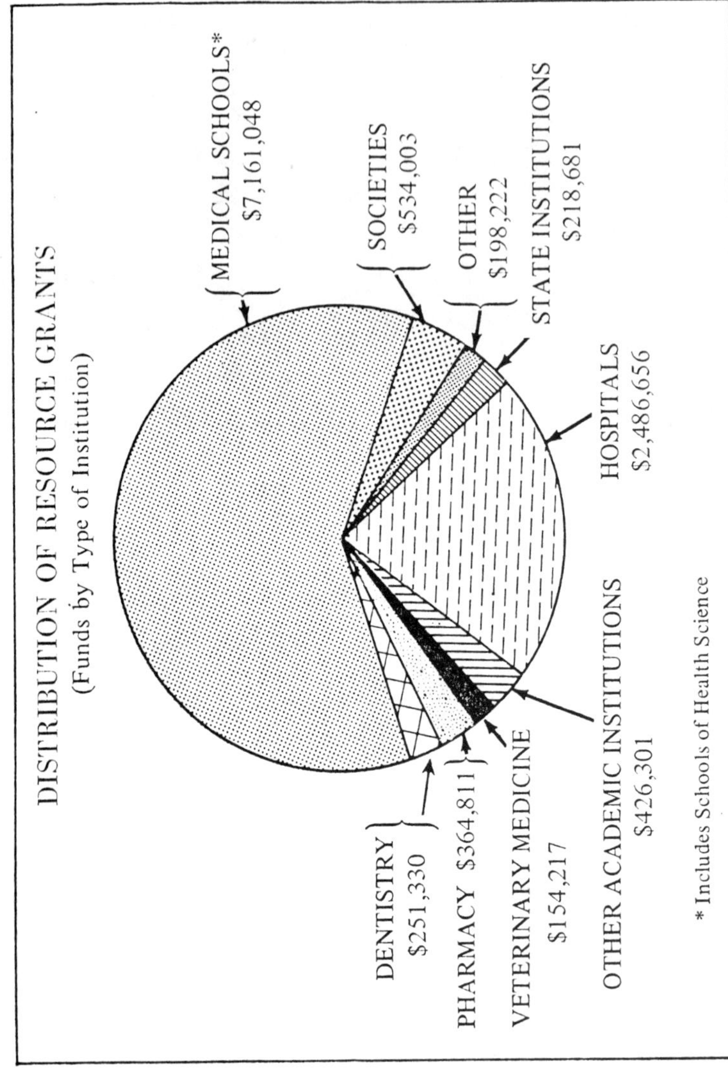

FIG. 5. The funding distribution of resource grants by type of institution.

and a good record of providing medical library services. The first Regional Medical Library was established at Harvard in 1967. Today there are eleven such Regional Medical Libraries, with the National Library of Medicine, itself, designated as a Regional Library for a geographic area in the mid-Atlantic United States (Table 6).

TABLE 6
LIBRARIES RECEIVING NLM GRANTS TO SERVE AS REGIONAL MEDICAL LIBRARIES IN ELEVEN GEOGRAPHIC REGIONS

	States	Funds (Million $)	Operational
#1—New England New England Regional Medical Library The Francis A. Countway Library of Medicine Boston, Massachusetts	Connecticut Maine Massachusetts New Hampshire Rhode Island Vermont	1.020	10/1/67
#2—New York New York & Northern New Jersey Regional Medical Library New York Academy of Medicine New York, N. Y.	New Jersey (Northern Counties: Bergen, Essex, Hudson, Hunterdon, Middlesex, Morris, Passaic, Somerset, Sussex, Union, & Warren) New York	.336	2/16/70
#3—Mid-Eastern Mid-Eastern Regional Medical Library College of Physicians of Philadelphia Philadelphia, Pennsylvania	Delaware New Jersey (Southern Counties: Atlantic, Burlington, Camden, Cape May, Cumberland, Gloucester, Mercer, Monmouth, Ocean, & Salem)	.715	7/1/68
#4—Mid-Atlantic Mid-Atlantic Regional Medical Library P. O. Box 30260 Bethesda, Maryland—(NLM)	Maryland North Carolina Virginia Washington, D. C. West Virginia		
#5—East Central Kentucky-Ohio-Michigan Regional Medical Library Wayne State University Detroit, Michigan	Kentucky Michigan Ohio	.256	4/1/69

TABLE 6—*Continued*

	States	Funds (Million $)	Operational
#6—Southeastern Southeastern Regional Medical Library A. W. Calhoun Medical Library Woodruff Research Building Emory University Atlanta, Georgia	Alabama Florida Georgia Mississippi Puerto Rico South Carolina Tennessee	.470	1/2/70
#7—Midwest Midwest Regional Medical Library The John Crerar Library Chicago, Illinois	Illinois Indiana Iowa Minnesota North Dakota Wisconsin	.325	11/18/68
#8—Midcontinental Mid-Continental Regional Medical Library University of Nebraska Medical Center Omaha, Nebraska	Colorado Kansas Missouri Nebraska South Dakota Utah Wyoming	.228	7/1/70
#9—South Central University of Texas Southwestern Medical School at Dallas Dallas, Texas	Arkansas Louisiana New Mexico Oklahoma Texas	.178	2/1/70
#10—Pacific Northwest Pacific Northwest Regional Health Sciences Library University of Washington Seattle, Washington	Alaska Idaho Montana Oregon Washington	.639	10/1/68
#11—Pacific Southwest Pacific Southwest Regional Medical Library, Center for Health Science University of California Los Angeles, California	Arizona California Hawaii Nevada	.512	9/1/69

The hierarchical concept for the Medical Library Network (Figure 6) is as follows:

1. The NLM is the comprehensive national resource which can assist other medical libraries in terms of material not in their collection, as well as serving as the medical indexing and cataloging center for the nation.
2. The Regional Libraries are to improve and expand their reference and interlibrary loan services to medical and hospital libraries in a broad geographic area, and
3. The local libraries are to assist individual health professionals as the closest point for library service.

MEDICAL LIBRARY NETWORK PLAN

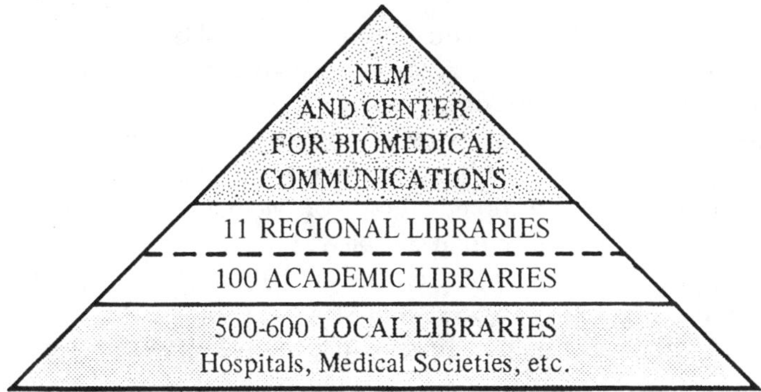

RELATIONSHIPS

- COMPATIBLE WITH NATIONAL INFORMATION SYSTEMS.
- COMPATIBLE WITH OTHER NATIONAL LIBRARIES.
- ASSIST SPECIALIZED INFORMATION CENTERS.
- ASSIST MISSION ORIENTED GROUPS, FEDERAL AND PRIVATE.

FIG. 6. Hierarchical structure of Medical Library Network Plan.

Designation as a Regional Medical Library required the recipient institution to increase its scope and nature of services to health professional users in a broader geographic area. Since the operation of the first Regional Medical Library in 1967, 4.7 million dollars have been expended and all eleven of the Regional Medical Libraries are in various stages of operational activity. If one examines the last year of operations for seven Regional Medical Libraries (with four of them operational for less than one year), the distribution of 1.65 million dollars in grant funds in terms of service is:

42% for Interlibrary Loan Services
17% MEDLARS Demand Search Services
9% Education and Consultation primarily for local hospital libraries
7% Preparation of Union Lists
6% Orientation and Information Programs
4% Reference Services
15% Other (Management and Overhead)

Prior to the establishment of the Regional Medical Libraries in 1967, the National Library of Medicine was receiving on a national basis approximately 175,000 interlibrary loan requests annually (Figure 7). In the subsequent three years, with the Regional Medical Libraries in various stages of operational capability, the total national interlibrary loan activity for both the National Library of Medicine and the Regional Medical Libraries has more than doubled. This is a real measurement of successful performance. If one excludes interlibrary loan requests which NLM receives in its role as a Regional Medical Library, and from foreign sources, then the level of interlibrary loan requests NLM receives in its capacity as a national resource has dropped to approximately 48,000. Although fewer in number, these requests are for the most inaccessible and rare items in the medical literature. Overall, however, we still provide more than 100,000 loans annually.

The establishment, in 1964, of the NLM's computer-based bibliographic storage and retrieval system, MEDLARS, generated considerable demand for MEDLARS demand searches throughout the U.S. and abroad. Accordingly, decentralized MEDLARS Centers were established in the United States. Some of these centers are part of the Regional Medical Libraries; others are located in different institutions in the same region and they work cooperatively with the Regional Medical Library. In the last year, there were 22,000 MEDLARS demand searches released. Of these, approximately 16 percent were performed by NLM, 48 percent by U.S. Centers, and 36 percent by Foreign Centers. The interlibrary loan and the demand search services are thus two functions of the National Library of Medicine which have been decentralized successfully in an effort to make these services available more efficiently to the professional health user. We

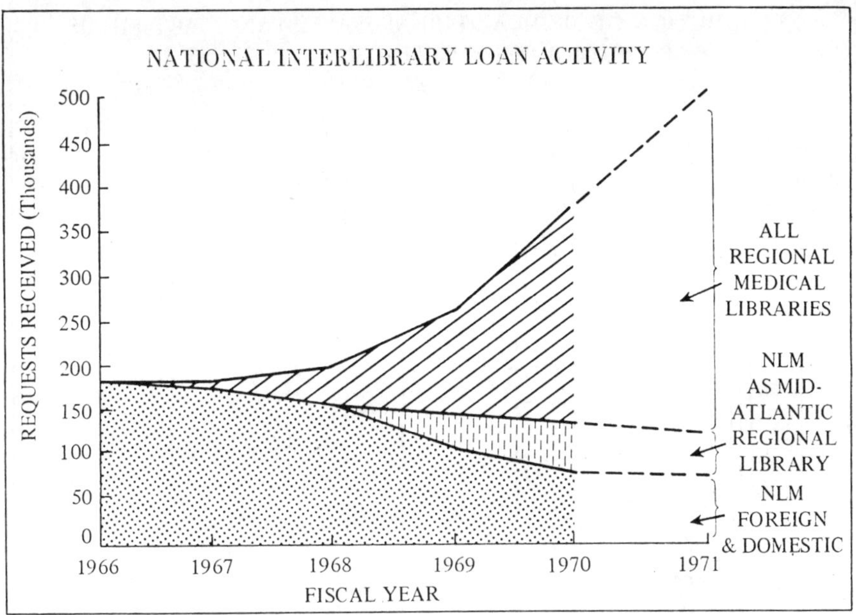

FIG. 7. A comparison of the distribution of national interlibrary loan activity before and after the establishment of Regional Medical Libraries.

are now planning to decentralize AIM—TWX, our successful on-line bibliographic service in a similar way.

An analysis of distribution of funds by program, according to regions presently defined for the Regional Libraries (Figure 8), indicates that each of the regions was funded in the 3.4—4.4 million dollar range, with two exceptions, Region VI (Southeastern) and Region X (Pacific Northwest). Although the funding would appear to have a fairly consistent distribution overall, the constituent elements vary considerably from region to region.

Construction funds increase the level of funding for each region. However, Regions VII (Midwest) and XI (Pacific Southwest) which had no construction monies still maintain a high overall figure because of emphasis on research and training. In these two areas only, the research and training funds totaled more than resource funds. By contrast, in Regions I (New England), II (New York), and VI (Southeast) the sum spent for both research and training was less than one-half that spent for resources.

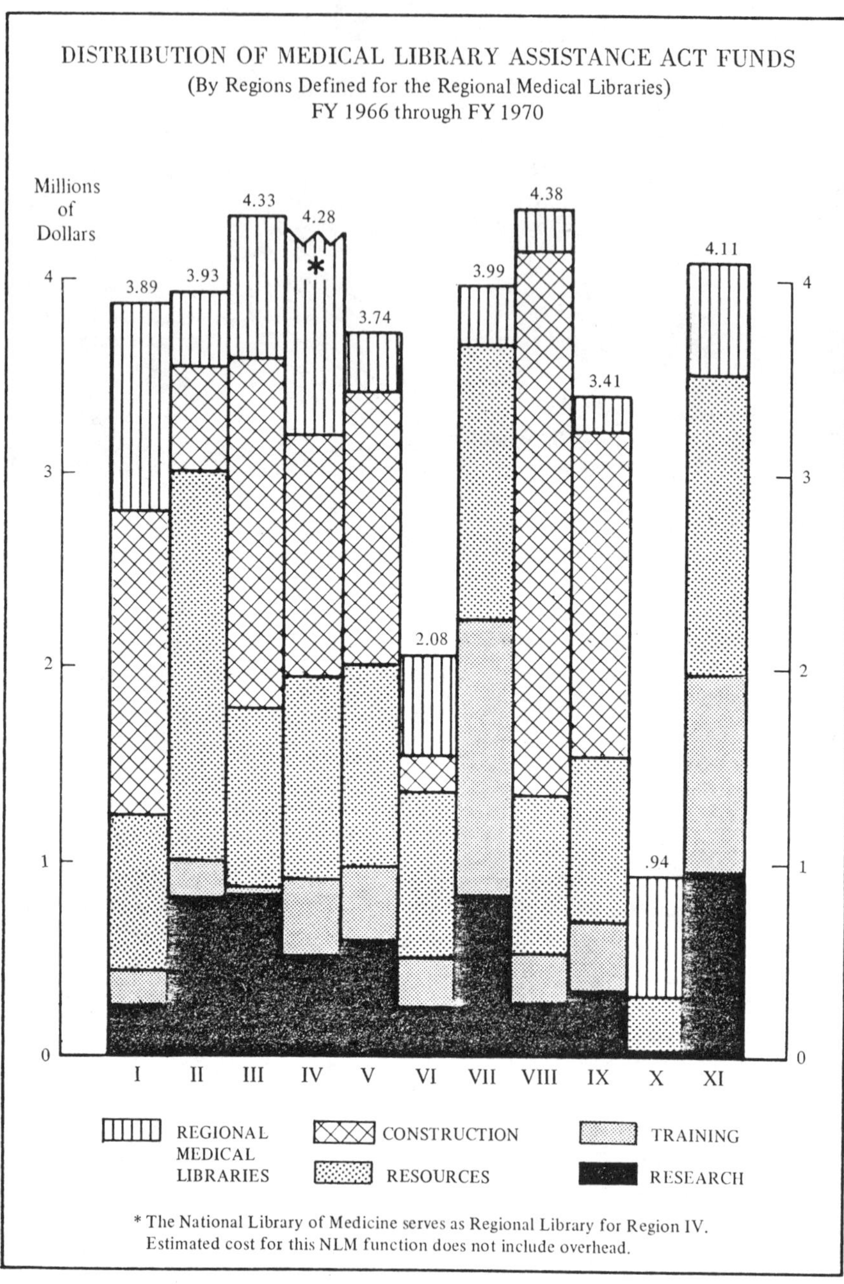

FIG. 8. Regional distribution of MLAA funds in terms of Research, Training, Resource, Construction and Regional Medical Library Programs of the NLM.

Assessment of the Medical Library Assistance Act

Fundamental Concepts Embodied in the Act

The fundamental concept of the Medical Library Assistance Act is to develop a cooperative sharing of resources in order to improve library and information services to the health community. The Act provides the mechanism and the authorization for funding to achieve this goal. We continue to believe that this is a firm and constructive basis for developing a national medical library network with clearly delineated responsibilities at the national, regional, and local levels.

Allocation of Resources

The appropriation of resources to fulfill the expectations of the Act has been 39 percent of what had been authorized. Accordingly, we have fallen short of goals which we had originally identified. For example, we had hoped to reach 600-700 medical libraries through our resource program; instead, we were able to assist only 400. We were informed in 1964 of immediate construction needs for eighty-six health sciences libraries, but we have been able to assist only eleven. Our training program has served to stimulate and encourage specialization in medical librarianship, but it cannot begin to fulfill overall manpower requirements. Thus, in both the specific and overall programs we have made a beginning, but the limited availability of funds has prevented more substantial accomplishments.

Impact on the National Library of Medicine

The MLAA has affected NLM both organizationally and functionally:

1. NLM has become part of a national medical library network instead of serving as every institution's library.
2. NLM has decentralized, to date, two information service functions (Interlibrary Loans and MEDLARS) to regional centers, with an accompanying provision of funds to these regions for increased resources.
3. NLM has expanded its efforts to identify not only the needs of the professional health user, but also of the medical library community and to seek appropriate solutions.
4. Considerable NLM staff time and resources are devoted not solely to the NLM daily operations but to the administrative support of programs directly relating to the medical library community.

It was anticipated that the development of a national medical library network would indeed shift workloads so that maximum efficiency would be achieved. This in fact has occurred, with NLM assuming greater workloads in some technical areas and lesser ones in others. NLM's service level in 1964 is compared with 1967 and 1970 in Table 7. The MLAA programs have reduced interlibrary loan and MEDLARS demand services from NLM, but they have altered significantly the kind and scope of other services provided by NLM. This is reflected in new products such as *Current Catalog, Abridged Index Medicus (AIM),* the on-line time-sharing system of AIM—TWX, and audiovisual services.

Impact on the U. S. Medical Library Community

It is true that the period of our experience with "regionalism" is short. However, definitive trends are becoming evident. Medical libraries seem to have been most interested in improving their collections or physical resources before improving medical library services. This appears logical if one has clearly in mind the level and scope of the services to be performed.

TABLE 7
COMPARISON OF SCOPE AND LEVEL OF NLM'S SERVICES
FY 1964, 1967, 1970

	1964	1967	1970
Interlibrary Loans	130,555	175,000	100,611
Reference Requests	20,154	25,514	21,702
Technical Services			
Items Catalogued	14,157	14,529	17,767
Publications Added	91,105	112,301	121,942
History of Medicine Services			
Reference	281	1,338	1,461
Index Medicus			
Articles Indexed	144,057	168,310	210,000*
Subscriptions	7,600	4,757	5,151
Abridged Index Medicus			1,924
MEDLARS Searches	586	4,733	22,000†
Recurring Bibliographies		10	18
Literature Searches Distributed		19,177	23,351
Audiovisuals Distributed			72,865**

* Includes NLM and U.S. and foreign sources under contract.
† NLM: 3,520; U.S. Centers: 10,560; Foreign Centers: 7,920.
** National Medical Audiovisual Center.

However, the time has come for primary emphasis on providing improved service.

We are not convinced that there is a sharp delineation of functions at the national, regional, and local levels (as portrayed in Figure 6), nor does there seem to be a clear understanding of this division of responsibilities. In some cases we find a "local" library with "regional" aspirations and a "regional" library with "national" inclinations. With limited resources, every library cannot be of equal size and status.

The National Library of Medicine has unique national responsibilities not only to serve as a resource library but to acquire, index, and catalog comprehensively. It should also encourage the establishment of library standards, union serial lists, and cooperative cataloging. Some of these tools and procedures are best developed cooperatively on an overall basis with subsequent availability to all. Otherwise, uncorrelated independent efforts will consume the limited available resources and produce few overall advances.

Impact on the User

Our experience with the Regional Library Network has convinced us that a medical library network is no longer a concept but a reality. This is particularly important now when the workloads continue to increase at national, regional, and local levels without a corresponding increase in fiscal and personnel resources. Conceptually, we believe that the value of the network is clearly demonstrated by the rising number of service requests made to local and regional libraries and by the increasing number of responses made by these libraries. We do not have, however, a quantitative measure of user reaction.

Practically, the linkage aspect of the network should permit a more effective redistribution of functions and workloads at all levels and an overall increase in both the number and kinds of services to users. The most tangible evidence we have noted is in the shift from the national level to the regional level in the provision of interlibrary loan and MEDLARS demand services to the individual. The NLM's role, particularly with regard to interlibrary loan service, is not primarily to respond to those interlibrary loan requests which the Regional Medical Libraries cannot fill.

We are disappointed, however, that there have not been adequate funds for an increase in reference services, for emphasis on consultation and educational programs, and the inclusion of multi-media informational services. The consultation and educational role of the Regional Medical Libraries should be developed so that they become demonstration and training centers. This does not mean that Regional Medical Libraries will vie with academic institutions for formal training programs, but they can be a unique resource for internships and specialized work experiences.

We are convinced that audiovisual materials as well as the printed word are important media to convey medical information. It must be determined whether the Regional Medical Library can become a multi-media information center to serve as a depository for the collection and dissemination of audiovisual materials.

Conclusions

We believe that, in the aggregate, the Medical Library Assistance Act and the extramural programs of the National Library of Medicine have had a significant beneficial effect on the improvement of library and information services to physicians, scientists, and other related health personnel. The impact of these programs obviously would be more profound had the appropriations been larger. This is particularly true with respect to medical library construction, where the funds made available were only sufficient to support the building of eleven new medical libraries. Funds invested in support of research were probably the least rewarding for several reasons: (1) Most medical librarians were not trained in the scientific method nor had they had a previous experience with research, (2) the so-called "information scientist" competed most successfully for the lion's share of these funds and thus made contributions which were only peripherally relevant to the improvement of library services. Funds appropriated for training of medical librarians have been well spent. Graduates from these programs may well be our library leaders of the future. More emphasis on retraining of existing librarians seems indicated. Resource grants have expanded the collection of many small libraries but there remains a need to use these funds for improved services. Historical studies and special publications have enriched the literature of medicine. Eleven Regional Medical Libraries (including NLM) are now operational as the first step toward a medical library network.

In summary, the MLAA has done much to upgrade medical library services to the nation's health community. However, we have not done well enough. There is a need for financial resources to reach all medical libraries who lack personnel to serve adequately health personnel requiring medical information. We believe that through creative resource sharing we can improve our collective performance. As the NLM now enters the period of administering extramural programs under a three-year extension of this Act, we shall be in a better position to allocate resources which are more realistically attuned to library performance and user needs.

REFERENCES

1. DEITRICK, J. E., AND BERSON, R. C. Medical Schools in the United States at Mid Century. New York, McGraw-Hill, 1953.
2. BLOOMQUIST, HAROLD. The status and needs of medical school libraries in the United States. J. Med. Educ. 38: 145-163, March 1963.
3. Surgeon General's Conference on Health Communications, November 1962. Washington, D.C., U.S. Department of Health, Education, and Welfare, Public Health Service, Feb. 1963.
4. National Academy of Sciences—National Research Council. Division of Medical Sciences. Communication Problems in bio-medical research: report of a study. Washington, D. C., Oct. 1963; supplement, Washington, D. C., March 1964.
5. President's Commission on Heart Disease, Cancer and Stroke. A national program to conquer heart disease, cancer and stroke. Volume I, Dec. 1964; Volume II, Feb. 1965. Washington, D. C., U.S. Government Printing Office.
6. Bull. Med. Libr. Ass. 52: 148-180, 414, 545, 645, 1964.
7. Bull. Med. Libr. Ass. 52: 442, 795, 1964.
8. DATAGRAM. Medical Library needs. J. Med. Educ. 40: 396-397, April 1965.
9. Guidelines for Medical School Libraries (Special Issue) J. Med. Educ. 40: 5-64, 1965.
10. Library Study Committee of the Association of American Medical Colleges. MERLIN K. DUVAL, M.D., Director, and SEYMOUR ALPERT, M.D., Co-Director. The health sciences library: its role in education for the health profession. J. Med. Educ. Part 2, Aug. 1967.
11. Committee on Surveys and Statistics of the Medical Library Association. Library statistics of schools in the health sciences: Part I. Bull. Med. Libr. Ass. 54: 206-229, July 1966; Part II. Bull. Med. Libr. Ass. 55: 178-206, Apr. 1967.
12. CUMMINGS, MARTIN M. The edge of husbandry: the role of the National Library of Medicine. Biblioteca Medica: Physician for Tomorrow, Ed. by David McCord. Boston, Harvard Medical School, 1966.

The Pacific Northwest Regional Health Sciences Library: A Centralized Operation*

BY GERALD OPPENHEIMER, *Librarian*

Health Sciences Library, University of Washington
Seattle, Washington

ABSTRACT

The Pacific Northwest Regional Health Sciences Library is described in relation to its health manpower and library population. Among the services which it provides are a document delivery service. A computer system provides a reporting system which analyzes trends in the borrowing pattern; these patterns are discussed, and some unusual features explained. Publicity campaigns have been conducted. The influence of a centralized library service on other libraries is discussed.

IN spite of apparent similarities of Regional Medical Library Programs, the differences caused by geography, population size and distribution, health care activity and health manpower ratios, and bibliographic resources are far more significant in the eventual determination of the program, in setting priorities, in the pace of development, and the cost of projects. These factors will also influence the particular type of structure in which the Regional Medical Library is imbedded and the amount of formal or informal cooperation which develops. In a subtler vein, perhaps, it guides the attitudes of the Regional Library towards its own admittedly experimental policies, rules and regulations and the degree of acceptance which may be expected from individuals and institutions served.

Region X, the Pacific Northwest, covers five states—Alaska, Idaho, Montana, Oregon, and Washington. The program of its Regional Library was indeed influenced considerably by the geographic and demographic character of this part of the country. Its most noticeable feature is its size.

*Delivered as part of the General Session on "Contrast in Patterns of Regional Medical Library Service" at the Sixty-ninth Annual Meeting of the Medical Library Association in New Orleans, Louisiana, May 20, 1970.

Originally published in *Bulletin of the Medical Library Association,* Volume 59 (April, 1971), pp. 237-241. Reprinted by permission.

The total area of Region X is 1,000,000 square miles or almost 30 percent of the total land mass of the United States. Perhaps even more startling are the distances of this region which covers five time zones.

Seattle itself has a fairly central location: 200 air miles to Spokane, 120 to Portland, 500 to Pocatello, 625 to Billings, 1450 to Anchorage. Yet the distance between Seattle and Attu is about the same as that between Seattle and Havana, and from Seattle to Point Barrow is about as far as between Seattle and New Orleans. In view of such distances travel is mostly by air, particularly since the Region is also poor in roads. Consider, for example, the difference between Alaska's 6,500 miles of paved roads and Texas, the state nearest in size, with 240,000. The total population of the Region is approximately 7 million or about 3.5 percent of the population of the United States.

Consider also the distribution of this population. Over half of Alaska's people live in the vicinity of Anchorage, and the rest in widely scattered and isolated towns and villages. Idaho has one city with a population exceeding 50,000, Montana two, Oregon and Washington three each.

As regards health resources of the Region there are about 350 nonfederal hospitals ranging from 150 in Washington to thirty in Alaska. The number of physicians ranges from 4,500 in Washington to 175 in Alaska, with a total of almost 8,800, or approximately one physician for 800 persons compared to the national average of 1 to 700. In Alaska there are only two communities with more than ten physicians, and out of a total of 434 towns, 412 have no local physician at all. Its active nurses live in fifty-eight different communities, leaving 376 localities bereft of even such elementary health care. In the total Region, health-related personnel, including public health officials, technicians, hospital administrators, and pharmacists amounts to 45,000, or about 3 percent of the health manpower of the Nation.

Among the institutional health resources of the Region there are only two medical schools, two dental schools, five schools of pharmacy, and three postbasic and postgraduate schools of nursing plus thirty-three NLN approved basic schools and only one firm as far as we have been able to discover which is a member of the American Pharmaceutical Manufacturers Association.

An appreciation of the Region must take into account bibliographic resources as well, and, specifically, health-related ones.

The 1968/1969 *American Library Directory* lists only three health-related libraries in Alaska, one for Idaho, eight for Montana, thirteen for Oregon and twenty-four for Washington. There are only seven of all of these libraries which exceed the 10,000 volume mark.

The question whether this area constitutes a natural region in some sense must, I believe, be answered affirmatively. On the whole there has always existed some cohesiveness, particularly in the area of health and library affairs. Both Portland and Seattle are referral centers of long standing, the latter particularly in relation to Alaska, and both medical schools have mounted continuing medical and paramedical education efforts for neighboring states, much accelerated recently, of course, by the Regional Medical Program.

Bibliographically the region has had a long history of cooperation. The five states and in some cases also the Province of British Columbia are those which are covered by the Pacific Northwest Library Association, the first regional library association in the country, by the Pacific Northwest Chapter of SLA, by the Pacific Northwest Regional Group of MLA and by the Pacific Northwest Bibliographic Center housed at the University of Washington.

Full operation of PNRHSL began on October 1, 1968. The cordial and uncomplicated relationship with the University of Oregon and the absence of any other library with which cooperative arrangements were to be made allowed the PNRHSL to concentrate on developing its service program.

Among these services there was first of all document delivery service. Next in importance we felt was the counterbalance to the "central resource" role, the stimulation of local self-reliance through resource development. We did not take resource development, however, as being synonymous with collection building. Major emphasis in this part of the program was placed on consultation in the field with library supervisors, hospital administrators, and chairmen of library committees, on training library personnel, primarily through workshops, at various locations in the region, on bringing the existence of the Library to the attention of potential users, and on gathering information about available resources. Other activities which had priority were a fully responsive reference service strengthened by MEDLARS search capability, and finally the production of a distributable Union List of Serials.

Since the responsibility for the Program in our centralized operation was not formally shared, our immediate attention had to be directed towards discovering ways and means of acquiring knowledge about the region and our users.

This requirement led us very early to the use of an automated reporting system developed by our systems analyst which would allow us to obtain the necessary data on all document delivery transactions. This system also produces as a subset of its total reporting capability the data required by the National Library of Medicine.

Each month the computer prepares a list of borrowers who have been active since the beginning of the report year. For each the tally will show the monthly figure and cumulative total for number of requests received, the number of requests not accepted, the number filled, the performance ratio, the number of photocopy sheets, and the number filled by loan and by photocopy.

These monthly reports are studied carefully, especially with an eye toward trends and changes in performance. Variations which are of particular interest to us are activity levels by state and for localities contacted by our field team. Another item which is scrutinized carefully is our performance ratio. In the original grant application we expressed confidence that the Health Sciences Library of the University of Washington would be a 90 percent library. Whatever criticism may be levelled against this concept, we would regard a decline from this figure as a cause of concern because this would demonstrate that for over 10 percent of requests regional resources are inadequate, delays would be inevitable, and the cost of operation would increase. The latest cumulative figures indicate an overall performance ratio of 91 percent for the second year. It might be true of course that as local libraries come into existence and others build up their holdings, users will no longer approach us for the same high percentage of the mundane, and as the proportion of more exotic requests increases our performance ratio will drop. Should such a drop occur, our reporting system will allow us to test this hypothesis. This information and my regular inspection of unfilled transaction records and of those transaction records not filled through Health Sciences Library holdings are used as guides for acquisition of monographs or journals on a selective basis. This is done because here also we have in mind our role as regional resource library. It should be noted that these additions are not charged to the Regional Library budget, which is only tapped for duplication made necessary by regional demands

Most of the data on journal titles requested is derived from another portion of the computer output which on a quarterly basis lists journal titles by CODEN, year, and requester. An annual printout arranged by requester, title, and frequency allows us without additional effort to determine the request patterns of any of our institutional borrowers. This listing has enabled us, for example, to assert that the frequency of requests per title has not exceeded for any user the degree which could reasonably suggest that placing a subscription rather than borrowing would be advisable. This device, of course, is not only helpful to us but also to the requester, who may obtain a copy of the printout from us for his own purposes.

Another data element in this monitoring system should be described. Flow through time is determined for filled and unfilled requests and reasons for delay are specified when processing time exceeds three days. The latest cumulation shows that 77.6 percent of filled requests are processed within two days, but that 5 percent take more than ten days and that 80 percent of unfilled requests required more than three days before their fate is determined. The last two figures require some explanation. Neither should simply be ascribed to the proverbial reluctance of librarians to give up. Our willingness to fill requests after ten days, and sometimes considerably longer, and to try to fill other requests (unsuccessfully as it may turn out) stems from the relative absence of other easily available sources and the fact that bibliographic searching is best conducted at PNRHSL short of sending the request on to the referral library, NLM, for example. There are several factors which tend to lengthen the processing time. The first has to do with the fact that we treat the whole University of Washington Library system rather than just the Health Sciences Library as our base of operation. This means that a PNRHSL searcher consults the bibliographic apparatus of the Main Library and, if the item is located, retrieves the material for loan or copying. I should add that the University has become the willing partner in our service in line with long established attitudes about its obligation to the Pacific Northwest.

Secondly, we occasionally also rely on the cooperative spirit exhibited by such a library as that of the King County Medical Society. Thirdly, we will in many cases hold requests for material not immediately available. It is our experience that claims for the universality of the need for urgency have been exaggerated. To be certain, however, we have developed a notification procedure which allows requesters to indicate their choice of courses of action for us to take. Our following up and responding definitively, even if late, has increased the feeling of confidence and reliability for the regional operation on the part of the user.

The centralized position of PNRHSL and the dearth of bibliographic tools in the Region led us to adopt a policy which is as free of restrictions as is compatible with efficient functioning in-house. We reject, for example, requests for reasons of lack of verification only when absolutely necessary and when our own efforts of identification have been fruitless.

As mentioned earlier and in contrast with other regional libraries operating in a different milieu we honor requests for any journal title and do not anticipate that we will be issuing a list of forbidden titles in the foreseeable future.

Within our particular configuration it is obvious that much care must be given to the development of avenues of communication. Our efforts in this direction have so far been mainly confined to attempts to stimulate the establishment of TWX units, to find means of connecting to the Advanced Record System employed by the General Services Administration which would allow direct contact with the Veterans Administration installations, and even establish contact in similar fashion to the state most in need of such a link, Alaska.

In addition to this method of communication, PNRHSL is engaged in an effort to contact in person, through field representatives, each of the hospitals and hospital libraries in the Region. The frequency with which this needs to take place has still to be determined.

What are the impressions that we have gained after a year and a half of operating this program?

One should take a look first of all at the user of PNRHSL. The first progress report showed that out of 12,000 ILL requests received, approximately 25 percent were from federal hospitals, 30 percent from other public and private hospitals, 10 percent from academic institutions, less than 5 percent from commercial enterprises including pharmaceutical companies, and 5 percent from individuals. It remains to be determined whether the surprisingly low figure of 4.3 percent direct requests from practitioners is due to the fact that more health professionals than expected do have access to an institution or whether a substantial number of this group are unaware of our existence or other means to satisfy their informational needs.

Another unanticipated result was the distribution of requests from the various states. While the pattern for Montana, Idaho, and even Washington is fairly straightforward, i.e., percentage of requests and percentage of health manpower running parallel, Oregon with 31 percent of all practitioners accounted for only 7.4 percent of requests, and Alaska with 2 percent of physicians was responsible for 11 percent of requests. The following hypotheses are offered in explanation of these apparent discrepancies.

First, the relatively high number of physicians in Oregon combined with a relatively low number of requests tends to show that where there is a good medical library like that of the University of Oregon Medical School with a well-established service pattern, the existence of the Regional Library appears not to disrupt this service, but to furnish a readily approachable resource whose response time, as acknowledged by the requesting library, is indeed satisfactory.

Second, the relatively low number of physicians combined with the relatively high number of requests from Alaska, particularly via the Alaska Health Sciences Library, seems to point up the effect of a small library with only a basic collection but with an aggressive and responsive service program.

This phenomenon provoked the question whether our obviously centralized pattern was not already on the road, in a natural and informal manner, toward decentralization by way of subregionalization. If this were true, the PNRHSL would still be the resource library but would relate differently not only to Idaho and Montana as compared to Oregon and Alaska but it could be expected that its service to Oregon would take on a different form from its assistance to the Alaska Health Sciences Library. Without going into details at this time, it may perhaps be summarized by saying that in the case of our neighbor to the south we shall continue to act as last regional resource library and to plan for cooperative service, using as partners the excellent staff of the University of Oregon Medical School Library. For our neighbor to the north it is perhaps more important that the Regional Library find ways and means of making the Alaska Library more self-sufficient in terms of its own well thought out program. The problems there center around increasing its staff and its collection, and supporting and augmenting services already under way on a minimal scale but with highly effective results, and those yet to be offered.

A look at the trip reports of our field librarians may provide partial answers to two further questions about the experiences gained during the operation of PNRHSL: first, the question of the effectiveness of the publicity effort undertaken to draw attention to PNRHSL services, and second, the question of whether or not, particularly in a strongly centralized set-up, the avowed intent of stimulating local initiative is not thwarted by the very existence of the Regional Medical Library. To answer the first, let me give you a very typical quote from the report of a trip in Washington State.

> This hospital library did not know of us and they were glad to hear of the PNRHSL. Since the Library is just getting under way, many questions arose. There is much interest and they want the Library to succeed and to be used.

Our publicity effort consisted of several mailings, one of which in particular we regarded as well designed and attractive. This literature was sent to every physician in the region, every hospital administrator, every state health department, all health-related and major other libraries, and all members of the Pacific Northwest Group of the Medical Library Association. It consists of editorials and articles in local medical journals and newspapers, of appearances before annual conventions of state medical associations and other professional groups. We occupied booths at some of these meetings. The yield of this effort, we must conclude, has been low. Perhaps not lower than any other such publicity campaign, but low enough to convince us that field contact is absolutely indispensable.

Has the existence of the Regional Library harmed local development? Because the elapsed time is still relatively short and conditions are still fluid it may perhaps be too sanguine to assume that all the buds our field librarians saw will turn into flowers, yet far from encountering the discontinuance of local service, which was sporadic at best, we find ourselves cast in the role of catalyst. Particularly in Idaho and Montana efforts are under way to build resources, to establish communication links, and to upgrade the quality of personnel and services, relying of course heavily on the backstopping function of PNRHSL.

In trying to anticipate what trends may establish themselves as far as features of the program are concerned, I believe that PNRHSL may become even less of a first-contact library and that reliance will be placed on the small hospital library which should gradually become more adequate. In a larger sense this process will of course be accelerated should subregionalization occur which would, in effect, create a middle layer of service. Even then I do not expect the number of interlibrary loans to diminish. We all know very well that as library service grows, it outpaces resources and we look forward to increased demands on us from this direction.

I see a continuing need for field visits to hospital libraries on a rotating basis. Not only is this a conviction based on the needs as observed by our field librarians but on the excellent results which can be demonstrated by a similar operation of the neighboring British Columbia Medical Library Service.

Workshops and continuing education opportunities for library supervisors will be prominent in the years ahead. We see possibilities however even in our region for a sharing of this burden and the feasibility that in some cases our participation will be minimal.

We also expect an extension of the TWX network which may reach Alaska in 1970 or 1971.

When I try to speculate what the Regional Medical Library Program might be some years from now, I encounter questions rather than visions.

Let me briefly indicate what some of these questions are. The National Library of Medicine in pursuing the objectives of the Medical Library Assistance Act has quite properly assumed responsibility for the Regional Medical Library Program, including plans for the development of a biomedical communications network. Yet at the same time, perhaps, equally properly, it is asserted that by this is not meant total responsibility. This is sometimes defended on philosophic grounds as when it is said that this attitude is necessary so that none of the interests of the other sectors will be compromised. More frequently however it is limitations of funding which, it is asserted, require multiple sources rather than a single source of revenue for full regional medical library service. The question then arises: How can the development of the subunits of the great network be secured? Even where enthusiasm runs high, are local resources sufficient to provide the links? When demonstration and persuasion have failed, is there another way in which priorities of other potential funding organizations can be altered in favor of library development? If local support is meager or nonexistent does this mean that the need is nonexistent? It will be of great interest to all of us how future goals are to be realized.

The whole staff of PNRHSL are extremely gratified in being part of an enterprise which one of our grateful users claimed to be the "single most effective piece of health legislation yet." We ourselves can from our corner of the country only think of the Regional Medical Library Program as a permanent federal obligation towards increasing the spread of knowledge which hopefully will lead to better health care. Whatever evidence we have been able to gather at least points in this direction.

Medical School Libraries in the United States 1960 through 1975

SUSAN CRAWFORD, PhD

FOR ALMOST two decades subsequent to World War II, federal supportfor science and technology in the United States reached a magnitude never before equalled. Especially during the period 1953 to 1965, there occurred a sharp and sustained increase of huge proportion. While total expenditures by all sectors of the economy increased at an average rate of 13% per year, the contribution of the federal government to science grew at the rate of nearly 20% per year[1]. It was in this period that a great national research program in the health sciences developed, followed by public demand for increasing services in health, education, and welfare.

Health sciences libraries, as strategies in attaining the objectives of research, teaching, and health care provision, were in turn affected by increased production of information and began to experience difficult problems in its handling and control. In the early postwar period, they were still relatively isolated units developed for local or specialized audiences. Cooperation existed among medical school, hospital, and medical society libraries, but relationships were informal rather than by integrated, national design[2]. In 1960, therefore, the National Library of Medicine (NLM) commissioned a study by Harold Bloomquist of the Harvard Medical School Library to investigate the status and needs of medical school libraries in the United States. This investigation, which was published in the *Journal of Medical Education*[3], was instrumental in adoption of the Medical Library Assistance Act in 1965 and subsequently led to a planned effort to improve biomedical communication on a national scale.

The objective of this communication is to trace, within the context of

From the Division of Library and Archival Services, American Medical Association, 535 N Dearborn St, Chicago.

Reprint requests to the Division of Library and Archival Services, American Medical Association, 535 N Dearborn St, Chicago, Il 60610 (Dr Crawford).

Originally published in *Journal of the American Medical Association*, Volume 237 (January 31, 1977), pp. 464-468.

environmental changes, the development of medical school libraries from the Bloomquist study in 1960 through the mid-1970s. The survey draws heavily on statistics developed by the American Medical Association Department of Medical Education, the Medical Library Association Committee on Surveys and Statistics, and the NLM Extramural Programs[2, 4-12]. The integration of data from these sources provides the first longitudinal perspective of medical school libraries in the United States that is supported by hard data.

Changes in Environmental Context

During the 15 years studied, a number of changes took place—sociopolitical, technological, and organizational—that have profoundly affected the development of health sciences libraries in the United States.

Growth of Medical Schools.—During the period 1960 through 1975, the number of accredited schools increased by 31%, from 87 to 114 schools (Table 1). These include fully accredited medical schools, medical schools with provisional approval, and schools accredited to offer basic science courses. Student enrollment increased by 75%, from some 30,000 students to 53,000. Growth in number of full-time faculty increased by more than 300%, from 11,000 faculty members to more than 36,000. But the most extensive increase was in the rise in financial support, from around $371,000,000 in 1960-1961 to more than $2,417,000,000 in 1973-1974, reflecting a 551% increase. These statistics do not include some 11 developing medical schools that have not as yet attained provisional approval and which had no students enrolled in 1974-1975. Clearly, the data indicate that, during the past 15 years, medical schools have grown dramatically in number, size, faculty, support, and student population.

Table 1.—Growth of Medical Schools, 1960-1975: Selected Years[18-21]

	No. of Schools*						
Academic Year	Fully Accredited	Developing, Provisional Approval	Accredited Schools of Basic Sciences	Total	Student Enrollment†	No. of Full-Time Faculty	Total Financial Support (Thousands of Dollars)‡
1960-1961	81	2	4	87	30,388	11,111	370,880
1963-1964	84	3	1	88	32,001	14,468	603,184
1966-1967	84	3	2	89	33,423	19,296	1,010,327
1969-1970	87	8	6	101	37,669	24,706	1,549,514
1972-1973§	98	6	8	112	47,546	33,550	2,110,247
1973-1974	104	5	5	114	49,808‖	33,172¶	2,417,219
1974-1975	107	5	2	114	53,143	36,336	...

*Number of schools include fully accredited medical schools, medical schools with provisional approval, and accredited schools of basic medical sciences. The difference in number of libraries for a given year reflects a population in transition, as the survey period does not always coincide with that of library surveys.

†Student enrollment is given for fully accredited, developing, and basic science schools.

‡In earlier years, amount of expenditures is reported; in later years, total financial support is reported.

§Missouri-Kansas City did not provide statistics in 1972-1973; it is excluded from the data.

‖Harvard did not report 1973-1974 statistics; it is excluded from data.

¶Yale did not report number of full-time faculty in 1973-1974.

Medical Library Assistance Act.—Passed in 1965, the Medical Library Assistance Act provided perhaps the greatest impetus for change in the history of the health sciences library community[13]. The Act designated the NLM as agent for development of biomedical communication to meet the needs of health care in the last third of the 20th century. In particular, the Act authorized funds for development of resources in medical libraries, construction of facilities, manpower training, support of research and publications, and establishment of regional medical libraries.

Table 2 indicates funds awarded by the NLM for support of medical libraries, which totalled some $30.5 million during the period 1968 through 1975. Support categories include construction of facilities, resource projects, resource improvements, and regional medical library development. The figures do not include indirect contributions, such as development of the Medical Literature Analysis and Retrieval System (MEDLARS), research in application of computer and other technologies, or extensive staff support services provided to the health sciences library community[14].

As indicated in Table 2, 11 construction grants totaling $11,250,000 were awarded by NLM to nine medical school libraries, one school of optometry, and one school of veterinary medicine. Construction support was provided by NLM in 1968-1969 and was continued by the Bureau of Health Manpower from 1970 to date. During the past decade, 86 new library buildings were constructed by medical schools[15].

Resource project grants provide for the support of specific projects within an institution, eg, development of an audiovisual resource center, compilation of a union list of serials, renovation of a facility, or reclassification of a collection. They are especially helpful to institutions that require some outside funding for development of a needed program or facility. During the period 1971 through 1975, 148 institutions received grants totaling some $7,478,000 (Table 2). Resource grants were provided to a variety of health sciences libraries, including research foundations, medical societies, voluntary health organizations, hospitals, and schools of

Table 2.—Support Awarded by the National Library of Medicine, 1968-1975*

Support Category	Time Period Covered	Total Funds Awarded	No. of Institutions
Construction grants	1968-1969	$ 11,250,000	11
Resource projects	1971-1975	7,478,143	148
Resource improvement	1971-1975	1,138,967	381
Regional medical libraries	1971-1975	10,707,397	10
Total	1968-1975	**$ 30,574,507**	...

*Data from the National Library of Medicine, Extramural Programs Division.

medicine and allied health sciences. Medical school libraries received 55% of the resource grant funds, for a total of some $4,155,000.

Resource improvement grants are directed toward better distribution of library resources, especially to hospitals. During the period 1971 through 1975, 381 institutions received a total of $1,138,967 (Table 2). Of this amount, $993,328 (or 87%) was awarded to general, psychiatric, or special hospitals to strengthen their basic collections for educational programs or practice. Although medical schools were not awarded funds under improvement grants, as their specific needs fell within the category of resource projects, the great impact of this program on the entire medical library community has been well documented by Matheson and West[16].

Construction, resource project, and resource improvement awards relate to specific institutions. The Medical Library Assistance Act also provided for their organization into a nationwide medical library network, which is described later in this communication.

Technological Changes.—In 1958, electronic data processing was first applied on a massive scale for bibliographic control of medical literature. Prior to this time, the *Quarterly Cumulated Index Medicus,* which provided the major access to medical journals, was manually produced by typewritten entries filed by hand, as had been the *Index Medicus* (first series) in 1879.

The first punched-card-produced *Index Medicus* was developed through the NLM's new Medical Literature Analysis and Retrieval System (MEDLARS) in 1960. Succeeding generations of MEDLARS brought the capability of storing data on tape, computer-driven typesetting, and finally, direct, on-line access to the computerized data base of the NLM. The latter, MEDLINE, enabled medical libraries the world over almost instantaneous access to medical references as well as computer-assisted searches capable of scanning millions of entries within fractions of a minute. This breakthrough has revolutionized the retrieval of information, which, less than five years ago, was accomplished by manual scanning of published indexes. Today, all major health sciences libraries have access to MEDLINE and its associated data bases.

Clearly, MEDLARS is one of the most noteworthy achievements in bibliographic control in the health sciences during recent times. Other technological advances include the development of innovations in learning, such as audiovisual media and experiments in transmission of data by television and satellite. These have also had great impact on libraries and their capability for providing information in practice, teaching, and research.

Organization of a Medical Library Network

As early as 1963, Bloomquist observed the waste and duplication of isolated libraries and recommended the development of a "reservoir" of medical libraries from which local units may draw resources[3] (p 162). It was obvious that coordination of library activities in the health sciences was a sound concept, and the Medical Library Assistance Act provided for the development of a library network.

The country was divided into 11 regions, each with a regional medical library serving as resource and coordinator for local libraries as well as link with the NLM. Eight of the regional medical libraries are medical school libraries, two are professional society libraries, and one is the NLM (which also acts as the regional medical library for its own Mid-Atlantic region). Table 3 lists the regional medical libraries and the regions under their jurisdiction.

Funds awarded to regional medical libraries during the years 1971 through 1975, through contracts and grants, are summarized in Table 2. More than $10.7 million were awarded to the 11 regional medical libraries. From the start, networking was community-directed, so that each regional medical library developed according to the needs of the respective region and at different rates. The New England regional medical library was the first to be operational (October 1967), and the Midcontinental regional medical library was the final one to be developed (July 1970). By 1975, the network was an operating reality, and efforts were made, through appointment of coordinators, to organize consortia of local libraries within the regions. Medical school libraries have served as resource libraries for their regions and have played an active part in development of the network.

Resources

By consensus of the directors of three large medical libraries (Harvard University, Medical Library Center of New York, and NLM) it was estimated in 1960-1961 that approximately 100,000 volumes and 1,200 to 1,500 current journals would be required "to meet the needs of a medical school community of good quality"[3] (p 148). Although subjectively conceived, this standard has been used as a baseline for measurement of growth. In 1960, less than 24% of the libraries met the suggested standard for number of volumes, and only 25% met the standard for current journals.

As indicated in Table 4, the median number of bound volumes in 86

Table 3.—Regional Medical Library Programs and Services in the United States

Regional Library Programs	States Within Region	Office Address
New England Regional Medical Library Service (NERMLS)	Conn, Mass, Me, NH, RI, and Vt	Francis A. Countway Library of Medicine, 10 Shattuck St Boston, MA 02115
New York and New Jersey Regional Medical Library	NY, NJ	New York Academy of Medicine 2 E 103 St, New York, NY 10029
Mid-Eastern Regional Medical Library Service (MERMLS)	Del, Pa, and ten southern NJ counties	Library of the College of Physicians of Philadelphia 19 S 22 St, Philadelphia, PA 19103
Mid-Atlantic Regional Medical Library	Washington, DC, Md, NC, Va, and WVa	National Library of Medicine 8600 Rockville Pike Bethesda, MD 20014
Kentucky-Ohio-Michigan Regional Medical Library Program (KOMRML)	Ky, Mich, and Ohio	Wayne State University Medical Library, 4325 Brush St Detroit, MI 48201
Southeastern Regional Medical Library Program (SERMLP)	Ala, Fla, Ga, Miss, SC, Tenn, and PR	AW Calhoun Medical Library Emory University, Atlanta, GA 30322
Midwest Health Science Library Network (MHSLN)	Iowa, Ill, Ind, Minn, ND, and Wis	John Crerar Library 35 W 33 St, Chicago, IL 60616
Midcontinental Regional Medical Library Program	Colo, Kan, Mo, Neb, SD, Utah, and Wyo	Library of Medicine University of Nebraska Medical Center, 42nd St and Dewey Ave Omaha, NE 68105
South Central Regional Medical Library Program (TALON)	Ariz, La, NM, Okla, and Tex	University of Texas Health Science Center, 5323 Harry Hines Blvd, Dallas, TX 75235
Pacific Northwest Regional Health Sciences Library (PNRHSL)	Alaska, Idaho, Mont, Ore, and Wash	University of Washington Health Sciences Library Seattle, WA 98195
Pacific Southwest Regional Medical Library Service (PSRMLS)	Ariz, Calif, Hawaii, and Nev	Biomedical Library, Center for the Health Sciences University of California at Los Angeles (UCLA), Los Angeles CA 90024

medical school libraries was 54,779 in 1960-1961, and the median number of current serials received was 992. Statistics over the past 15 years are not entirely comparable, since averages rather than medians were computed in subsequent years. However, they do provide an indicator of change over these years. When 1965-1966 is used as a baseline, the average number of bound volumes showed an increase of 47% by 1973-1974, from 76,312 to 112,014 volumes. During the same period, the average number of serial titles increased by 23%, from 1,698 to 2,096 titles.

In summary, by 1973-1974, the baseline of 100,000 volumes was attained by the average accredited medical school library, compared with fewer than 25% of libraries in 1960-1961. By number of current serial titles the average medical school library exceeded the upper limit of 1,500 required titles by 500.

Operating Expenditures

There is a dramatic increase over the 15-year period in the average library budget, as indicated in Table 5. Again, there is some variation in the basis for calculation, since for all years except 1973-1974, the figures were computed on the basis of library budget rather than operating expenditures, as well as combined budget for approved and developing medical schools and schools of the basic sciences. In 1960-1961, the average library budget was $57,471, in comparison with $328,093 in 1973-1974 for approved medical schools, an increase by a factor of 5.7.

Table 4.—Average No. of Bound Volumes and Current Serial Titles Received by Medical School Libraries, 1960-1974: Selected Years

Academic Year	No. of Libraries*	Average No. of Bound Volumes	Average No. of Serial Titles
1960-1961[3]	86	...	...†
1965-1966[10]	88	76,312	1,698[22]
1969-1970[23]	103	95,357	1,882
1973-1974‡ Accredited medical schools	99	112,014	2,096
Accredited schools of the basic medical sciences	3	37,265	781
Developing medical schools, operational (not yet eligible for approval)	3	26,167	773

*Statistics given are for fully accredited medical schools, schools with provisional approval, and accredited schools of the basic medical sciences.

†The Bloomquist study[3] does not indicate averages, but reported a median of 54,770 bound volumes and 992 current serial titles.

‡Data from the Survey of Health Sciences Libraries, 1973-1974.

Table 5.—Average Budget-Operating Expenditures of Medical School Libraries, 1960-1974: Selected Years

Academic Year	No. of Libraries*	Expenditures, $†
1960-1961[3]	86	57,471
1965-1966[10]	88	112,313
1968-1969[23]	99	193,896
1969-1970[24]	103	233,448
1973-1974‡		
Approved medical schools	99	328,093
Approved schools of the basic medical sciences	3	83,549
Developing medical schools, operational (not yet eligible for approval)	3	170,367

*The 1973-1974 survey data provides separate statistics for three types of schools that train medical students.

†The 1973-1974 survey requested statistics for operating expenditures. Previous surveys indicated the amount budgeted for the academic year.

‡Data from Survey of Health Sciences Libraries, 1973-1974.

Table 6.—Medical School Library Personnel, 1960-1961 and 1973-1974*

Personnel Category	Range		Median		Total	
	1960-1961†	1973-1974‡	1960-1961	1973-1974	1960-1961	1973-1974
Professional§	1-11	1-60	3	8	324	986
Nonprofessional‖	0.5-20.5	1-41	4	13	...	1,556
Part-time (including student assistants)	...	0-58	...	8	...	1,070

*For the academic year 1960-1961, number of libraries (n)=79; in 1973-1974, n=105.

†Data for 1960-1961 includes the total number of full-time equivalents for professionals or nonprofessionals derived from Bloomquist.[3]

‡Data for 1973-1974 distinguishes the number of full-time professionals or nonprofessionals and the number of full-time equivalents for part-time staff.[9(p25)]

§"Professional" is defined in the 1960-1961 survey as "an employee who performs work requiring education, training, and skill in theoretical or scientific aspects of library work." In the 1973-1974 survey, the definition was "persons performing functions requiring a graduate degree or its equivalent in experience."

‖"Nonprofessional" is defined in the 1960-1961 survey as a person performing "merely mechanical and clerical aspects" of library work; in 1973-1974, as "persons performing job tasks of a routine nature, not requiring specialized training, degree."

Personnel

In 1961, the Bloomquist study identified 324 professional librarians employed in 79 medical school libraries in the United States. The median number of professional librarians employed in medical schools was three, a level that had not changed from the findings of a study made in 1951[3] (p. 148). By 1973-1974, the total number had increased by a factor of three, to 986 professional librarians in 105 medical schools (Table 6). The median number of professionals also increased by more than a factor of three during this 15-year period. The threefold increase in personnel correlates with the doubling in number of students and tripling in number of faculty. No data are available comparing the changes in functions of personnel during this period.

Conclusion

We have traced the development of medical school libraries in the United States from 1960 through 1975, an era of great social and technological change. Federal support for science and technology reached a magnitude never before equalled. The number of medical schools increased by 31%, the number of students by some 75%, and expenditures by over 500%. The Medical Library Assistance Act laid the groundwork for massive research and development in biomedical communication. Manual manipulation of data in bibliographic control was converted to computerized searching and transmission of data by a wireline system. Health sciences library resources became organized into a nationwide network.

Bloomquist observed, in 1960-1961, that medical school libraries double in size every 12 years. As we view their development during the past 10 to 15 years, we find that, in terms of bound volumes, his estimate is a close approximation. The median number of bound volumes in 1960-1961 was some 54,700; the average in 1973-1974 was more than 112,000. Average operating expenditures increased by a factor of more than five, and the median number of professional personnel increased by a factor of three. The medical school library emerged during this period as the leading center of growth, by all variables measured in the 1973-1974 survey of health sciences libraries in the United States[2].

As we enter the fourth quarter of the century, however, there are signs that the growth is levelling off as a response to what appears to be a period of stability for medical schools. It is the consensus of medical school educators that the growth we have witnessd in the past 15 years will not continue at the same rate[17]. In this longitudinal study, we have captured medical school libraries in a stimulating and expansive period. The process is continuous, and the shape of the growth curve will be revealed to us over the perspective of time.

This study was supported in part by grant R01-LM0064 from the National Library of Medicine.

REFERENCES

1. WOLFE D: The support of science in the United States. Sci Am 213:19, 1965.
2. CRAWFORD S: Directory of Health Sciences Libraries in the United States, 1973. Chicago, American Medical Association, 1974, p vii.
3. BLOOMQUIST H: The status and needs of medical school libraries in the United States. J Med Educ 38: 145-168, 1963.
4. Medical Education in the United States: Medical school libraries. Department of Medical Education. *J.A.M.A.* 190: 614-615, 1964.
5. Medical Education in the United States: Medical school libraries. Department of Medical Education. *J.A.M.A.* 194: 758-759, 1965.
6. Medical Education in the United States: Medical school libraries. Department of Medical Education. *J.A.M.A.* 198: 858-859, 1966.
7. Medical Education in the United States: Medical school libraries. Department of Medical Education. *J.A.M.A.* 202: 735-736, 1967.
8. Medical education in the United States: Medical school libraries. Department of Medical Education. *J.A.M.A.* 214: 191-192, 1970.
9. Medical education in the United States: Medical school libraries. Department of Medical Education. *J.A.M.A.* 231 (suppl): 25-26, 1975.
10. Library statistics of schools in the health sciences, Committee on Surveys and Statistics. Bull Med Libr Assoc 54: 207-299, 1966.
11. Library statistics of schools in the health sciences, Committee on Surveys and Statistics. Bull Med Libr Assoc 55: 178-190, 1967.
12. SCHICK F, CRAWFORD S: Directory of Health Science Libraries in the United States, 1969. Chicago, American Medical Association, 1970.
13. Medical Library Assistance Act of 1965, Public Law 89-291.
14. CUMMINGS MM, CORNING ME: The Medical Library Assistance Act: an analysis of the NLM extramural programs 1965-1970. Bull Med Libr Assoc 59: 375-391, 1971.
15. HUANG CK: Physical facilities of medical school libraries in the United States, 1966-1975: A statistical review. Bull Med Libr Assoc 64: 173-178, 1976.
16. MATHESON N.W., WEST R.T.: NLM Library Resource Improvement grant program: an evaluation. Bull Med Libr Assoc 64: 309-319, 1976.
17. KEYES J.A., WILSON M.P. BECKER J: The future of medical education: Forecast of the Council of Deans. J Med Educ 50: 310-327, 1975.
18. International education exchange in medicine, Council on Medical Education and Hospitals. J.A.M.A. 178: 604, 1961.
19. Medical education in the United States, Council on Medical Education. *J.A.M.A.* 190: 597-620, 1964.
20. Medical education in the United States Council on Medical Education. *J.A.M.A.* 202: 725-762, 1967.
21. Medical education in the United States, 1974-1975, Council on Medical Education. *J.A.M.A.* 234: 1333-1351, 1975.

22. Medical education in the United States, 1966-1967, Council on Medical Education. *J.A.M.A.* 198: 186, 1966.
23. CRAWFORD S. Health science libraries in the 1960s: an overview. Bull Med Libr Assoc 60 (suppl): 9, 1972.
24. Medical education in the United States: Medical school libraries. Department of Education. *J.A.M.A.* 214: 1492, 1970.

V
INNOVATIONS AND SERVICES

Introduction

"But, my dear," said the Hatter, "Was there progress?"
"Well," said Alice earnestly, "There was change[1]."

John Shaw Billings, librarian of the Library of the U.S. Surgeon-General's Office, 1865-1895, and "author" of the *Index Catalogue* of the Surgeon-General's library and the *Index Medicus*, summarized his lifelong work philosophy in a comment he once made to the librarian of the Royal Society of Medicine:

> ... I'll let you into the secret—there's nothing really difficult if you only *begin*—some people contemplate a task until it looms so big, it seems impossible, but I *just begin* and it gets done somehow. There would be no coral islands if the first bug sat down and began to wonder how the job was to be done[2].

With imagination and hard work, medical librarians have accomplished much in resolving problems in common and doing so in economical ways. They have creditability in the eyes of their colleagues in medicine. This creditability was earned and is the product of the achievements of all who are or have been involved in this exciting adventure in a very special profession. Over the years, medical librarianship has changed; and it continues to change, so that an important part of the adventure now rests in ensuring that change is improvement. The factors of accountability are increasingly more evident. It is also apparent that our future developments will be influenced greatly by the efficiency with which we can manage the information needs of our users and by the cost savings that can be developed through continuous planning and modification. We can build on the successes of our collective experiences and avoid costly mistakes encountered with the realities of innovation.

The articles included in this chapter are from the literature of persons who have contributed to solving the problems of library services and techniques.

A historical review of users and user services of health sciences libraries is presented by Mildred Langner. Her paper outlines the traditional services offered users by health sciences libraries from 1945 to 1960.

Helen Crawford shares the results of a survey, made by formal query of members of the Medical Library Association, on library extramural services. She summarizes her findings and enumerates several practical suggestions for persons interested in the mechanics of extension services.

The technical report, a widely neglected source of recent and current data for the medical library, is the topic reported on by Dr. Charles Sargent. He discusses how to acquire, process, and use the tools that abstract and index this literature.

Jack Key and Katherine Sholtz describe a service useful at the Mayo Clinic library involving a comprehensive computerized method for identifying research and for identifying and indexing publications of Mayo Clinic staff members. The end product—the Mayo Clinic Author Catalog—has proved itself such a useful tool that other libraries, large and small, may wish to consider adopting such a service.

Teletypewriter communication between medical libraries, today so commonplace, was initially given much impetus by Warren Bird. He outlines the background of library applications of teletypewriter systems, the advantages, types of use, cost factors, and experiences of some user groups, and he notes the impact of the "network concept" on library service.

Dr. Wilhelm Moll reviews and evaluates a project during which the Medical Library of the University of Virginia experimented with a remote-access bibliographic control and retrieval system via its teletypewriter machine. The system was called AIM-TWX and utilized a time-shared IBM 360/67 computer in Santa Monica, California. Citations from 109 clinically oriented journals from 1966 to 1970, including those in *Abridged Index Medicus,* could be retrieved on- or off-line.

Keys to the doors of medical literature are provided by William Beatty, who comments on the major secondary sources of biomedical information.

What can the librarian do today when faced with providing better services to more patrons while operating on shrinking dollars in a field where prices continue to rise? Advice on how to cope when budgets falter, at least in the selection process for health sciences library collections, is the subject of Stanley Truelson's article. He suggests that "the challenge to the librarian is to optimize the insufficient" and that the expertise of the librarian "is more needed and has more impact in times of trouble than in times of plenty."

REFERENCES

1. DUNKIN P.S.: From the editor's desk: progress is our most important product. Libr Resour Tech Serv 12: 367, 1968.
2. MACALISTER J.Y.W.: John Shaw Billings (obituary). Br Med J 1: 642, 1913.

User and User Services in Health Sciences Libraries: 1945-1965

MILDRED C. LANGNER

THE LITERATURE on health sciences libraries in the United States and Canada from 1945 to 1965 reveals a vast amount of activity in the field of user services and shows that, despite the almost insurmountable problems encountered due to unprecedented increases in the literature and in use of libraries, many goals were reached and important results were realized.

While endeavoring to point out these developments, this review will not dwell upon the basic reference and fact-location assistance with which many library users are the most familiar. These services, perhaps because they are so universally expected and accepted, have not been emphasized in the literature, consequently, it is difficult to document them.

Attention here will be directed to discussions of those important behind-the-scenes, reference-related activities—such as special and interlibrary cooperative services—to which there are many references in the literature. Not considered are selection, acquisition, cataloging and classification, which fit more pertinently within the realm of technical services. Circulation procedures also will be omitted.

The year 1945 introduced the tumultuous period immediately following World War II when unbelievable developments in the fields of research, education and technology were demonstrating the overwhelming results which could be achieved when massive research and development funds were applied to predetermined objectives, and when the need for worldwide cooperation was strongly manifesting itself. When UNESCO was chartered in this momentous year it had as its principal aim the attaining of international cooperation on a huge overall scale. With government

---

Mildred C. Langner is Director, Louis Calder Memorial Library, University of Miami School of Medicine, Miami, Florida.

Reprinted from *Library Trends,* Volume 23, Number 1, July 1974, pp. 7-30, by permission of the publisher.

programs—particularly in the fields of defense and space exploration—leading the way, society as a whole began to devote gigantic sums to scientific research and technical development. "For the first time in the history of the world a nation deliberately mobilized all its relevant resources to achieve radical and comprehensive technological innovation as rapidly as possible."[1]

One of the most noticeable results of this research was the fantastically rapid increase in the amount of recorded information produced, especially in the fields of medicine, biological and physical sciences, and engineering. The number of books published in these fields increased from approximately 1,500 in 1940 to nearly 5,000 in 1965, the publication of new journals grew by large numbers, and countless unpublished research reports multiplied astronomically, setting the trend for the "information explosion."

Throughout all this turbulence, librarians attempted to give the scientific research worker the best possible service, but neither they, nor perhaps even the researcher himself, knew exactly what was needed from the library. The war, however, had clearly demonstrated to many scientists the vital place of an efficient information service. Their experience, together with the much wider range over which research now had to be carried out and the necessity for scientists to familiarize themselves with entirely new and multifaceted subjects, had put a premium on information gained from libraries rather than from means such as slowly acquired experience, conferences and personal correspondence. With this understanding came the realization that the complexity of science had grown to such a degree that library and information service was an important key to the world of advancing knowledge.

How the health sciences libraries responded to this challenge is vividly described by Friedrich:

> The war had demonstrated how inefficient were many of the peacetime methods of medical libraries. For example, where the medical librarian once probably seemed to rely largely upon memory and often to make somewhat vague generalizations, a need for speed and accuracy under heightened war pressure necessitated more accurate record-keeping and prompt, specific information. Details of record-keeping became streamlined; time required for library operations was now of first importance. Duplication of effort had to be eliminated. As demands for reference service increased, short cuts of all kinds were utilized.

> Service, unlimited service, became the slogan of medical libraries. The more work that was done for people and for agencies, the more they demanded. What formerly was given as an occasional favor was now demanded and was expected as if it were a long-established right. Dormant powers and potentialities of medical librarians sprang to life when the entire medical and governmental staff turned to them for help.[2]

Marshall, too, pointed out the extended service which librarians would be called upon to give. She outlined new programs in education and research that would make extensive demands upon medical librarians and urged them to be prepared to face the future.[3]

Forewarned both by exhortation and personal experience, librarians endeavored to meet the deluge of requests that poured in upon them, but finding the means to answer these requests was most difficult because, although millions of dollars had been allocated to research, very little had been provided for the correlation of research, and the need for library support in this field had hardly even been recognized.[4]

It was time, therefore, to look at the entire health sciences libraries picture. It was not a particularly bright one. Faced with the need to provide increased services, yet well aware of the deficiencies in number and size of the existing health sciences libraries, librarians and administrators began concerted studies to meet this crisis. A study by Deitrick and Berson in 1953 pointed out that the plight of the medical library was serious.[5] In 1963 Adams said:

> Today, ten years and some hundreds of millions of research dollars later, [than the Deitrick report] it is stated with increasing frequency that the medical libraries are worse off than ever before. Last November the National Advisory Health Council submitted a resolution to the Surgeon General. "The medical library network," the resolution reads, "which has been designed to make the published record of medicine available, is in dire trouble. During a period of intensive development of research institutions, medical schools, and other medical facilities, their essential library support has been seriously neglected. In recent years the needs for adequate library working and storage space, for more trained library personnel, and for new methods of handling and disseminating the growing scientific medical literature have become acute."[6]

Meanwhile the National Advisory Health Council and other professional science groups became increasingly alarmed concerning medical libraries' ability to provide comprehensive service for education and research. The National Library of Medicine had long been concerned with this problem. Consequently it determined that data on medical school libraries which would show most clearly what research facilities were available, should be collected in order that the overall condition could be assessed. Harold Bloomquist was asked to survey these libraries and to prepare a report of his findings. His account appeared in 1963 and showed what services were actually being performed and what special services librarians wished to provide but could not because of lack of funds.[7]

It was obvious from the report that in individual library collections varying from 12,000 to 340,446 volumes with a median of 54,779 volumes, very little support was generally available to provide any but the most basic reference service. It was also clear that with a total of only 324 professional librarians employed in U.S. medical school libraries in 1961, only a small percentage were strictly reference librarians available to serve on a full-time basis as members of the health research teams of their parent institutions. It was evident that such a situation could not continue in face of the great demands made upon libraries beginning in 1945 and accumulating explosively every year since then.

Awareness of the plight of libraries led the scientific community to wonder if they could rise to the challenge to meet the demands of the research community. Some scientists thought not and felt that other types of institutions for supplying information should be found, thus ignoring the fact that the library has proved that it is as efficient an institution for storing and retrieving information as society has yet devised, and that reinforcing the foundation and types of services already supplied by libraries would enable them to meet demands as they always have.[8]

In the meantime, health sciences librarians were quickly adjusting to the new era and were busy providing the different approach to services necessitated by changing trends. Many of them had had very little specialized training but, filled with the willingness to serve, they had developed a sophistication in the area of user services in response to the need for these services in their libraries. Bloomquist, despite the gloomy results revealed by his survey, could still say: "The best medical librarians are virtuosos in the area of services to readers. Training, the desire to serve, and imagination are the prime requisites."[9]

Arturo Castiglioni, the famous historian, in recognition of the medical librarians' philosophy of service, gave this unusually fine tribute to them:

> I think it is possible and obvious to discuss and disagree on different ways of education in different schools and countries, on various tendencies and various degrees of humanistic or historical trends in medical studies. But there is one subject on which, I am quite sure, all those who are able to pass judgment on the evolution of medical thought must agree, that is the remarkable, decisive influence that the splendid organization of the American medical libraries and the work of their librarians has had in the progress of medical science in this country.[10]

Types of Health Sciences Libraries

What were the libraries like in this particular period? What user services were they giving? What users frequented those libraries? Health sciences libraries were of many types: government, professional school, society, hospital, state, industrial and divisions of public libraries.

GOVERNMENT

The largest library of this important group was the national library, which finally received its proper title as the National Library of Medicine. From its very beginning it had rendered generous reference services on a national and international basis. Its activities have been thoroughly described through the years in its annual reports as well as in other articles, and its importance as one of the great libraries of the world is fully recognized and appreciated. (See Additional References.)

The Veterans Administration also carried on an extensive library program featuring a Central Office Reference System.[11] Other forms of government libraries were those connected with state, county and regional departments of public health.[12]

SOCIETY

Society libraries have long been noted for special services to their patrons. The specifically unusual activity which first comes to mind is the "package library" sponsored by the American Medical Association, the American Dental Association and the American College of Surgeons. As early as 1934 as many as six staff members were employed in this service at the American Medical Association Library.[13]

The largest society libraries were the New York Academy of Medicine, the Kings County Medical Society, the College of Physicians of Philadelphia and the Boston Medical Library, later to be incorporated with the Harvard Medical School Library and renamed the Francis A. Countway Library of Medicine.[14] This amalgamation was one of several brought about during this period by the financial plight of rising costs. Medical societies could no longer carry the heavy burden of a separate library, and even though their members feared that many special services would be lost to them, there was no alternative but to combine with medical school libraries. A symposium on this newly developing pattern appeared in 1962.[15]

PROFESSIONAL SCHOOL AND RESEARCH

Professional school libraries and research libraries such as the Mayo Clinic Library and the John Crerar Library formed the largest group. Their collections covered areas of medicine, dentistry, pharmacy and nursing, and were usually more extensive than those of hospitals and of society libraries. Their staffs and user groups, too, were larger and so was their group of users. Some of them provided extensive bibliographic research and other special reference services.

From the 1940s to the early 1960s there were many articles describing the multitudinous approaches to provision of service in the various school libraries: Troxel and Robinson debated the advantages and disadvantages of a combined medical-dental-pharmacy library.[16] Lentz described medical school library service, saying: "The library is an integral part of the medical school and though some may think it is quite removed from the drama of medicine, one soon finds that there is much here related to the battle to save and prolong human life.[17]

Morrisey discussed the library's place in the nursing school, pointing out the responsibility of the librarian: "Her imagination must constantly be at work and she must always be willing to employ all of her resources both native and acquired for the good of the family, which in this case is the faculty and the students in the school of nursing.[18]

HOSPITAL

Hospital libraries during this period were usually associated with the larger hospitals. Only later would many small-to-medium sized hospitals develop libraries of their own. The literature of 1945-65 depicts the special services for which the hospital libraries were noted and shows why this type of library rapidly became more important to the health sciences community and why more emphasis would be placed upon it by leaders in the field of medical education. (See Additional References.)

Many public libraries were also active in carrying on extensive medically related programs for the blind and handicapped.[19] Many specialized in work with children in hospitals and institutions.[20]

INDUSTRY

Descriptions of the special reference services offered by pharmaceutical company libraries clearly show why they have always been considered leaders in this area. (See Additional References.) Bloomquist states that:

> They are financially better supported. There are funds for more and better trained personnel, for mechanized devices to streamline routines, and funds simply to turn into action those ideas which will meet the assessed needs of the community to be served. The motivation in pharmaceutical houses is neither benevolence nor extravagance; it is simply a matter of economic self-interest. To them cost studies have indicated that money spent in library services saves money elsewhere or makes money elsewhere.[21]

UNIVERSITY AND PUBLIC

Health sciences libraries, university libraries and public libraries have been closely associated throughout the years. A study of the literature shows that the main projects connected with bibliography, bibliographic control and interlibrary loan procedures have been cooperative ones with leaders in all three fields displaying great interest in improvements which would be of help to all.

Reference methods were approximately the same in the three

types, except that perhaps the health sciences libraries maintained stronger and more sustained emphasis upon personal assistance. This emphasis was especially evident in clinical areas where emergency, "spoon-fed" service was offered to busy practitioners in their patient care activities.

Long ago Garrison pointed out that: "the university librarian and his medical librarian, can exist and function side by side without friction and with mutual benefit. In the case of the individual medical library of a community, the chief will find himself continually in need of cooperation with his colleagues of the municipal or university library and *vice versa*."[22]

Librarians of public and academic libraries usually directed professional and technical medicine-related requests to the medical library, and they have long felt that the assembling of an extensive medical collection should be left to the large medical library of the community.

Radmacher, however, questioned how far the public library should go in selecting medical material. She pointed out that the public library's book selection policy must make available works representing conflicting points of view to enable the reader to broaden his scope and to form his own opinions, but wondered about this in relation to medicine and disease. She states that as a public librarian she would welcome more help from medical librarians.[23]

Relegating questions to the medical libraries, however, did not mean that the other libraries relinquished all activities in the health sciences fields. Indeed, because of their broader coverage they were much better able to serve the peripheral areas such as behavioral and social sciences than was the medical library.

Library Users

Users of the health sciences libraries were as varied as the types of libraries they patronized, and each group required special attention.

Classification of users was made in the 1940s by Cunningham who stated:

> Reference aid in a medical library is needed by individuals who can be roughly grouped into four categories:
>
> 1. Professional.
>
>   This group includes: (a) members of university faculties, scientists and research workers accustomed to doing

bibliographic research; (b) patrons who know scientific literature and its scope thoroughly but are unaccustomed to the bibliographic tools; (c) busy practitioners who are often unfamiliar with the literature or tools, but who are faced with the problem of writing a paper or making a case report; (d) interns, young research workers engaged on their first original problems, and post-graduate students who have not had access to a library for a long time.

2. Semi- and pre-professional.
   This group consists primarily of: (a) medical and pre-medical students; (b) student and graduate nurses; (c) dental students; (d) technicians; (e) free lance bibliographers; (f) ghost writers; and (g) secretaries working for doctors and scientists. Some of the individuals in this group will be comparatively unfamiliar with the medical literature or terminology, and they will frequently need to be shown how to use the books.
3. Professional laity.
   This class is represented by: (a) lawyers; (b) industrial and sanitary engineers; (c) reporters; (d) clergymen; and (e) social service workers. They know little of medical literature or medical bibliographic tools, but their interest is of a technical nature. They are accustomed to gathering information from various sources, and therefore have the bibliographic approach.
4. Non-professional laity.
   This group consists of: (a) readers sent by physicians with requests for specific books; (b) those who wish to study some particular diseases because they themselves or some member of their families are sufferers; (c) the small group of the morbidly curious; (d) the usual casual inquirers who wish the addresses of physicians, the names of hospitals or institutions; and (e) individuals who are writing papers for presentation before non-professional groups, women's clubs, etc.[24]

PROFESSIONAL, STUDENT AND LAYMAN

Needs and demands of the professional clientele have been emphasized throughout the literature. (See Additional References.)

Student needs, too, have always been a most important

consideration in health sciences libraries and the students themselves have been eager to list their observations. (See Additional References.)

Service to the layman in health sciences libraries varied from none through guarded to full recognition of the need. The Medical Library Association devoted a session of its annual meeting to this important subject in which Biehler pondered "Who Is the Lay Public?" and King asked if lay material should be purchased and to what extent. Monahan narrated policies that society libraries have established to regulate use, while Clark described the services given and Chambers questioned what services *should* be given.[25]

Library Services

The term services covers a wide range of activities. Its whole concept, however, was succinctly, clearly and perceptively described long ago by a famous librarian, Samuel Green: "The more freely a librarian mingles with readers and the greater the amount of assistance he renders them, the more intense does the conviction of citizens, also, become, that the library is a useful institution, and the more willing do they grow to grant money in larger and larger sums to be used in buying books and employing additional assistants."[26] This idea has been reiterated *ad infinitum* throughout the years.

The areas of service which were covered, however, may be different and more inclusive than generally realized. It is certain that in some cases the desire to be helpful had reached the ultimate as exemplified in the statement made in 1896 by one of the founders of the Medical Library Association: "I take no credit for special fitness for the position except that I could fill the requisite that I must reside in the library building."[27] Evidently either this twenty-four-hour-a-day service was not terribly difficult or Marcia Noyes was of an extremely strong constitution because she lived a long life and left the memory of her devotion to her library engraved on the hearts of its users. Fundamentally, however, library service boils down to the provision of complete back-up support for the teaching, research and patient care needs of the environment served. Needless to say, all types and sizes of health sciences libraries are involved to some extent with these three basic interests of their users. This back up for the programs of the sponsoring institutions consisted mainly of provision of information or fact location, bibliography and interlibrary loans. However, librarians continued to extend the scope of their reference services whenever possible and important trends were revealed.

SOME SPECIAL SERVICES

In the 1950s there appeared articles on changing concepts,[28] on present and potential services,[29] on the library research assistant,[30] and on the librarian as a member of the health research team.[31] Suggestions were made that the reference librarian should be initially consulted when a book or article is contemplated and then expected to supply bibliographic references, abstracts, editorial and transation services, and to be involved with the project until publication.[32] Protest to such active participation, however, rose to a crescendo with Goodall's article "The Place of the Librarian in the Medical Team."[33] There was some discussion that too much service was provided.[34] Most librarians, however, were undaunted by this reaction because the majority of their own patrons showed the desire and need for much additional help, including extension and bookmobile service.[35]

TEACHING

Scores of articles were written on teaching the use of the library. Articles from a 1952 panel on the teaching of medical bibliography to medical, dental, pharmacy and graduate students pointed out the importance of teaching activity.[36] The panel advocated that time be alloted to teaching because of its value both to the students, who afterwards would become able to use the library with more skill and understanding, and to the library staff, who would not have to give so many separate instructions. The last article in this panel concerned on-the-job teaching of medical bibliography to medical librarians.[37]

Other articles on teaching described orientation programs and teaching the use of the library in many types of health sciences libraries. (See Additional References.) Truelson pointed out that it was also the responsibility of the faculty to teach students the use of the library. He emphasized that: "Using the library is not a goal in itself; it is simply a necessary step to far higher and more exciting accomplishments. The librarians and the faculty, working together, can help to create both of the conditions for learning library skills: motivation and practice."[38]

EXHIBITS

Exhibits formed an important part of the library's service to its users as they presented a visual means of imparting information over a period of time to many people. So important did the *Bulletin of the Medical Library Association* consider this subject of displays that prominence was given to many articles in its pages. For a time it designated a special section in its issues to this subject. (See Additional References.)

An important development in the exhibit area was the traveling exhibit, a spendid innovation which enabled the small libraries to reap the benefit of the extensive display material provided by one of the large medical center libraries.[39]

TRANSLATION

Health sciences librarians were particularly concerned with the provision of translation services. Many libraries kept lists of local translators available for assistance, and some who had linguists on their staffs offered either long or short translations. Several articles pointed out important services and indexes available (see Additional References), and Parker and Hawkins prepared an important guide to sources and services.[40] Far reaching international scientific translation programs were carried on throughout this era by the National Library of Medicine, the National Institutes of Health, the National Science Foundation and other organizations.

EDITING

Editing was one of the services which all librarians could not give, even though most of them would have liked to do so. Among those who did offer this service were librarians who, in addition to teaching and lecturing on the subject, aided their readers by compiling instructions on scientific writing.[41]

BIBLIOTHERAPY

Bibliotherapy was a user service carried out more often in hospital libraries. The Veterans Administration and the American Hospital Association particularly have shown great interest in this subject. Reviews throughout the 1950s and 1960s gave prominence to accounts of this activity, and in 1958 an important development occurred.

The Bibliotherapy Committee, Association Hospital and Medical

Librarians, a division of the American Library Association has recently received the approval of the ALA executive board to proceed on the research project which will outline basic questions and identify areas worthy of research regarding the effects of reading in hospitals and institutions. Various foundations are interested in this project which will take about 18 months to complete.[42]

Important Interlibrary Cooperative Services

INTERLIBRARY LOANS

Among the earliest interlibrary cooperative activities was that of interlibrary loans or document delivery service. That this activity was alive and flourishing in the 1930s is revealed by reading Archibald Malloch, one of the leading physician-librarians of this time: "The librarian of old would probably hold up his hands in horror at the thought of inter-library loans of which we hear so much. Many librarians now lend all but their oldest and best books to almost any other library in the country in this way, and very few volumes are lost in the express or mails. This is really lending a helping hand as well.[43]

Long before this date, however, interlibrary loan service was carried out by many institutions. Samuel Green in 1876 had suggested that it would be a good and helpful thing if libraries would lend books to each other.[44] Later in 1891, in his presidential address to the ALA, he again advocated this action and noted that the library of the Surgeon General's office was already lending widely.[45]

This library, later called the Army Medical Library, the Armed Forces Medical Library and finally the National Library of Medicine, remained the leader among health sciences libraries in lending its material. Its generosity was practically boundless, and thousands of libraries all over the world profited from its wonderful source of supply. Rogers expressed its generous lending policies when he said: "As one of the earliest American libraries to allow items in its collection to go beyond its own walls, and as a library which had raised its photocopying service to a high level, the N.L.M. has demonstrated time and again its concern with getting its holdings to the people who need them, wherever they may be."[46] He sorrowfully noted, however, that this bountiful policy could not continue forever, because the demand throughout the years had become so insistent that it could not be fulfilled. Therefore in 1957 the National Library of Medicine was forced to change its lending policy.

The VA also had provided a generous interlibrary loan policy. Its Medical and General Reference Library served as its central office both lending to and borrowing for its field stations throughout the country. It also maintained reciprocal borrowing and lending policies with libraries outside the VA.[47]

Many articles testify to the fact that interlibrary loan services were vitally important to health sciences libraries. Some of these showed the need for a uniform code. Some were pleas for service, usually from the smaller libraries, and some were justifications when curtailments were considered necessary by the lending—usually the larger—libraries.[48]

Even though interlibrary loan service was most active and libraries were profiting by this exchange of material, it was obvious that lending of the actual original material was placing undue strain on the libraries involved. Various means of photocopy had been tried, but had been found time-consuming and expensive. These difficulties, however, did not daunt Atherton Seidell, a forward-thinking honorary consultant of the Army Medical Library and one of the foremost proponents of the importance of microfilm for document delivery service. While complimenting the work being done by health sciences librarians, he also chided them, stating that whereas they had in the first edition of the *Handbook of Medical Library Practice* placed strong emphasis upon taking care of the needs of their readers, they had not mentioned "the particular application of microfilm copying by which persons at a distance may be supplied with miniature photographic copies of the separate original articles in periodicals."[49] At the time of Seidell's initial efforts, he suffered the fate of most innovators because many individuals found microfilm processing inconvenient and cumbersome. By 1962, however, photocopy procedures had improved greatly. In that year the definitive publication on NLM's vast interlibrary loan program appeared.[50] Two years later an account depicting the photocopy experiences of the NLM's neighbor, the National Institutes of Health Library, was presented by Martin and Ferguson.[51]

Even with the advent of dry-process photocopy and the establishment of interlibrary loan codes it was clear that all was not functioning as smoothly as desired in this area of librarianship. At the time when the NLM stated that it would no longer lend to individuals, its director laid down the policy which was to lead later to regionalization and to the establishment of a network of libraries for document delivery.[52]

The abundance of literature on the important subject of interlibrary loans revealed that it was a formidable part of reference librarianship. It also emphasized that cooperation between health sciences libraries in the field of document delivery was a flourishing and most comprehensive activity.[53]

REGIONALIZATION

Other library areas, however, were becoming more actively involved with interlibrary coordination. Amalgamation of society libraries with professional school libraries has already been mentioned. Regional activities including cooperative acquisitions programs and the centralized storing of esoteric resources began to increase in number. An important advancement toward cooperation took place when the Midwest Inter-library Center was established " '(1) To provide more adequate research materials for the needs of midwestern scholarship and research; and (2) To provide for economical and efficient utilization of resources to avoid needless duplication and expense.' These objectives go beyond the functions of any cooperative library now existing, and, thereby, offer the greater challenge to the librarians who determine whether the objectives of such an institution are successfully realized."[54]

Later, members of the New York Medical Community gathered together for a conference on coordination among libraries of the area in which they found: "The time has come when a route must be chosen leading either forward to co-operation or backward to chaos."[55] Fortunately, the step forward was taken leading to the establishment of the Medical Library Center of New York.[56]

BIBLIOGRAPHY AND RESEARCH

It was in the fields of cooperative bibliography and research, however, that the health sciences librarians were working most feverishly to supply the broadened approaches to and the centralized control of the vast literature now being produced so that they might more quickly and more comprehensively serve the needs of their library users. Morse, in reporting on the International Conference on Scientific Information, recognized their efforts by stating that the person expecting the ICSI to provide answers to most of the problems of scientific literature would be disappointed because there is no foreseeable substitute for the imagination and experience of energetic librarians and information specialists.[57]

In 1949 the Medical Library Association invited the then Librarian of Congress, Luther Evans, to address its membership on the important subject of cooperative bibliography. He admitted the immensity of the problem and pointed out that in a period which had witnessed rapid and extensive developments in the preparation of bibliographic tools the problem still remains. Evans deplored that adequate bibliography continued to be the principal obstacle in the realization of UNESCO goals: the promotion of knowledge and education; the dissemination of information; and the provision of understanding among the peoples of the world. Evans concluded with this pertinent call for cooperation: "Every library, whether it is called a bibliographic center or not, is one in reality; and I look forward to a time when the libraries of the nation and indeed of the world, will be recognized as a system of bibliographical centers, each contributing to the vital bibliographic organization of the world's knowledge and each drawing upon the entire system for the benefit of its clientele."[58]

Health sciences librarians increased their cooperation activities by continuing their earlier successful efforts and pursuing many new projects. The important bibliographies produced and the accomplishments realized in improving, encouraging and coordinating indexing and abstracting services were many. Indeed the support given to the better integration of the total research effort was outstanding. A partial list of achievements includes:

1. the bibliographic control exercised from the beginning of its existence by the Army Medical Library, later the National Library of Medicine;
2. the Herculean efforts in coordinating indexing and abstracting services by the Medical Library Association in conjunction with other library and scientific organizations;
3. the publication of the excellent first edition of the *Handbook of Medical Library Practice* containing the impressive comprehensive "Annotated List of Reference Books;"
4. valuable contributions to bibliography and research by persons actively engaged in health sciences librarianship. These included special volumes of learned bibliographies and other reference tools such as histories, directories and dictionaries;

5. the day-by-day reference assistance and guidance extended wholeheartedly to their users by librarians of all types of libraries. This significant back-up support and participation in the educational, research and patient care activities of their users contributed greatly to the success of these projects throughout the years 1945-65.

The New Era in Information Retrieval

SELECTIVE DISSEMINATION OF INFORMATION PROGRAMS

At the same time that cooperative activities in the areas of abstracting and indexing were proceeding at a great rate, close attention was also being focused directly on the difficult problem of basic information retrieval both on a demand and continuing basis. Efforts to carry on selective dissemination of information programs were being made in some libraries. That these programs were facing a losing battle is obvious in retrospect, but the absolutely desperate attempt to supply what was so needed by library users is agonizingly delineated by Thomson, who describes the arduous ordeal endured in establishing a collection containing 80,000 papers and abstracts on cancer. He says that:

> I have been slowly losing ground with masses of material waiting to be dealt with. I have no time for original research, and I feel that I am fighting a losing battle with the Frankenstein monster which I have created. To add to these difficulties I urgently need more room and more steel cases, but neither of these is available. . . . Now [the library] has reached important dimensions I fell that it should be kept up to date. Therein lies my difficulty. I am now very forcibly driven to the conclusion that this is not a task for one man with little assistance, but that it is an international affair, requiring much money and a number of highly qualified workers.[59]

Fleming, discussing his more limited but more numerous SDI programs, called attention to their success and added: "The conclusion is inescapable that the libraries of the world must in the future play a far more decisive role than at present in increasing the productivity of research. One of the major ways in which university libraries can contribute is through the establishment of a continuous bibliographic service for the scholars requiring their active support."[60]

Fleming's point was an excellent one and one with which librarians firmly agreed. That such a continuous bibliographic service in the face of the literature explosion could not possibly proceed was becoming more evident as each day's mail delivery was received by the libraries of the world. Overwhelmed with the deluge, they sought new ways out of the difficulty. The most significant among these approaches was that to be soon realized in *mechanization*. This term, awesome in its primary implications, was to become one of the most important words in all activities connected with information retrieval during the coming years.

MECHANIZATION

The Army Medical Library, with its vast responsibilities for service, was among the first to consider automation. Its director asked the Surgeon General to appoint a committee of consultants for the study of the indexes to medical literature published by the library. This committee soon saw the hopelessness of manual retrieval and recommended that mechanization be investigated. Subsequently the NLM arranged for Sanford Larkey, under a contract between the NLM and the Johns Hopkins Institute for Cooperative Research, to conduct a research project at Welch Medical Library in Baltimore on problems of medical indexing, the evaluation and study of present indexes, the study of subject headings and the possibility of using machine methods in indexing.

In his first report in 1949 on this project to the MLA, Larkey stated: "There are many problems to be solved before final decisions can be reached as to the best and most efficient means of bibliographic control of our vast medical literature. The aim of the research project is to supply some factual answers to these questions."[61]

Factual answers regarding mechanization did come, and quickly, and for the next two years articles and reports continued to appear, detailing progress and pointing out the widespread participation by scientists and librarians in all aspects of the project.

A complete report entitled "The National Library of Medicine Index Mechanization Project" appeared in 1961, showing that computer indexing of medical serials was well on its way, and that the new bibliographic retrieval system, if not exactly the librarian's perfect dream, was at least nearing that point.[62] In 1963 "The MEDLARS Story"[63] appeared as well as Seymour Taine's comprehensive article on this new system.[64] By this time many users of libraries were beginning to take advantage of this much improved means of searching and retrieving the literature. Another long-sought goal of bettering service to library patrons had materialized and was functioning.

References

1. Lacy, Dan. "Social Change and the Library: 1945-1980." *In* Douglas M. Knight and E. Shepley Nourse, eds. *Libraries at Large.* New York, R.R. Bowker, 1969, p. 6.

2. Friedrich, Dorathea W. "The Effect of the War upon Medical Libraries and Their Probable Trends," *Bulletin of the Medical Library Association,* 34:60, April 1946.

3. Marshall, Mary Louise. "The Library and Medical Education in Postwar Years," *Bulletin of the Medical Library Association,* 32:407-10, Oct. 1944.

4. Larkey, Sanford V. "The Medical Library Association and Medical Research," *Bulletin of the Medical Library Association,* 38:291-95, Oct. 1950.

5. Deitrick, John E., and Berson, Robert C. *Medical Schools in the United States at Mid-Century.* New York, McGraw-Hill, 1953.

6. Adams, Scott. "Medical Library Resources and Their Development," *Journal of Medical Education,* 38:20, Jan. 1963.

7. Bloomquist, Harold. "The Status and Needs of Medical School Libraries in the United States," *Journal of Medical Education,* 38:145-63, March 1963.

8. Adams, *op. cit.,* p. 123.

9. Bloomquist, *op. cit.,* p. 155.

10. Castiglioni, Arturo. "Libraries and Librarians," *Bulletin of the Medical Library Association,* 34:182, July 1946.

11. Gartland, Henry J. "The Veterans Administration Medical Library Program, 1946-1956," *Bulletin of the Medical Library Association,* 45:389-98, July 1957; and Ricker, Eleanor L. "The Hospital Librarian in a Large Organization," *Special Libraries,* 48:455-57, Dec. 1957.

12. Poliakoff, Augusta. "Functional Medical Libraries for Medical Districts," *Bulletin of the Medical Library Association,* 33:473-81, Oct. 1945; Crawford, Helen. "Medical Library Extension Service," *Bulletin of the Medical Library Association,* 37:15-22, Jan. 1949; and Herman, Flora E. "The Public Health Library," *Bulletin of the Medical Library Association,* 43:212-16, April 1955.

13. Wilson, Harriet. "The Package Library," *Bulletin of the Medical Library Association,* 22:133-37, Jan. 1934.

14. Colby, Charles C., and Esterquest, Ralph T. "The Francis A. Countway Library of Medicine, Harvard Medical Library-Boston Medical

Library," *Bulletin of the Medical Library Association,* 48:121-24, April 1960.
15. "The Medical Society in a Changing World; A Symposium," *Bulletin of the Medical Library Association,* 50:214-23, April 1962.
16. Troxel, Wilma, A. "Library Service for Modern Dental Education in a Combined Medical-Dental-Pharmacy Library," *Bulletin of the Medical Library Association,* 40:21-25, Jan. 1952; and Robinson, Arline. "The Separate Dental School Library," *Bulletin of the Medical Library Association,* 40:26-29, Jan. 1952.
17. Lentz, Robert T. "The Medical School Library," *Bulletin of the Medical Library Association,* 43:92, April 1955.
18. Morrisey, Mary. "Relation of Librarian to Nursing School Staff," *Bulletin of the Medical Library Association,* 44:454, Oct. 1956.
19. Greenaway, Emerson. "Library Services to the Blind and Other Handicapped Groups," *ALA Bulletin,* 55:320-23, April 1961.
20. Lunper, Hilda K. "The Public Library at Work With Children in Hospitals and Institutions," *ALA Bulletin,* 55:329-31, April 1961; and Sharp, E. Preston. "Philadelphia Team—Free Library and Youth Study Center," *ALA Bulletin,* 55:324-28, April 1961.
21. Bloomquist, *op. cit.,* p. 155.
22. Garrison, Fielding H. "The Medical Library in Relation to the University Library." In *Essays Offered to Herbert Putnam by His Colleagues and Friends. . . .* William W. Bishop and Andrew Keogh, eds. New Haven, Conn., Yale University Press, 1929, p. 167.
23. Radmacher, Mary. "Questionable Medical Literature and the Library: A Symposium; The Public Library," *Bulletin of the Medical Library Association,* 51:463-66, Oct. 1963.
24. Cunningham, Eileen R. "Reference Work." *In* Janet Doe, ed. *A Handbook of Medical Library Practice.* Chicago, ALA, 1943, pp. 373-74.
25. "Service to the Lay Public," *Bulletin of the Medical Library Association,* 43:241-61, April 1955.
26. Green, Samuel S. "Personal Relations Between Librarians and Readers," *Library Journal,* 1:81, 1876.
27. Noyes, Marcia. *Celebration of the Centennial of the Library of the Medical and Chirurgical Faculty of the State of Maryland.* Baltimore, 1931.
28. Keys, Thomas E. "Changing Concepts in Library Services," *Bulletin of the Medical Library Association,* 45:5-13, Jan. 1957.
29. Crowe, Mildred R. "The Medical School Library: Its Present and Potential Services," *Journal of Medical Education,* 30:497-503, Sept. 1955.
30. King, Henry H. "Assistance to the Faculty in Library Research: Report from Cornell University," *College & Research Libraries,* 9:227-30, July 1948.
31. Leake, Chauncey D. "Ideals for a Community Health Library," *Texas Reports on Biology and Medicine,* 13:420-33, Fall 1955.
32. Emery, Verna M. "The Medical Librarian's Role in Chronic Disease Research," *Libri,* 3:356-62, 1954.
33. Goodall, Archibald L. "The Place of the Librarian in the Medical Team," *Bulletin of the Medical Library Association,* 42:19-22, Jan. 1954.
34. Forscher, Bernard K. "Faculty Comments on the Dental School Library," *Bulletin of the Medical Library Association,* 49:83-90, Jan. 1961.

35. Crawford, *op. cit.;* and King, Louise D.C. "Availability of Medical Library Service" [Letter to the Editor]," *Bulletin of the Medical Library Association,* 44:488-89, Oct. 1956.
36. "Teaching of Medical Bibliography: Panel Discussion," *Bulletin of the Medical Library Association,* 40:355-68, Oct. 1952.
37. Brodman, Estelle. "Teaching Medical Bibliography to Medical Librarians," *Bulletin of the Medical Library Association,* 40:366-68, Oct. 1952.
38. Truelson, Stanley D. "Needed: Curriculum Reform [Guest Editorial]," *Bulletin of the Medical Library Association,* 49:635, Oct. 1961.
39. "UCLA Biomedical Library Traveling Exhibits," *Bulletin of the Medical Library Association,* 51:283, April 1963.
40. Parker, Sheila M., and Hawkins, Miriam. *Scientific Translations: A Guide to Sources and Services.* U.S. Department of Health, Education and Welfare, Public Health Service, 1959.
41. Crowe, Mildred R. "An Introduction to the Preparation and Writing of Articles for Medical Journals," *The Jefferson Hillman Hospital Bulletin,* 4:60-98, April 1950.
42. O'Toole, Margaret M. "Annual Administrative Reviews: Library Service," *Hospitals,* 32:55, April 16, 1958.
43. Noyes, *op. cit.*
44. Green, Samuel S. "The Lending of Books to One Another by Libraries [Letter]," *Library Journal,* 1(1):15-16, 1876.
45. ________. "Address of the President," *Library Journal,* 16(12):1-9, Dec. 1891.
46. Rogers, Frank B. "The Loan Policy of the National Library of Medicine," *Bulletin of the Medical Library Association,* 45:487, Oct. 1957.
47. McKenna, Muriel R. "The Veterans Administration and Interlibrary Loans," *Bulletin of the Medical Library Association,* 41:140-43, April 1953.
48. Ballard, James F. "Co-operation and Co-ordination in Special Library Work," *Bulletin of the Medical Library Association,* 24:149-54, Feb. 1936; Raymond, Jurgen G. "Interlibrary Loans," *Bulletin of the Medical Library Association,* 34:189-93, July 1946; and Ballard, James F. "Interlibrary Loans," *Bulletin of the Medical Library Association,* 34:196-97, July 1946.
49. Seidell, Atherton, "The Aims of Medical Library Service," *Bulletin of the Medical Library Association,* 34:336-37, Oct. 1946.
50. Kurth, William H. *Survey of the Interlibrary Loan Operations of the National Library of Medicine.* U.S. Department of Health, Education and Welfare, Public Health Service, April 1962.
51. Martin, Jess A., and Ferguson, M.S. "Photocopying in a Research Library," *Bulletin of the Medical Library Association,* 52:410-13, April 1964.
52. Rogers, *op. cit.*
53. Kennan, Elizabeth L. "Interlibrary Loan, 1952-62: Ten Years of Progress?" *Bulletin of the Medical Library Association,* 52:307-15, Jan. 1964; Esterquest, Ralph T. "Co-Operative Control of Library Resources: The Realities of Co-Operation," *Bulletin of the Medical Library Association,* 47:369-74, Oct. 1959; and Orr, Richard H., and Pings, Vern M. "Document Retrieval: The National Biomedical Library System and Interlibrary Loans," *Federation of American Societies for Experimental Biology Proceedings,* 23:1155-63, Sept. 1964.

54. Minsk, Gertrude G. "Implications of the Midwest Inter-library Center for Medical Librarians," *Bulletin of the Medical Library Association,* 40:43, Jan. 1952.

55. Craig, Howard, and Felter, Jacqueline W. "Co-Operation or Chaos; A Summary of the Problems Confronting the Medical Libraries of Greater New York," *Bulletin of the Medical Library Association,* 46:381, July 1958.

56. "Co-Operative Control of Library Resources: A Symposium," *Bulletin of the Medical Library Association,* 47:369-86, Oct. 1959; and "Regional Plans for Medical Library Service," *Bulletin of the Medical Library Association,* 52:497-523, July 1964.

57. Morse, Kenneth T. "International Conference on Scientific Information: A Brief Report," *Bulletin of the Medical Library Association,* 47:170-71, April 1959.

58. Evans, Luther H. "Bibliography by Cooperation," *Bulletin of the Medical Library Association,* 37:197-212, July 1949.

59. Thomson, David. "A Highly Organized Medical Library," *Journal of Documentation,* 2:59, Sept. 1946.

60. Fleming, Thomas P., *et al.* "A Continuous Bibliographic Service in University Libraries," *College & Research Libraries,* 8:328, July 1947.

61. Larkey, Sanford V. "The Army Medical Library Research Project at the Welch Medical Library," *Bulletin of the Medical Library Association,* 37:124, April 1949.

62. "The National Library of Medicine Index Mechanization Project, July 1, 1958-June 30, 1960," *Bulletin of the Medical Library Association,* 49(2):1-96, Jan. 1961.

63. *The MEDLARS Story at the National Library of Medicine.* U.S. Department of Health, Education and Welfare, Public Health Service, 1963.

64. Taine, Seymour I. "The Medical Literature Analysis and Retrieval System," *Bulletin of the Medical Library Association,* 51:157-67, April 1963.

ADDITIONAL REFERENCES

Adams, Scott. "The Office of Science Information Services, National Science Foundation," *Bulletin of the Medical Library Association,* 47:387-92, Oct. 1959.

Bolef, Doris. "An Orientation Program for Student Nurses," *Bulletin of the Medical Library Association,* 38:1-8, Jan. 1950.

Brodman, Estelle, *et al.* "The National Medical Library; The Survey and Ten Years' Progress," *Bulletin of the Medical Library Association,* 43:439-46, Oct. 1954.

Brown, Alberta L. "The Relation of the Librarian to Management, to the Patron and to the Library Staff," *Bulletin of the Medical Library Association,* 46:82-90, Jan. 1958.

———. "Survey of Translation Activity in the United States and Canada," *Special Libraries,* 53:34-36, Jan. 1962.

Brown, Amy F. "The Importance of Hospital and Nursing School Libraries to the Nursing Profession," *Bulletin of the Medical Library Association,* 47:258-63, July 1959.

Cavanagh, G.S.T. "Medical Travel Books," *Bulletin of the Medical Library Association,* 47:315-18, July 1959.

Clopine, John J. "Translation Programs," *Bulletin of the Medical Library Association,* 50:188-95, April 1962.
Coffyn, Eleanor N. "Medicine's 'Information Please,' " *Bulletin of the Medical Library Association,* 36:184-89, July 1948.
Crandall, Ella J. "The Hospital Medical Library," *Bulletin of the Medical Library Association,* 43:184-87, April 1955.
Darling, Louise. "Darwin and Evolution," *Bulletin of the Medical Library Association,* 47:510-14, Oct. 1959.
Davis, Lora-Frances. "Helping the Smaller Library," *Bulletin of the Medical Library Association,* 52:202-06, Jan. 1964.
__________. "The Simple Exhibit," *Bulletin of the Medical Library Association,* 48:91-95, Jan. 1960.
Esterquest, Ralph T. "Medical Library Service in the Hospital," *Bulletin of the Medical Library Association,* 52:253-61, Jan. 1964.
Flandorf, Vera. "A Library for Students and Staff," *Nursing Outlook,"* 9:288-89, May 1961.
Foregger, Richard. "What the Physician Expects of the Librarian," *Bulletin of the Medical Library Association,* 40:283-87, July 1952.
Foulke, Jean E. "The Young Student and the Scientific Library," *Bulletin of the Medical Library Association,* 51:489-98, Oct. 1963.
Fraser, M. Doreen. "Canadian Medical School Libraries and Their Collections; A Brief Review," *Bulletin of the Medical Library Association,* 48:149-61, April 1960.
Gilman, Henry. "What the Scientist Expects of the Librarian," *College & Research Libraries,* 8:329-32, July 1947.
Gorlin, Robert J. "Dental Research in a Medical Center Library," *Bulletin of the Medical Library Association,* 46:503-05, Oct. 1958.
Gruen, Sonia L. "Establishing a New Medical School Library," *Bulletin of the Medical Library Association,* 52:684-91, Oct. 1964.
Hallam, Bertha B. "Finding Your Way Around a Library," *American Journal of Nursing,* 61:108-09, Oct. 1961.
Hawkins, Miriam, and Parker, Shiela M. "Scientific Translations: Sources and Services," *Bulletin of the Medical Library Association,* 48:199-202, April 1960.
Heatherman, Mary E. "How the Medical School Library Can Better Serve the Graduate Student," *Bulletin of the Medical Library Association,* 40:13-15, Jan. 1952.
"The Hospital User," *Bulletin of the Medical Library Association*, 44:57-64, Jan. 1956.
Ingersoll, C. F. "The Responsibility of the Library to the Faculty," *Bulletin of the Medical Library Association,* 40:16-20, Jan. 1952.
Johnson, Barbara C. "The Context of Reference Work in the Hospital Professional Library," *Special Libraries,* 53:141-44, March 1962.
Kennedy, Catherine E. "Medical Translation Service and Index," *Bulletin of the Medical Library Association,* 41:132-37, April 1953.
Keys, Thomas E. "Research Libraries in Medicine," *Bulletin of the Medical Library Association,* 43:207-11, April 1955.
Klumpp, Theodore G. "What Scientific Libraries Can Do for Industry" *Bulletin of the Medical Library Association,* 37:35-45, Jan. 1949.
Lewis, Robert F. "From the Mountains to the Moon: Some Historical Aspects

of Survival at Great Heights," *Bulletin of the Medical Library Association*, 49:212-17, April 1961.

Long, E. Croft, and Miller, Polly G. "The Medical Library and the Medical Student," *Bulletin of the Medical Library Association*, 52:568-74, July 1964.

McCann, Alice M. "The Value of Exhibit Material to the Professional School Library," *Bulletin of the Medical Library Association*, 34:22-25, Jan. 1946.

McClure, Cuvier D. "A Medical Student Views the Medical Library," *Bulletin of the Medical Library Association*, 40:10-12, Jan. 1952.

MacWatt, J. Alan. "The Pharmacy Library," *Bulletin of the Medical Library Association*, 43:203-06, April 1955.

Martin, Jess A., *et al.* "Twenty-five Years of Translating Service at NIH," *Bulletin of the Medical Library Association*, 53:422-25, July 1965.

Mettler, Frederick A. "What Does a Research Man Want of a Medical Library?" *Bulletin of the Medical Library Association*, 36:28-33, Jan. 1948.

Meyers, Lawrence. "The Clinician and the Medical Library," *Bulletin of the Medical Library Association*, 36:210-13, July 1948.

Norris, Helen H. "Serving the Professional Public," *Bulletin of the Medical Library Association*, 34:219-20, July 1946.

Osborne, George E. "Faculty and Student Use of the Library," *Bulletin of the Medical Library Association*, 41:405-09, Oct. 1953.

Parker, Sheila M. "War and its Aftermath—Some Medical Aspects," *Bulletin of the Medical Library Association*, 49:100-01, Jan. 1961.

Parker, Sheila M., and Purtle, Helen R. "A Guide to the Planning and Development of Exhibits for Medical Libraries," *Bulletin of the Medical Library Association*, 46:335-43, July 1958.

Pizer, Irwin. "The Doctor's Bag: Past and Present," *Bulletin of the Medical Library Association*, 51:250-55, April 1963.

Pulaski, Edwin J. "The User Looks at the Library," *Bulletin of the Medical Library Association*, 42:421-25, Oct. 1954.

Rogers, Frank B. "The Army Medical Library—Problems, Plans and Possibilities," *Bulletin of the Medical Library Association*, 38:145-51, April 1950.

Shaver, Mary C. "The Library's Contribution to Nursing Education," *The Canadian Nurse*, 57:553-55, June 1961.

Southern, Walter A. "Information Service at Abbott Laboratories," *Illinois Libraries*, 45:493-98, Nov. 1963.

Strieby, Irene M. "Reference Files in a Pharmaceutical Library," *Bulletin of the Medical Library Association*, 35:107-15, April 1947.

Swift, Helen P. "Trends in Library Service," *ALA Bulletin*, 55:338-40, April 1961.

Walker, Mabel. "Research Problems in Dentistry: The Role of the Dental Library in Dental Research," *Journal of Dental Education*, 27:74-80, March 1963.

Wiles, Juanita Z. "The Case for a Hospital Library," *ALA Bulletin*, 55:341-44, April 1961.

Yast, Helen T. "The Library's Integral Services," *Hospital Progress*, 43:142-46, Sept. 1962.

Zachert, Martha Jane K. "The Use of Reference Service Records in Pharmacy Library Development," *Bulletin of the Medical Library Association*, 48:331-38, July 1960.

Medical Library Extension Service*

By HELEN CRAWFORD, *Librarian,*
University of Wisconsin Medical School.

WHENEVER I am speaking on a topic that may perhaps be of less interest to my audience than it is to me, I remember the story of the small boy who belonged to a children's book club. The agreement was that any book not wanted could be returned to the company on condition that the recipient explain his reasons. So his young man wrote: "Dear Sirs: I am returning your book because it is about penguins and it tells me more about penguins than I care to know." I hope that my topic this morning is not in the class of penguins.

The preliminary survey of the extension activities of medical libraries reported here had a personal as well as a professional basis. Any library conducting an extension service has had inquiries from former residents of the state or from alumni asking for continued service, or for information on similar services available in their own regions. Failing to find any general description of these extension services, I was driven to asking the members of this Association for the information. Questionnaires concerning the extra-mural services, both interlibrary loans and loans made directly to individuals, were distributed to nearly 300 members of the Association in the United States and Canada. Returns were secured from better than 60 per cent, in 39 states and 6 provinces. Nearly three-quarters of the medical schools and most of the major reference libraries responded, nearly 60 per cent of the county and association libraries, and nearly half the hospital libraries and the libraries of private clinics and commercial organizations. Knowing the high sedimentation rate of questionnaires on my own desk, I am particularly grateful for the generous assistance, and apologetic that the results are not more impressive.

Interlibrary loans and direct lending to the individual borrower are two approaches to the same purpose: getting the publication needed into the hands of the inquirer. The interlibrary loan is best suited to localities with either a public or a special library suffciently staffed to take on the rather demanding work of identifying, locating, and safely handling

***Read at annual meeting of the Medical Library Association, Philadelphia, May 30, 1948**

Originally published in *Bulletin of the Medical Library Association,* Volume 37 (January, 1949), pp. 15-22. Reprinted by permission.

material borrowed from another library. Extension service is designed for the speedier supply of material, often in its more economical unbound form, direct to the user, although it also aids the smaller library with material not available locally. The general state extension agency, the library commission or traveling library, is rarely well enough equipped with medical books to supply even the lay demand. Medical extension service has therefore grown up apart from these agencies, but for essentially the same purpose: to provide book service to residents without adequate library facilities.

I shall not trouble you with a detailed analysis of the answers to the questionnaire but shall give a running account of the problem and the various methods of meeting it. The major defect of an inquiry such as this, directed to existing medical libraries is that they represent the well populated areas, or at least the major cities of more rural states. The physicians in these centers have access to the necessary books and journals, either through direct consultation or through the generous interlibrary loan practice of the large libraries in the city. They deal with librarians accustomed to interlibrary borrowing and not intimidated by unfamiliar references.

The development of interlibrary loan service in this country has been notoriously haphazard and unplanned, placing too heavy a burden on the nearest large library that is known to be a generous lender and perhaps too little on the collections of moderate size. It is, however, infinitely better established among medical libraries than medical extension service, which is developing gradually as the result of the effort of various agencies to meet a need with whatever resources they have available. Without exception, medical librarians in the large metropolitan areas expressed themselves as well satisfied with, and grateful for, the assistance given them by such libraries as the Army Medical Library, the New York Academy of Medicine, the College of Physicians of Philadelphia, the Boston Medical Library, the John Crerar, the Lane Medical Library, and local medical school libraries. The librarians of county, hospital, and clinic libraries in smaller communities and more sparsely settled states, and provinces, while acknowledging the help of interlibrary loan, more generally felt the need for an extension service.

The physician in the small town or rural area is glimpsed only occasionally in the bare returns from a questionnaire, but he is really the crucial character in this study. The availability of medical literature is undoubtedly one of the attractions of medical practice in a city. The rural physician is faced with stagnation unless he can keep up with his profession through reading as well as through refresher and graduate courses. He cannot afford to subscribe to all the journals he may wish to consult, nor does he have access to indexes to guide his requests for material from the nearest medical library. I cannot state his case better than the hospital librarian in a large mid-western city has done it for me. Although nearby medical libraries enable her to give adequate service to her own clientele, she is touched by the "hopeless letters received from some of the former residents of the hospital:"

> I do think that after these young doctors have been taught to use and depend upon a library, it is too bad to have them find no library facilities where they locate. Many of them have located in these out-of-the-way places because of the urging of all the medical associations, from the A.M.A. down; so that the people in these places may have the advantage of good medicine and surgery. They need something quicker than inter-library loan from a university library. The hospitals to which they take their patients are too small ever to have a library of even 500 volumes.

Let us follow one of these ambitious young physicians into his small community. How is he to go about getting even an interlibrary loan of, say, a recent book on Hodgkin's disease? He may, perhaps, apply to the medical school or the hospital in which he trained, but it may not be able to assume the burden of service to all its graduates, particularly in other states. If the community is large enough to support an active public library, he may persuade the librarian to apply to the nearest medical school library, only to learn that the volume is on reserve or in too much demand to be sent out of town. If, as happens too often in our rural areas, the library is a hopeful product of local pride with a budget of a few hundred dollars a year, what help may he expect in the intelligent use of interlibrary loan techniques? Besides, interlibrary loan is cumbersome and rightly surrounded with safeguards for material available only through the generosity of the lender. Finally, since fully half the larger libraries reporting limit their lending of current issues of journals, and a fourth restrict the lending of recent books, interlibrary loan would not fill the doctor's need for up-to-date material.

Let us follow our persistent young physician farther. If he is a member of the American Medical Association or a subscriber to one of its journals, he may write to the A.M.A. Library for recent journals or a selection of reprints on a topic of interest and receive prompt service. However, the loan period from a library with a nationwide coverage and 12,000 loans a year is necessarily brief. The American College of Surgeons also offers a reference and loan service in this specialty, sending out some

1500 packets a year on subjects requested, in addition to translation, abstracting, and bibliographic service offered at cost.

If our young doctor settles in certain states, he may find that his needs are being met by any of a number of agencies. The one most specifically designed for the purpose is the state medical library, of which the first, the New York State Medical Library, was founded in 1891 as part of the thorough library coverage of New York State. It and the Iowa State Medical Library are both somewhat above the size of the average medical school collection and have a circulation comparable to that of the medical school library. The reference load of the state library varies somewhat, depending on the number of local physicians who can do their own searching, but it may range above a thousand requests a year. With smaller collections, the library of the Florida State Board of Health offers an extensive loan, bibliographical, and reference service to physicians in the state, and the Mississippi State Board of Health Library serves laymen as well.

Another statewide service is that offered to its members by the state medical association library as in Maryland, Rhode Island, and Texas. The medical society of Pennsylvania maintains a large collection of reprints and tear-sheets for this purpose. Other state societies may provide a similar service on a more limited basis.

Several state medical schools have developed, in practice if not in name, the functions of an extension service. The University of Oregon Medical Library is the official medical library for Oregon physicians, receiving financial support through an annual registration fee paid to the state board of examiners, and fees paid to the city and county medical associations. The Medical Library Service of the University of Wisconsin is supported by the Medical School, with extensive contributions of books and journals from the State Medical Society and the use of almost any publication in the Medical School Library collection. It mails specific titles and answers reference questions for physicians, nurses, laymen, and libraries, and accepts requests on medical subjects transferred to it from the state traveling library. The University of California Medical School Library is continuing, on a more limited basis, the statewide service originally supported in part by a grant from the State Board of Medical Examiners.

The medical school libraries, both state and private institutions, in some other states where medical libraries are few, as in Georgia and

Louisiana, often feel a responsibility to a wider public than the local staff and student body and give what state-wide and regional service they can. Emory University, for instance, is generous with its resources, and Jefferson County and University of Louisville Medical Library lends widely in its area. The University of Nebraska Medical School Library extends full library facilities to members of the state medical association, although the use is not at present extensive. Some medical school libraries, such as Vanderbilt, are already sufficiently taxed by the demands of other medical, hospital, and V.A. hospital libraries in their metropolitan areas.

The larger county and academy libraries often serve a more than local public. The Cleveland Medical Library Association, for instance, gives the same service to its non-resident as to its local members. On the other hand, physicians in outlying areas, perhaps unaccustomed to the advantages of library facilities, are not always willing to contribute even a fraction of the fee assessed upon local members in order to obtain service. For instance, the offer of the Tulane and Orleans Parish Medical libraries to serve the membership of the state society at $1.00 per member was refused, whereas a county association library in another southern state assesses a membership fee of $60. The unwillingness to contribute for mail service is a curious and apparently rather general phenomenon, and a fee once granted may be subject to revocation.

The medical school libraries of Canada, particularly in the less populated areas, have taken the responsibility for lending material requested by physicians in their regions. The University of Alberta Medical Library and the University of Western Ontario Faculty of Medicine Library do an extensive loan service to individuals. The University of Manitoba attempts to answer or to transfer to the appropriate agency all questions received. Queens University and McGill likewise have a considerable extra-mural loan. Membership in the Academy of Medicine of Toronto or a deposit paid to the University of Toronto Medical Reading Room gives physicians in this area library privileges. Dalhousie serves as the medical library center for the Maritime Privinces.

What are the prospects for the future? No consistent opinion on the need for a state-wide service where it does not exist could be extracted from the answers to the questionnaires. Four medical school libraries in rural states, Alabama, South Carolina, South Dakota, and Utah, anticipate extending their services as demand develops. Scattered expressions of interest were received from libraries in Illinois, Michigan, Minnesota, Missouri, New Jersey, Ohio, Tennessee, and Vermont, as well as some from states where an organized service is already available. Several replies indicated an interest in, but an inability to take on, a larger responsibility with the available staff.

To summarize the evidence from the questionnaires: the large metropolitan areas, particularly in the East, are adequately served by interlibrary loan. In perhaps a fourth of the states, by virtue of a state medical library, a medical school extension service, a state association lending library, or the generosity of a large metropolitan association library, the rural physician has reasonably good access to medical literature. Another twenty states have one or more libraries willing to lend to residents outside their own cities, although hampered by lack of staff and funds. Four medical school libraries anticipate expanding their coverage as demand increases.

Extension service is a problem for all medical libraries in a state, regardless of their direct need. In the first place, it is unwise to infer that the existence of a good medical library in a city entirely satisfies a doctor's need. Because the material he wants is in use in his local library, or simply because less effort is required, the physician will often prefer to write for a publication and have it delivered to him. As much as a fourth of the annual out-of-town loans of the service with which I am most familiar may go to a nearby city, which has an excellent medical library but a large physician population.

In the second place, the extension service can provide the basic modern books and the standard American journals, releasing the larger medical school and reference libraries to concentrate on the unusual titles, the foreign books and journals, and the historical volumes. Few libraries have such an even balance of interlibrary borrowing and lending that they can escape guilt feelings on the one hand or, on the other, an occasional twinge of annoyance at the magnitude of the demands on them. One of the most heartfelt endorsements of the need for an extension service came from a library which lends a thousand times what it borrows. Physicians and smaller libraries feel freer to call for loans and reference service on an agency organized and properly staffed for their use, equipped to send material promptly in its lightest form and by the cheapest means.

An extension service is, by the nature of the distribution of the calls on it, a function of a state or of some organization with statewide membership. However, although availability of extension facilities is by no means in direct relation to the economic ability of the state, there are large areas of the country in which a regional arrangement would be necessary because of the paucity of medical books and medical libraries: the upper New England states and large areas of the northwest and southwest. Some of the larger states in these areas have no medical libraries, or at best only an occasional small clinic collection with no responsibility to the profession at large.

Dr. H. B. Mulholland, Chairman of the Committee on Rural Medicine of the American Medical Association, has expressed his interest in the extension of medical library service, probably through state medical associations and medical school libraries, and with the proposed networks of regional hospitals in mind.

In conclusion, I should like to pass on a few practical suggestions for the benefit of those who may be interested in the mechanics of service-by-mail.

1. Try to secure an affiliation with some association receiving publications in exchange for its own journal and review copies of books. Our Medical Library Service receives from the Wisconsin Medical Journal a few dozen volumes a year, most of the state journals, and some from abroad. With the exceptions of a few from Great Britain, the foreign titles are of little use for the extension work and are transferred to the Medical School Library.

2. Maintain files of unbound duplicates for mailing. Removal or obliteration of the advertisements permits mailing at a special library rate much less than the temporary second-class rate. The unbound copy is also valuable to supplement the permanent copy for local use when the latter is in circulation or at the bindery. Sending material by mail, at least within the state, has proved entirely satisfactory. The losses do not average one in 10,000 loans.

3. Extension service is not inexpensive. Intelligent reference assistance and speedy mailing are important. Unless sufficient personnel is available, the extension work may take to wagging the dog.

4. Gifts from staff members and other doctors are useful, but it is almost essential to have the major clinical journals available, and available promptly. Our duplication of 46 American and British journals costs more than $500 a year. In general, the titles most in demand locally are also those needed for the extension work. On the other hand, we have found it an economy to maintain only the one unbound file of most of the state journals and certain ephemeral titles, accessible to both libraries.

5. Requests for material on identical topics are so infrequent that ready-made packets have not, in our experience, been practicable except for popular material. We have discontinued our reprint files in favor of direct use of unbound journals. Unless a deliberate effort is made to request the reprints needed, the collection will be unbalanced and inadequate, and the labor of recording and filing them is far from trivial. Some extension services, however, prefer to maintain subject files of reprints and tear-sheets and find them adequate.

6. The routine mailing of each issue of a journal to any physician requesting it sounds attractive, but it takes an undue proportion of the time of the staff (usually to serve a very small proportion of the borrowers), and requires duplication of some expensive journals.

7. The question of service to laymen is a troublesome one. Over two-thirds of the medical school libraries reporting make no loans to laymen except when referred by a physician, or through interlibrary loan to a public library. Some, of course, lack facilities to accomodate a larger clientele. Admittedly, it is easier to select material suitable for a medical man than to find appropriate material for a laymen on multiple sclerosis, or on what one of our correspondents (a thorough Wisconsonian) called "cheesofrania." However, in these days when many physicians are concerned over public mis-information on medicine and the need for accurate interpretation of the profession to the public, the medical extension service may feel that it has a responsibility to supplement the scanty material in public libraries. For this reason we send what we can to the mother with a spastic child or the student writing a paper on plastic surgery.

Extension work can be an eye-opener to the medical librarian, increasing her respect for the alertness of the doctors with whom she deals. The range of questions, the occasional urgency of the need, and the interest in new developments are a challenge to her skill and her knowledge of the literature. The occasional unintentionally cryptic question or garbled term tests her ingenuity as well. If she sometimes feels that she is diagnosing without a license, she is also touched by the confidence placed in her omniscience. I hope that an increasing number of my fellow medical librarians will be privileged to experience this satisfaction.

Handling Technical Reports in the Medical Library*

BY CHARLES W. SARGENT, PH.D.

Deputy Librarian and Assistant Professor†
Library of the Medical Sciences
University of New Mexico School of Medicine
Albuquerque, New Mexico

ABSTRACT

One of the most widely neglected sources of information in the medical library is the technical report. Often this bibliographic form is ignored because there is a general lack of information on the part of the librarian concerning its mysteries. In many cases the technical report provides the most recent and current information on a given subject, and to ignore it or wait for its appearance in the published literature could prove costly to a research project.

Technical reports have reached flood proportions since World War II, and are issued from many diverse sources. Means of acquiring, processing, and using the tools which abstract and index this literature are discussed.

IF we were to look at the category of literature variously referred to as technical reports or documents, and the treatment of this literature in medical libraries, we would soon see that we are dealing with a kind of literary pariah. Most medical libraries prefer to ignore them, while others are in a somewhat ambivalent position as to whether or not they should have them. Some libraries treat them as pamphlets and file them in vertical files, whereas in other libraries, they are given full book treatment. *The Handbook of Medical Library Practice* gives little attention to the problem beyond mentioning that they do exist and that "close attention needs to be paid to the identification of the author ..."[1]. It is hoped that the third edition of the *Handbook* will give more space and treatment to this subject.

*Presented as part of a general session on "Current Cataloging Problems" at the Sixty-seventh Annual meeting of the Medical Library Association Denver, Colorado, June 13, 1968.

†Presently Assistant Director, Medical Center Computer Program, University of Missouri School of Medicine, Columbia, Missouri.

Originally published in *Bulletin of the Medical Library Association*, Volume 57 (January,1969), pp. 41-46. Reprinted by permission.

The basis for the cavalier treatment with which technical reports have been treated in medical libraries is the idea that most of them will appear in the open literature at some future date. In 1952 Dwight E. Gray wrote that in a survey he had made of eighty-four technical reports only one should have been published that was not. There were actually nineteen that did not appear in some journal or book, but "the concensus of the authors and of NSF scientists who studied these documents is that eighteen were unsuitable for journal publication"[2]. This is a rather strange conclusion to reach in light of the fact that one technical report in the sample gave birth to four published papers, one submitted for publication. and seven others in preparation[3]. One wonders if the one report that never did get published, and should have, was one which might have greatly accelerated a medical breakthrough such as a vaccine for polio. Mr. Gray closed his short paper with the statement that plans were being made to extend this survey to cover a larger sample of unclassified reports. I was not able to find this extension, but I hope that some day it will be published.

Herner and Company issued a report under contract to the National Science Foundation in 1961, in which they showed that of a base number of 276 reports in medicine and biology, only 38.5 percent was announced in various abstracting publications. One of the largest percentages listed was from the *Current List of Medical Literature* with 12.3 percent. The report found that there was a tendency for the Department of Defense to strive for publication of their reports, whereas the Atomic Energy Commission's policy has been one of announcement. The authors concluded that they preferred 100 percent announcement to 25 or less percent publication, and probably the costs were a great deal less[4].

In another report, also by now dated, Mary M. Cobb surveyed six months of the *Current List of Medical Literature* (October 1950-April 1951) for technical reports[5]. A total of 239 reports apeared in the *Current List* in this six-month period. Of these, fifty-six, or 22.5 percent appeared later as articles in scientific journals. Miss Cobb found that the average time lapse between the date of a research report's release and its appearance in a journal was seven months. One was delayed for eighteen months.

Dr. Richard Orr and Alice Leeds, writing in 1964, noted that roughly 2,000 United States technical reports on biomedical subjects were being issued each year and that most of these were, for all practical purposes, not available to the scientist[6]. He did find that of the approximately 16,000 reports in all subject areas issued in 1961/1962 by authors whose research was supported by NIH grants, 90 percent appeared at some later date in journals. It was interesting to note that 100 core journals contained two-thirds of these articles and that ten accounted for over one-quarter of all the publications[7]. This signifies something about the rapidity with which the report literature finds its way into the journal literature.

Research report literature is far from a new phenomenon, as its issue has been noted for centuries. It has only been in the past few decades, with particular emphasis during World War II and the years following, that "technical reports" as a term has come into common usage. During this period the increase in this type of literature was quite marked. Because of the difficulty in obtaining this literature, libraries and many researchers have avoided what often has proved to be the most current information on a given subject.

A number of government agencies have been founded to deal with the technical report. Their primary functions have been to collect, announce, store, and retrieve this literature, and in this way perform for report literature the same services that the traditional publishers and abstracting-indexing services maintain for books and journals. Unfortunately for the library, these services have operated independently and often unknown to each other.

In the main, three government agencies issue the majority of technical reports: National Aeronautics and Space Administration (NASA), Atomic Energy Commission (AEC), and the Department of Defense (DOD). Each of these agencies has established a central clearinghouse for its own reports, which are generated as a result of contractual arrangements with various industrial firms and research institutions. Each agency issues its own announcement bulletin in which, initially, only reports generated under contract to that agency were included. NASA issues *Scientific and Technical Aerospace Reports* (STAR); AEC issues *Nuclear Science Abstracts* (NSA); and the Department of Defense Documentation Center (DDC) issues the *Technical Abstract Bulletin* (TAB). Orr and Leeds were able to identify 1,615 reports dealing with biological subjects which were announced in these three abstracting journals for the period of their research[8].

Any researcher, preferably through his library, may obtain unclassified reports. This is assuming that the organization for which he works or he himself has a government contract. Those who are not eligible can obtain them in various ways, primarily through the Clearinghouse of the Office of Technical Services, for a fee. This is the most direct route, but there are various devious ways to obtain certain reports if the library wishes to make the effort. The Atomic Energy Commission has in the past few years begun to make charges for its reports to those not in the initial distribution list (TID—4500).

What has actually developed has been, to some extent, confusion. Whereas the initial intent was that each agency would list only those reports which were the by-products of its own contractual research, the tendency has been to list everything which has come to hand and been cataloged in their respective technical service centers. This has resulted in a duplication of effort and in bulkier issues of the announcement journals. It has, also, resulted in some confusion for the user of the announcement journals; many of the reports found listed are not available from the listed agency. Orr and Leeds found that for various reasons, not always explained, fully two-thirds of the reports listed in the three major announcement periodicals were unavailable to the general scientific community[9]. The fate of these reports has been mentioned in Cobb's article, but another report shows that only 28 percent of the biomedical reports issued in 1957 appeared as journal articles within three and one-half years. The fate of all technical reports was about the same, with 22 percent published at a later date as journal articles[10]. Nothing that I have seen in recent years has measurably altered any of the above statistics. It can be assumed that biomedical literature has been on the increase rather than on the decrease, with a rather static statistic relative to publication in journals.

For some time it has been the considered opinion of many medical librarians that, because of a misconception that most technical reports appear in the published literature at some future date, there was little need to acquire them as they were initially issued. In addition, faced with staff shortages, especially of persons trained in processing this type of literature, combined with space restrictions, most libraries have ignored the technical report and have failed to alert their clientele of the existence of this literature. However, this is not an opinion shared by all, as witnessed by the appearance of a new section in the *Current Catalog* for 1968, which lists selected technical reports. This event was forecast in the MLA/NLM Liaison Committee's report which appeared in the October 1967 issue of the *Bulletin of the Medical Library Association*. Evidently the National Library of Medicine decided that there was some merit in listing these reports. The basis of this selection is not clear to me, however.

If a library decides that it does wish to collect technical reports, there are several considerations that must be taken under advisement by the librarian. On what basis will technical reports be obtained? How will they be cataloged? What tools are available to aid in this cataloging? How and where will the reports be housed?

Probably the first, and thereby the most important, decision which a library must make is whether to build a collection of technical reports. If, for the sake of argument, many of these reports find their way into the journal literature at some later date, upon what basis would a library consider building a collection of reports? The only defensible answer would be one based on better service. Most of the clientele of a library are not too concerned with the form in which their information comes as long as the library supplies it. Aside from the general resistance (fast evaporating) to microprint, the user wants his information portable, easy to read, and authoritative.

Medical research is by nature expensive, and any lead time that a scientist might get would benefit his project and carry with it a general benefit to all concerned, especially to the potential patient. If the technical report, by its very nature, can be issued several months to several years in advance of its appearance in a journal, then it seems to me that we are not doing a thorough job of making available all the known literature to the requester. There can be grievous results from not having all the facts, and if all researchers waited until those facts appeared in a journal or a monograph, it might well be too late to eliminate duplication of effort or to avoid a serious error. There was a technical report, "Fire and Blast Hazards in Space Cabins," which had been published prior to the tragic accident at Cape Kennedy, but was not, for various reasons, heeded. It may not have been known to the individual whose responsibility it was to make certain design decisions. It is a known fact, moreover, that many medical discoveries were based on previous research, the results of which were available in some form. The Salk vaccine is an example. Many libraries will want to be highly selective of which technical reports they obtain, whereas others will collect on a broader scope. As many of the unclassified reports are available by one means or another, acquiring them should put little additional burden on the acquisition facilities of the library.

Organization of the collection, however, will take some consideration and will depend on several factors. The first should be the availability of space within the library to shelve the reports. I have already indicated the rapidity of growth shown by this literature. Some libraries with report collections prefer to shelve them separately, segragated from both the monographic and serial collections. This is advisable if the document number or "short title" is used as a shelving device. The approach to this arrangement would have to be through the library catalog. It is possible to do some browsing in this arrangement, but only if one knows the corporate entry, as the call number is often based on an abbreviation or acronym designation of the corporate entry.

On the other hand, some libraries wish to arrange reports in a subject or classified manner similar to the monograph collections, and indeed, some shelve reports with monographs. This seems to be the approach that the National Library of Medicine is using in cataloging those reports that are now being listed in the *Current Catalog*. This arrangement has certain advantages over the first discussed, since no separate section of the library need be set aside for future growth of the collection; the reports may be intershelved with the monographs as they are acquired. One disadvantage, or it seems to me to be a disadvantage, is that if technical reports are treated as monographs, the tendency is to use the same subject headings as are used for the books. Technical reports are usually of a more definitive nature than monographs. The contents of a given report may be extremely difficult to describe in one or two subject headings. In some report libraries an average of ten subjects per report seems to be the rule rather than the exception. Segregating reports in a library and filing by report number leaves a greater freedom in subject indexing because classification often binds too rigidly the subjects that the cataloger must use. In many libraries with large report collections, new subject listings have been developed which have been called "thesauri" in most instances.

Many libraries which have large report collections rely heavily on the announcement journals mentioned above in place of their own library catalogs. If the collection of reports is segregated, use of these journals becomes maximal, for the reference given is to the document number. If a monographic subject approach is used, the facility of retrieval using the announcement journals is restricted and sometimes nullified.

Until recently most government reports were cataloged in various ways. The AEC probably issued the most comprehensive aids to their contractors for cataloging and indexing their reports: such tools as TID—5059, which was a listing of corporate entries established by AEC with cross references from older designations or allied corporate bodies. In another section of this manual were the rules for establishing corporate authors. It was an extremely useful tool and many non-AEC libraries used it to establish consistency of entry. AEC discontinued new editions of this publication as the corporate bodies increased in number and changed with such frequency as to make TID—5059 out of date before it was printed.

Because of the "information explosion" which has faced the scientific community for some time, the federal government has become acutely aware, since the fall of 1957, of the importance and effect of efficient information networks. From 1957 to 1965, $100 billion have been expended by the government to support science and technology, with a resultant outpouring of information which had to be controlled. Various committees have been assigned to study the problem and have published their findings and recommendations. Some of these were the Baker, Crawford, and Weinberg reports[11]. The most recent and far-reaching study and resultant report was that of the Committee on Scientific and Technical Information (COSATI)[12]. As a result of this report, most of the government agencies issuing reports have moved toward uniformity of corporate entries as well as of other aspects of bibliographic control. This entry remains, as it has for years, the main entry, with the personal author as an added entry. The corporate entry is followed by the geographical location of the corporate body and then by subdivisions of that body. The title then follows, with the author or authors next. In some cases only the senior author is listed, if known, otherwise the first author listed on the title page. The date of the report is rather important and follows the personal author(s). Often there are two dates: one, the date that the report was written, and the other, the date that the report was issued. The date that the report was issued usually takes precedence. Pagination is usually the next item. The contract numbers almost always are included. An exception is that, with AEC prime contractors, some libraries elect to omit them since they seldom change. This is not necessarily true of DOD or NASA reports. The contract number of an Air Force contract, for instance, may be parcelled out to various industrial or research firms. The first part of the contract number remains constant, with the last set of digits being peculiar to a particular organization (AF30(602)-1900).

If a report number is assigned by the library, a bibliographic tool which has proven useful is the *Dictionary of Report Series Codes,* issued by the Rio Grande Chapter, Special Libraries Association, in 1962. A new edition is in preparation. This is an alphanumeric arrangement of report codes or numbers in one column with the name of the organization in an opposite column. Another section of the volume is the reverse arrangement. Many of these numbers are not assigned by the issuing agency but are supplied by one of the libraries which has cooperated in the compilation of the *Dictionary*. One method which has proven successful in assigning new report numbers, when none has been assigned by the issuing agency, is to create one from an abbreviated form of the corporate body (SC for Sandia Corporation, UNM for the University of New Mexico) plus a series of numbers which often come from the contract number plus another alpha series which indicate the type of report. There are a number of these two- or three-letter designations which further explain the report. Some are: TR, technical report; RR, research report; RP, reprint report; PR, progress report; FR, final report; AR, annual report; etc. Thus UNM—4565—PR—5 would indicate that this was progress report number five which was done under some contract, probably an Air Force contract, at the University of New Mexico. This is a rather safe method since the contract numbers are very seldom duplicated from one agency to the other.

Most AEC and NASA reports have preprinted codes already on the cover or title page of each report. With the AEC, these are usually made up of an acronym designation of the contractor plus a serial number, the exception to this being those reports which are originated within the Technical Information Division at Oak Ridge, Tennessee. These are prefixed by the letters TID followed by a serial number. NASA reports are usually issued in designated series and are, with almost no exception, prefaced by the letters NASA. These series are: TR, technical reports; TP, technical paper; CR, contract report; TN, technical note; etc.

Bibliographic control is somewhat easier than subject control. AEC and DOD through DDC have had for several years a subject authority listing.

With DDC it has been a thesaurus which was available to requesters with government contracts. Recently NASA has compiled and released its own thesaurus. The *Current Catalog* of the National Library of Medicine is using *MeSH* terms, but not in great depth in most cases. In one issue which I examined, the median number of terms used was from three to four with one report receiving one term and another, seven. An indexer in a technical report library expects to assign a median of ten with the upper limits unrestricted. I realize that in any cataloging situation the cataloger has to use his judgment in the selection and number of subjects. The major decision, so it seems to me, is whether to build a new subject authority or to use one that is already in existence in the library.

Because report literature adapts itself to automatic systems, a number of libraries have devised computer-based systems for subject control. This is true of both DDC and NASA and a number of other corporation libraries with large report collections. Because of the desire in government libraries for uniformity, several of the subject systems are either based on each other or are a result of cooperative efforts. Project LEX, sponsored by DOD, was an attempt to standardize the language of all DOD contractors so that the various libraries would be using the same term which would have the same meaning in every case. NASA's thesaurus purports to be based on the LEX efforts.

If the report collection is to be segregated, then it becomes almost mandatory to build a separate catalog and shelflist. If a manual system is employed, the catalog must be divided into the following components: (1) corporate authors, (2) personal authors, (3) titles, (4) subjects, and (5) shelflist. Some report libraries find it necessary to have one more section, contract numbers. If the subjects are to be retrieved by some automated system, it has been the practice not to duplicate the subjects in the card catalog. Some libraries, however, use both, one as a backup for the other. In one library with which I have intimate knowledge, the computer would print out the terms with the documents listed under each term. This program was run once every two or three months to provide the means for doing a subject search when the computer was not available for various reasons and the requester did not wish to wait. This method was eventually abandoned as too costly when the total number of listings became too bulky, and the library reverted to computer search only.

If the collection is not segregated, no separate catalog would be needed. The cards for the reports could then be interfiled with the book cards. If this method were used, it would mean that the same subjects used to describe the monograph collection would be used for the report collection. This could create some problems since many subject systems do not lend themselves easily to the report literature. The *MeSH* headings could well prove to be the exception. No doubt this is the reason that the major government report collections have their own subject thesauri and do not use those which have been developed for monographic collections.

The final decision of how to handle technical reports is, after all, the librarian's. Many factors, as I have previously mentioned, must be weighed very carefully, and the final decision may very well be not to build a technical report collection. If this is the case, then I feel that that library is not giving the best service to its clientele. Every medical library, however, should be acutely aware that this literature exists, that in the majority of cases it is the most current information on a given subject, and that most of it is available to the enterprising librarian.

REFERENCES

1. DOE, JANET. Handbook of medical library practice. 2nd ed. Chicago, American Library Association, 1956, p. 164.
2. GRAY, DWIGHT E. Is the technical report an information tomb? Physics today 5: 4, Dec. 1952.
3. *Ibid.*
4. HERNER AND COMPANY. Factors governing the publication of United States government research reports. Dec. 1961. (AD—290-208.)
5. COBB, MARY M. Publication of medical research reports in scientific journals. Bull. Med. Libr. Ass. 41: 154-155, Apr. 1953.
6. ORR, RICHARD H., AND LEEDS, ALICE A. Bio-medical literature: volume, growth, and other characteristics, Fed. Proc. 23: 1310, 1316-1331, 1963.
7. *Ibid.*, p. 1310.
8. *Ibid.*, p. 1317.
9. *Ibid.*, p. 1318.
10. HERNER AND COMPANY, *Ibid.*
11. MLA/NLM Liaison committee report. Bull. Med. Libr. Ass. 55: 472, Oct. 1967.
12. BAKER, W. O., et al. Improving the availability of scientific and technical information in the United States. Panel report of the president's science advisory committee, Dec. 7, 1958; CRAWFORD, J. H.; ABIDAN, G.; FAZAR, W.; PASSMAN, S; STEGMAIER, R. B., JR.; AND STERN, J. Scientific and technical communications in the government. Task force report to the president's special assistant for science and technology. Apr. 1962. (AD—299-545); WEINBERG, A. M., et al. Science, government and information: the responsibilities of the technical community and the transfer of information. Report of the president's science advisory committee, Jan. 10, 1963.
13. Systems development corporation. Recommendations for national document handling systems in science and technology, 1965.

The Mayo Clinic Author Catalog: A Living Repository of Medical Knowledge

By Jack D. Key, *Librarian*
Katherine J. Sholtz, *Associate Librarian*
Mayo Clinic
Rochester, Minnesota

ABSTRACT

Since 1907 records have been kept of publications by staff members of the Mayo Clinic, and this information has been invaluable. The Author Catalog has proved itself such a useful tool for the Mayo Clinic that other libraries, large and small, may wish to consider adopting such a service.

The Mayo medical complex is a large institution with more than 500 staff and faculty members engaged in the publication of clinical, educational, and research findings. The great amount of cross-disciplinary cooperation and interdepartmental research makes essential an up-to-date record of what is going on.

The Mayo Clinic Library developed a comprehensive computerized method for identifying research and for identifying and indexing publications of Mayo staff members. At the end of 1971 more than 25,000 citations had been stored on computer tape.

LIBRARIANS are being challenged to meet the information needs of a clientele which is constantly becoming better educated, better prepared, and more sophisticated. Modern applications of library techniques are required. One innovation, a computerized catalog of all publications by staff members of the Mayo Clinic, is the subject of the paper. A catalog of staff publications would be useful in any institution, although smaller institutions will not need to avail themselves of the computer as the Mayo Clinic does. Even a regular check of *Index Medicus* against a list of staff members could serve for a small hospital library. Record-keeping of this sort is recommended in *Standards for Library Services in Health Care Institutions*, 1970[1].

More than 25,000 citations to papers by members of the staff of the Mayo

Originally published in *Bulletin of the Medical Library Association*, Volume 61 (April, 1973), pp. 228-237. Reprinted by permission.

Clinic are now stored on computer tape. Certainly, it is impossible for any man to master the vast store of knowledge reflected in these 25,000 contributions to literature. But, happily, he can, in a matter of minutes, ask and receive printed analyses of the subject matter, authors concerned, and time periods encompassed in this impressive store of information.

The enabling agency is the Mayo Clinic Library Author Catalog, a continuing apparatus in which citations to books, journal papers, abstracts and contributions in nonprint media are preserved on magnetic tape for computer retrieval by author or subject.

This broadly inclusive system offers (1) speedy answers to questions from any quarter about work done by Mayo Clinic physicians; (2) the ability to provide a quick survey to acquaint residents in the Mayo Graduate School of Medicine with work done by members of the staff; (3) ready access to vital information needed in the preparation of applications for grants; (4) instant data about published works of individual members of the faculty for evaluation of prospects for promotion; (5) invaluable indications of the directions which both research and medical care are taking at any given time at the Mayo Clinic; and (6) statistical summaries about educational matters which are of concern to the Mayo Graduate School of Medicine and the Mayo Foundation.

The system indeed constitutes a living body of medical and scientific knowledge which the two founding brothers recognized as a need and sought to maintain.

Origin and Development

On March 1, 1907, Mrs. Maud H. Mellish was taken on the staff of the Drs. Mayo, Stinchfield, and Graham to organize and develop a library and to undertake editorial work in connection with the publication of papers[2]. From a small beginning the editorial work increased. Most members of the staff began to refer their books and papers to the editorial section for revision before submitting them for publication. At the end of each year the papers were assembled and republished in full, in abridgment, or in abstract as the *Collected Papers of the Mayo Clinic*. From this time, therefore, it was necessary to keep a file of the articles and books as they were published. Also, there was the problem of retrieval of the articles written by the Drs. Mayo and their associates prior to 1907. In 1912 this resulted in the publication of two volumes entitled *A Collection of Papers: Published Previous to 1909*[3]. These volumes, classed under appropriate subject headings arranged alphabetically, include some of the publications of Dr. William Worrall Mayo and also a complete file of the writings of William James Mayo and Charles Horace Mayo from the time of their graduation from medical school to February 1909, which was the date of publication of the first volume of the *Collected Papers by the Staff of St. Mary's Hospital*[4]. This volume reprinted in their entirety the papers which had emanated from the Clinic between 1905 and 1909. In other words, it included papers written by the Mayos and by the twelve staff members associated with them in the practice of medicine: Drs. H. G. Andrews, E. H. Beckman, W. F. Braasch, H. Z. Giffin, C. Graham, D. Guthrie, M. S. Henderson, E. S. Judd, W. C. MacCarty, H. S. Plummer, and L. B. Wilson, and Miss Alice Magaw, anesthetist. Mrs. Mellish is listed as the editor. Publication of the *Collected Papers of the Mayo Clinic and the Mayo Foundation* was discontinued with Volume 60, 1969.

In 1919, *The Clinic Bulletin* was issued. In it for the first time (vol. 1, no. 6, Aug. 9, 1919) were listed "Recent Articles by Members of the Staff." From this time on, staff publications were listed at frequent intervals in the *Bulletin*. In 1926, the *Proceedings of the Staff Meetings of the Mayo Clinic* began publication. Later, the staff publications were listed in these volumes.

It is difficult to determine whether a member of the library staff or of the editorial department did this work at first. The question is really academic, since the two originally were combined. At first, the bibliographic elements provided were author, title, name of journal, year, volume number (in roman), and pagination. Beginning in 1931, the journal articles were cited according to the procedure of the *Journal of the American Medical Association*. The items were as follows: author, title, name of journal, volume number (in arabic), pagination, month, and year.

Miss Violet Vihstadt began to work for the Library in 1920. As mentioned in the first typewritten "Report of the Mayo Clinic Library"[5], one of the routine duties of the Library was the compilation of current bibliographies of staff members. Miss Vihstadt helped in the compilation of these current bibliographies—one of her responsibilities as Reference Librarian. Her procedure was as follows. She scanned the table of contents of the current journals and placed a pencil check mark next to each Mayo Clinic article. She also checked for obituaries of deceased members of the staff and reviews of books written by Mayo Clinic authors.

The medical staff was small enough at that time so that this was a fairly reliable procedure. After the checking, bibliographic data were typed on 3" x 5" paper slips. Then subject headings were assigned and cards were retyped for each entry chosen. These cards were filed in the Mayo Clinic Author Card Catalog.

The card catalog has always been arranged in two categories: author and subject. Authors' names are in alphabetic order. Cards under names of authors are filed in chronologic order by year, and within each year in alphabetic order by title. The subject file is in alphabetic order, under headings that conform with the entries used in indexes to periodical literature.

Before 1952 the Mayo Clinic Author Catalog included only articles from medical periodicals. Since January 1952, this catalog has covered articles in journals, proceedings (including the *Proceedings of the Staff Meetings of the Mayo Clinic*), reports, and so on; chapters or contributions to books, loose-leaf systems, or encyclopedias; separate monographs or textbooks which Mayo Clinic authors have written or to which they have contributed as coauthors or editors. Pre-1952 catalog contents have since been expanded to include as much as possible of the material falling under post-1952 criteria. Writings published in the period between 1936 and 1952 can be found by consulting the textbook catalog and the indexes to the *Proceedings of the Staff Meetings of the Mayo Clinic.* Items published prior to 1936 are listed in excellent bibliographies that appear at the close of each biographical sketch in the *Physicians of the Mayo Clinic and the Mayo Foundation* (1937)[6].

Miss Vihstadt was responsible for the author catalog and bibliography as well as for the Reference Department until each was made a separate library department on Oct. 1, 1964. From that date until her retirement in 1966 (after forty-six years of continuous service in the Mayo Clinic Library), Miss Vihstadt continued as head of the Reference Department, and Mrs. Margaret Ford became the Mayo Clinic Library Bibliographer, a position that she held until her retirement on June 30, 1971. This new arrangement permitted expansion of bibliographic services. It made it possible to keep the catalog more up-to-date and to make changes consistent with the recommended library service. It soon became apparent, however, that the assignment of subject headings was one very time-consuming responsibility of the Bibliographer.

In early 1966 the decision was made to computerize the complete bibliographies of authors on the Mayo Clinic staff as of that year and thereafter. Writings published prior to a staff member's joining the Mayo Clinic were also included as part of his bibliography. Figure 1 shows the listing of types of publications appropriate for a bibliography and those not to be included. Additional part-time employees were hired to complete the checking and adding of entries on forms for machine manipulation. By January 1, 1971, the data file for this catalog contained bibliographic information for approximately 25,000 items, including journal articles, books, chapters in books, and motion pictures by staff members and others as well as nonprint media such as Wisconsin Regional Medical Program Dial Access Library Service cassettes.

The following are included in Mayo Clinic bibliographies:

1. Books.
2. Chapters or sections in scientific books.
3. Scientific papers.
4. Letters to Editors when these are original contributions similar to those found in Nature, Science, Journal of Clinical Endocrinology, Metabolism, Lancet, etc.
5. Abstracts covering scientific presentations prepared for scientific societies. Example: Abstracts in Federation Proceedings, Journal of Laboratory and Clinical Medicine, etc.
6. Editorials with medical or scientific contributions.
7. Films and other non-print media when these are available for distribution outside the Clinic.

The following are not to be included in the bibliography:

1. General editorials.
2. Questions and answers.
3. Book reviews.
4. Unsigned obituaries.
5. References in programs.
6. Letters to the Editor not containing original contributions.
7. Discussions of scientific papers.
8. Non-scientific material. Examples: Articles in Atlantic Monthly, Wall Street Journal, Saturday Evening Post, etc.
9. Mayo Clinic Seminars.
10. Translations of articles previously appearing in the bibliography unless translated by the author(s).
11. Compiled lists, such as bibliographic and similar lists with no original material.
12. Exhibits, unless published in a journal.
13. Third-person accounts or report of a presentation made by another at a meeting.
14. Introduction of a speaker.
15. Condensations of published material appearing in digest-type publications and not prepared by author(s): Example: Modern Medicine.

FIG. 1.—Types of publications included in bibliographies.

Since January 1, 1971, the Mayo Clinic Author Catalog has been maintained only in book catalog format. This book catalog, printed and cumulated monthly, consists of three listings: (1) publications by Mayo Clinic staff authors arranged alphabetically (Fig. 2), (2) a key-word index to these publications (Fig. 3), and (3) publications by accession numbers giving full bibliographic information (Fig. 4). A final cumulation is published for each calendar year. Cumulated volumes of both author and key-word indexes are available at several locations within the Library and also are supplied to the Division of Education, the Department of Biomedical Communications, and the Department of Laboratory Medicine.

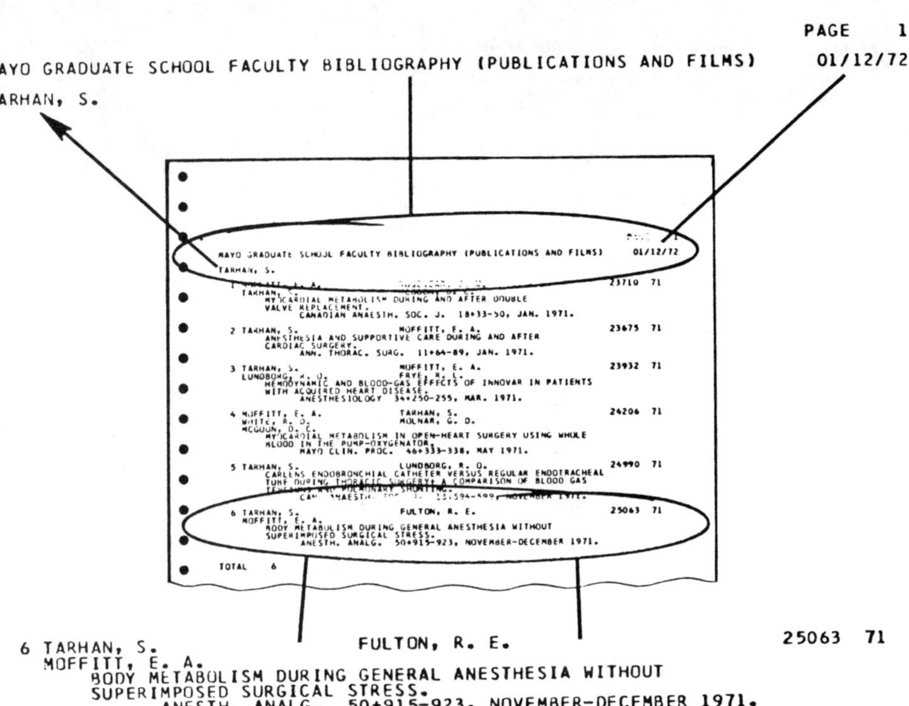

FIG. 2.—Author index.

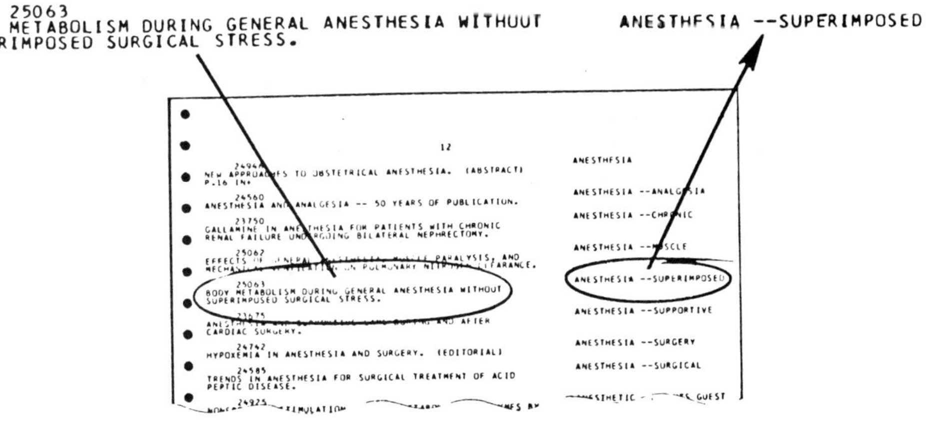

FIG. 3.—Key-word subject index.

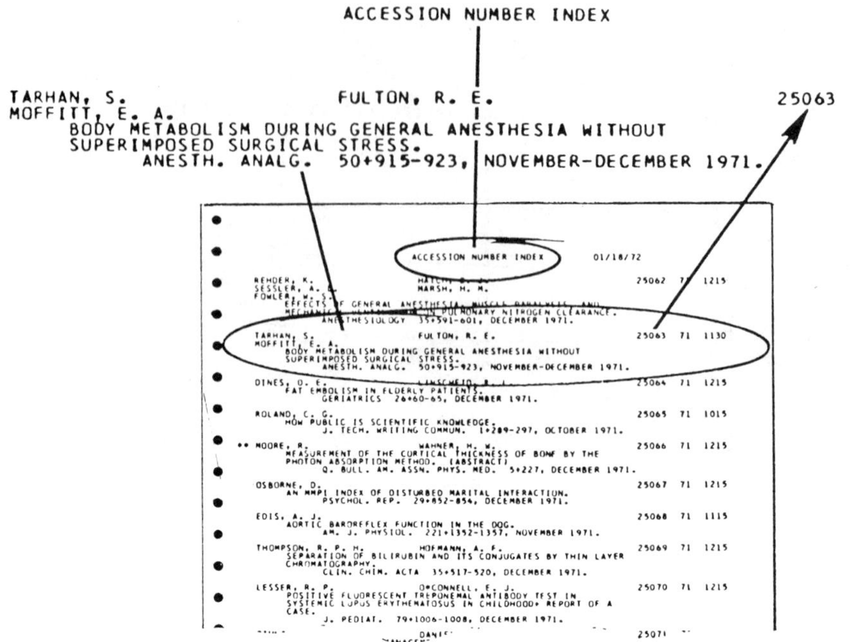

ACCESSION NUMBER INDEX

TARHAN, S. FULTON, R. E. 25063 71
MOFFITT, E. A.
BODY METABOLISM DURING GENERAL ANESTHESIA WITHOUT
SUPERIMPOSED SURGICAL STRESS.
ANESTH. ANALG. 50+915-923, NOVEMBER-DECEMBER 1971.

ACCESSION NUMBER INDEX 01/18/72

REHDER, K. 25062 1215
SESSLER, A. MARSH, H. M.
FOWLER, W. S.
EFFECTS
IN PULMONARY NITROGEN CLEARANCE.
ANESTHESIOLOGY 35+591-601, DECEMBER 1971.

TARHAN, S. FULTON, R. E. 25063 71 1130
MOFFITT, E. A.
BODY METABOLISM DURING GENERAL ANESTHESIA WITHOUT
SUPERIMPOSED SURGICAL STRESS.
ANESTH. ANALG. 50+915-923, NOVEMBER-DECEMBER 1971.

DINES, D. E. 25064 71 1215
FAT EMBOLISM IN ELDERLY PATIENTS.
GERIATRICS 26+60-65, DECEMBER 1971.

ROLAND, C. G. 25065 71 1015
HOW PUBLIC IS SCIENTIFIC KNOWLEDGE.
J. TECH. WRITING COMMUN. 1+289-297, OCTOBER 1971.

** MOORE, R. WAHNER, H. W. 25066 71 1215
MEASUREMENT OF THE CORTICAL THICKNESS OF BONE BY THE
PHOTON ABSORPTION METHOD. (ABSTRACT)
Q. BULL. AM. ASSN. PHYS. MED. 5+227, DECEMBER 1971.

OSBORNE, D. 25067 71 1215
AN MMPI INDEX OF DISTURBED MARITAL INTERACTION.
PSYCHOL. REP. 29+852-854, DECEMBER 1971.

EDIS, A. J. 25068 71 1115
AORTIC BAROREFLEX FUNCTION IN THE DOG.
AM. J. PHYSIOL. 221+1352-1357, NOVEMBER 1971.

THOMPSON, R. P. H. HOFMANN, A. F. 25069 71 1215
SEPARATION OF BILIRUBIN AND ITS CONJUGATES BY THIN LAYER
CHROMATOGRAPHY.
CLIN. CHIM. ACTA 35+517-520, DECEMBER 1971.

LESSER, R. P. O*CONNELL, E. J. 25070 71 1215
POSITIVE FLUORESCENT TREPONEMAL ANTIBODY TEST IN
SYSTEMIC LUPUS ERYTHEMATOSUS IN CHILDHOOD+ REPORT OF A
CASE.
J. PEDIAT. 79+1006-1008, DECEMBER 1971.

25071

Fig. 4.—Accession number index.

Random or manual query instructions suggest that for citations prior to 1971 one must consult the card catalog and that for citations dated January 1971 or later one must consult the book catalog. On demand, an individual's bibliography can be retrospectively retrieved complete by computer. Normally these "on demand" bibliographies are retrieved with complete citation information printed in chronologic sequence from the earliest entry through the latest entry.

Worthy of brief note is the fact that the computer-produced key-word index has eliminated the need for a bibliographer to assign subject headings. The position of Bibliographer was discontinued with the incumbent's retirement.

Description and System Design

Under favorable conditions the Library early becomes aware of a research or clinical project which will lead to a publication. When a physician or researcher first conceives of a project, he fills out a Registration of Subject card (Fig. 5), obtains approval of the head of his department, enlists coauthors if necessary, and prepares a tentative title and abstract. This card is submitted to the Committee on Medical Relations and Publications for approval. After approval the item appears on a weekly list of newly registered titles and authors which is prepared and distributed throughout the Clinic (Fig. 6). The Registration of Subject cards (about 900/year) are filed in the Library by authors and broad subject fields. This card file is kept current by weekly elimination of cards for published articles. Any card remaining after three years is returned to the first author with a note asking him to resubmit if the work is still in progress.

A

THIS SPACE FOR COMMITTEE USE

Subject Code ANESTHESIOLOGY Med. Rel. Comm. Approval Date

Signature of First Author Sait Tarhan, M.D. Head of Section E.A. Moffitt, M.D.

Co-Authors Richard E. Fulton, M.D. 2 E.A. Moffitt, M.D.

(type name below signature) Chairman: A. Faulconer, M.D. 4

Title: Body Metabolism during General Anesthesia Without Superimposed Surgical Stress

Abstract: Twenty patients having renal arteriograms for investigation of hypertension were studied. They were anesthetized by four combinations of agents with Halothane, Nitrous Oxide, Thiopental and Innovar as major agents. No evidence of stress to the body elicited, and these anesthetic agents per se did not alter body metabolism.

Check Research ☐ Study ☐ Publication ☒ Presentation ☐ Grant ☐ No

Registration of Subject MC 495—Rev. 8-66

B

Please indicate material required for this registration and obtain signature of appropriate consultant approving use of the material.

Check material needed	Appropriate signature	Consultant check if paper is to be seen before publication
☐ Computer		
☐ Necropsy Material		
☐ Surgical Specimens		
☐ X-Ray Films		
☐ Laboratory Aid		
☐ Animals		
☐ Histories or Follow-Up Letters		

Lists supplied by Dates

Signatures of other consultants concerned with this subject (not co-author)	Check if you wish to see paper before publication

FIG. 5.—Registration of subject card. A: Front. B. Back.

WEEKLY REPORT OF REGISTRATION OF SUBJECTS
Submitted to
The Committee on Medical Relations and Publications

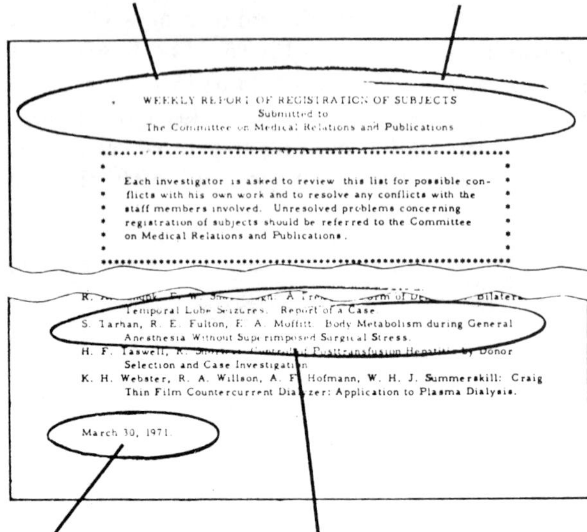
WEEKLY REPORT OF REGISTRATION OF SUBJECTS
Submitted to
The Committee on Medical Relations and Publications

Each investigator is asked to review this list for possible conflicts with his own work and to resolve any conflicts with the staff members involved. Unresolved problems concerning registration of subjects should be referred to the Committee on Medical Relations and Publications.

Temporal Lobe Seizures. Report of a Case.
S. Tarhan, R. E. Fulton, E. A. Moffitt: Body Metabolism during General Anesthesia Without Superimposed Surgical Stress.
Selection and Case Investigation
K. H. Webster, R. A. Willson, A. F. Hofmann, W. H. J. Summerskill: Craig Thin Film Countercurrent Dialyzer: Application to Plasma Dialysis.

March 30, 1971.

S. Tarhan, R. E. Fulton, E. A. Moffitt: Body Metabolism during General Anesthesia Without Superimposed Surgical Stress.

March 30, 1971.

FIG. 6.—Weekly report of registration of subjects.

On registration of the first draft of a paper in the Section of Publications, a duplicate copy (Fig. 7) of the registration card is prepared. The duplicate registration slips are sent to the Library weekly and are attached to the corresponding Registration of Subject cards. (About 850 papers are registered each year.) After final editing and acceptance of the paper by a publisher, a copy of the final proof card (Fig. 8) is sent from the Section of Publications to the Library. These proof slips (numbering about 500/year) indicate where articles will be published. Those for journal articles are filed alphabetically by journal title in the Serials Department; those for monographs are kept in a special file in the Order Department.

As books and journals are checked in daily, they are cross-checked against the files of articles awaiting publication. Proof slips are matched with published articles and separated from the file, first pages of articles are photocopied (Fig. 9), and bibliographic data are entered on the copy. The first pages are attached to the proof slips and utilized daily to type citations onto key-punch sheets (Fig. 10). The key-punch sheets are sent weekly to

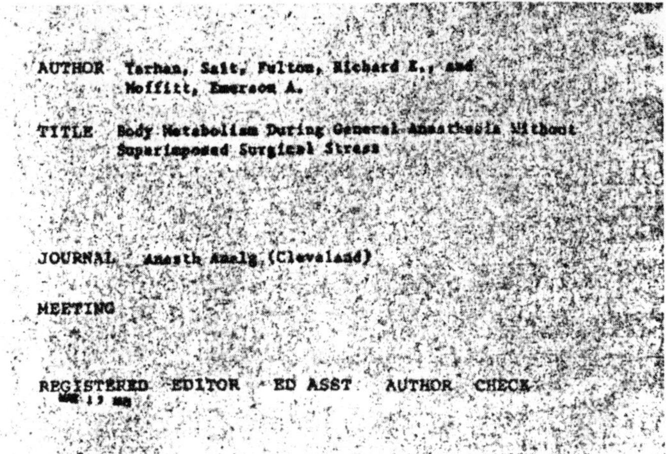

AUTHOR Tarhan, Sait, Fulton, Richard E., and
Moffitt, Emerson A.

TITLE Body Metabolism During General Anesthesia Without
Superimposed Surgical Stress

JOURNAL Anesth Analg (Cleveland)

MEETING

REGISTERED EDITOR ED ASST AUTHOR CHECK

FIG. 7.—Duplicate registration slip from section of publications.

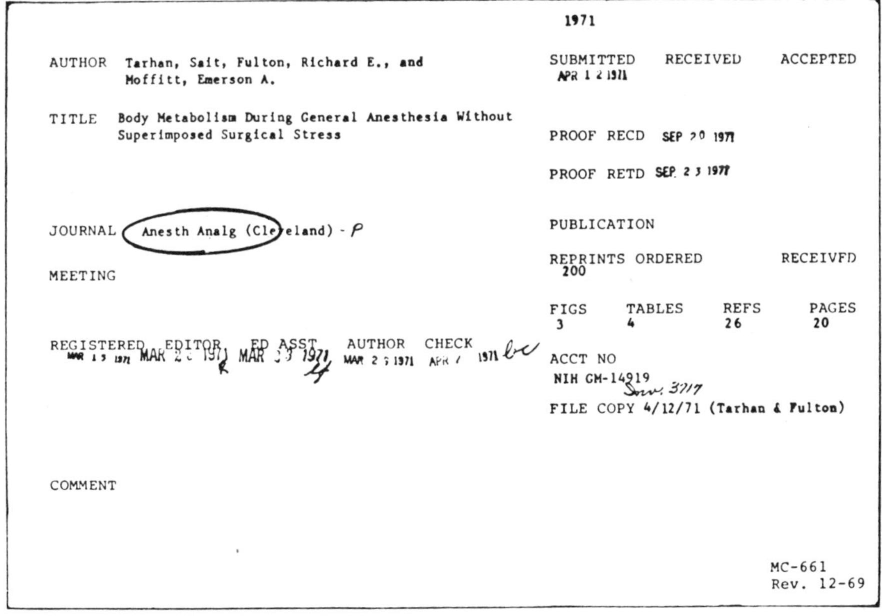

1971

AUTHOR Tarhan, Sait, Fulton, Richard E., and
Moffitt, Emerson A.

TITLE Body Metabolism During General Anesthesia Without
Superimposed Surgical Stress

JOURNAL Anesth Analg (Cleveland) - P

MEETING

REGISTERED EDITOR ED ASST AUTHOR CHECK
MAR 1 5 1971 MAR 2 1971 MAR 1971 MAR 2 5 1971 APR 1971

SUBMITTED RECEIVED ACCEPTED
APR 1 2 1971

PROOF RECD SEP 20 1971

PROOF RETD SEP 2 3 1971

PUBLICATION

REPRINTS ORDERED RECEIVED
200

FIGS TABLES REFS PAGES
3 4 26 20

ACCT NO
NIH GM-14919
Serv. 3717

FILE COPY 4/12/71 (Tarhan & Fulton)

COMMENT

MC-661
Rev. 12-69

FIG. 8.—Final proof card.

Data Processing for punching, and the photocopied first pages are sent with the attached proof slips to the Section of Publications for completion of its records.

The computer system for updating the master tape and producing individual bibliographies consists of seven programs, all written in common business-oriented language (COBOL). Currently the system is being run on an IBM 360/40 with operating system (OS) and 256 K memory. The minimal core requirement for the largest program is 56 K memory. The key-word index program, written in COBOL, calls for an

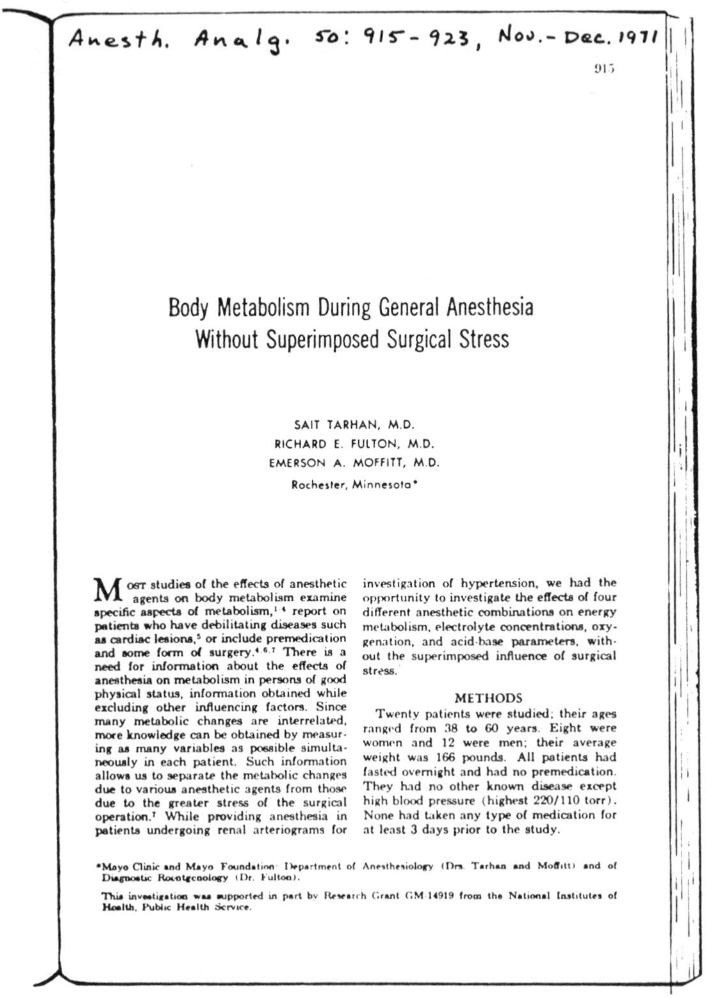

Anesth. Analg. 50: 915-923, Nov.-Dec. 1971

915

Body Metabolism During General Anesthesia Without Superimposed Surgical Stress

SAIT TARHAN, M.D.
RICHARD E. FULTON, M.D.
EMERSON A. MOFFITT, M.D.
Rochester, Minnesota*

Most studies of the effects of anesthetic agents on body metabolism examine specific aspects of metabolism,[1-4] report on patients who have debilitating diseases such as cardiac lesions,[5] or include premedication and some form of surgery.[4,6,7] There is a need for information about the effects of anesthesia on metabolism in persons of good physical status, information obtained while excluding other influencing factors. Since many metabolic changes are interrelated, more knowledge can be obtained by measuring as many variables as possible simultaneously in each patient. Such information allows us to separate the metabolic changes due to various anesthetic agents from those due to the greater stress of the surgical operation.[7] While providing anesthesia in patients undergoing renal arteriograms for investigation of hypertension, we had the opportunity to investigate the effects of four different anesthetic combinations on energy metabolism, electrolyte concentrations, oxygenation, and acid-base parameters, without the superimposed influence of surgical stress.

METHODS

Twenty patients were studied; their ages ranged from 38 to 60 years. Eight were women and 12 were men; their average weight was 166 pounds. All patients had fasted overnight and had no premedication. They had no other known disease except high blood pressure (highest 220/110 torr). None had taken any type of medication for at least 3 days prior to the study.

*Mayo Clinic and Mayo Foundation: Department of Anesthesiology (Drs. Tarhan and Moffitt) and of Diagnostic Roentgenology (Dr. Fulton).

This investigation was supported in part by Research Grant GM-14919 from the National Institutes of Health, Public Health Service.

FIG. 9.—First page of published article showing bibliographic data.

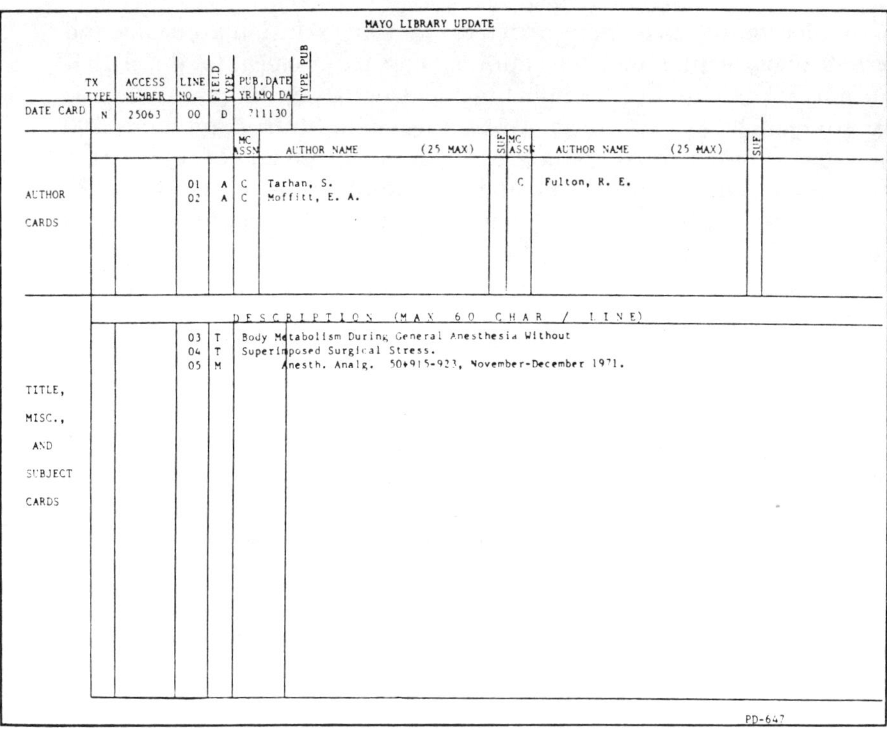
MAYO LIBRARY UPDATE

	TX TYPE	ACCESS NUMBER	LINE NO.	FIELD TYPE	PUB. DATE YR MO DA	TYPE PUB
DATE CARD	N	25063	00	D	711130	

	LINE NO.	FIELD TYPE	MC ASSN	AUTHOR NAME (25 MAX)	SUF	MC ASSN	AUTHOR NAME (25 MAX)	SUF
AUTHOR CARDS	01	A	C	Tarhan, S.		C	Fulton, R. E.	
	02	A	C	Moffitt, E. A.				

	LINE NO.	FIELD TYPE	DESCRIPTION (MAX 60 CHAR / LINE)
TITLE, MISC., AND SUBJECT CARDS	03	T	Body Metabolism During General Anesthesia Without
	04	T	Superimposed Surgical Stress.
	05	M	Anesth. Analg. 50+915-923, November-December 1971.

PD-647

FIG. 10.—Key-punch sheet.

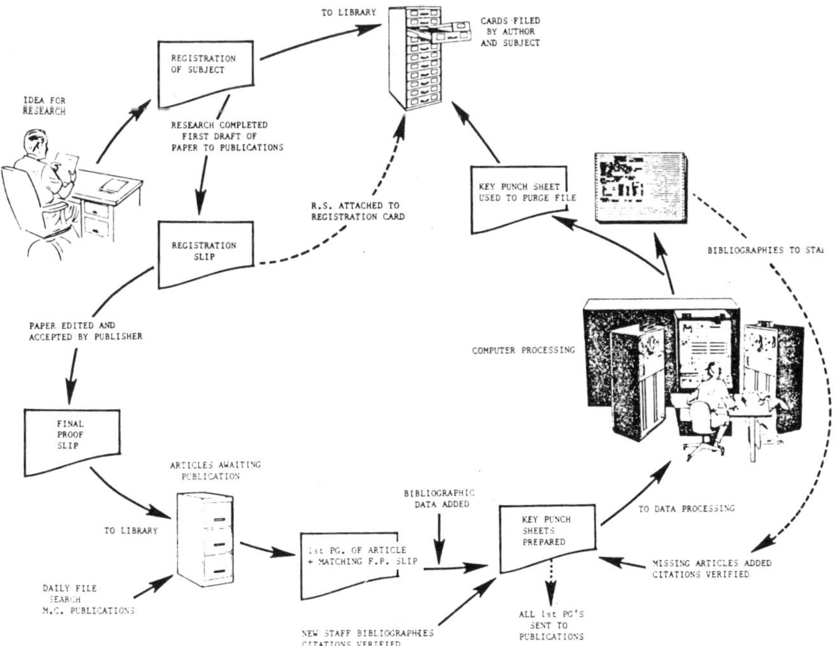

FIG. 11.—Flowchart of Author Catalog process.

assembler routine for a binary search to check an exclusion word table and to re-format the title lines. The minimal core requirement for this is 40 K memory. The cost for key-punching and updating the master tape is approximately $1 per entry. An average monthly run produces 100 bibliographies at a cost of about $2 each. Monthly costs rise throughout the year on the cumulated key-word and author indexes. The November 1971 cumulated key-word index, for example cost $53 and the corresponding author index, $33.

When the key-punch sheets are returned from Data Processing, they are used to purge the Registration of Subject File.

Annually, each staff member receives a copy of his own bibliography and is asked to report omissions. The missing citations are verified and key-punch sheets are prepared as usual. Each *new* staff member is called and asked for a copy of his bibliography. The citations are verified and prepared for computer processing. More than 1,500 citations were added to the data base in 1971.

Figure 11 is a flowchart depicting the process which has been described.

The Mayo Clinic Library Author Catalog has proved itself such a viable reference tool for our library and institution that we hope, by sharing of our experiences, to encourage our colleague libraries, large or small, to adopt such a service.

REFERENCES

1. American Library Association. Association of hospital and institution libraries. Hospital library standards committee. Standards for library services in health care institutions. Chicago, American Library Association, 1970, p. 9.
2. Mayo Clinic. Division of publications. Sketch of the history of the Mayo Clinic and the Mayo Foundation. Philadelphia, Saunders, 1926, p. 106.
3. Mayo, W. J., and Mayo, C. H. A collection of papers: published previous to 1909. Philadelphia, Saunders, 1912. 2 v.
4. Collected papers by the staff of St. Mary's Hospital. Philadelphia, Saunders, 1911. 603 p.
5. Report of the Mayo Clinic Library. 1924, p. 3 (Typewritten).
6. Physicians of the Mayo Clinic and the Mayo Foundation. Minneapolis, The University of Minnesota Press, 1937. 1,575 p.

TWX and Interlibrary Loans*

BY WARREN BIRD, *Associate Director*

Duke University Medical Center Library
Durham, North Carolina

ABSTRACT

Libraries now have available to them a variety of ways of speeding the flow of information among widely scattered locations. One of the means for the improvement of interlibrary loan service is the use of the teletypewriter, and the use of Teletypewriter Exchange Service (TWX) by medical libraries during the past three years is described. The background of library applications of teletypewriter systems is outlined, and the advantages, types of use, cost factors, and experiences of some groups are discussed, as well as the impact of the "network concept" on library service.

ON September 2, 1965, the medical librarians of Duke University, Bowman Gray School of Medicine, and the University of North Carolina met to seek ways of broadening the base of medical library collections and services in the three institutions. The question of communications methods was raised early in the discussions, and a decision was made to investigate various possibilities of speeding up the transmission of procedural information among libraries. It was immediately evident that any degree of sophistication in communications would be more attractive with more participating libraries, and the medical libraries of the University of Virginia and the Medical College of Virginia were invited to join the group. Representatives of the common-carrier communications companies were contacted later that month, and formal proposals for several systems were prepared. TWX, or Teletypewriter Exchange Service, on the national dial network, was chosen after careful study showed the following advantages:

(1) As many libraries as wished to join the system could do so by simply

*Presented as part of a general session on "National and Regional Library Systems" at the Sixty-seventh Annual Meeting of the Medical Library Association, Denver, Colorado, June 11, 1968.

Originally published in *Bulletin of the Medical Library Association*, Volume 57 (April, 1969), pp. 125-129. Reprinted by permission.

installing TWX equipment, and the service was readily available in all parts of the country.

(2) There were already several libraries using TWX service.

(3) The equipment was simple and straightforward in operation.

(4) It was not necessary to have an operator in attendance in order to receive a message.

(5) A written record, or even a multiple-copy written record, was made available at both the transmitting and receiving stations.

(6) Message costs were reasonable, and each station would be billed individually for the calls it originated. Collect messages could also be handled with operator assistance.

TWX was installed at Duke on January 11, 1966, and at Chapel Hill and Bowman Gray shortly thereafter. The Medical College of Virginia was already a participating member of the state-wide Virginia Libraries network, and the University of Virginia School of Medicine installed their TWX late in the spring. The Universities of Kentucky and Louisville became affiliated with the group, and each installed equipment at its medical library, effectively completing a three-state medical library network upon which to build. Soon after, the National Library of Medicine joined us, agreeing to accept interlibrary loan requests via TWX in their efforts to improve their increasingly overloaded loan service. As of November 1968, there were seventy-two medical libraries on the TWX network.

It must be remembered that TWX was installed by these libraries as a tool, primarily an adjunct to their interlibrary loan service. Realizing that TWX communication increases only the communication speed, and not the loans themselves, we undertook to accelerate the handling of interlibrary loan requests within the library and to streamline the provision of material by using photocopy, first-class mail, and by providing prompt reporting of exceptions when an item is not held. In addition to this means of enhancement of interlibrary loan service, the libraries also found themselves with an advanced communications medium available for almost unlimited applications.

The Teletypewriter Exchange Service network is very similar to our Long Distance Dial Telephone System. A teletypewriter is a machine much like an electric typewriter, which may be connected by ordinary telephone wires, through a dial exchange, to any other teletypewriter in the system. When two stations are connected, any message typed on the keyboard of one machine appears printed out, not only at the sending station, but also at the receiving station. If the receiving, or called, station wishes to respond, it is only necessary for the operator to type on the keyboard, and the message again appears on both machines. Most machines are equipped with a paper-tape punching and sending unit, which permits the operator to prepare a coded punched paper tape when typing on the machine, before actually dialing another station. While punching the tape, typing may be done carefully and slowly if desired, and corrections are easily made. When the tape is completely and correctly prepared, it may be sent automatically by the machine to the called station, thereby permitting full utilization of the 100-word-per-minute speed of the teletypewriter, and ensuring accuracy of the transmission. The message paper normally used is a continuous roll and consists of two sheets with an interleaving carbon sheet, providing two copies of the message at both the sending and receiving station. The arrangement of the keyboard is like that of a standard typewriter, and there are only a few additional controls to be mastered. A good typist can be instructed in the use of the equipment very quickly.

Teletypewriters have been in use for a long time. Western Union has used them for the transmission of telegrams, and the news services transmit to radio and television stations and newspapers via various teletypewriter services; also the military and industry have long been active users. The medium has been in use in libraries in this country since 1927, with most of the early installations found in public library systems. TELEX, as the service is known in Europe, has been used quite extensively by continental libraries, with some 700 installations noted in 1966[1]. At that time there were 120 libraries in the United States using TWX; this number has since tripled. Some installations have been private-line systems connecting a few nearby institutions or connecting several locations within a single library. Several installations are parts of networks of libraries, more or less formally structured. Many of these are TWX-linked, such as those in the states of Indiana, Texas, Virginia, Pennsylvania, Utah, Vermont, and New York; and some are closed-circuit systems, with a central point being used for access to the TWX network, as in Connecticut, Rhode Island, Maryland, and Oklahoma. The literature relating to reports of TWX operations has recently been reviewed by Herbert Poole[2] and Brigitte Kenney[3]. An extensive bibliography has been maintained by the Systems Division of the Duke University Medical Center Library, covering the literature on use of TWX by all types of libraries, and we have been in correspondence with most of the groups making, or planning, new teletypewriter installations. The Library also publishes, in cooperation with the Library Mechanization Committee of the Canadian Library Association, a directory of all libraries in the United States and Canada known to be using exchange service telecommunications. The *Library Telecommunications Directory: Canada—United States* is computer produced and updated, and a new edition is prepared every few months, with supplementary pages distributed as needed[4].

As with any means of communication, the need for standards rapidly became obvious. Many libraries in the past which had used teletypewriter systems found themselves either with no control of any sort over message format and transmission techniques, or severely hampered with complex coding systems and extensive abbreviations. We felt that there must be some systematization provided, but that plain language text should be the form of choice within the body of any message. The ALA Interlibrary Loan Code had long ago made provision for standardized forms for interlibrary loan. Formats were developed for TWX use which made it possible to record all of the essential information normally included on the ALA form, and it was found that the data could be arranged on the page in such a way that the finished message could be used interchangeably with the old form—even to the point of having the name and address of the requesting library in a location properly aligned for use in window envelopes or photocopy mailers. The use of two-part paper provides the requisite four copies, as prescribed by the ALA Code, of a request, all generated at the location desired. In order to formalize these points, a procedures manual, *Teletypewriter Exchange System for Interlibrary Communications*[5], was designed by the group from operating experience in such a way that the other libraries using TWX could adopt it, usually without altering their own internal procedures. It specifies standards for message conventions, permissible abbreviations, operating procedures, rationale and instructions for formats, sample messages, and other applicable information. In addition, the Interlibrary Loan Policy Statement of the five libraries was included, indicating the how, when, and why of our request handling. The manual has been revised three times, and several hundred copies are now in circulation.

In addition to interlibrary loan requests, the system provides a good medium for searching, or polling, several libraries for a given item and permits rapid responses and exception reporting to requests. Unusual or difficult reference questions and cataloging problems may be referred to the appropriate expert at another library. Information notes on new serials acquisitions may be exchanged, providing an efficient updating system to previously published journal lists. Assuming that the vendors with whom a library deals also have TWX service, rush orders and tracers on past orders may also be handled. For the traveling librarian, transportation and accommodation reservation service via TWX is rapid, positive, and almost universally available. National Union Catalog search requests are usually answered within twenty-four hours. In fact, any general interlibrary correspondence is capable of transmission via TWX. In all of these applications, the combination of speed and a positive written record of the message at both stations, thus insuring accuracy and minimum misunderstanding in interpretation, is very effective.

Of the advantages offered by the use of TWX, the most obvious is the rapid speed of communication. Added to this, and perhaps more important to libraries, are the opportunities for better readers' service and public relations, increased library cooperation and use of local resources, and the general increase in communications efficiency. We have experienced definite improvement in all interlibrary communications with the advent of TWX. Especially in the processing of interlibrary loans, TWX, together with a conscious effort to streamline the provision of loans, has enabled us to give and receive much better service. In the instance of a search for a given item, the old expected delays of several weeks have been cut to a few days at the most—and a few hours at best—since negative reports are transmitted within twenty-four hours. We have found a distinct advantage over the telephone: the provision of a written record, eliminating misunderstanding when dealing with foreign languages, exotic medical terms, and complex citations; and the possibility of receipt of a message even if no one is in attendance at the receiving end. Costs have been quite reasonable (Table 1), even discounting the fact that it is difficult, if not impossible, to put a price tag on the savings in time, or on the goodwill engendered by improved service. Reactions of operating personnel have been excellent. Interlibrary loan clerks find, and report, that "cutting a tape" is no more difficult than typing a standard ALA form, and some even prefer to initiate TWX requests than to use the old forms.

Six of the medical libraries of the North Carolina—Virginia—Kentucky group were asked to submit figures on their interlibrary loan traffic. The study[6] shows the quantitative shifts in the areas supplying loan material to a given library and indicates the increased speed in filling requests. The

TABLE 1

COMPARATIVE MESSAGE COSTS:
JANUARY–JUNE, 1968

LIBRARY	NUMBER OF MESSAGES	AVERAGE COST PER MESSAGE
KYU-M	292	$1.76
KYLU-M	301	$1.92
NCBG	364	$1.32
NCU-H	438	$1.25
NCD-M	608	$1.01
VIU-M	626	$ .90

geographical pattern of the libraries lending to members of the group shifted away from the predominance of the National Library of Medicine and resulted in increased use of locally available resources. Table 2 shows the number of loans obtained by the six reporting libraries from all others in the group and from NLM, for three six-month periods in 1965 (without TWX), 1966 and 1968. In 1965, 58 percent of the loans to the group was supplied by NLM; in 1966 and 1968, while TWX was being used, this percentage dropped to 34 and 32, respectively. These figures also reflect a substantial increase in the number of loans obtained from within the group. The average time required to obtain materials from another library in the group decreased from eight days to three and one-half days; the latter figure has remained essentially constant since the fall of 1966. Negative reports were generally received within the agreed-upon twenty-four hours.

Future uses of the system are still to be fully exploited. The possibility of remote inquiry of computer-stored information for journal location, with automatic switching and initiation of interlibrary loan requests according to the dictates of the stored listings, will probably become feasible. Work on similar systems is already in progress. The use of TWX as a remote computer terminal is already a reality, and access to several time-sharing installations affords the opportunity for experimenting with computer-oriented projects. Since the TWX system is not dedicated, that is, it is not a privately leased and controlled system, expansion is quite simple, and

TABLE 2

NUMBER OF LOANS RECEIVED: SIX-MONTH SAMPLE PERIODS

BORROWING LIBRARY	LENDING LIBRARY																						
	1965 (No TWX)								1966 (TWX)								1968 (TWX)						
	VIU-M	NCBG	NCD-M	NCU-H	KYLU-M	KYU-M	VIR-M	DNLM	VIU-M	NCBG	NCD-M	NCU-H	KYLU-M	KYU-M	VIR-M	DNLM	VIU-M	NCBG	NCD-M	NCU-H	KYLU-M	KYU-M	DNLM
KYU-M			5		19	x		48	6	4	30	13	29	x	1	38	1	1	5	12	29	x	23
KYLU-M	1	4	4	3	x	66		56	4	3	15	6	x	52		61	1	1	13	4	x	29	56
NCU-H	4	6	75	x			1	80	9	26	149	x	6	6	11	93	30	78	147	x		11	24
NCD-M		10	x	90	4	17	7	65	6	7	x	82	5	10	5	32	3	29	x	103	3	5	71
NCBG		x	49	5				98	18	x	55	65	13	11	10	55	28	x	79	56			73
VIU-M	x		5	2			20	211	x	3	26	19		11	14	90	x	70	42	44	2	2	139
Total lent by each	5	20	138	100	23	83	28	558	43	43	275	185	53	90	41	369	63	179	286	219	34	47	386
Total	955								1099								1214						

more important, the system exists in the here and now. While the use of an electronic medium for message transmission hardly represents the ultimate sophistication of computer-controlled switching networks, library use of TWX has afforded an opportunity to utilize a readily available medium in the alleviation of communication problems. At the same time, experience can be gained immediately with such a system, and insights can be gained into the solution of more far-reaching problems in biomedical communications.

REFERENCE

1. WOLK, L. J. VAN DER. Teletype and the telecode for libraries. UNESCO Bull. Libr. 20: 170-176, 1966.
2. POOLE, HERBERT. Teletypewriters in libraries: A state of the art report. Coll. Res. Libr. 27: 283-286, 290, 1966.
3. KENNEY, BRIGITTE L. A survey of interlibrary communications systems. Biomedical communications Project Research Memorandum No. 3, Apr. 26, 1967.
4. BIRD, WARREN, AND SKENE MELVIN, DAVID. Library telecommunications directory: Canada—United States, 2d ed., rev. Durham, N. C., Duke University Medical Center Library, 1968.
5. BIRD, WARREN, AND CAVANAGH, G. S. T. Teletypewriter Exchange System for interlibrary communication. Durham, N. C., Duke University Medical Center Library, 1966, 1967, 1968.
6. BROWN, MARY ANN AND BIRD, WARREN. Effectiveness of cooperative Loan Agreement and Teletype use on interlibrary loan service within the North Carolina—Virginia—Kentucky Medical Library Group. Durham, N. C., Duke University Medical Center Library, 1967.

AIM-TWX Service at the University of Virginia: A Review and Evaluation

By Wilhelm Moll, J.D., *Director*

University of Virginia Medical Library
Charlottesville, Virginia

ABSTRACT

The paper reviews the highlights of a four-week trial period (November 19-December 18, 1970) during which the Medical Library of the University of Virginia experimented with a new remote-access bibliographical control and retrieval system via its TWX machine. The system, called AIM-TWX, was sponsored by the Lister Hill National Center for Biomedical Communications and utilizes a time-shared IBM 360/67 computer in Santa Monica, California. Citations from 109 clinically-oriented journals from 1966 to date, including those currently included in the *Abridged Index Medicus,* may be retrieved either on- or off-line.

Various aspects of this service are described, including problems of staffing, training, and record keeping, as well as the role of the *MeSH* vocabulary which is the principal "language" of the man-computer dialog.

The statistical results indicated that the system was used for approximately 200 minutes on nineteen days and that an average of sixteen searches were run on any given day, or about 4.6 searches per hour of use. In spite of an inexperienced staff who had little knowledge of the *MeSH* vocabulary and whose training schedule was limited to one four-hour session, the experiment was highly successful in terms of searches and citations.

At the end of the period, 298 searches had been run for 114 requestors, and 5,343 citations had been produced. Only fifty-five searches yielded no citations. The experiment generated a great deal of excitement and interest among the staff of the Library and of the Medical Center. Moreover, a large number of medical practitioners in large and small communities of Virginia participated in this experiment, indicating that there exists a great demand for this type of literature searching which AIM-TWX is able to provide with great rapidity.

On November 6, 1970, Mr. Davis B. McCarn, then Deputy Director of the Lister Hill National Center for Biomedical Communications,

Originally published in *Bulletin of the Medical Library Association,* Volume 59 (July, 1971), pp. 458-462. Reprinted by permission.

informed the Medical Librarian of the University of Virginia that the Library would have on-line access to the files of the AIM-TWX system for a two-week trial period from December 7 through December 18, 1970. Service was to be available for four hours daily from Mondays through Fridays. Thus began one of the most stimulating and exciting periods in the history of this library, whose major accomplishments form the basis of the following report.

AIM-TWX

As is probably well known, the AIM-TWX system, which utilizes a time-shared IBM 360/67 computer, was developed by the System Development Corporation at Santa Monica, California, for the Lister Hill Center. Its files are a subset of the *Index Medicus* data bank; namely, citations, including author, title, and source information, from 109 English language journals, beginning with 1966. The data can be retrieved on-line through a TWX (teletype) terminal which the Medical Library has had on its premises since early in 1966.*

As soon as formal approval for the two-week trial period was received, announcements were printed and disseminated to all Virginia hospitals and to the medical and nursing staffs of the Medical Center. Moreover, a press release was issued about one week after the beginning of the trial period which was featured in several media, including the Charlottesville *Daily Progress*. These announcements resulted in a rash of bibliographical search requests being submitted which kept the Library staff working overtime. The prospect of having rapid literature searches done free of charge may have been, in part, responsible for this tremendous demand. Although the "official" trial period was limited to the two weeks of December 7 through 18, actual use of the system began on November 19, as Mr. McCarn gave permission to "log in" for experimentation and demonstration purposes.

Training of Operators

Inasmuch as the Medical Library does not have a regular Reader Services Department, it was decided to train four staff members in AIM-TWX methodology, including two professionals (Head Cataloger and Director of the Virginia Medical Information System—U. Va. Center) and two subprofessionals who had all been involved in interlibrary loan work and who knew how to operate the TWX machine.

At first the staff studied the various user manuals which were received about two weeks before the library had access to the computer. These

*The system can also be used with various acoustic-coupled terminals, including the teletype (TTY) and the wired IBM Selectric typewriter (2741).

manuals ("User's Manual for the ELHILL Program, Gamma Version, May 1970," "Introductory User Packet for the Experimental *AIM-TWX* System," and "Questions and Answers About AIM-TWX") were very helpful, but not quite understood at first reading. The staff kept referring to the manuals throughout the trial period, and every one of the operators was under strict orders not to remove the booklets from a shelf near the teletype machine.

The second training experience was a face-to-face tutorial session conducted by Miss Kay Mayfield, a young, intelligent, and enthusiastic librarian who divides her time between work at the Lister Hill Center and at the National Library of Medicine. Miss Mayfield did a splendid job during the four-hour session, and no further formal training was necessary. This does not mean that "the system" was used to full effectiveness from the very beginning. Many small details had to be learned by working with the computer day by day, and frequent telephone calls had to be made to officials at the Lister Hill Center to iron out various problems which seemed to defy solution as they arose.*

Operating Procedures

A detailed description of the various operating procedures of the information and retrieval system would go beyond the confines of this paper. In essence, the program manipulating the bibliographic files (called ELHILL) requires the issuance of certain commands and messages which must be properly understood by the operators. These communications are typed on the TWX keyboard and fed into the computer by striking the carriage return key. The program, in turn, searches the files for unit records that match the specifications that have been included in the search statement. It reports back on the number of citations which have or have not been retrieved, and print commands must then be issued in order that all or parts of the retrieved records may be printed out.

MeSH (Medical Subject Headings)

Probably the most difficult, and at the same time interesting, aspect of the job of processing search requests for a variety of users was the search formulation. Like MEDLARS, the AIM-TWX system employs the

*One of these calls, for example, concerned the input of the *MeSH* term CONDITIONING (PSYCHOLOGY) which was rejected by the computer. The staff was told that the proper way of entering this term is not to use parentheses but the character # instead.

network of *MeSH* descriptors and subheadings, and none of the staff was really well acquainted with the terminology and "trees" of *MeSH*. It became obvious from the beginning that the success or failure of a search depended heavily on the formulation of the search statements which were fed into the computer. Fortunately, the system is designed in such a way that even without access to the full printed *MeSH* vocabulary formulations can be made. Nevertheless, as any cataloger knows, the formulation of search statements came to be regarded as the most difficult, as well as challenging, aspect of the man-computer dialog.

It was also noted that much costly time could be spent developing search formulations while being "logged into" the machine, and every effort was made to prepare the searches on the day before they were actually "run." Two request forms were developed locally on which prospective patrons listed their search topics and parameters. Many search requests were called in on the telephone, however, or came by letter. Probably the very best results were achieved when the requestors couched their requests either in *MeSH* terminology which presumed a familiarity with *MeSH*, or when they were physically present when the search was run and could overview the citations as they came off the machine. In the latter case, they had an opportunity of advising the operators on means of either enlarging or narrowing the topics, or of introducing other subject terms and term combinations which would produce results.

Record Keeping

A daily log was kept in a three-ring notebook on which the various searches were recorded. The log proved essential for any evaluation of the system because it not only provided detailed information for every search, but also data on the number of searches run each day, and on the length of time the machine was in actual contact with the computer.

Working the System: The Team

Another decision made after some experimentation related to the staffing of the project. It was decided that a continuous four-hour stretch was too long for one person. A team effort evolved according to which two persons staffed the machine for the first two hours and another two for the second two. One of the two would always be working on the teletype; that is, doing the actual "input" or transmitting, while the other would record the findings on the log, keep the various papers (search requests and results) in some order, and most important of all, being equipped with a copy of *MeSH*, would reformulate search statements as seemed necessary from time to time. The latter was an essential operation and became an important part of the work even if the initial search formulation had been carefully prepared the day before.

Results

Although better results could have been obtained through greater familiarity with the system and, in particular, with *MeSH*, the overall results were most gratifying. AIM-TWX represents a unique, rapid method of retrieving bibliographical citations, especially for the clinically oriented user. Patrons who desired materials in the preclinical sciences or areas not specifically covered by the 109 journals in the system were disappointed, but the fact that the data base had been limited was pointed out in all presearch request discussions and in the publicity. Similarly, the limitations of *MeSH* had to be taken into account in evaluating the results of any particular search.

In the table below, statistical data are presented regarding the type of user, the number of searches, and the number of citations retrieved or not retrieved.

TABLE 1
AIM-TWX Service at U. Va. Medical Library
November 19–December 18, 1970

	Total Requestors	Individual Searches			Citations Retrieved		
		Total	Successful	Unsuccessful	Total	On Line	Off Line
Virginia Practitioners	50	103	83	20	2,013	381	1,632
U. Va. Medical Faculty	32	84	62	22	1,655	302	1,353
U. Va. Nursing Faculty	7	64	57	7	802	261	541
U. Va. House Staff & Students	17	39	36	3	756	250	506
MCV Faculty & House Staff	8	8	5	3	117	4	113
Totals	114	298	243	55	5,343	1,198	4,145

Users of the System

A total of 114 individuals requested 298 searches during the nineteen-day trial period, and a total of 5,343 citations were retrieved.

The users ranged from practitioners in various communities of the state to medical and nursing school personnel, including teaching staff, specialists, house staff, and students. A few requests came from hospital administrators, nursing staff supervisors, and members of the paramedical professions.

Many of the requests originated in small communities such as Bloxom, Christiansburg, Galax, Radford, Wise, and Wray. Not all of the practitioners could be identified since some of the search requests were mailed or telephoned in by local secretaries or community hospital librarians, and time did not permit verifying the source of every request.

Search and Citation Findings

The survey indicates that fifty practitioners used the system, representing 44 percent of the total number of users. They requested 103 (or 35 percent) of all searches and obtained 2,013 (or 38 percent) retrieved citations.

University of Virginia Medical School and Nursing School faculty comprised the second largest user group. There were thirty-nine requestors (or 34 percent) in that category. They asked for 148 (or 49 percent) searches and obtained a total of 2,457 (or 46 percent) retrieved citations.

The remaining users were University of Virginia house staff and students and a few Medical College of Virginia faculty whose requests were forwarded by the MCV reference staff.

"Successful" Versus "Unsuccessful" Searches

The term "successful" is used here only in the sense that a search formulation produced citations. Accordingly, the vast majority of search requests (243, or 82 percent) resulted in citations being furnished. Only fifty-five searches (or 18 percent) out of the total of 298 produced no citations and were, therefore, termed "unsuccessful."

"On-Line" Versus "Off-Line" Printouts

According to ELHILL, citations may be printed on- or off-line. Our findings show that a substantial majority of searches (160) was done on-line, while seventy-three were printed off-line. In ten cases both on- and off-line citations were printed. However, the largest number (4,145) of all citations retrieved (5,343) was printed off-line, while only 1,198 were printed on-line.

In reviewing the findings, it should be considered that not *all* possible citations in the system were retrieved in *all* cases. The prime object of the searches was to produce quick and reasonable results which may explain the fact that many more on-line printouts were made.

The printing of large numbers of citations was only attempted in cases when the requestors desired "everything published." On such occasions, the "Print Off-Line" command was given, and the citations were printed in Santa Monica and mailed (air mail), arriving usually two to four days later.

On the whole, an attempt was made to keep the number of citations retrieved to a reasonable level, and it was found that the majority of requestors favored such a policy also. "Some of the latest papers" was a frequently heard request, especially on the part of the busy practitioner. In accordance with these policies, various qualifying elements were introduced whenever the computer reported an unduly large number of citations. They included time limitations (e.g., 1970 only), or subheadings which would bring the topic into sharper focus.

Another method designed to speeding up the compilation of citations was the practice of excluding authors' names from the printouts. It was found that the printing of many authors' names extended the printout time and did not add materially to the findings. Many users evaluated an item in a bibliography primarily on the basis of titles of articles rather than authors' names.

Interruptions, Cut-Offs, Etc.

Although the library had been promised a four-hour period daily from Monday through Friday, the periods of actual use were shorter due to many "cut-offs" which separated the user from the system either temporarily or permanently for that day. The causes cannot be explained entirely. They may have been due to machine, line, or computer malfunctioning, but the staff suspected that most of the difficulties originated with the computer in Santa Monica. Most of the interruptions were temporary, and it was possible to get back into the system, or "logged in," after a short break. Nevertheless, it should be stressed that interruptions were quite frustrating, especially when a physician had taken time off from patient care or other duties to be present in the library while the search was conducted.

Hopefully, some of these problems will be ironed out in the not too distant future to guarantee an uninterrupted service.

Time Factors

Inasmuch as time is money in a very real sense when one is hooked into a computer network, the following findings may be of special interest.

According to a review of the AIM-TWX log, the AIM-TWX system was in use during nineteen days—or less than three weeks. During that period, the average number of minutes of computer time on any given day was 200; the average number of searches, sixteen; and, the average number of searches per hour, 4.6.

It would be premature to make definitive statements on the basis of this very short experience. However, a tentative conclusion would be that given more expertise and know-how in terms of *MeSH* terminology and man-machine dialog, six searches could be carried out during one hour of uninterrupted service. Excluded from this estimate would be the time that it takes to dial into the system, to "call in" the program, and possible delays caused by accidental interruptions and "number of users exceeded" messages.

Conclusions

From November 19 to December 18, 1970, the Medical Library of the University of Virginia had on-line access to the AIM-TWX computer at Santa Monica, California. Although actual contact with the computer was to be had for four hours daily on five days a week, the average use per day was a little over three hours. During that time, the operators in the Library were able to run a total of 298 searches for 114 individual requestors which resulted in the printout of 5,343 citations from the current (1966 onwards) medical literature. Only fifty-five searches did not produce any citations, a fact which must not be regarded as a total failure, however, since some of these searches dealt with topics which may not have been reported on in the recent literature.

The fact that this mass of bibliographical output could be produced by an inexperienced staff—in terms of the vital *MeSH* terminology and in the use of on-line computers—with only minimal instruction speaks highly for the system. A few of the searches could have been handled in a manual way. The overwhelming majority of the searching, however, involved multi-concept requests which was greatly speeded up by the use of the machine. The experience indicated that AIM-TWX is a viable and productive system which, it is hoped, will soon be a permanent feature in most of the larger medical libraries serving a clinically-oriented clientele.

The Lister Hill Center staff and their California systems and development satellites must be congratulated on having produced a fully automated storage and retrieval system which should go far toward improving access to data in the vast biomedical literature of today.

Keys to the Medical Literature

By William K. Beatty

In the field of medical literature the reader's problem is seldom that of finding material, but rather of winnowing pertinent articles, books, and reports out of a vast mass of information which seems to be increasing exponentially.

The old invitation to "Come you now and sit with me, Underneath the medlar tree" has taken on a less romantic tinge in the 1960's. The quiet country landscape has been stripped of its trees to provide paper for the burgeoning medical literature, and the medlars themselves have turned into a whirring blinking computer system. The *Med*ical *L*iterature *A*nalysis and *R*etrieval System at the National Library of Medicine lies at the core of much of the practice and most of the theory of modern bibliographic control of the medical literature. The reader's problem is no longer that of finding material, but rather of winnowing pertinent articles, books, and reports out of the vast mass that is piling up both in this country and abroad. There are several "keys," physical and mental, that will help to accomplish this. The physical "keys" include an up-to-date medical library, and the mental "keys" include a logical mind, a good imagination, and an awareness of the basic methods for searching the literature.

Before you start your search you should sit down and think. Do you have a clear picture of just what is involved in the subject? Are you interested in etiology, medical or surgical treatment, complications, or some other particular aspect of the subject? Are you going to be dealing with humans, animals, or both? Do you want only English language articles, or can you use one or more foreign languages? Will you cover only the current literature, or will you go back five or more years? The answers to these questions will help to define your problem and make your search more effective. You will want to take advantage of both the mental and physical keys, so keep in mind the help that your reference librarians can give you. Dragons are almost as extinct on library staffs as they are in the outside world, and you may be pleasantly surprised by the interest and usefulness of your librarian.

If you want two or three good, recent articles on a subject, for basic information or for preparing a report, you would probably not be

Originally published in *The New Physician,* Volume 18 (August, 1969), pp. 634-641. Reprinted by permission.

overjoyed to have the current issue of each of the 19,000 medical and related journals that are now pouring out of almost a hundred different countries dumped in your lap. What you want are references to two or three articles in English, in journals that are in the library of your school or hospital. The best guide for this is the "new" *Index Medicus.*

Index Medicus is your first "key" to current medical articles, and you will find it a great time-saver. This monthly index to 2,300 journals is one of the products of Medlars. Each issue is divided into five parts. The first, the introduction, is short, clear, and informative. The second and third parts contain the subject and name sections of the *Bibliography of Medical Reviews.* The fourth and fifth parts contain the subject and name sections for the body of the *Index Medicus* itself, and it is in the fourth part that you will look for your two or three articles.

If your subject is retinal detachment the pertinent page in a recent (October, 1967) issue of *Index Medicus* would look like this (Fig 1). Depending on your requirements you can select your articles from the general heading or one of the subheadings. English articles appear at the head of each subject or subheading. These are followed by the foreign-language articles which have not only the square bracket preceding them but an abbreviation for the language given at the end of each citation. If you are looking for recent articles on therapy of retinal detachment you will find one by Cox under the subheading "therapy" (Fig 1). If you want more references on this subject you would go back to the September, August, etc, issues.

If you had heard, on the ward or in the lecture room, that Cox had recently written a good article on retinal detachment, you would go directly to the Name section and find the citation (Fig 2) under the author. The attending physician or the lecturer might have remembered the name of the second or third author rather than of the first, and then you would have found a cross reference (in the Name Section) that would have referred you to the senior author and the citation.

The term "Name Section" is used here, rather than "Author Section," because this section includes more than authors. If you are seeking an obituary or biographical article on a particular person you would locate it in the "Name" section.

If you have to do some further searching, and have exhausted the monthly issues of the current year, you would turn to the *Cumulated Index Medicus.* This cumulates the 12 monthly issues for each year into one annual arrangement for subjects and another annual arrangement for names. Here (Fig 3) you will find a much larger number of articles, and two additional elements of the arrangement will become evident. Under the subheading "Etiology" you will see that the English language articles, at

INDEX MEDICUS

studied with linearly p...
Bell Soc Ital Biol Sper 42:1420-2, 31 Oct 66 (It)
[Fractional sleep in the monomodal canal of the information transmission system and the role of the feed-back in the control of afferent pulses of the input system] Ataev MM.
Izv Akad Nauk SSSR [Biol] 2:230-43, Mar-Apr 66 (Rus)
[Macular representation in the visual cortex. Electrophysiological analysis in man] Aranda L, et al.
Neurocirugia 23:41-3, Jan-Dec 65 (Sp)

PHYSIOPATHOLOGY

Studies of dark adaptation of discrete paracentral retinal areas in glaucomatous subjects. Zuege P, et al.
Amer J Ophthal 64:56-63, Jul 67

RADIATION EFFECTS

Retinal lesions produced by Q-switced lasers. Bergqvist T, et al. Acta Ophthal (Kobenhavn) 44:853-63, 1966
Alterations in the fine structure of the mature retina of dogs irradiated as neonates. Shively JN, et al.
Exp Eye Res 6:278-82, Jul 67
Provitamin A2: electroretinographic measurements of its effect on photopic sensitivity in chicks. Auerbach E, et al. Nature (London) 211:77-8, 2 Jul 66
Molecular and thermal origins of fast photoelectric effects in the squid retina. Hagins WA, et al.
Science 157:813-6, 18 Aug 67

X RETINAL DETACHMENT (C11)

[Postoperative detachment of the retina. Mechanism and prospects of prevention] Bessière E.
Annee Ther Clin Ophtal 17:209-18, 1966 (Fr)

COMPLICATIONS

Homocystinuria and ocular defects. Presley GD, et al.
Amer J Ophthal 63:1723-7, Jun 67
Vitreoretinal traction in serous and hemorrhagic macular retinopathy. A biomicroscopic study. Tolentino FI, et al.
Arch Ophthal (Chicago) 78:23-30, Jul 67
[Malignant melanic tumor of the choroid revealed by a spinal metastasis] Auvert B, et al.
Ann Oculist (Paris) 199:1079-87, Nov 66 (Fr)

Annee Ther...

THERAPY

X The manifestations and current therapy of the retinal detachment disease. Cox MS Jr.
Amer J Med Sci 254:236-42, Aug 67
[Current status of photocoagulation in the therapy of diseases of the fundus oculi] Meyer-Schwickerath G.
Annee Ther Clin Ophtal 13:55-67, 1962 (Fr)

RETINAL HEMORRHAGE (C8, C11)

[Hyperuricemia and gout in retinal vascular accidents. New etiological and therapeutic data] Bourde C.
Annee Ther Clin Ophtal 14:91-113, 1963 (Fr)

ETIOLOGY

Hyperviscosity syndrome in multiple myeloma. Kopp WL, et al. Amer J Med 43:141-6, Jul 67
Hemorrhage in hyaline bodies (drusen) of the optic disc during an attack of migraine. Gaynes PM, et al.
Amer J Ophthal 63:1693-6, Jun 67
Dermal vasculitis with retinal involvement. McCarthy JT, et al. Arch Derm (Chicago) 96:109-10, Jul 67
[Anomalies of platelet aggregation during Waldenström's disease. (Apropos of 3 cases)] Doumenc J, et al.
Nouv Rev Franc Hemat 6:734-8, Sep-Oct 66 (Fr)

RETINAL PIGMENTS (D10)

Rhodopsin kinetics and rod adaptation in Oguchi's disease. Carr RE, et al. Invest Ophthal 6:426-36, Aug 67
A thermal component of excitation in the lateral eye of Limulus. Srebro R.
J Physiol (London) 187:417-25, Nov 66
[Life and death of the pigmented epithelium of the retina] Hervouet F.
Annee Ther Clin Ophtal 14:115-22, 1963 (Fr)

ANALYSIS

Pigmented iris and retrocorneal membrane simulating an iris melanoma. Haver RP.
Arch Ophthal (Chicago) 78:55-7, Jul 67

Laser photocoagul...
al.
Trans Amer Acad Op... ...43,
Nov-Dec 66

RETINITIS PIGMENTOSA (C11)

COMPLICATIONS

[Neuromuscular syndromes in so-called atypical retinitis pigmentosa as a hint to a fat metabolism disorder] Dieckmann H, et al.
Verh Deutsch Ges Inn Med 71:634-7, 1965 (Ger)

DIAGNOSIS

Pigmentary degeneration of the retina: early diagnosis and natural history. Sunga RN, et al.
Invest Ophthal 6:309-25, Jun 67

URINE

[Studies on a melanocyte-stimulating hormone-like substance in the urine, with reference to retinitis pigmentosa] Aonuma S, et al.
Folia Endocr Jap 42:512-20, 20 Aug 66 (Jap)

RETINOBLASTOMA (C2, C11)

COMPLICATIONS

Invasion of choroid and sclera by retinoblastoma following photocoagulation. Howard GM.
Trans Amer Acad Ophthal Otolaryng 70:984-9, Nov-Dec 66

RADIOTHERAPY

Retinoblastoma, megavoltage, therapy and unilateral disease. Bagshaw MA, et al.
Trans Amer Acad Ophthal Otolaryng 70:944-50, Nov-Dec 66

SURGERY

Invasion of choroid and sclera by retinoblastoma following photocoagulation. Howard GM.

Part 2 of the January issue contains a categorized list of subject headings, including cross references. Their location in the categorized list is indicated by the letter-number designations (A1, B1, etc.), following each subject heading.

677

Fig 1—Page from Subject Section, Oct, 1967, issue of Index Medicus, showing section on "Retinal Detachment," and reference to article by Cox under subheading "Therapy."

INDEX MEDICUS

Cortese I, Macri G, Rubino M: Influenza dell'enteramina sulla stimolazione della sete nell' uomo, nella cavia, nel topo e nella rana. Arch Ital Sci Farmacol 15:177-82, Jul-Oct 65 (It)
Cortese I see Zamboni P
Cortesi S, Fontanin O, Xodo P, et al: Influenza della circolazione extracorporea sulle resistenze osmotiche e termiche eritrocitarie. Minerva Med 58:2153-5, 9 Jun 67 (It)
Cortesi S, Vettore L, Ancona G, et al: Comportamento della colinesterasi plasmatica in corso di emodialisi. Minerva Med 58:2103-5, 6 Jun 67 (It)
Cortesini R: Problemi organizzativi di un reparto dialisi e trapianti renali. Minerva Med 58:2068-71, 6 Jun 67 (It)
Cortiñas JJ see Murphy G
Corwin JH, Ferguson EF Jr, Moseley T, et al: Carcinoma of the male breast. Southern Med J 60:777-80, Jul 67
Cory RP, Wold F: Isolation and characterization of enolase from rainbow trout (Salmo gairdnerii gairdnerii). Biochemistry (Wash) 5:3131-7, Oct 66
Cosar C see Bénazet F
Coscas G, Halimi G: La correction optique des aphaques. Arch Ophtal (Paris) 26:599-608, Sep 66 (Fr)
Coscas G see Bouniq C
Coscia L, Causa P, De Natale G: A new synthetic analgesic drug, p-phenetidine-alpha-N-n-propylpropionamide (FC 379). Arch Int Pharmacodyn 164:331-9, Dec 66
Coscia L, De Natale G, Causa P: General pharmacological properties of p-phenetidine-alpha-N-n-propylpropionamide (FC 379). Arch Int Pharmacodyn 164:340-4, Dec 66
Coscia L see Causa P
Cosemans J see Gyselen A
Cosgrove JB see Murphy BE
Coskey R, Huldin R, Pinkus H: Lupus vulgaris. Arch Derm (Chicago) 96:107-8, Jul 67
Coskey RJ, Mehregan AH: Granuloma pyogenicum with multiple satellite recurrences. Arch Derm (Chicago) 96:71-3, Jul 67
Coskey RL, Magidson O: Electrocardiographic response to selective coronary arteriography. Brit Heart J 29:512-9, Jul 67
Cossa GA see De Marchi F
Cossart YE: Marker studies of poliovirus. Nature (London) 211:1432, 24 Sep 66
Cossins EA see Wong KF
Cosson G see Leclerc M
Costa A, Cottino F: An epidemic of acute nodular goitre. Lancet 2:50, 1 Jul 67
Costa AL, Spadaro M, Mundo A: Sui rapporti tra lisozima e tasso di colesterolo surrenale nei ratti pan-irradiati. Boll Soc Ital Biol Sper 42:1280-3, 15 Oct 66 (It)
Costa AL see Spadaro M
Costa C see Zappia V
Costa E see Boullin DJ
Costa LD, Horwitz M, Vaughan HG Jr: Effects of stimulus uncert[illegible] ...atibility on speed [illegible] ...66

Cottier H see Wagner HP
Cottino F see Costa A
Cottino F see Magro G
Cottle MK, Mitchell R: Degeneration time for optimal staining by Nauta technique. A study on transected vagal fibers of the cat. J Comp Neurol 128:209-22, Oct 66
Cotton DW see Mier PD
Cotton WR: Pulp response to an airstream directed into human cavity preparations. Oral Surg 24:78-88, Jul 67
Cotton WR see Russell JR
Cottrell GA: Occurrence of dopamine and noradrenaline in the nervous tissue of some invertebrate species. Brit J Pharmacol 29:63-9, Jan 67
Couch NP: Supply and demand in kidney and liver transplantation: a statistical survey. Transplantation 4:587-95, Sep 66
Couch NP, Wheeler HB, Hyatt DF, et al: Factors influencing limb survival after femoropopliteal reconstruction. Arch Surg (Chicago) 95:163-9, Aug 67
Coughlan MP see Winder FG
Coughlin CA: Spheroplast production in thymine starvation. Nature (London) 212:633-5, 5 Nov 66
Coul AA op de: The effect of ACTH and corticosteroids on the brain. Psychiat Neurol Neurochir 69:385-98, Nov-Dec 66 (66 ref.)
Coules J, Avery DL: Human performance and basal skin conductance in a vigilance-type task with and without knowledge of results. Percept Motor Skills 23:1295-302, Dec 66
Coullaud D, Lévêque J: Action du métoclopramide sur différentes portions de l'intestin isolé de lapin, et sur l'intestin "in situ". Path Biol (Paris) 14:963-5, Oct 66 (Fr)
Coulombe MJ see Spencer RP
Coulshed N see Epstein EJ
Coulson RA, Hernandez T: Changes in free amino acids of caymans after feeding. Amer J Physiol 212:1308-12, Jun 67
Coulson RA see Hernandez T
Coultate TP see Dennis DT
Coulter NA Jr see Kunz AL
Coulter SK see Hingtgen JN
Counsell LA: Inverted premolar. Oral Surg 24:210, Aug 67
Counsell RE, Adelstein GW: Anabolic agents. 19-Nor-and 19-substituted 5alpha-androst-2-ene derivatives. J Med Chem 9:685-9, Sep 66
Counsell RE, Klimstra PD, Elton RL, et al: Chemical and biological properties of some 17-substituted estradiol derivatives. J Med Chem 9:689-92, Sep 66
Counsell RE, Willette RE: Synthesis of 14-C-labeled isomers of dichlorodiphenyldichloroethanes (DDD). J Pharm Sci 55:1012-5, Oct 66
Counsell RE see Klimstra PD
Counts RM: Family crises and the impulsive adolescent. Arch Gen Psychiat (Chicago) 17:64-7[illegible]
Courbier R see Gérard R
Coursin DB see Lowe C[illegible]

Cowden JE: Institutional and post-release adjustment of neurotic and social delinquents. J Clin Psychol 22:477, Oct 66
Cowden RR see Alvarez MR
Cowden RR see Levi JU
Cowden RR see Malzone WF
Cowell TK, Marsden CD, Owen DA: Objective measurement of parkinsonian tremor. Lancet 2:1278-9, 18 Dec 65
Cowen DL, Burtis B, Youmans J: Prolonged coma after acetohexamide ingestion. JAMA 201:155-6, 10 Jul 67
Cowie AT see Watson SC
Cowie V, Gammack DB: Serum proteins in Huntington's chorea. Brit J Psychiat 112:723-6, Jul 66
Cowley JJ, Griesel RD: The effect on growth and behaviour of rehabilitating first and second generation low protein rats. Anim Behav 14:506-17, Oct 66
Cowsert MK Jr, Carrier O Jr, Crowell JW: The effect of hemorrhagic shock on blood uric acid level. Canad J Physiol Pharmacol 44:861-4, Sep 66
Cox AG see Abernethy RJ
Cox AJ, Reaven EP: Histidine and keratohyalin granules. J Invest Derm 49:31-4, Jul 67
Cox CP, Leaverton PE: Statistical procedures for bioassays when the condition of similarity does not obtain. J Pharm Sci 55:716-23, Jul 66
Cox CS: Bacterial survival in suspension in polyethylene glycol solutions. J Gen Microbiol 45:275-81, Nov 66
Cox CS: The survival of Escherichia coli in nitrogen atmospheres under changing conditions of relative humidity. J Gen Microbiol 45:283-8, Nov 66
Cox DR: The null distribution of the first serial correlation coefficient. Biometrika 53:623-6, Dec 66
Cox EF: Hemobilia following percutaneous needle biopsy of the liver. Arch Surg (Chicago) 95:198-201, Aug 67
Cox FE: Acquired immunity to Plasmodium vinckei in mice. Parasitology 56:719-32, Nov 66
Cox FE, Vickerman K: Pinocytosis in Plasmodium vinckei. Ann Trop Med Parasit 60:293-6, Sep 66
Cox FE, Voller A: Cross-immunity between the malaria parasites of rodents. Ann Trop Med Parasit 60:297-303, Sep 66
Cox FE see Vickerman K
X Cox MS Jr: The manifestations and current therapy of the retinal detachment disease. Amer J Med Sci 254:236-42, Aug 67
Cox PA, Keshishian JM, Blades BB: Traumatic arteriovenous fistula of the chest wall and lung. Secondary to insertion of an intercostal catheter. J Thorac Cardiov Surg 54:109-12, Jul 67
Cox PJ see Adels BR
Cox R see Demott BJ
Cox RM see Fay P
Cox RP see Griffin MJ
C[illegible] RW, Grant RA, Horne RW: The assembly of macromol[illegible] to form native

Fig 2—Page from Name Section, Oct, 1967, issue of Index Medicus, showing reference to article by Cox.

the top of the subsection, are arranged alphabetically by journal title. The foreign language articles are arranged alphabetically by language, and, within each language, alphabetically by journal title. This format can be helpful if you want to limit your searching to one or two specific journals, or if you read a foreign language and want to coordinate your subject search with some practice in that language.

With the aid of the current issues of *Index Medicus* and a year or two of the *Cumulated Index Medicus* you will probably be able to dig out as many references as you need. You could then jot these citations down on the backs of old grocery lists or whatever scraps of paper you may have in your pocket, or you might try a reference slip (Fig 4). Such a slip will remind you to copy down all the data you need in order to locate the article. A group of such slips forms a handily managed packet that will fit easily into a pocket, whereas grocery lists, etc, are usually of different sizes and are quite likely to be thrown away if you happen to look at the wrong side first when you take one out of your pocket.

Review articles are among the most important and useful in the literature. If you want a picture of the current state of a particular subject, or if you want to find out how a certain therapy or operative procedure has developed, you will stand a good chance of finding the information you want in a review article. The only problem, then, is to find that review article.

"BMR" are easy initials to remember. Bibliographically speaking, they stand for another "key," the *Bibliography of Medical Reviews,* which makes up the second and third parts of the monthly issues of *Index Medicus.* These pages are also published as a separate monthly journal, and are cumulated into an annual arrangement with the same title.

The BMR has the same basic arrangement as the *Index Medicus.* For example, if you look under "Retina" in the October, 1967, BMR subject section of *Index Medicus* you will find a reference to an article by Campbell. To give you an idea of the depth of the review the index entry gives the number of references cited by the author; in this case, 206. This bit of information not only gives you a clue as to the coverage of the article but also, where several reviews are listed on the same subject, permits you to choose a review by size. If you have an author of a specific review article, you would go first to the Name rather than the Subject Section.

Review articles generally require some time for digestion. If your library has a photocopier you might consider having a copy made of the review you have found. You will then take only those pages from the journal that you need, read them at your leisure, and, possibly, check off appropriate references in the article's bibliography as you follow up on them later.

The symbols following the subject headings in *Index Medicus* and its

RETINAL DETACHMENT **CUMULATED INDEX MEDICUS**

deficiency] Yano T
Acta Soc Ophthal Jap 68:1502-20, Oct 64 (Jap)

RADIATION EFFECTS

Observations on early pathologic effects of photic injury to the rabbit retina. Fine BS, et al
Acta Ophthal (Kobenhavn) 43:684-91, 1965
Chorioretinal lesions produced by laser on monkeys and rabbits. Santos R, et al
Amer J Ophthal 61:230-40, Feb 66
The threshold of the retina to damage by laser energy. Campbell CJ, et al
Arch Ophthal (Chicago) 76:437-42, Sep 66
Is there a hazard in laser photocoagulation? Mellerio J
Brit Med J 5489:719, 19 Mar 66
Quantum energy specificity of simple photoreceptor units. Dawson WW
Nature (London) 208:589-90, 6 Nov 65
Effects of laser radiation on the mammalian eye. Ham WT Jr, et al
Trans NY Acad Sci 28:517-26, Feb 66 (32 ref.)
Eclipse burns in humans and laboratory threshold measurements in rabbits SAM-TR-66-45. Allen RG Jr, et al **US Air Force Sch Aerospace Med 1-5, May 66**
[Radiation injury of the retina induced by roentgen rays in newborn mice] Fischer H
Radiobiol Radiother (Berlin) 6:439-45, 1965 (Ger)
[Retinal metabolism and ionizing radiation. I. Modifications of protein synthesis in elements of centripetal conduction] Maraini G, et al
Ann Ottal 91:583-9, Jul 65 (It)
[Retinal metabolism and ionizing radiations. II. Modifications of protein synthesis in sensorial elements] Maraini G, et al
Ann Ottal 91:590-7, Jul 65 (It)

SURGERY

Transscleral freezing of the retina: an experimental study. Archambeau PL, et al
Invest Ophthal 4:885-93, Oct 65
[On some conditions for the use of lasers in photocoagulation of the retina] Blabla J, et al
Cesk Oftal 21:281-91, Jul 65 (Cz)

RETINAL DETACHMENT (C11)

Rhegmatogenous retinal detachment? What is the evidence? Potts AM
Amer J Ophthal 61:1264-71, May 66
The effects of detachment of the retina on the induced and resting ocular potentials in the rabbit. Foulds WS, et al. **Invest Ophthal 5:93-108, Feb 66**
Clinical study of lattice degeneration of the retina. Byer NE
Trans Amer Acad Ophthal Otolaryng 69:1065-81, Nov-Dec 65
An unusual form of glaucoma in aphakics. Roberts W
Trans Amer Acad Ophthal Otolaryng 69:1024-8, Nov-Dec 65
A clinical classification of retinoschisis with a preliminary report of three unusual fundus appearances. Crock GW
Trans Ophthal Soc New Zeal 17:18-24, 1965
[Bilateral annular detachment of the retina] Michiels J, et al. **Bull Soc Belg Ophtal 141:581-90, 1965 (Fr)**
[Aspect of the dysproteinemic fundus oculi (microaneurysms and retinal detachment) in a case of Waldenstrom's disease] Ardouin M, et al
Bull Soc Ophtal Franc 66:129-32, Jan 66 (Fr)
[Retinal detachment following psychic trauma?] Munchow W
Klin Mbl Augenheilk 147:580-7, Nov 65 (Ger)
[A case of retinal detachment occurring in flight] Terrana C, et al **Minerva Med 56:3963-4, 14 Nov 65 (It)**
[Retinal detachment in Charlin's syndrome] Mazza C, et al **Riv Otoneurooftal 41:53-62, Jan-Feb 66 (It)**
[Prurigo, cararact and retinal ablation--a rare oculo-cutaneous syndrome] Kozmińska A, et al
Przegl Derm 52:589-92, Nov-Dec 65 (Pol)
[Ophthalmologic observations following retinal coagulation by means of optic quantum generator] Puchovskaia NA, et al **Oftal Zh 20:428-31, 1965 (Rus)**
[Retinoschisis] Pavia JJ, et al
Arch Oftal B Air 40:97-105, May 65 (Sp)

COMPLICATIONS

Intra-ocular pressure in retinal detachment. Linnér E
Acta Ophthal (Kobenhavn) Suppl 84:101-6, 1966
Retrolental membrane associated with Bloch-Sulzberger syndrome (incontinentia pigmenti) Jones ST **Amer J Ophthal 62:330-4, Aug 66**
[Annular chorio-retinal detachment or exudative annular cyclitis. Reflections apropos of a further case] Paufique L, et al
Bull Soc Ophtal Franc 65:532-5, May 65 (Fr)
[Unrecognized intra-orbital foreign body and retinal detachment] Voisin J, et al
Bull Soc Ophtal Franc 65:864-6, Oct 65 (Fr)
[Observations on changes in the vitreous body and the extreme retinal periphery in normal elderly persons, in aphakic subjects and in patients with retinal detachment] Sanna G, et al
Ann Ottal 91:1031-8, Nov 65 (It)
[On a particular aspect of spontaneous resolution of retinal detachment: reattachment with amaurosis] Proto F, et al **Boll Oculist 44:725-33, Oct 65 (It)**
[Uncommon postoperative complications in cases of retinal detachment] Hirose K, et al
Folia Ophthal Jap 16:740-2, Oct 65 (Jap)
[Lens opacities in cases of retinal detachment] Yoshioka H, et al
Folia Ophthal Jap 16:739, Oct 65 (Jap)

DIAGNOSIS

Visual field examination in retinal detachment. Enoksson P
Acta Ophthal (Kobenhavn) Suppl 84:93+, 1966
Intra-ocular pressure in retinal detachment. Linnér E
Acta Ophthal (Kobenhavn) Suppl 84:101-6, 1966
The electroretinogram in retinal detachment. Rendahl I **Acta Ophthal (Kobenhavn) Suppl 84:107-9, 1966**
Choice of surgical technique. Rosengren B
Acta Ophthal (Kobenhavn) Suppl 84:163+, 1966
The search for retinal ruptures. Rosengren B
Acta Ophthal (Kobenhavn) Suppl 84:61-9, 1966
Some clinical types of retinal detachment. Tornquist R
Acta Ophthal (Kobenhavn) Suppl 84:87-91, 1966
Retinal detachment surgery. Diagnosis and treatment. Biomicroscopy of the fundus. Tornquist R
Acta Ophthal (Kobenhavn) Suppl 84:71-6, 1966
Coats' disease. Natural history and results of treatment. Gomez Morales A
Amer J Ophthal 60:855-65, Nov 65
Rhegmatogenous retinal detachment. Pilkerton R, et al **Med Ann DC 35:481-5 passim, Sep 66**
Twin subretinal cysticerci simulating posttraumatic detachment of the retina. Radian AB, et al.
Rum Med Rev 19:56-9, Oct-Dec 65
Recent developments in the management of retinal detachment. Schepens CL
Trans Amer Acad Ophthal Otolaryng 69:896-911, Sep-Oct 65
The clinical significance of the fundus periphery. Shanahan LF **Trans Ophthal Soc Aust 24:15-20, 1965**
[Bilateral retinal pseudo-detachment caused by posterior uveitis during pregnancy] Hugonnier R, et al. **Bull Soc Ophtal Franc 65:1103-5, Dec 65 (Fr)**
[ERG and postoperative reapplication in retinal detachment] Jayle G, et al
Bull Soc Ophtal Franc 65:827-9, Sep 65 (Fr)
[Use of the suction cup in the diagnosis of idiopathic detachment of the retina] Tieri O, et al.
Ann Ottal 91:875-8, Nov 65 (It)
[Prognostic value of some functional investigation methods in retinal detachment] Filatova ZA.
Oftal Zh 20:496-500, 1965 (Rus)

X **ETIOLOGY**

Acute posterior vitreous detachment and its retinal complications. A clinical biomicroscopic study. Linder B
Acta Ophthal (Kobenhavn) Suppl 87:1-108, 1966
Chorioretinal lesions predisposing to retinal breaks. Dumas J, et al. **Amer J Ophthal 61:620-30, Apr 66**
Spontaneously reversible retinal detachment occurring during renal insufficiency. Lapco L, et al.
Ann Intern Med 63:760-6, Nov 65
Experimental retinal detachment. Freilich DB, et al.
Arch Ophthal (Chicago) 76:432-6, Sep 66
Retinal detachment in the retinopathy of prematurity. Tasman W, et al
Arch Ophthal (Chicago) 75:608-14, May 66
Retinal detachment in prosthetophakia. Tasman W, et al. **Arch Ophthal (Chicago) 75:179-88, Feb 66**
Retinal detachment with spontaneous regression in renal failure. Sharpstone P, et al.
Brit Med J 5505:92-3, 9 Jul 66
Rhegmatogenous retinal detachment in Filipinos. I. Site and types of breaks and other associated findings. Espiritu RB, et al. **Philipp J Surg 20:158-63, May-Jun 65**
Retinal dialysis as the cause of a special type of retinal detachment. Hagler WS.
Southern Med J 58:1475-82, Dec 65
New retinal tears following photocoagulation. Byer NE, et al. **Trans Pacif Coast Otoophthal Soc 46:237-59, 1965**
[Clinical aspects and treatment of retinal detachment] Seedorff HH
Maanedsskr Prakt Laegegern 43:261-9, Jun 65 (Dan)
[Ablatio retinae] Hagedoorn A
Nederl T Geneesk 109:1741-3, 11 Sep 65 (Dut)
[Apropos of traumatic retinal detachment in young subjects] Braun-Vallon S, et al.
Bull Soc Ophtal Franc 65:171-7, Mar 65 (Fr)
[Bilateral detachment of the retina during eclampsia] Duhamel E, et al
Bull Soc Ophtal Franc 65:644-6, Jul-Aug 65 (Fr)
[Choroiditis in multiple sclerosis and so-called uveoencephalomeningitis] Bammer H, et al.
Deutsch Z Nervenheilk 187:300-16, 2 Jul 65 (Ger)
[Retinal detachment, cataract, keratoconus as ocular symptom complex in endogenous eczema] Jutte A, et al. **Klin Mbl Augenheilk 147:12-25, Sep 65 (Ger)**
[Eye symptoms as first manifestations of bronchial

Fig 3—Page from Cumulated Index Medicus, 1966, showing subject arrangement under "Retinal Detachment," and subheading "Etiology."

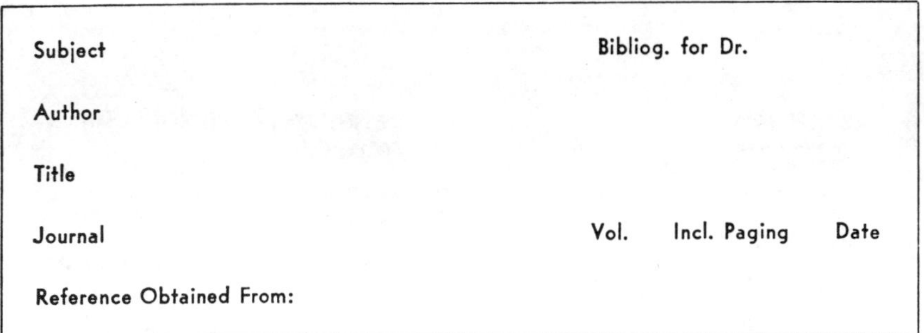

Subject

Bibliog. for Dr.

Author

Title

Journal

Vol. Incl. Paging Date

Reference Obtained From:

Fig 4—Reference Slip. Note headings for each part of citation, and space for notes by reader.

annual cumulation are guides to the Medlars list of subject headings. This list, called *Me*dical *S*ubject *H*eadings (MeSH), will be useful in helping you to understand the production and arrangement of *Index Medicus*. MeSH is published each year as part 2 of the January issue of *Index Medicus*. It consists of three parts: an introduction, an alphabetical list and categorized lists. This introduction is worth a few minutes of your time since it explains the purposes, cross references, subheadings, and other elements of the list. The final section of the introduction draws attention to headings that have been added or deleted during the past year. Medical terminology is always growing and changing, and the subject headings appropriate for today may very well not have been the ones used for that subject 10 or 20 years ago. Whenever you make a subject search for articles or books you will want to be sure that you are searching under the terms in use at that time. Textbooks and dictionaries, contemporaneous with the period of your search, can be helpful in providing subject headings under which material was indexed.

The alphabetical list of subject headings shows you which headings are used in *Index Medicus* and under what heading you should look if the term you are using is not used as a separate subject. If you look at the appropriate page (Fig 5) in the 1967 MeSH you see that "Retinal Detachment" is a separate subject, so that you don't need to look under any other subjects in this particular search. Looking higher up on the page you will see that if you wanted articles on "Angioid Streaks" you would want to look under both "Retina" and "Angioid Streaks." Further down in the same column you will see that if you were searching for articles on "Retrograde Degeneration" you should look under the heading "Nerve Degeneration," or moving further down, both literally and figuratively, if you wanted articles on "Retroperitoneal Fibrosis" you would also find articles dealing with "Ormond's Disease" under the same heading. A few minutes spent with MeSH before you start a search will enable you to cover the ground much more thoroughly and quickly than if you jumped right into *Index Medicus*.

X RETINA (A9)
see also related
ANGIOID STREAKS (C11)
ELECTRORETINOGRAPHY (E1)

X RETINAL DETACHMENT (C11)

RETINAL HEMORRHAGE (C8, C11)

RETINAL PIGMENTS (D10)
XU RHODOPSIN (D10)
XU VISUAL PURPLE (D10)
XR RODS AND CONES (A8, A9)

RETINAL VESSELS (A7)

RETINITIS (C1, C11)

RETINITIS PIGMENTOSA (C11)

RETINOBLASTOMA (C2, C11)

RETIREMENT (I)
XR GERIATRICS (G1, G2)

RETORTAMONAS (B1)
XU EMBADOMONAS (B1)

RETROGNATHISM (C3, C4, C16)

X RETROGRADE DEGENERATION see under NERVE DEGENERATION (G1)

RETROGRADE OBTURATION (E6)

RETROLENTAL FIBROPLASIA (C11, C16)

X RETROPERITONEAL FIBROSIS (C4)
X ORMOND'S DISEASE (C4)

RETROPERITONEAL NEOPLASMS (C2, C4)

RETROPERITONEAL SPACE (A3)
XR ABDOMEN (A1)

RETROPNEUMOPERITONEUM (E1)

RETROSPECTIVE STUDIES (E5)

REVERIN see ROLITETRACYCLINE (D3)

REVERSAL LEARNING (F)

REVONAL see under TRANQUILIZING AGENTS (D6)

REWARD (F)

RH FACTORS (D12)
XR ERYTHROBLASTOSIS, FETAL (C9, C14, C16)

RHABDITOIDEA (B1)

RHABDITOIDEA INFECTIONS see under NEMATODE INFECTIONS (C1)

RHABDOMYOMA (C2, C3)

RHABDOMYOSARCOMA (C2, C3)

Fig 5—Page from Medical Subject Headings (MeSH), 1967, showing that part of the Alphabetical List which contains "Retinal Detachment" and three other headings referred to in text.

The other major part of MeSH, the "Categorized Lists," gives you a broad picture of the arrangement of the headings themselves. The "C11" after "Retinal Detachment" (Fig 1) refers you to the section of "Diseases" which covers specifically the "Sense Organ Diseases" (Fig 6). Here you find part of the subject headings used in *Index Medicus* for these diseases. A glance over this may give you clues for other pertinent headings for your searching and it will also give you an indication of the thinking behind the choice of these headings.

Your searching of *Index Medicus* may have turned up several excellent references on your exact subject, but these references may have been to articles in Bulgarian, Portuguese, or some other language you do not read fluently. If this happened (and, since much of *Index Medicus* deals with foreign language material this is quite likely) your natural inclination might be to toss these references aside. Don't, at least not until you have taken several additional steps. First, if the reference is to a journal that is available in your library go and take a look at it. More and more foreign language journals are printing English summaries and such a summary may give you sufficient information. The summary sometimes appears at

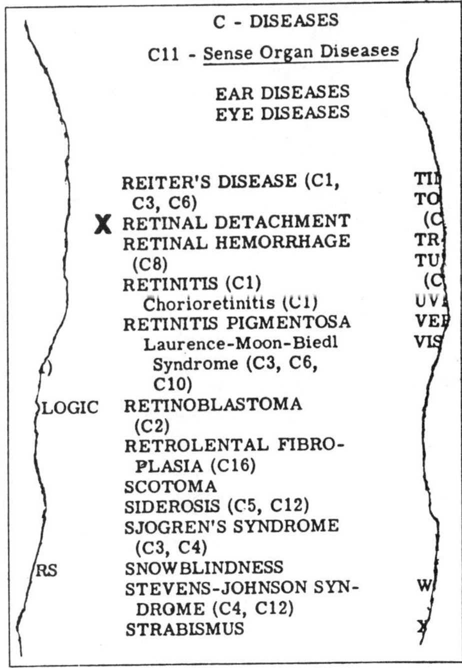
C - DISEASES

C11 - Sense Organ Diseases

EAR DISEASES
EYE DISEASES

REITER'S DISEASE (C1, C3, C6)
X RETINAL DETACHMENT
RETINAL HEMORRHAGE (C8)
RETINITIS (C1)
Chorioretinitis (C1)
RETINITIS PIGMENTOSA
Laurence-Moon-Biedl Syndrome (C3, C6, C10)
RETINOBLASTOMA (C2)
RETROLENTAL FIBROPLASIA (C16)
SCOTOMA
SIDEROSIS (C5, C12)
SJOGREN'S SYNDROME (C3, C4)
SNOWBLINDNESS
STEVENS-JOHNSON SYNDROME (C4, C12)
STRABISMUS

Fig 6—Page showing C11, "Sense Organ Diseases," in "Categorized Lists" part of Medical Subject Headings, 1967.

the beginning or end of the article, or sometimes they are all grouped together in one place near the front or back of the journal issue. If the article you are looking for does not fall into this category of journals, or if it is in a journal not immediately available, you still have another printed possibility. If you are searching for an English summary of an article on retinal detachment, you might turn to an English abstracting journal in the subject field. Bear in mind that it takes longer to produce an abstract than it does to index an article: there will often be a six to 12 months' lag before an English language abstract of a foreign language article appears.

The major English language abstracting journal is the series entitled *Excerpta Medica*. This is published in Amsterdam, in 33 subject sections. Each month an issue is produced in each of these subject areas: anatomy, ophthalmology, cancer, geriatrics, etc. *Excerpta Medica* covers several thousand journals from all over the world, and provides fairly detailed English abstracts for these articles.

In addition to *Excerpta Medica* many specialized abstracting journals exist and a few moments spent with the reference librarian in your library will acquaint you with the titles pertinent to your interests.

All of these abstracting journals serve several purposes. Not only will they furnish you with an English abstract of a specific article, but they are also useful for retrospective and "current awareness" searches.

A retrospective search is an extension in time of the original search you started out with, the one for "two or three good recent articles" on a specific subject. You can make a basic retrospective search by going back through several years of the *Cumulated Index Medicus* or you can expand this retrospective search both in number of journals covered and in immediately available information by using several years of one of the pertinent English-language abstracting journals. You will often be able to judge the pertinence of an article more readily from an abstract than from the index entry.

The "current awareness" search is one that keeps you up with the current articles in your field. If you want to know what is happening throughout the medical world in, for example, pediatrics, you would skim through each monthly issue of the section of *Excerpta Medica* on that subject as it comes in to your library. With a relatively small expenditure of time you will be able to keep up (taking into account the time-lag involved in writing and publishing abstracts) with the current work in your field.

After you have found some useful articles you will want to make notes of them. You can keep all of your information together by using your reference slip (Fig 4) for your notes as well. The references the author lists at the end of the article may be useful if you wish to pursue this subject further or if you want to check a specific point the author has mentioned.

Most authors are careful to list only those references that proved helpful or directly pertinent. Occasionally, however, an author will just amass a list of references to make his paper look impressive. This is one of the cardinal sins of medical writing, and such authors soon become well-known for this "inflation."

Computers have made possible one of the most intriguing indexing tools now available. The *Science Citation Index*, produced by the Institute for Scientific Information in Philadelphia, covers some 1,600 journals and indexes the references cited in them alphabetically and chronologically by author to show who has cited whom (Fig 7). Such an index would simply not be possible without a computer to manipulate the millions of references involved. There are many potential uses for "SCI" and as you become acquainted with it you will find productive possibilities. Basically, you will be able to pursue a specific method, test, operative procedure, etc, and see who has referred to this same item.

If your search of the literature takes you back before the Second World War—and one or two important things did happen in medicine prior to 1940—you will find the *Index-Catalogue of the Library of the Surgeon-General's Office* useful. This monumental bibliography of 61 volumes was called by William Welch the greatest contribution to medicine by the United States after the development of surgical anesthesia. The *Index-Catalogue* lists books and journal articles by subject and books by author as well. It was issued in five alphabetical series which are gold-mines of references for the deep digger.

The front-line of medical science appears in the journals. However, books, reports, and other types of medical publications are also helpful, and if you need to cover these as well there are "keys" to this store of information. Currently, there is a branch of Medlars that presents a subject and author approach to recently published books and other nonjournal materials. The *Current Catalog* lists material recently catalogued by the National Library of Medicine. This comes out twice each month, and there are quarterly cumulations.

The best immediate source for available books on a particular subject is the card catalogue of your library. Here you will find books arranged by subject as well as by author. These cards will carry a "call number" derived from the subject classification system your library uses, and this will be helpful in locating the book on the library's shelves.

Medicine has a long and fascinating history, and if your interests are historically inclined you will find three "keys" that will be of special value. The first of these is a quarterly index produced in England, *Current Work in the History of Medicine*. This comprehensive index covers articles of medicohistorical interest that have appeared in both medical and nonmedical journals. The second, and newest, of these keys is an annual index to the history of medicine. Now in its third volume the *Bibliography of the History of Medicine*, another product of Medlars, will increase in usefulness as the years pass. The third key is a small book, *Garrison and Morton's Medical Bibliography: an Annotated Check-List of Texts Illustrating the History of Medicine*. The compilers have arranged the important books and journal articles chronologically within each subject. Many of the entries are annotated. *Garrison-Morton* will give you a panoramic view of how the knowledge of a particular medical subject has developed over the years and centuries, and will also acquaint you with the names of the important individuals in each field.

Computers have become useful tools in the bibliographic control of the medical literature. Types of indexes are now possible that could not have been produced by manual methods, and the production of most of the "old"indexes has been considerably speeded by automation. At the base of all of these "keys," however, are the qualified and experienced individuals who do the indexing and abstracting before the machine takes over for the mechanical processing. Keeping this in mind, and the immediately available assistance of the reference librarian in your own library, you should find that a search of the literature is not only a productive but a stimulating affair.

Annotated List of Major Indexing and Abstracting Tools

Index Medicus. New Series. Vol. 1- , 1960- . This is the major current medical index. It indexes 2,300 journals from 69 countries by subject and author. The *Cumulated Index Medicus* arranges the 12 monthly issues into one alphabet for subjects and one alphabet for authors each year.

Current List of Medical Literature. Vols. 1-36, 1941-1959. This predecessor of the "new" *Index Medicus* is especially useful for the period 1952-1959 when it was issued with semiannual cumulative indexes. Each issue lists articles alphabetically by journal title, and contains author and subject indexes.

Quarterly Cumulative Index Medicus. Vols. 1-60, 1927-1956. The "QCIM" is a useful index in "dictionary" form which should be used with *Current List of Medical Literature* since each of these indexed journals not covered by the other.

Index Medicus. Ser. I, Vols. 1-21, 1879-Apr., 1899; Ser. II, Vols. 1-18, 1903-

1920; Ser. III, Vols. 1-6, 1921-June, 1927. Each issue gives an author and a subject approach, but the arrangement varies. This contains some material not found in the Index-Catalogue.

Quarterly Cumulative Index to Current Medical Literature. Vols. 1-12, 1916-1926. Should be used with the *Index Medicus* for this period.

Bibliographia Medica. Vols. 1-3, 1900-1902. A French publication, this attempted to fill part of the gap between the first and second series of *Index Medicus.*

Index-Catalogue of the Library of the Surgeon-General's Office. Ser. I, Vols. 1-16, 1880-1895; Ser. II, Vols. 1-21, 1896-1916; Ser. III, Vols. 1-10, 1918-1932; Ser. IV, Vols. 1-11, 1936-1955; Ser. V, Vols. 1-3, 1959-1961. This monumental work contains millions of references to books and articles. Anyone doing a comprehensive or historical search of the literature will find this an invaluable tool. Books are listed both under the author and the subject; journal articles are listed under the subject. The introduction to each series should be checked to find out what period is covered and what special material is contained in that series.

Bibliography of Medical Reviews. Vol. 1- , 1956- . Annual. This gives a subject and an author listing of recent review articles. Each entry gives full bibliographic citation and the number of references cited in the article. Beginning with 1968 BMR was published as a separate monthly journal as well as in the front of the monthly *Index Medicus.*

Excerpta Medica. Monthly. This is the major English-language abstracting journal. It is produced in 33 subject sections which cover the major preclinical and clinical fields. Fifteen of the sections began in 1947 or 1948. Each issue has author and subject indexes, and each volume has cumulated author and subject indexes.

Abstracts of World Medicine. Vol. 1- , 1947- . Monthly. This British publication provides "selective coverage of the important world literature" in all major subjects. Each issue has author and subject indexes, and each volume has cumulated author and subject indexes.

Science Citation Index. 1961, 1964- . The 1961 index was an annual; from 1964 on SCI has appeared quarterly with annual cumulations. This is an exhaustive index to references cited in some 1600 journals (many of them medical).

Biological Abstracts. Vol. 1- , 1926- . This major abstracting tool covers many fields related to medicine. It has a variety of up-to-date indexes.

Chemical Abstracts. Vol. 1- , 1907- . This is another major abstracting tool of considerable interest to those working in medicine. 10-year and 5-year cumulative indexes make searching quick and efficient.

Morton, Leslie T. Garrison and Morton's Medical Bibliography; An Annotated Check-List of Texts Illustrating the History of Medicine. 2nd ed., rev. London, Deutsch, 1965. "Garrison-Morton" is the basic handbook for the history of medicine.

Bibliography of the History of Medicine. No. 1- , 1965- . National Library of Medicine, Bethesda, Maryland. Annual. This indexes articles of medicohistorical interest, from medical and nonmedical journals, by subject and author.

Current Work in the History of Medicine. Quarterly. No. 1- , 1954-. The Wellcome Historical Medical Library produces this comprehensive index to articles in medical and nonmedical journals. It also gives the addresses of the authors, and lists new books and journals in the field.

Current Catalog, National Library of Medicine. Biweekly, with quarterly cumulations. Vol. 1- , 1966- . *Current Catalog* lists, by subject and author, monographs, new serial titles, and audiovisual materials catalogued by the National Library of Medicine. Information on prices and publishers is given when available.

Selecting for Health Sciences Library Collections When Budgets Falter

By Stanley D. Truelson, Jr., *Librarian*

Yale Medical Library
New Haven, Connecticut

ABSTRACT

The economic plight of the 1970s often limits the librarian, who should be the final selector, to insufficient funds for acquiring essential publications. The librarian, in addition to making every effort to acquire the best possible collection, must provide access from other libraries, within and outside one's parent institution, to materials not acquired; for this purpose, an effective document delivery network has proved more significant than formal plans for shared acquisitions. Too much is published, but the choices become more manageable with selection criteria that include limiting subject scope and keeping within the English language. In regard to journals, new titles should be added only reluctantly; cancellation lists compiled with the help of selective lists, the librarian's judgment, and users' responses; and newsletters and state journals pruned to a minimum. As to books, selective lists should be consulted; congress proceedings generally ignored; and reprinted collections, multiple copies, and gifts considered with care. Book reviews are more useful selection aids now that lack of funds causes delays in purchasing than when new titles were acquired promptly with less discrimination. Audiovisual media, although widely pushed, do not replace printed materials, are not of central importance to many faculties, are expensive, and thus comprise a bandwagon which the impoverished library cannot afford to board without extra funding. The less money there is, the more need for a librarian's selection skills.

Budget

Recent Trends

THE 1960s were good years for library budgets, as for most other budgets, but the 1970s are a letdown all around. When the nation cannot afford to expand social and educational services, libraries suffer.

The passage of the Medical Library Assistance Act of 1965 was a political breakthrough which could have happened only when the economy was

Originally published in *Bulletin of the Medical Library Association,* Volume 64 (April, 1976). pp. 187-195. Reprinted by permission.

favorable. Federal support for health sciences libraries is a result of political concern for better health care, just as federal support for other libraries results from national interest in education in general. In the 1960s the federal government heavily funded basic science research, but today such funding has been reduced drastically and attention turned to using better what we already know, to applying existing knowledge so as to provide health care most efficiently and economically, an alternative emphasis which is clearly an effect of inflation, depression, and unemployment as much as a deliberately planned change of the nation's social goals.

While both research and application require library service, and some aspects of the 1965 Medical Library Assistance Act continue to be funded, federal support for health sciences libraries is now concentrated on seed money for demonstration projects or new libraries, which the recipient is expected to find other funds to continue, rather than on operating subsidies such as in the 1960s permitted the accelerated strengthening of research collections. At the same time, private institutions now lack the funds to maintain routine operations, let alone continue new projects seeded by federal grants. The demise of health sciences library resource grants ironically paralleled the decline of the private sector's ability to take up the slack.

Fight or Facilitate?

It is difficult for a librarian to accept that the mission of his or her library should not be an exception to the general trend. We librarians entered the field of librarianship believing that rendering library service to society is a sacred cause, whether society wants to pay for it or not. The librarian who did not stand up for library programs and fight without letup for the money to fund them was supposed to feel guilty for being passive, lacking in initiative, and failing his present and future clientele. There is some truth to the charge that librarians should be more effective in the power struggle for program priority and funding, but the issues are not so simple as to call merely for crusading; there is that other matter of facing reality. When, for example, a long established private university, which always has prided itself on the magnificence of its libraries, finds itself, along with the rest of the country, unable to pay its fuel bills and at the same time carry on its activities in accustomed style, someone with overall responsibility has to decide how to match expenditures with income. If these highest officials, in full recognition of the consequences of their decisions, regretfully decree that their libraries, along with all other units, must share in budget retrenchments, it then becomes the librarian's duty, not to fight, but to facilitate the program cutbacks in the best possible way in order to accomplish the mission of both the library and the parent institution.

One major program area which budget cuts are likely to affect is the acquisition of library collections. Even though the acquisitions budget is not reduced, it often fails these days to increase with the same speed as inflation. In addition to such direct reduction in annual purchasing power, libraries face the need to reduce their growth rate in order to lessen the pressure for continually expanding stack space, which generates another cost that institutions are becoming unable to fund as the years go by[1]. Even the largest of the nation's libraries are now urgently seeking ways to avoid continued growth at a pace which they can no longer afford[2-3]. A library that does not aim, at least in theory, to acquire all the books and journals its readers want? As a matter of fact, yes. The problem and the solution, of course, is to select wisely and to obtain alternative access for the less-needed materials not acquired.

Who Selects?

Some nonlibrarians are reluctant to admit that the most logical and effective agent to select a library collection is the librarian. The originator of the famous Project INTREX wrote:

> It is neither fair nor sensible to assign to libraries the total responsibility for scholarly communications. Quality judgments concerning the substance of the printed record are essential elements of the total task. Such judgments will be accepted by scholars only if they are made by recognized authorities in the various fields. . . . once that decision is made, it becomes the responsibility of the library profession to provide the best possible access to each item in the total record. . . . The task of controlling the holdings of central libraries and departmental book rooms at universities will be regarded as a responsibility deserving the close and continuing attention of the best available talent in each department[4].

Skepticism about the ability of librarians to build library collections usually is accompanied by an unstated assumption that subject experts are more capable than librarians of balancing the need for materials in their own field against the needs in other fields or by an assumption even more remarkable that such experts will get together regularly to coordinate their requests after having taken the time to keep up with all new publications in their own field. It just doesn't happen that way very often.

This is not to say that the librarian will not need to consult subject experts on occasion, and happy is the librarian who finds experts who will respond promptly and cheerfully when asked. But in the end it is the librarian at whose desk the buck stops, or he is not fully the librarian. When there is more than one librarian on the staff, the head librarian may want to delegate selection duties, but few health sciences libraries are so large that the head librarian is forced to relinquish all participation in what is perhaps one of the most important and professional aspects of his job, shaping the collections.

Alternative Access

Shared Acquisitions

Within the Institution. In times of plenty, when a title was of interest to more than one of the various specialized libraries of a large institution, they would tilt the balance in favor of duplicate purchasing. Convenience to readers was worth the cost. In times of scarcity it is necessary to decide that the institution generally can afford only one copy and that readers will have to learn to use the several library facilities more fully. The medical library thus buys fewer chemistry, general biology, or social sciences titles than it did formerly, leaving their provision solely to the science or social science libraries.

Outside the Institution. It has been fashionable to believe that libraries can achieve significant savings and at the same time insure full access to the literature by formal commitments for dividing among themselves the responsibility for acquiring all relevant publications. This achievement may be possible, but there are many problems in attempting to demonstrate it.

One of the major efforts of the Research Libraries Group, a formal consortium of four of the nation's largest libraries (New York Public, Harvard, Yale, and Columbia) is to share the acquisition of serials and expensive monographs. An elaborate petitioning process, coordinated by a bibliographic center (which also performs various other services), has been established to keep the records and nudge the decisions necessary.

Jones has proposed a regional program for cooperative purchasing of serials whereby each medical library would commit itself to continue a portion of the titles previously shared by all in common (presumably the most important ones) as well as a number of titles not held elsewhere in the region[5]. The theory is that each library can cancel some subscriptions to titles provided by the others and thus save enough to more than afford the less needed titles for which it has assumed responsibility.

The chief difficulty when budgets are pinched is that a library needs to cancel every title it possibly can, regardless of whether the title remains in the consortium or region. Consequently, no funds are freed up to cover the less needed titles which are being divided among the cooperating libraries—the money freed is already needed elsewhere. Furthermore, it is difficult to justify cancelling needed titles and relying on an outside library for access to them merely in order to free money to acquire less needed titles assigned under a cooperative agreement.

The assumption that it is important to keep a little used title somewhere in the consortium or region is the weak link in the theory of shared acquisitions. In view of the technology and functioning arrangements for shared access to collections, at least among health sciences libraries, it often is likely that one or a very few copies are enough in the entire country, and for this purpose the comprehensive collecting activities of a National Library of Medicine or a Center for Research Libraries offer a reasonable degree of security.

There is, no doubt, a danger, when only one or a few copies of little used titles are maintained in the entire country, that such unique material may get lost or destroyed. If the National Library of Medicine should lose part or all of its collections through disaster, the absence of back-up duplicates would constitute a second disaster. Perhaps it is fear of such an occurrence that makes it seem useful to insure comprehensive collecting within each and every region or consortium. The sorry fact, however, is that this kind of insurance is too expensive; the institutions that have to pay the bills cannot afford today to buy the little used titles and hardly the moderately used titles which shared acquisitions plans would require.

Network Access

The premise upon which this questioning of shared acquisitions rests is an effective system for borrowing or obtaining reproductions of those one or very few copies of a title, wherever they may be. In effect, a comprehensive document delivery network is far more significant in providing alternative access to publications than is formal sharing of acquisitions responsibility. That such an effective network among health sciences libraries is alive and well, copyright law revisers willing, does not need demonstrating here.

Any network is in danger of overloading its apex with too many requests. It is necessary to spread the load, which usually is concentrated on a well-known body of common titles rather than on a wide range of little-used titles. The natural needs of network members tend to insure that within any region the heavily requested titles are sufficiently available so as not to require their provision from the major back-up collection. Sometimes contractual arrangements for spreading government subsidies for document delivery are important to bring about necessary spreading of the service load.

The Proliferation Problem

The complaint that too much is published is not new, but an echo from the beginning of publishing history which will only be touched on here.

JAMA in 1966 quoted a 75-year-old passage mentioning "these days of numerous medical journals," while one of its 1966 editorials stated: "It is our credo that vastly too many books are being published"[6]. The soon-to-be editor of the *New England Journal of Medicine* addressed the Medical Library Association earlier that same year with a proposal that librarians hasten the elimination of poor quality journals by relegating them "to an inconspicuous area" of the library—"it would really be a boycott"[7]. And in 1974 the President of the International Union of Pure and Applied Chemistry wrote about "the fragmentation of science through the mushroom growth of new journals" and the concern of three colleagues whose memorandum on "the rapid and undesirable increase in number of commercial journals" proposed "that *libraries should be urged to show more reluctance in buying new commercial journals*" (italics in original)[8]. That is indeed a good suggestion, which will be explored more fully below.

Selection Criteria

Some of the steps proposed here may involve going out on a limb, but then, it is necessary to take drastic steps to cope with a budget crisis. What else can one do but make judgments and take chances?

General Principles

Several general principles immediately reduce the universe of choices.

Subject Scope. One already has been implied, that subject scope be limited mainly to fields of direct interest to the library and not of primary concern to libraries serving other types of clientele. Thus, while the behavioral sciences in all their branches of psychology, sociology, anthropology, management, and so on are sometimes essential for the health sciences, the health sciences library cannot afford to collect widely in these peripheral areas and regularly must refer its clientele to resources of other libraries. Even within the health sciences, subjects which are not taught, practiced, or investigated in one's own institution or which are done so only as adjuncts to primary interests cannot be covered except in a cursory way. If an academic health center has no dental, pharmacy, or veterinary school, even though its hospital may operate a dental clinic and an active clinical pharmacy service and its medical school a large laboratory animal care section, the library should not build a major collection in dentistry, pharmacy, or veterinary medicine. In all such cases, however, the existence of special gifts, such as annual allocations from the local dental society, can increase the degree of coverage possible.

Language. A second general principle is that most selection should be limited to the English language. The major foreign-language journals of international reputation will be continued by the academic health center library, but seldom should it consider new journals or books not in English when budgets are inadequate. It used to be preached that the best publications in all languages should be collected in order to avoid provincialism and achieve scholarly balance. In practice there is no money for such luxury. The health sciences library must invest its funds on publications which its clients can and will read. Fortunately for us, in all our parochialism, the English language is becoming more and more the international language of science, as witnessed, for example, by the number of changes of journal title and content from German to English and by the practice of new European journals of adopting English as their "sole language of publication" in order "to assure the widest readership"[9].

Journals

New Titles. As already mentioned, the choice of new journals should be made reluctantly. Instead of rushing to add every new title that comes along, fearful that early issues will go out of print or that clients will be impatient at a seeming unawareness of what is new, it is better to consider carefully the quality, relevance, and need for a new title; to ask for advice as to whether the title is really top priority, merely an essential addition (in which case, funds still may not permit its purchase), or an obvious loser; and to keep listening for the clamor of unsatisfied clients or the silence which implies no great loss. It might be argued that library users cannot be expected to know what they are missing if the library does not call it to their attention, but beyond searching continuously for the truly important new title the library cannot afford to be a showcase for new publishing ventures.

Cancellations. A library's existing subscription list must not only be pruned of dead wood but also trimmed of live branches when inflationary increases in journal prices race ahead of the conservative increases of most budgets. Various facts can help identify the most important titles and thus by a process of elimination the candidates for cancellation: whether a title is indexed by relevant indexing services, such as *Index Medicus, Abridged Index Medicus,* or the several selective services of the Institute for Scientific Information[10] or Information Retrieval Limited[11]; whether it is included in relevant selective lists[12-23]; or how high it may be ranked in studies of circulation[24] or citation[25] counts. When all this information has been gathered and the librarian's personal judgment based on experience and intuition has been applied, a list of low priority titles will have developed which can be circulated to department heads and/or other experts with an explanation of the urgent need to reduce expenditures. Sometimes all or most objections to cancelling specific titles can be honored and still leave sufficient room for the needed cost saving; at other times, particularly when more than just obscure titles are being proposed for elimination, the librarian will have to cut where it hurts but hurts the least. The reality which strengthens the librarian's resolve is the realization that if not everything needed can be afforded, then for a reader to assert merely that a title is essential is not sufficient justification to prevent its being cancelled. If the clamor continues, reconsideration *may* be appropriate, but one approach is to ask the petitioner to find the money for his request, whether through new income or suggestions of other titles to cancel.

Newsletters. In compiling a cancellation list, entire categories of journals may be included with few exceptions. One is newsletters, particularly those prolific and expensive services which purport to keep one up to date with what is going on in Washington or wherever. If the grants officer or hospital administrator needs any of these, he is likely to have his own copy, anyway. One or two of these services may be worth the cost to a limited number of readers, but many of them seem to be serving up generally available information, even if from scattered sources otherwise slower to report, at an enormous price as a quick moneymaker for the publisher, and libraries should be wary of them.

State Journals. Another category for arbitrary cancellation is the state and local medical (or other health field) journal, except for one's own. It has been long recognized that the substance of most of the state journals has been thin. A few outstanding exceptions, like the *New England Journal of Medicine,* do not alter the fact that the state journals usually are not basic sources of research information. The Editor of the *New York State Journal of Medicine* describes well the useful role which state journals could play:

> The state journals should . . . become an important asset in continuing medical education. . . . That is their true mission. . . . the state journals can do a better job than the 'throwaways' in keeping physicians abreast. . . . The state journals are not appropriate vehicles any longer for primary publication of experimental or even outstanding, esoteric clinical research. Such material now goes to the specialty and basic science journals. The state journals should stress continuing medical education; that they can and should do[26].

It is not essential for most health sciences librarians to buy or give stack space to this kind of repackaged information, when there is not money or space enough to acquire the basic sources.

Books

Textbooks and Monographs. When I first began choosing books for a health sciences library, some faculty members advised that research monographs be favored over textbooks. In an active research environment where in-house library resources were relatively minimal, they were hungry for in-depth reports rather than the often too brief surveys that are the content of teaching tools. If book purchases are cut to the bone, however, it turns out that research monographs are too numerous to be covered equitably, while a look at any "core list" will show that the books considered most essential by experts in all fields are usually textbooks or other works of summary or encyclopedic nature. It is the textbook, after the "revolutionary new concepts" in a field have "become consolidated," which "attempts to contain the avalanche of recent information under one roof"[27]. As with journals, a number of selected or core lists of varying authoritativeness exist to guide in the most important purchases[12-14, 16, 18, 20-21, 28-32], including reference aids[33-34].

Congresses. One entire category of publication may *a priori* be treated as low priority and its acquisition, with few exceptions, postponed until, if ever, a reader asks for a particular title. That category is the proceedings of meetings, whether called symposia, conferences, workshops, or, as the National Library of Medicine's subject headings identify them with a subheading, "congresses." The reason that congresses are arbitrarily suspect is that as a class the proceedings of congresses are routinely published without referring of individual papers or an evaluation of the need to publish even the overall results: the meetings often are held mainly to give colleagues an opportunity to keep in touch with each other, without regard to whether the papers will be important; the papers often report the authors' work in progress at preliminary stages where it would not otherwise warrant a paper; and the one advantage of timely reporting usually is lost through the year or two's delay in publishing.

> Is it really worth all the effort and cost to produce...all these contributions which, if valuable enough ought to be made more readily available in regular journals, and if not, ought to sink unobtrusively into oblivion? Short conference contributions are not usually, and certainly should not necessarily be, as complete as papers published in the normal way, and one is never certain when referring to them that they are quite reliable. If they are complete and reliable, and are not published elsewhere because the authors consider them to be published already as proceedings, they are often ignored or forgotten[35].
>
> The contemporary symposium has become the spawning ground of many books in the biological and social sciences. Symposiogenesis usually entails a short breeding period, and it presents scientific hemlines in the passing fashion. Symposiogenetic offspring usually are snuffed out in a short period of time—frequently only after begetting another symposium—ad infinitum. Symposiasts on the other hand, are a more durable kindred...[36].

> ... why bother to publish the proceedings from such a gathering ...? Much of what was presented summarized material that the speakers had published previously elsewhere. That which was new, is new no longer. The subjects themselves span such a wide range that to compress them between the covers of a single volume ensures that no one will read the entire work (except, perhaps, the editors and an occasional reviewer).
>
> Unorthodox as it might sound, perhaps such symposia could simply be attended, enjoyed, and learned from. Whatever insights they might provide would then live on in the minds of the participants, rather than becoming entombed on the shelves of their institutions' libraries[37].

It surely seems as if publishing the proceedings of congresses has become an unthinking routine, whether for the profit of commercial publishers or the vanity of the congress participants. It is amazing how many standing orders for serials can be cancelled by identifying the serial as a succession of congress proceedings, whether of the same or various groups. Some congresses are outstanding exceptions, of course, and even some series of congresses should be continued, such as the *Cold Spring Harbor Symposia* or the various *CIBA Foundation Symposia*. But a book selector immediately can reduce the quantity of his selection with reasonable assurance that quality is receiving due consideration if he automatically passes over those titles which are "congresses."

Reprinted Papers. What to do about collections of reprinted papers can be a dilemma. While it seems most economical to rely on the original papers if they appear in the journals a library already owns, there are instances where the new physical arrangement in one place, by suggesting relationships and saving access time, may be worth the cost of what ordinarily would constitute unwarranted duplication. If the collected papers are revised or are supplemented by new introductory material, there may be added reason to acquire them. The importance of the material to the library's readers must guide the selector in balancing convenience versus cost.

Multiple Copies. It may be more important to acquire multiple copies of a few heavily-used works than to buy additional new titles. As funds become scarcer, however, multiple copies become less important in the overall picture, and most of them, too, have to be gone without, in spite of the decreased availability that results. While the percentage of readers' unfilled requests for books in the collections but off the shelves may be high, as engineering studies of library circulation alarmingly indicate[38], this unavailability at least may be corrected upon the return of the circulated volume, in conjunction with an effective system for holding the book for successive requesters. It is helpful to welcome gifts of duplicate current volumes, perhaps of the latest five years, to increase general availability of volumes most likely to be used. (As a parallel practice, it is desirable to weed all duplicates older than five years unless they show signs of active, *recent* use.)

Gifts. Even gifts, which seem to be free, must be carefully screened, however. Most libraries have never had space to accept everything in scope, but those few which have been building large historical collections have tried to keep all editions of all substantive works. When the future of stack expansion becomes bleak, even those libraries must pass up superseded editions (except the first) and those other outdated books of the current century which are not of mainstream importance.

Using Book Reviews

The usefulness of book reviews in guiding selection is much greater in times of restricted budgets than when the typical large library strives to acquire all relevant new titles as soon as they are published, sometimes through automatic approval shipments from a dealer. Automatic approval shipments cease to be sensible for libraries which can buy very few of the newly published titles. For these libraries, the delays in receiving reviews of new titles can be tolerated more easily than before, because they are withholding action on most new titles anyway.

Reviews can help distinguish very important or very poor titles from the majority. The unusual titles can be acted on immediately, while the majority become for the impoverished library a pool from which to fish only as bait becomes available.

In the press of daily activity the librarian cannot read every word of a review. In many cases the subject complexities described will be beyond him, as also beyond the library users whose expertise is not in the field in question. What the librarian looks for is the reviewer's overall judgments of the book, which often can be ascertained by scanning merely the first and last paragraphs of the review.

If the review states that a book is useful or contributes new information, the book is a candidate for the holding pool from which possible future selection may be made. It is only when the review is ecstatic and uses phrases such as "the best present text on the subject," "it has no equal," "should become the standard work" that the librarian is prompted to buy immediately. Even a title from arbitrarily excluded categories such as congresses may rise on the selection scale when a review describes it as "a monumental effort. . .the most ambitious publication in the field so far."

The selector has to choose first the review media at which he can take the time regularly to look. Among the general titles which warrant top attention are *Nature, Science, Journal of the American Medical*

Association, New England Journal of Medicine, Lancet, British Medical Journal, and, for nursing, *American Journal of Nursing.*

Audiovisual Media

In all this discussion there has been a decided silence about audiovisual media: motion pictures, audiotapes, videotapes, slides, filmstrips, and the like. It is not because there is any slackening in the volume of such material being produced. Nor is it because of any lack of publicity, pressure, or even euphoria regarding the merits of AV. Rather, it is because these media do not replace but only supplement printed materials; are not, in spite of current fashions, regarded at all institutions as of overwhelming importance; and are very expensive.

AV media are undeniably useful in enriching the effect of the printed word with motion and sound or at least in reproducing the color and form of the still picture for group viewing. It is generally accepted that the multisensory stimulation provided by such media facilitate the processes of teaching, persuading, and entertaining. They are particularly useful in introducing a new concept and in creating a sense of the whole situation. Some teachers skillfully exploit AV media to save time in the presentation of often repeated segments of lectures or demonstrations and to permit their review on demand. Just as lecture hall and laboratory are the first focus of most courses, with the library as a backup facility, so AV media can replicate or supplement what goes on in the lecture hall and laboratory, as well as the world outside, and add to the background provided by the book or journal. But, on the other hand, for intensive study or reference purposes, the printed word is usually the most efficient medium for recording and conveying the message. It would be very difficult, for example, to convert the contents of Goodman and Gilman to a color videotape performance.

Teacher demand for AV media is widely different from one institution to another, as well as within any single institution. Some faculties are reluctant by tradition or training to use someone else's product in their courses. The particular films or tapes available do not accomplish what they want, and it is a costly nuisance to produce one's own AV materials. Overcoming this lethargy is a constant battle for the media man in some schools, yet in others he cannot keep up with the demands for his services. Certainly at an institution where apathy toward media predominates over enthusiasm, the librarian is advised to think more than twice before boarding the AV bandwagon out of a sense of duty or zeal to convert.

And the clinching reason, again, is cost: AV media are very expensive. It is good practice for an administrator not to embark on new programs unless they either replace the need for old programs or bring new funding; otherwise, the old but still needed programs are in trouble.

For the school or hospital that wants an AV operation, it makes sense to set up the AV unit administratively separate from the library, not only because of the different technical skills required, but also because library funds are most likely to be safeguarded by a clear separation of library and AV budgets; fiscal policy makers may then be less likely to lull themselves into dreaming that AV allocations make up for weaknesses in library budgets.

Coordination between the library and the AV unit is undeniably important in cataloging AV materials so that users may be able to find them and in providing central facilities such as wet carrels for their use in conjunction with printed materials. But all of this coordination should presuppose a commitment of the parent institution to fund the AV program without taking money from other needed programs.

No matter the supposed expectations of the television generation of students (who might surprise us by revealing that AV media sometimes can bore them and books turn them on), the missionary appeals of AV devotees to get something going somewhere, the "every library should do it" stance of grant purveyors (who want to withdraw their money as soon as the seed is planted), or the fond wish of higher administrators to save money by merging AV media in the library (if not submerging the library in AV media), it remains true that libraries in budget trouble cannot afford to be distracted by pressures to invest in what are for them not the primary media. After all, in spite of far-reaching proposals to centralize in the library such diverse materials as pathological slides, radiology films, patient records, and every other kind of record or artifact used to convey knowledge, there really is no more reason to insist that all media belong in the same unit than to insist that all physicians serve in the same department—there is such a thing as useful specialization.

For the library to try to stretch insufficient acquisitions funds for books and journals to buy into the vast, complementary field of AV media and machines would be disaster.

The Art of Selecting

If libraries had enough money, they could expand instead of retract in many of these areas. Perhaps then there would be overwhelming tages in combining AV operations with libraries that could also buy all needed books and journals, as well as explore many other dreams for information processing and transfer[39]. Then the librarian's challenges would be in exciting new directions. But now the challenge to the librarian is to optimize the insufficient.

Perhaps it is consoling that it is more of an art to select library materials when money is scarce than when one can obtain everything wanted. The librarian's selection expertise is more needed and has more impact in times of trouble than in times of plenty. Let us take heart that although we are poorly funded at least we are greatly needed.

REFERENCES

1. GORE, DANIEL. The view from the Tower of Babel. Libr. J. 100: 1599-1605, Sept. 15, 1975.
2. ROGERS, RUTHERFORD D. New approaches to old problems. In: Yale University Library. Report of the University Librarian, July 1971-June 1972. New Haven, 1973. p. 5. Bulletin of Yale University, ser. 69, no. 2, 15 Jan. 1973.
3. DEGENNARO, RICHARD. Austerity, technology, and resource sharing: Research libraries face the future. Libr. J. 100: 917-923, May 15, 1975.
4. OVERHAGE, CARL F. J. Science libraries: Prospects and problems. Science 155: 802-806, Feb. 17, 1967.
5. JONES C. LEE. A cooperative serial acquisition program: Thoughts on a response to mounting fiscal pressures. Bull. Med. Libr. Assoc. 62: 120-123, Apr. 1974.
6. Books and book reviewing (editorial). *J.A.M.A.* 198: 1118, Dec. 5, 1966.
7. INGELFINGER, FRANZ J. Austere librarians—Volteface! Bull. Med. Libr. Assoc. 55: 1-4, Jan. 1967.
8. THOMPSON, HAROLD W. Proliferation of journals in chemistry. Spec. Libr. 66: 172, March 1975. Reprinted from Chem. Eng. News 52: 2, Oct. 7, 1974.
9. To our Readers. Eur. Urol. 1: 1, 1975.
10. Institute for Scientific Information: List of Journals covered by Current Contents. List of Journals covered by Scisearch. Source Publications, Automatic Subject Citation Alert (ASCA) and ASCATOPICS. Source Publications, Science Citation Index (SCI). All: Philadelphia (updated annually).
11. Information Retrieval Limited. Primary Journals monitored and abstracted by IRL and Associated International Organizations. London, Nov. 1971 (updated annually).
12. ALLYN, RICHARD, AND STEARNS, NORMAN S. A library for internists. Ann. Intern. Med. 79: 293-322, Aug. 1973.
13. BRANDON, ALFRED N. Selected lists of books and journals for the small medical library. Bull. Med. Libr. Assoc. 63: 149-172, Apr. 1975.
14. ENNIS, BERNICE. Guide to the Literature in Psychiatry. Los Angeles, Partridge Press, 1971. 127 p.
15. FELTER, JACQUELINE W. 500 selected periodicals for the Medical Library. Teaneck, N.J. Franklin Square Subscription Agency, n.d.
16. Library Association. Medical Section. Books and Periodicals for Medical Libraries in Hospitals. 4th ed. London, 1973. 53 p.
17. MOLL, WILHELM. Basic journal list for small hospital libraries. Bull. Med. Libr. Assoc. 57: 267-271, July 1969.
18. STEARNS, NORMAN S. AND RATCLIFF, WENDY W. An integrated health-science core library for physicians, nurses and allied health practitioners in community hospitals. New Engl. J. Med. 283: 1489-1498, Dec., 1970.
19. TIMOUR, JOHN A. Selected lists of journals for the small medical library: A comparative analysis. Bull. Med. Libr. Assoc. 59: 87-93, Jan. 1971.
20. U.S. Veterans Administration. Central Office Library. Basic list of books and journals for Veterans Administration Medical Libraries. 1971 revision. Washington, 1972, 35 p. (Department of Medicine and Surgery Program Guide, G-14, M-2, part XIII, revised July 31, 1972.)
21. ——. Medical and General Reference Library Staff. Medical Specialty Checklist for

Veterans Administration Medical Libraries. Washington, 1968-70. (Department of Medicine and Surgery Program Guide, G-15, parts 1-11; M-2, part XIII.) (Eleven subject parts published Sept. 1968-Sept. 1970.)

22. WENDER, RUTH, AND LEHR, KAREN. Study of medical journals used by individual Oklahoma physicians. J. Okla. State Med. Assoc. 66: 426-429, Oct. 1973. As cited in: MOLL, WILHELM. A Comment on Another Core List. Bull. Med. Libr. Assoc. 62: 327-328, July 1974.
23. YAST, HELEN T. 90 recommended journals for the hospital's health science library. Hospitals 41: 59-62, July 1, 1967.
24. KOVACS, HELEN. Analysis of one year's circulation at the Downstate Medical Center Library. Bull. Med. Libr. Assoc. 54: 42-47, Jan. 1966.
25. GARFIELD, EUGENE. Citation analysis as a tool in journal evaluation. Science 178: 471-479, Nov. 3, 1972.
26. ANGRIST, ALFRED A. A plea for Selective Library Service: to bring advances in library science to the practitioner. New York State J. Med. 74: 2055-2058, Oct. 1974.
27. AUGUSTIN, R. (Review of) Immunological Aspects of Allergy and Allergic Diseases. Edited by E. Rajka and S. Korossy. Nature 257: 342, Sept. 25, 1975.
28. INKE, GABOR. A list of most frequently recommended medical textbooks. Bull. Med. Libr. Assoc. 59: 589-598, Oct. 1971.
29. KERKER, ANN E., AND MURPHY, HENRY T. Biological and biomedical resource literature. Lafayette, Ind., Purdue University, 1968. 226 p.
30. LAROCCO, AUGUST, AND JONES, BARBARA. A Bookshelf in Public Health, Medical Care, and Allied Fields. Bull. Med. Libr. Assoc. 60: 32-101, Jan. 1972.
31. MENNINGER, KARL. A Guide to Psychiatric Books in English. 3d ed. New York, Grune & Stratton, 1972. 238 p. (Menninger Clinic Monograph Series, no. 7.)
32. WEST, KELLY M., WENDER, RUTH W., AND MAY, RUBY S. Books in Clinical Practice 1971-1975; a selected and annotated list for medical practitioners, indexed by subject and author. Postgrad. Med. 56: 60-81, Dec. 1974.
33. DUNCAN, HOWERTINE FARRELL. Selected reference aids for small medical libraries. Bull. Med. Libr. Assoc. 58: 134-158, Apr. 1970.
34. Interagency Council on Library Resources for Nursing. Committee (8th rev.). Reference sources for nursing. Nurs. Outlook 22: 331-337, May 1974.
35. BREWER, D. F. Weighing words in conference proceedings. Nature 253: 666, Feb. 20, 1975.
36. HAASE, GUNTER R. (Review of) Epilepsy: Its Phenomena in Man, edited by Mary A. B. Brazier. *J.A.M.A.* 229: 339, July 15, 1974.
37. CALLAWAY, WAYNE. (Review of) Nutritional Problems in a Changing World, edited by Dorothy Hollingsworth and Margaret Russell. *J.A.M.A.* 229: 1664, Sept. 16, 1974.
38. TRUESWELL, R. W. Analysis of library user circulation requirements, final report, January 1968. NSF Grant GNO 435. As cited in (1).
39. MILLER, JAMES G. Design for a University Health Sciences Information Center. J. Med, Educ. 42: 404-429, May 1967.

VI
TECHNOLOGIES

Introduction

Richard de Bury[1] (1281-1345) wrote in his *Philobiblon,* "Whosoever, therefore, acknowledges himself to be a zealous follower of truth, of happiness, of wisdom, of science, or even of the faith, must of necessity make himself a lover of books." Given a 20th-century perspective, he might have written that those who build and maintain our medical libraries play a most significant role in the development, progress, and welfare of the whole of medicine.

Writings included in this chapter are examples of efforts to reduce the gap between the source of information and its destination—to provide desired resources within economic and human limitations, where needed, when needed, and in whatever format is most useful.

Few, if any, good anthologies of readings for medical librarians could overlook the work of Dr. Eugene Garfield. Genius, pioneer, and entrepreneur, Garfield has made many significant contributions to the world of information science. Two of Garfield's articles are reproduced herein for the reader. The first represents his early thoughts, which later became centrally embodied in *Science Citation Index,* the cornerstone to an industry for which Garfield is president—the Institute for Scientific Information. The second is Garfield's formal description of the *Permuterm Subject Index,* an epochal paper for those interested in information science.

The Welch Medical Library Indexing Project reported on by Dr. Sanford Larkey was an early effort in the development of machine-based indexes to the medical literature for the Army Medical Library (now the National Library of Medicine).

Space does not permit the inclusion of the lengthy acounts that would be needed to pay adequate tribute to MEDLARS or to that great medical librarian Brad Rogers, who shepherded it from infancy to the largest openly available information retrieval system dealing with science in the world. The reader is referred to *The MEDLARS Story at the National Library of Medicine* by Frank B. Rogers, U.S. Department of Health, Education, and Welfare, Public Health Service, 1963. This 74-page publication describes the history, objectives, and characteristics of MEDLARS—an epochal bibliographic breakthrough for the medical library world. Adequate for our purposes with this book is Scott Adams' "Janet Doe Lecture" in chapter I, which deserves special attention from the reader to more readily appreciate the significance of MEDLARS for medical librarianship. The pervasive importance of this information-processing system was highlighted by Adams when he commented, "Not only in the world of medical libraries, but in that of research libraries, of information science, of information systems nationally and internationally, MEDLARS was the rock which raised the level of the ocean."[2] The impact of MEDLARS will be felt for a very long time.

Intralibrary tasks that computers can perform, of value to library administration, are discussed by Dr. Estelle Brodman. Her comments are based on much personal experience in this field.

Glenn Brudvig summarizes "The Minnesota Experience" in the development of a library minicomputer system. The project, funded by the National Library of Medicine, is charged with developing a low-cost, stand-alone, library-controlled computer system that medium and large medical libraries could afford. There should be tremendous potential for the use of minicomputers and software dedicated specifically to libraries.

Looking forward in 1936, Eileen Cunningham examined problems associated with the increasing quantity of material available for publication, the complexities involved with abstracts, the increasing number of journals, the difficulties of information dissemination, and, in general, the accelerating problem for the harassed investigator to keep abreast of knowledge in his field.

The articles by Dr. Vern Pings, Alderson Fry, and Alderson Fry and Scott Adams provide excellent advice to those planning and designing libraries. Not to be overlooked and certainly to be enjoyed are Fry's random thoughts on weeding.

Erich Meyerhoff closes out this chapter with a synopsis of the proposed program of the Medical Library Center of New York. The progress of this project after 4 years of experience was reported on by Felter in Chapter IV and is a tribute to the foresight, imagination, and hard work of Meyerhoff.

REFERENCES

1. De Bury R: Philobiblon. San Francisco, Edwin and Robert Grabhorn, 1925, p 6.
2. Adams S: The way of the innovator: notes toward a prehistory of MEDLARS. Bull. Med. Libr. Assoc. 60: 523-533, 1972.

Citation Indexes for Science: A New Dimension in Documentation Through Association of Ideas

By Eugene Garfield

"The uncritical citation of disputed data by a writer, whether it be deliberate or not, is a serious matter. Of course, knowingly propagandizing unsubstantiated claims is particularly abhorrent, but just as many naive students may be swayed by unfounded assertions presented by a writer who is unaware of the criticisms. Buried in scholarly journals, critical notes are increasingly likely to be overlooked with the passage of time, while the studies to which they pertain, having been reported more widely, are apt to be rediscovered"[1].

In this paper I propose a bibliographic system for science literature that can eliminate the uncritical citation of fraudulent, incomplete, or obsolete data by making it possible for the conscientious scholar to be aware of criticisms of earlier papers. It is too much to expect a research worker to spend an inordinate amount of time searching for the bibliographic descendants of antecedent papers. It would not be excessive to demand that the thorough scholar check all papers that have cited or criticized such papers, if they could be located quickly. The citation index makes this check practicable. Even if there were no other use for a citation index than that of minimizing the citation of poor data, the index would be well worth the effort required to compile it.

This paper considers the possible utility of a citation index that offers a new approach to subject control of the literature of science. By virtue of its different construction, it tends to bring together material that would never be collated by the usual subject indexing. It is best described as an association-of-ideas index, and it gives the reader as much leeway as he requires. Suggestiveness through association-of-ideas is offered by conventional subject indexes but only within the limits of a particular subject heading.

If one considers the book as the macro unit of thought and the periodical

Originally published in *Science*, Volume 122 (July 15, 1955), pp. 108-111. Reprinted by permission of author and publisher.

article the micro unit of thought, then the citation index in some respects deals in the submicro or molecular unit of thought. It is here that most indexes are inadequate, because the scientist is quite often concerned with a particular idea rather than with a complete concept. "Thought" indexes can be extremely useful if they are properly conceived and developed.

In the literature-searching process, indexes play only a small, although significant, part. Those who seek comprehensive indexes to the literature of science fail to point out that such indexes, although they may be desirable, will provide only a better *starting point* than the one provided in the selective indexes at present available. One of the basic difficulties is to build subject indexes that can anticipate the infinite number of possible approaches the scientist may require. Proponents of classified indexes may suggest that classification is the solution to this problem, but this is by no means the case. Classified indexes are also dependent upon a subject analysis of individual articles and, at best, offer us better consistency of indexing rather than greater specificity or multiplicity in the subject approach. Similarly, terminology is important, but even an ideal standardization of terminology and nomenclature will not solve the problem of subject analysis.

What seems to be needed, then, in addition to better and more comprehensive indexes, alphabetical and classified, are new types of bibliographic tools that can help to span the gap between the subject approach of those who create documents—that is, authors—and the subject approach of the scientist who seeks information.

Since 1873 the legal profession has been provided with an invaluable research tool known as *Shepard's Citations,* published by Shepard's Citations, Inc., Colorado Springs, Colo.[2]. A citation index is published for court cases in the 48 states as well as for cases in Federal Courts. Briefly, the Shepard citation system is a listing of individual American court cases, each case being followed by a complete history, written in a simple code. Under each case is given a record of the publications that have *referred* to the case, the other court decisions that have affected the case, and any other references that may be of value to the lawyer. This type of listing is particularly important to the lawyer, because, in law, much is based on precedent.

Citation indexes depend on a simple system of coding entries, one that requires minimum space and facilitates the gathering together of a great volume of material. However, a code is not absolutely necessary if one chooses to compile a systematic listing of individual cases or reports, with a complete bibliographic history of each of them. Thus, it would be possible to list all pertinent references under each case with sufficient completeness to give the index more of the appearance of a bibliography. However, this would result in an extremely bulky volume.

There are analogies in bibliographic operations. For example, in cataloging books for booksellers' or library catalogs, an attempt is made to find references to each book in one or more authoritative bibliographic sources, such as the catalogs of the British Museum (BM), Bibliotheque Nationale (BN), or the Library of Congress (LC). The "authority" card used in cataloging sometimes looks like a Shepard entry.

Another example is a book-review digest, in which one finds for each book title a series of references and selections from published reviews, critical and otherwise. Certain indexing publications perform a similar function.

Some time ago I became concerned with the problem of developing a citation code for science. This was necessary for the efficient manipulation by mechanical devices of entries to scientific indexes. In the course of this research I developed a very simple system for identifying an individual scientific article that had appeared in the periodical press. The resulting numerical code consisted of two parts. The first part was a serial number, used instead of an abbreviation, to identify each periodical; it was similar to the serial numbers employed in the *World List of Scientific Periodicals,* by no means a new idea. For example, *Die Bibliographic der fremdsprachigen Zeitschriften Literatur* has for many years used such a system to save space.

The second part of the code number was also a serial number, assigned to each article in a particular publication, starting with 1 and continuing throughout all volumes. The code thus gives no indication of year or volume number, a serious shortcoming. The article number is also not unique, having been used by the *Proceedings of the Society for Experimental Biology and Medicine* since its inception. These two serial numbers taken together, it can be seen, can identify any published periodical article. It soon became apparent, after such codes had been utilized on an experimental basis, that the use of the codes would facilitate the compilation of a citation index. (Other coding systems would be equally applicable.)

A citation index to science would have the following main characteristics. First there would be a complete alphabetic listing of all periodicals covered, in addition to the code number for each periodical. This list would be similar to the *World List,* but without the library holdings information. The main portion of the citation index would list in straight numerical order the code numbers for all the articles covered. Under each code number, for example, 3001-6789, there would be listed other code numbers representing articles that had *referred* to the article in question, together with an indication of whether the citing source was an original article, review, abstract, review article, patent, or translation, and so forth. In effect, the system would provide a complete listing, for the publications covered, of all the original articles that had referred to the article in question. This would clearly be particularly useful in historical research, when one is trying to evaluate the significance of a particular work and its impact on the literature and thinking of the period. Such an "impact factor" may be much more indicative than an absolute count of the number of a scientist's publications, which was used by Lehman[3] and Dennis[4]. The "impact factor" is similar to the quantitative measure obtained by Gross[5] in evaluating the relative importance of scientific journals, a method later criticized by Brodman[6] but used again by Fussler[7].

Other advantages would also obtain. In a way such listings would provide each scientist with an individual clipping service. By referring to the listings for his article, an author could readily determine which other scientists were making reference to his work, thus increasing communication possibilities between scientists. It is also possible that the individual scientist thus might become aware of implications in his studies that he was not aware of before.

Most authors like to see how their works are received. Bringing together all book reviews and abstracts is very important, for it is not possible for an author to keep up with the thousands of publications in which his contribution might be reviewed. This applies equally to publishers. It would not be impossible to include books in the citation index. Indeed, as a first suggestion, the use of Library of Congress card numbers as the identifying code for books would seem appropriate.

It is necessary next to discuss some realistic questions concerned with the realization of such an index. Bitner[8] has estimated that 30,000 cases are covered by *Shepard's Citations* in 1 year, the cases and articles appearing in not more than a few hundred publications. In 1953 about 1 million citations were added—close to 40 citations per case.

What is the prospect in scientific literature? The last published edition of the *World List of Scientific Periodicals* contained more than 50,000 titles in science and technology. It is variously estimated that between 1 and 3 million new scientific articles are published each year. The *Journal of the American Chemical Society* alone publishes more than 3000 per year, including approximately 2000 original articles. The order of magnitude is therefore potentially from 50 to 100 times as great as it is for *Shepard's Citations*.

However, not all of these 50,000 publications are being covered in our present indexing activities, and yet this has not prevented us from continuing indexes of standard type or from starting new ones. Lack of complete coverage is not necessarily an argument against a citation index. It is in fact an argument in its favor. Coverage could perhaps be limited to the list of periodicals covered by one of the leading indexing services. This approach would, of course, have an immediate disadvantage. Such a *subject* selection would mean that less directly related subjects of interest would be excluded, and these are the publications that the individual is least likely to cover in his own research. It would be necessary to consider all the pros and cons in a selective approach and then to determine the possible utility of such a tool. For example, would a citation index to the 1500 periodicals covered by the *Current List of Medical Literature* be of real value, or, similarly, a citation index to the 5000 periodicals covered by *Chemical Abstracts*? The *Current List* would, in fact, offer a good starting point, since it already provides a unique code for the 100,000 items indexed by it each year. Presumably these are the most significant contributions in the covered fields for the year. If 10 is the number of references in the average article, then about 1 million citations would be involved. The preparation of that number annually is not unreasonable. Shepard's has already used well over 50 million citations in its publishing activities.

The ultimate success of a citation index would depend on many factors. For example, if each periodical would assign unique code numbers to the articles published, it would be possible for authors to list these numbers in their bibliographies and, thus, to save the work of coding on the part of the citation index staff. It is unlikely that such a development could take place in less than 5 or 10 years, but it is comparable to the problem of getting publishers to include Library of Congress card numbers in their publications.

When such a large volume of data is to be handled, mechanical devices of high speed and versatility could be used to great advantage and would probably determine success or failure. Once the coding is done, compilation itself is quite mechanical. This could be done by means of conventional filing slips; the Shepard organization itself has used them successfully for 80 years. However, it would be facilitated by a mechanical approach using punched cards.

The utility of a citation index in any field must also be considered from the point of view of the transmission of ideas. A thorough scientist cannot be satisfied merely with searching the literature through indexes and bibliographies if he is going to establish the history of an idea. He must obviously do a great deal of organized, as well as eclectic, reading. The latter is necessary because it is impossible for any one person (the indexer) to anticipate all the thought processes of a user. Conventional subject indexes are thereby limited in their attempt to provide an ideal key to the literature. The same may be said of classification schemes. In tracking down the origins of an idea, the citation index can be of real help. This is well illustrated by an example from my own experience.

Many years ago the Radio Corporation of America developed a reading-aid for the blind[9]. This device had an electronic system for converting printed letters into recognizable sound patterns. Using the device, a blind man could scan a printed page; in a set of headphones he could hear a series of sound patterns, each letter having its own recognizable sound pattern. In effect, the words were spelled out, letter by letter, in code. I was particularly interested in this device because I had been independently working on a device that would *copy* print, letter by letter, and reproduce it for bibliographic and other purposes. The two devices had something in common in that they both employed scanning devices. I then wanted to learn whether anyone had ever suggested that the RCA reading-aid could be used for this purpose. It will be apparent that if anyone had known of the RCA device and had thought of adapting it for copying purposes, a reference to the article might have been made. This reference could easily have been included in an article or patent that was not at all related to the problem of reading devices. A citation index would have given me just what I was after. Nothing could substitute for extensive reading, but a great deal of time could have been saved by bringing the appropriate works to my attention.

In the course of my reading I did find a few references to this device, one in a book[10], and several others in periodical articles, one of which was a German article on the mechanization of philological analyses and concordance building. The latter article[11] did not discuss my own special interest in copying devices but it did show the similarity between the author's and my own thinking from the point of view of letter-recognition devices, which is what the RCA device attempts to be. In other words, both of us were interested in this device as a letter-recognition device for the analysis of text.

In another instance the RCA article was unexpectedly cited in the journal *Electronic Engineering* in an article on information theory[12] that I was reading because of an entirely different interest. No subject indexer could have anticipated this crossbreeding of interests. Perhaps there are many other articles and books unknown to me that have made similar references to this device. How can they be located when the main subject matter of the article is, on the surface, so unrelated in nature?

One might say that it would be possible to index articles more thoroughly to achieve the same results. For example, the article on information theory, if thoroughly indexed, might have included an entry under reading devices for the blind. Yet if this were done, our periodical indexing services would clearly become hopelessly overloaded with material that is not necessary to lead us to the micro unit—the entire article or one of its major sections. Although it might be said that no scientist interested in the greater comprehensiveness to be found in a citation index would object to having such a great mass of references in a subject index, this is impracticable. It would require an army of indexers to read the articles and identify the exact subject matter of every paragraph or sentence. Yet this would be necessary. To illustrate, it is only in the very last paragraph of the article on information theory that one would find a reference to reading devices for the blind.

Were an army of indexers available, it is still doubtful that the proper subject indexing could be made. Over the years changes in terminology take place, that vitiate the usefulness of a standard subject index. To a certain extent, this is overcome through the citation approach, for the author who has made reference to a paper 40 or 50 years old has interpreted the terminology for us. By using authors' references in compiling the citation index, we are in reality utilizing an army of indexers, for every time an author makes a reference he is in effect indexing that work from his point of view. This is especially true of review articles where each statement, with the following reference, resembles an index entry, superimposed upon which is the function of critical appraisal and interpretation. To the indexer this has its advantages as well as its disadvantages[13].

To determine in a practical way what the citation index could offer, it was decided to track down the citations made in one journal to a single significant article, in order to compile a sample entry for the citation index. At the suggestion of Erich Meyerhoff, I selected Hans Selye's famous article on the general adaptation syndrome[14]. A systematic search was then made of all papers that were published in the *Journal of Clinical Endocrinology* subsequent to Selye's paper up to 1951—a period of 5 years, including well over 500 articles. Every bibliography in each of the 500 articles was checked for a reference to Selye's article. Twenty-three articles were found to make such reference; each of them was then checked for the character of the information provided.

Examination of the citation list (Table 1) shows the great variety of subject matter included. One thing became quite clear, even to the uninitiated—that is, the influence of Selye's article has been quite pronounced. Such evidence is extremely valuable to the historian.

It is interesting to note that, although all the articles cited were indexed in *Quarterly Cumulative Index Medicus*, not one is to be found there under the heading "Adaptation." In fact, it is surprising not to find any articles from this journal under this subject heading.

It also becomes quite obvious that many references to Selye's paper were general and contribute little or nothing to the readers' enlightenment, since exact page references are not provided. In several cases the Selye

Table 1. Index sample based on article by Hans Selye, "General adaptation syndrome" [*J. Clin. Endocrinol.* **6**, 117 (1946)]. The code number for this journal in the *World List* is 11.123a; the article number is arbitrarily taken as 687; and the code number for the article is 11123a-687. The 23 articles that cited Selye's article are listed, followed by *A hypothetical citation index entry for Selye's article. R,* review article; *A,* abstract; *O,* original article.

1. Williams, R. H.: Thyroid & Adrenal Interrelations, 7: 52–57 (1947).
2. Venning, E. H.: Glycogenic Corticoids, 7: 79–101 (1947).
3. Forbes, *et al.*: 17-Ketosteroids in Trauma and Disease, 7: 264–288 (1947).
4. Talbot, *et al.*: Excretion of 11-Oxycorticosteroids, 7: 331–350 (1947).
5. Castillo, E. B. del, *et al.*: Syndrome of Rudimentary Ovaries, 7: 385–422 (1947).
6. Forsham, P. H., *et al.*: Pituitary Adrenocorticotropin, 8: 15–66 (1948).
7. Pincus, G., *et al.*: Rhythm in Biped Excretion, 8: 221–226 (1948).
8. LeCompte, P. M.: Width of Adrenal Cortex in Lymphatic Leukemia, 9: 158–162 (1949).
9. Wolfson, W. Q.: 17-Ketosteroids in Gout, 9: 497–513 (1949).
10. Stein, H. J., *et al.*: Hormonal Response to Heat and Cold, 9: 529–547 (1949).
11. Davis, M. E.: Eosinophils in Pregnancy and Labor, 9: 714–724 (1949).
12. Conn, J. W.: Na and Cl of Sweat as Cortical Index, 10: 12–23 (1950).
13. Recant, L., *et al.*: Effect of Epinephrine on Eosinophils, 10: 187–229 (1950).
14. McArthur, J. W., *et al.*: Urinary Excretion of Corticosteroids in Diabetic Acidosis, 10: 307–312 (1950).
15. Bors, E.: Fertility in Paraplegic Males, 10: 381–398 (1950).
16. Grossman, S., *et al.*: Idiopathic Lactation following thoracoplasty, 10: 729–734 (1950).
17. Cooper, J. S., *et al.*: Metabolic Consequences of Spinal Cord Injury, 10: 858–870 (1950).
18. Hioco, D.: Adrenal Metabolites in Bronchial Asthma, 10: 1570–1578 (1950).
19. Jailer, J. W.: Pituitary-Adrenal System in Infants, 11: 186–192 (1951).
20. Deane, H. W.: The Adrenals in Experimental Hypertension, 11: 193–208 (1951).
21. Hioco, D., *et al.*: Epinephrine and ACTH in Bronchial Asthma, 11: 395–407 (1951).
22. Schaffenberg, C. A., *et al.*: p-Hydroxypropiophenone (PHP) and other so-called pituitary inhibitors, 11: 1215–1223 (1951).
23. Talbot, N. B., *et al.*: Urinary Water-Soluble Corticosteroids, 11: 1223–1236 (1951).

Citation Index Entry

11123s-687

464-9789(R)
869-3366(R)
1105-9876(A)
1123-4432(R)
a11,123-0752(O)
-0779(O)
-7264(O)
-7331(O)
-7385(O)
-0866(O)
-8221(O)
-9158(O)
-9497(O)
-9529(O)

article is even cited but not referred to in the text. Selye's influence on all of these authors is quite apparent. In particular instances the citations are of value in locating confirmatory evidence of some of Selye's claims.

Thus, in the case of a highly significant article, the citation index has a quantitative value, for it may help the historian to measure the influence of the article—that is, its "impact factor." With regard to a less significant work, one would suspect that the bibliographic advantages might be increased, because the scientist or librarian would be provided with references not to be found in conventional indexes. The preliminary evidence presented indicates that the citation index offers interesting possibilities for another approach to bibliographic control.

The next step in compiling the index for the Selye article would be to seek out additional references to it in more peripheral journals, but obviously the farther away you get from the immediate subject area of the main article, the fewer the references to it you will locate. Yet these may well be the most useful references of all, for the cross-fertilization of subject fields is one of our most important problems in science literature.

It will be well to close with a brief description of how the citation index might be compiled. The first step would be the selection of the particular group of periodicals to be covered; next, the period to be covered, say, only that since 1900.

The problem actually has two facets: the selection of periodicals to be covered in order to obtain citations, and the selection of those articles for which we want a citation record. For example, all *articles* in journals in the *Current List of Medical Literature* that have remained in continuous publication since 1900 might be coded, in which case the *Journal of Clinical Endocrinology* would not be included. However, we might include as citation sources all *journals* covered by the *Current List*. Thus, the bibliographies appearing in articles in the *Journal of Clinical Endocrinology* would supply references to the basic group of articles.

Each coder would be assigned a group of articles in a particular journal. The first step would be to number each article in the journal in ascending order, by utilizing a complete table of contents of that journal from its inception.

Once a code number has been assigned to each article, the proper codes may then be assigned to each periodical. This might be the number given in the *World List*, with new numbers for any periodicals not to be found there.

Actual coding starts with the first article in a particular periodical. The coder prepares a 3- by 5-in. card in each citation made in the article. Each card should give (i) the code number for the citing article, (ii) the code number for the article cited, and (iii) a classification of the citing article as an original contribution, review article, abstract, and so forth.

Many references will be excluded by the limits of coverage set up. Thus all references to articles not in the prescribed list of journals would be excluded.

All books would be excluded unless otherwise specified, in which case the reference card would carry the code for the citing article and the code for the book (its LC card number).

After all the articles had been coded, it would next be necessary to sort the cards by the code numbers for the items cited. This would yield a group of cards for each cited article. These would then be sorted by code numbers for the citing articles. This completes the coding and sorting. The next step would be preparation for the printer.

From this description it will be apparent that, although a great volume of material is to be covered, relatively unskilled persons can perform the necessary coding and filing. Professional supervision would still be required, because certain decisions require skilled judgment, for example, when *ibid.* or *loc. cit.* must be carefully interpreted. Footnotes tend to make coding somewhat cumbersome. The code I have described is merely an example used to illustrate the method in principle. If the system were adopted, then in the future every author ought to be required to include the serial number of each item he referred to, so as to facilitate not only the compilation of citation indexes but also other operations such as requests for reprints[15, 16].

In a certain sense a citation index is not very different from a compendium like *Beilstein,* which gives a rather complete record of a compound, compiled by a similar method. A citation index for the literature of chemistry would undoubtedly make the preparation of such works as *Beilstein* much easier than it is at present. The new bibliographic tool, like others that already exist, is just a starting point in literature research. It will help in many ways, but one should not expect it to solve all our problems.

REFERENCES

1. P. THOMASSON AND J. C. STANLEY. Science 121, 610 (1955). Thomasson and Stanley were commenting on C. Zirkle's discussion of the use of fraudulent data Science 120, 189 (1954).
2. W. C. ADAIR. Am Documentation 6, 31 (1955).
3. H. C. LEHMAN. SCI Monthly 78, 321 (1954).
4. W. DENNIS. *ibid.* 79, 180 (1954).
5. P. L. K. GROSS AND E. M GROSS. Science 66, 385 (1927).
6. E. BRODMAN. Med. Library Assoc. Bull. 32, 479 (1944).
7. H. H. FUSSLER. Library Quart. 19, 19 (1949).

8. H. Bitner. Personal Communication, April 1954.
9. V. K. Zworykin and L. E. Flory. Proc. Am. Phil. Soc. 91, 139 (1947).
10. R. R. Shaw. Machines and the Bibliographical Problems of the Twentieth Century (Univ. of Illinois Press, Urbana, 1951), p. 19. Reprinted from *Bibliography in an Age of Science* (Univ. of Illinois Press, Urbana, 1951).
11. R. Busa. Nachr. Dokumentation 3, 14 (1952).
12. A. M. Andrew. Electronic Eng. 25, 471 (1953).
13. E. Garfield. Review literature as a source of critical entries for scientific indexes. Unpublished paper. December 1952.
14. H. Selye. J. Clin. Endocrinol. 6, 117 (1946).
15. E. Garfield, Science 120, 1039 (1954).
16. J. A. Behnke, Science 120, 1055 (1954).

The Welch Medical Library Indexing Project*

By Sanford V. Larkey, M.D.

Director and Librarian, Welch Medical Library
Johns Hopkins University, Baltimore, Md.

I AM very happy to have this opportunity to report to the Association on some of the aspects of the Welch Medical Library Indexing Project, which has been going on now for about three and one-half years. This research program is supported by the Armed Forces Medical Library through a contract between it and the Johns Hopkins University.

The background of the project—how the Welch Library, after World War II, was interested in a program for training medical librarians with the necessary research aspects; the interest expressed by the then Army Medical Library in the research side of the program; and the eventual negotiation of a research contract—has already been given in the BULLETIN in the report of the meeting of the Honorary Consultants to the Army Medical Library of 1948[1]; so I will not repeat the details here.

Our own plans covered a fairly large area of medical bibliography, but with particular emphasis on the problems of indexing of periodical literature, including, by extension, the related aspects of abstract journals, review journals, etc. I believe the statement of the scope of the project, as given in the contract, will give some idea of the general picture:

"To study the problems of indexing medical literature.

To explore the theory and practice of subject heading (nomenclature) and classification (coding) as they concern medical literature.

To explore existing and projected methods, emphasizing machine methods, applicable to medical bibliography, operating such pilot projects as may be necessary, and to report on the suitability of machine methods in the bibliographic operations of the Army Medical Library."

* Read at the 51st Annual Meeting, Medical Library Association, Lake Placid, N. Y., June 24–27, 1952.

[1] Larkey, Sanford V. The Army Medical Library Research Project at the Welch Medical Library. BULLETIN, 37: 121–124, April 1949.

Originally published in *Bulletin of the Medical Library Association,* Volume 41 (January, 1953), pp. 32-40. Reprinted by permission.

As you can see, the first sentence covers a very large area and really states the whole problem. When taken in connection with the other two points, this charge has worked out in practice to mean the evaluation and study of present indexing and abstracting services, including studies of their coverage of the medical literature, of their methods of indexing, and of their use.

One way to learn something about how indexing and abstracting services are used is to ask those who use them. We decided to do this, asking directly through interviews rather than by questionnaires. We interviewed a fairly large number of medical librarians and scientists, and many of you generously took part in such interviews at the Galveston meeting. The analysis and study of these interviews gave us many valuable leads, but in the meantime there have been so many changes in the indexes and abstract journals, that further studies along these lines will be needed.

Studies have been made of the coverage of journals and of articles within journals by individual services, but a detailed analysis of the coverage of all or almost all medical literature requires a knowledge of what periodicals are available in the world in medicine and related fields. Since a principal objective of the project in this regard was to determine the scope and coverage desirable in a medical index, with special reference to one published by the Armed Forces Medical Library, it was decided to compile a list of the world's medical journals, on IBM punched cards, with facts included which would give information as to scope, coverage by indexing and abstracting services, and features for evaluation of the journals as to their possible inclusion in a medical index. Details of the present status of this part of the project will be given later in the paper.

Similarly, I will defer discussion of the other aspects, namely subject indexing and subject headings, and machine methods, although work on all phases has been proceeding simultaneously. Since progress reports on all aspects of the project have been given every year to the Honorary Consultants to the Army Medical Library and published in the BULLETIN[2], it is not intended to review these developments but to tell now only of the present status of certain things we are doing.

PSYCHOLOGY OF MACHINES

I think I should say something about "machines" themselves at this point. Since we are using machines in all the major phases of our work, I would like to describe the machines we are using and just how we are using them. I will discuss the present status of each phase of our work primarily on the basis of the machine operations involved. Another reason for this approach is that we

[2] BULLETIN, 38: 113–116, April 1950; 39: 87–89, April 1951; 40: 107–112, April 1952.

have found in discussing our program with others, our use of machines seems either to interest or worry people more than any other feature.

This brings me to what might be called the "psychology of machines." The very word "machines" seems to do things to people. We hear talk of "electronic robots," as though they were some sort of "men from Mars" who could take over all intellectual activities by merely pushing buttons. This sort of talk leads to excessive hopes or to inordinate fears and precludes objective thinking about the possible uses of machines. One should consider machines as practical adjuncts, as we do typewriters, 3 x 5 cards, and visible indexes. Machines are only doing very rapidly what one could do with his own eyes and brain if he had all the time in the world to do it and wanted to do it. There is no magic about it.

There is, however, a more valid psychological aspect to machines. Since machines operate on a strict yes-or-no principle, we must be rigidly exact in presenting a problem. Each step must be in the most precise logical form, since one rarely can stop to correct as one goes along. Each step must be gone over and over in relation to every other one. One has to think not once, but many times. Programming often takes almost as long as the machine operation itself, but the end result is still reached much more quickly than by manual operations.

These strict limitations of machines have been very useful to us. They not only have tightened up our own thinking processes, but their application has emphasized many semantic inconsistencies in our terminology and classifications. So, perhaps there may be a good psychological side to machines.

Machines and Our Use of Them

Our machines at least have a very respectable genealogy. As Raymond Pearl[3] has pointed out, it was John Shaw Billings, who, while working on the 1880 census, suggested to Mr. Herman Hollerith the idea of punching holes in cards for recording data and then sorting by mechanical means. Mr. Hollerith invented the basic IBM machines. It is not known if Billings ever thought of applying the principle to bibliographical work, but it would seem eminently fitting that it might be so utilized.

The machines we are now using in the project are all IBM equipment and I will confine myself largely to a description of these and of our uses of them. Most of these machines were designed primarily for statistical and accounting uses, including tabulating, and their application to or modification for our purposes is one of the tasks confronting us. There are, however, many operations which are applicable to our purposes, and we are trying to make the best use of them.

[3] Pearl, Raymond. Some contributions of Dr. John Shaw Billings to the development of vital statistics. Bull. Inst. Hist. Med. 6: 387–393, May 1938.

I think it will be well to describe what the machines can do in some detail, since it will make clearer what I will have to say about our application of them. I will speak of these functions in terms of the card, because cards are our units of information, on which have been punched items of information, either numerically or alphabetically as words or abbreviations. Codes could be either or both. Probably the basic thing a machine can do is to *sort*, that is, pick out cards which have a common characteristic or characteristics and put them together in packs. A machine can *count* these cards or certain points of information punched in the cards. Another machine, the collator, can *match* like cards or various punches in cards, and *merge* two decks of cards in a numerical or alphabetical sequence. Other machines, the tabulators and card-operated typewriters, can *print* what has been punched on cards.

A special type of sorting is what has been termed "searching." This involves the selecting out of cards which meet complex requirements of punches or combinations of punches. This procedure can be carried out with some of the ordinary standard machines, but would take so many steps that it would not be practical in point of view of time and effort except for very small files of cards. The problem is now being approached by means of much more elaborate IBM machines—the 101 and another designed especially for this purpose.

We are using or have some familiarity with all of these IBM machines. The first group of machines are those used for preparing the cards. Our cards are prepared with an interpreting punch which simultaneously prints on the card what has been punched. Cards are then checked on the verifier if necessary. A reproducer is used when duplication of a large number of cards is desired or when there is a common item to be punched into a number of cards. This latter operation is known as "gang punching." By use of prepared number decks or special attachments, continuous serial numbers can be punched in a file of cards. We have used other standard machines for sorting, collating, and printing. We are now using the IBM 101 electronic statistical machine for most of our sorting but particularly for searching.

IBM machines are activated by an electrical current set up by contact of brushes through the holes punched in the cards. The operation of the ordinary sorter is relatively simple. Operating on only one column at a time, an electric impulse is initiated by the brush contact through the hole in the card. The impulse travels through a set of electro-magnetic relays and causes a chute to open. This directs the card to a pocket corresponding to the punch in the column. But it is when more complex patterns are needed that the electronic element comes in, as in the 101; for here, a great number of matching operations, that is, matches between what is desired and what is punched in a card, are performed in an amazingly short period of time. This is accomplished by setting up on a wiring board, somewhat like a telephone switchboard, extensive and complicated selector circuits which send currents through series of electronically controlled relays. Such electronic set-ups are used in many of the more complicated IBM machines, and notably in the 101. Such a system is almost essential for any high speed searching device. Our work covers a wide range of these operations, from the simplest to some of the most complicated. In some phases we have used machines almost entirely as a research tool while in others the machine is the all-important or essential feature. I intend now to describe certain areas of our work, emphasizing the role of the machines, but also to tell you something of the overall status of our work in these areas.

Subject Heading Studies

One of the great difficulties in compiling and in using indexes of any kind has been that of the subject headings themselves, the essential key to the index. There has been little standardization of headings used by various indexes and even inconsistencies in usage within a single index. A great deal of this trouble stems from basic inadequacies and inconsistencies in medical terminology and nomenclature. Subject headings have attempted to keep up with changing terminology, but since the headings are usually in alphabetical lists, it is very difficult to work out relationships. It was our plan to transform alphabetical lists of subject headings to a categorized arrangement. We started by using conventional 3 x 5 cards, typing on these cards the headings and cross references with complete tracings, from *Quarterly Cumulative Index Medicus*, *Index-Catalogue*, and other sources. Category arrangements were then attempted. Preliminary results of these studies convinced us that we were on the right track. For instance, striking discrepancies were shown up in the field of chemistry.

It was not until last year that we began to use punched cards for this part of our work. We started then to put on punched cards all the headings used by *Current List* in the first five months of 1951. The actual heading was put down in full by alphabetical punching and code numbers punched for category sorting. As it turned out, we were very glad we had gone over to punched cards, for this file was the basis for the later studies for revision of the *Current List* headings now being used.

I am not going to say much about the basis for the revision since Mr. Seymour Taine will tell of that. I will only mention some of the machine features. By category sorting and then printing lists from the punched cards, we were able to study the terms used in restricted fields and to compare them against other authorities. For instance, having based our category code for diseases on the World Health Organization International Statistical Classification, we sorted on these code numbers and then could compare the terms used by *Current List* with all the terms in the WHO classification for each specific group of diseases.

The staff of the *Current List* and the project cooperated on similar studies for all of the categories, and the revised cards constituted the main subject heading deck.

See and *See also* references were punched on cards and by machine methods put in the proper order with the main subject headings. Lists were then printed from the cards. This was the tentative authority list. The next step was to add the tracings, *See from* and *See also from* cards. A good part of the compilation and punching of these was done by machine methods. The last printing was done directly onto Multilith mats, making it possible to produce a large number of copies of the list. Here we have made most extensive utilization of the ***printing*** function of the machines.

We will continue our category studies, with comparison of terms from many other sources. While we realize we can never have a permanent standard authority, we hope we can make an approach to something like this and to have a method for logical and fairly easy revision.

Journal List on Punched Cards

In the compilation of the list of the world's medical serials on punched cards, the machines were intended to be used primarily as research tools. Since analyses of scope, coverage by indexing and abstracting services, and evaluation of the thousands of titles require compilation and study from a number of different axes, it was believed that machines would be a great saving of time and would provide more extensive and accurate statistical data. At the same time, the sorting and printing features of the machines would enable us to have preliminary groupings or listings along any line desired. We now have about 7000 serial titles represented in our file.

The information about each journal has been taken from the journal itself, from the latest issue for current information (title, sponsorship, country, publisher, language, frequency, etc.) and from a whole volume for more general information (type, contents, and subject fields covered). To date, information has been assembled from the Armed Forces Medical Library, the Library of the American Medical Association, and the Welch Library. Preliminary checks have been made against the holdings of the New York Academy of Medicine and the Library of National Institutes of Health. The staff of the Armed Forces Medical Library is supplying us with data sheets of information on its holdings and we could not have done anything without its help.

After the information is collected, it is then punched on cards as follows: a number code for alphabetizing, abbreviation of the title, code numbers for language, country, frequency, type, contents, and major and minor subject fields. In addition to this information about the journal itself, other types of information are being assembled and punched in code on the cards. These include coverage by indexing and abstracting services, holdings by libraries, inclusion on selective lists, such as the MLA list of recommended periodicals.

We are thus able to make analyses from many different points of view. We have made a number of preliminary studies which have included statistical studies of coverage by *Current List*, *QCIM*, *Excerpta Medica*, *Biological Abstracts*, and *Chemical Abstracts*, comparative studies of the coverage by combinations of these, studies of coverage by country and by subject by *Current List* and by *QCIM*, and listing of indexing and abstracting services, and of other journals publishing indexes and/or abstracts. Some of the studies have been previously reported in the BULLETIN. I might say that one form of information most difficult to come by is that of coverage. Very few services publish lists of the journals they cover and we have been eagerly awaiting the publication of *Periodica Medica Mundi*. If it does not appear soon, we may have to go through the entire year's file of a service to pick out the journals covered. Even this might be worthwhile, for we believe an analysis of this coverage would be a valuable thing in itself and a factor in evaluation.

Our earlier analyses were done with a standard Sorter. Now that we are using the 101 machine, we will be able to make more complicated analyses, generally at one pass, and also have counts on all items registered by machine. At the present time we are working at bringing our file up to date, planning for adding information on additional items of information that we can dig out. We plan to set a deadline in the late fall and then to begin a series of detailed analyses, leading to evaluation studies.

One of the advantages of having such a file on punched cards is that it can easily be integrated with similar punched card files, such as those proposed by the Library of Congress. At present we have a limitation in the printing feature of the machine, in that we can print from our card only an abbreviated title. This is really all that is necessary for a research tool, but as the demand arises for printed lists with full title and publisher, we will have to provide additional cards to do this. We have worked out designs for these.

MACHINE INDEXING AND SEARCHING

The term machine indexing has acquired two rather different meanings. In the first place it may mean the preparing and printing of a printed index by machine methods, or it may mean an information searching system wherein the various subject concepts of a document are represented in code on punched cards, or on other media, and a machine is used to select out the desired items.

There are a number of instances of printed indexes produced by machines but not, so far as I know, in the field of medicine. We are considering, on an experimental basis, the possibilities of preparing the entire *Current List*, by machine methods. Mr. Eugene Garfield of the project has worked out a detailed procedure, utilizing a number of IBM machines. I want to emphasize that the machine cannot perform the intellectual side of reading articles and of subject indexing. The machines take over only after this has been done. All of the entries, as they now appear in the *Current List*, in the Register and in the Subject and Author indexes, will be on punched cards. All of the numbering, sorting, merging with subject and cross reference entries, and arranging in alphabetical and subject order will be done by machine. The copy for photo-offset printing, except at present for the Register entry, will be printed from the punches in the cards. I will not go into any details now, as we are just beginning our first pilot run. If the method appears to be practicable, we plan to study its application to other types and formats of indexes.

Because there has been a feeling that modern science demands a more rapid, a more thorough, and a more detailed correlation of the facts set forth in scientific literature than apparently is possible with present printed or card indexes, attention has turned to machines as a way of accomplishing this. In a machine searching operation, the facts or subject concepts of a document must be symbolized by codes which can then be represented by punches in a card. The fundamental practices of analysing a document, let us say a periodical article, are essentially the same as in present subject indexing. One must still read the article to find what it is about and what are its salient facts. Assuming this, the various subject concepts in the article are assigned code designations from a pre-arranged code. The code designations for all of the subject concepts in an article are then punched on a card or cards, along with a serial number identifying the document. It is the code numbers for which the machine searches, correlating those in the card or cards representing a single document for answers to a specific question requiring a certain combination of code numbers.

Suppose, for a simple example, the number 90015 represents the concept *pulmonary tuberculosis* and 35062 *Streptomycin*. If one wanted all articles on streptomycin treatment of pulmonary tuberculosis, the machine would be set to pick out all those cards which have both of these numbers punched in them. In our earlier work with a sorter and collator, it was necessary to have the code numbers for various categories in a fixed order and in a fixed place on the card. This was also true of earlier work with the 101 machine, but now Mr. Garfield has worked out an amazing but fundamental wiring system for the 101 which permits searching for any 5-digit number in any one of 16 five-column fields on a card. His system permits searching for up to 48 such 5 digit numbers in various combinations at one time. This will allow a number of separate questions to be asked at one time.

At present we are experimenting with arbitrary numerical codes but will soon use actual coding from indexing articles. I will not give any details since the project will prepare a comprehensive report. One should realize though what the machine is doing here. As described earlier, there is a very rapid matching operation going on for each card, correlating the desired combinations of all these 48 individual codes with those codes punched in the card. The cards are going through the machine at the rate of 450 a minute.

Machines may speed up searching operations; they should permit greater depth of indexing and possibly greater coverage of the literature; and there should be greater possibilities of correlation since the machine can search for any combination of concepts. Whether these advantages will outweigh the values of printed indexes or partially so, only time and more study will tell.

Summary and Conclusion

I have tried to tell you of some of the problems we have been working on and where they are leading us. I still believe, as I said almost four years ago, before the project started, "that our present indexes are extremely valuable bibliographical aids and that while a search is being made for new methods, including machine methods, the improvement of these indexes in something like their present form must be a primary consideration."[4] A great deal of our work has been along these lines. It is quite possible that machines will help in solving some of the problems. We have found that their practical application has been greater and more useful than we had anticipated. Familiarity has bred anything but contempt.

In conclusion, I should like to point out that, while our work and our findings are primarily for the use of the Armed Forces Medical Library, we feel that they will be applicable to other fields just as we have profited greatly from work others are doing. Coordination of research in bibliographical problems in all fields should benefit all.

[4] Larkey, S. V., op. cit.

Machines in Medical Libraries

By Estelle Brodman
The Library and the Department of Anatomy
Washington University School of Medicine
St. Louis, Missouri, U.S.A.

The tasks that computers can perform in the field of library administration are discussed in the light of the author's own experience in this field. The next few years should see the computer firmly ensconced in medical libraries and accepted with the same lack of surprise as copying machines and typewriters are at the moment. All in all, it is an exciting time to be connected with medical libraries.

MEDICAL libraries, especially medical school libraries, have come a long way from the situation described by John Shaw Billings in 1876,

"... almost all attempts to establish medical libraries in connection with medical schools have been failures. Commenced with enthusiasm, they soon become antiquated, are rarely consulted, except by one or two species of beetles, are never properly catalogued or cared for, and dust and mold reign in them supreme. Students and teachers want the newest books and journals only."

The reason has to do as much with the way in which medicine has changed in that period as with changes in medical libraries and librarians *per se*. In a world where medical and paramedical workers must continue to study for the whole of their lives, where advances in medicine are made more frequently in medical schools than in any other single class of institution, where the methods of teaching require constant recourse to published literature, the medical school library has become essential. One thing, however, has not changed; "students and teachers want the newest books and journals." It follows that they want them speedily and they want to find the data in them again when needed. To that end, medical libraries have begun to turn to machines for many routines, thus freeing their staffs for more individualized tasks.

Libraries are reflections of the culture around them, and it is inconceivable that any library in the western world today would be without typewriters, telephones, electric lights, inside plumbing, copying machines for users and staff, or a place for the staff to make morning coffee. When the discussion concerns "machines in medical libraries" today,

Originally published in *Medical and Biological Illustration*, Volume 16 (October, 1966), pp. 238-242. Reprinted by permission.

however, most people think of punched cards, computers, closed-circuit television, and apparatus which a few years ago would have been the province of the science fiction writer. The interest in data processing is intensified by the emergence of MEDLARS (Medical Literature Analysis and Retrieval System) developed by the National Library of Medicine in Bethesda, Maryland, U.S.A., and, in Great Britain, by the announcement that it will be made available in the United Kingdom through the offices of the National Lending Library. It seems appropriate, therefore, to discuss some facets of this work and to make cautious predictions of the impact which these machines will have on medical libraries and their users.

A good deal of the work of medical library staffs is connected with the routine of seeing that material is acquired, properly catalogued and indexed, and arranged physically so that it can be found when desired, and that records of its whereabouts are available at all times. All this is necessary before the more interesting task of extracting the data contained in the physical volumes can be carried out. Medical librarians have always

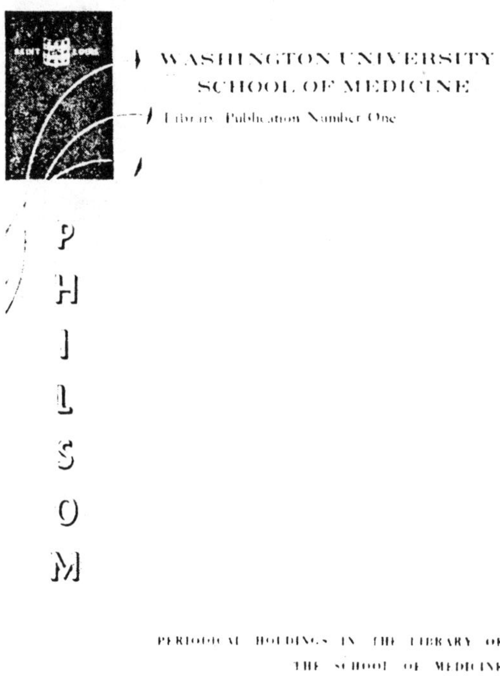

Fig. 1 *PHILSOM (Periodical Holdings in Library of School of Medicine, Washington University).*

tended to begrudge the time spent on these routine tasks, considering them as chores which kept them from undertaking the work for which they had entered the profession—helping the medical scientist to obtain the information he needs—but they were aware of the absolute necessity of carrying on these routines in order to serve their readers. They therefore appointed clerks to do the repetitive but exacting record-keeping.

Recently, as the volume of literature has expanded, the amount of such work has grown enormously and the work force of clerks has grown smaller and more expensive, so that some other way had to be sought to prevent the library's routine "underpinning" from collapsing. Punched card methods were first introduced into medical libraries in the 1940s and 1950s, but their help was only meagre. When electronic data processing machines, particularly computers, were developed in the 1960s and were made available to many of the institutions with which the medical libraries were associated (e.g., hospitals and universities), much more use began to be made of machines for performing routine library tasks. The pious hope that computers would free trained librarians to do research into the literature has, unfortunately, not yet turned out to be a reality. As one librarian wryly observed, "These labour-saving devices don't save the

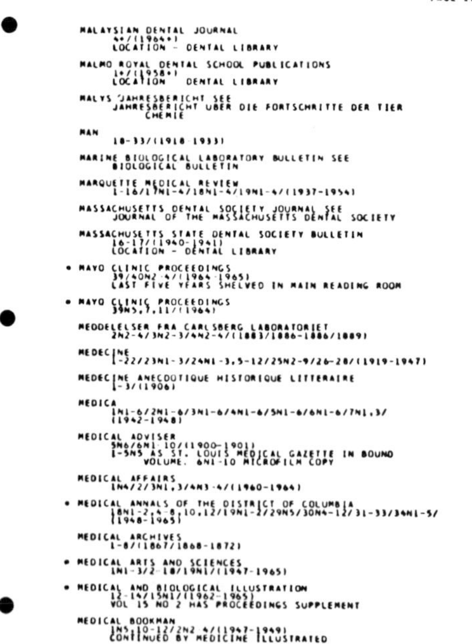

```
                                                        PAGE 119

  MALAYSIAN DENTAL JOURNAL
        4+/(1964+)
        LOCATION - DENTAL LIBRARY
  MALMO ROYAL DENTAL SCHOOL PUBLICATIONS
        1+/(1958+)
        LOCATION   DENTAL LIBRARY
  MALYS 'JAHRESBERICHT SEE
        JAHRESBERICHT UBER DIE FORTSCHRITTE DER TIER
              CHEMIE
  MAN
        18-33/(1918-1933)
  MARINE BIOLOGICAL LABORATORY BULLETIN SEE
        BIOLOGICAL BULLETIN
  MARQUETTE MEDICAL REVIEW
        1-16/17N1-4/18N1-4/19N1-4/(1937-1954)
  MASSACHUSETTS DENTAL SOCIETY JOURNAL SEE
        JOURNAL OF THE MASSACHUSETTS DENTAL SOCIETY
  MASSACHUSETTS STATE DENTAL SOCIETY BULLETIN
        16-17/(1940-1941)
        LOCATION - DENTAL LIBRARY
* MAYO CLINIC PROCEEDINGS
        39/40N2-4/(1964-1965)
        LAST FIVE YEARS SHELVED IN MAIN READING ROOM
* MAYO CLINIC PROCEEDINGS
        39N5,7,11/(1964)
  MEDDELELSER FRA CARLSBERG LABORATORIET
        2N2-4/3N2-3/4N2-4/(1883/1886-1886/1889)
  MEDECINE
        1-22/23N1-3/24N1-3,5-12/25N2-9/26-28/(1919-1947)
  MEDECINE ANECDOTIQUE HISTORIQUE LITTERAIRE
        1-3/(1906)
  MEDICA
        1N1-6/2N1-6/3N1-6/4N1-6/5N1-6/6N1-6/7N1,3/
        (1942-1948)
  MEDICAL ADVISER
        5N6/6N1-10/(1900-1901)
        1-5N5 AS ST. LOUIS MEDICAL GAZETTE IN BOUND
              VOLUME. 6N1-10 MICROFILM COPY
  MEDICAL AFFAIRS
        1N4/2/3N1,3/4N3-4/(1960-1964)
* MEDICAL ANNALS OF THE DISTRICT OF COLUMBIA
        18N1-2,4-8,10,12/19N1-2/29N5/30N4-12/31-33/34N1-5/
        (1948-1965)
  MEDICAL ARCHIVES
        1-8/(1867/1868-1872)
* MEDICAL ARTS AND SCIENCES
        1N1-3/2-18/19N1/(1947-1965)
* MEDICAL AND BIOLOGICAL ILLUSTRATION
        12-14/15N1/(1962-1965)
        VOL 15 NO 2 HAS PROCEEDINGS SUPPLEMENT
  MEDICAL BOOKMAN
        1N5,10-12/2N2-4/(1947-1949)
        CONTINUED BY MEDICINE ILLUSTRATED
```

Fig. 2 *Sample page from PHILSOM. Asterisks indicate that the title is indexed in* Index Medicus.

labour of librarians so much as the labour of the librarians' clerks." If anything, computers have required so many additional staff of so different a level of knowledge that the overall cost of running a library with computers is nearly the same, or possibly even greater, than with conventional methods. Money and the people to perform the more glamorous jobs connected with data processing equipment are somewhat easier to find than clerical staff. A further difference is that some by-products are obtained from the machine that are not economically available using manual methods.

Punched cards are the beginning, both historically and in today's schedule of operations, of data processing. Developed by Herman Hollerith, following a suggestion from John Shaw Billings in the 1870s, they were first used on a large scale in the 1880 Census of the United States to tabulate and count the census returns. Essentially, it is a system whereby holes are punched manually in the cards in a certain designated pattern. Later, the cards are sorted by passing an electrical circuit through the places where the holes might be: those which carry holes at certain points are shunted into one pocket and those without these holes into another pocket. It is then a simple matter to count the representatives in each pocket.

This was the incunabula period of data processing, and it should be noted that this system had a number of limitations. It was comparatively slow, in that each card had to be scanned by the machine, column by column. More important, it could not retain any of the data on the card; once the number of holes had been determined or the cards sorted into the various pockets, the work of the punched card machine was over. Further, the data recorded on any one card could only be equal to the number of columns in the card times the number of positions in that column (80 columns with 12 places in each column, or 960 variations in the common tabulating card configuration), so that many cards were needed for any comprehensive record. The punching of the cards themselves was a chore, especially at first, when the machines did not visually present to the operator the information being coded into the card.

It must not be concluded that these machines were totally useless for libraries. Many large university libraries in the United States used punched card machines, tied in with tabulators and accounting machines, which printed out (and sometimes even performed simple arithmetical operations like summing) in their fiscal accounting. Often the first experience librarians had with data processing was in the form of fund balances and cheques from their institution's business office, and many small department stores today still use a similar system for customer accounts.

These punched card systems are generally designated "unit card records" because each card or group of cards forming a single record can only be handled as a unit. They are not capable of storing or manipulating the information in the punched cards except in the most primitive fashion. The development of computers, which are capable of performing these tasks, changed the entire picture of record-keeping in business and made feasible the use of machines in medical research (such as computing electro-encephalographic data) and in medical libraries. These machines are very speedy, very accurate, and apparently tireless. On the other hand, they are not capable of varying the routines built into them in any way, and so when data are fed into them in a manner deviating even slightly from the established pattern, the computer is unable to process them and either stops altogether or rejects the data. At present, most computers still obtain their data from punched cards (or now, punched tapes), although methods to place the data in the computer in simpler ways are being investigated at the moment. Since the punched card is the mainstay of the computer process, and since the computer is rigid in what it will or will not manipulate, the demand for consistency and accuracy which it places on the human operator who prepares the punched cards is enormous. In this sense, the machine is a much more demanding "boss" than the most inflexible and rigid human supervisory martinet.

Another computer necessity, which is not so important in manual systems, is the need to map out each step of the work in great detail and to translate these verbal steps into a form on which the computer can act. This "programming" consists essentially of transforming conventional written language into the hybrid mathematical-verbal logical analysis with which the particular computer works. A number of differernt "languages" have been evolved, such as FORTRAN, COBOL, AUTOCODER, SPS; and people interested in linguistics, as well as those interested in mathematics, have been used to draft such languages. Not all computers can work with all of them, which adds somewhat to the difficulty, since a programme written in one language (say AUTOCODER or SPS, used in the Washington University School of Medicine Library for its Serials Control) may have to be partially or wholly re-written by another library whose computer cannot accept these languages. The National Library of Medicine, for example, had to let a several-year contract to the computer facilities at the University of California in Los Angeles to re-programme its MEDLARS tape from the Honeywell 800 computer for the IBM 7090 computer, now so much more frequently installed in the United States. The author's library, now using an IBM 7072 and a 360, expects to have to do some further slight programming when the Los Angeles tapes become available to it. Automatic translation of these languages by so-called machine "compilers" has helped in some cases, but not in all.

Computers are used most economically when large mounts of data are manipulated frequently. Most libraries, and certainly most medical libraries, are on the fringes of the benefit:cost ratio, and therefore most of them would have difficulty in justifying the great expenditure needed to purchase or rent the larger computers themselves, or to maintain the staffs of programmers, clerks, operators, and maintenance people who are vital to the success of such operations. Many medical libraries, on the other hand, are in institutions which have already installed this equipment and staff for other purposes, and in such a situation the library's share of the cost becomes reasonable. The Medical Library of the University of Louisville, where no institutional computer is available, has made arrangements to rent time on the local bank's machines. The results have been very satisfactory so far.

It was on the basis that a large number of medical libraries would be able to benefit from the use of computers, once the research and development work had been done, that the Library of the Washington University School of Medicine began a series of experimental projects in 1962. Since that time, under grants from the Public Health Service, methods have been worked out for employing a computer to keep the records of the 1,500 serials received there regularly, to prepare and produce overdue notices automatically, and (more recently) to produce a printed List of Selected Acquisitions, and an author-title-subject Book Catalogue which can be consulted in the office of every department in the Medical Center (Fig. 3).

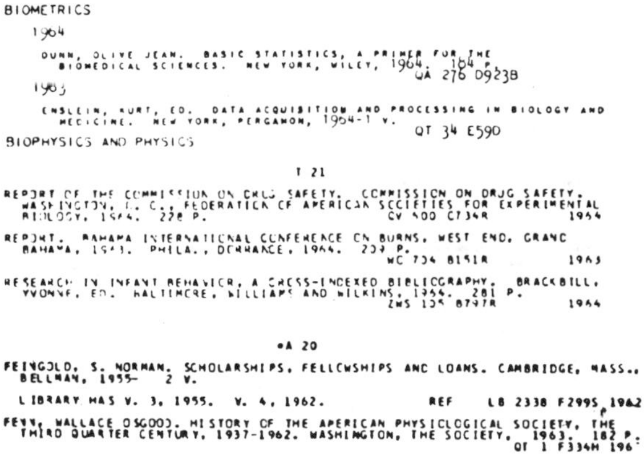

BIOMETRICS

1964

DUNN, OLIVE JEAN. BASIC STATISTICS, A PRIMER FOR THE BIOMEDICAL SCIENCES. NEW YORK, WILEY, 1964. 184 P.
QA 276 D923B

1963

ENSLEIN, KURT, ED. DATA ACQUISITION AND PROCESSING IN BIOLOGY AND MEDICINE. NEW YORK, PERGAMON, 1964-1 V.
QT 34 E590

BIOPHYSICS AND PHYSICS

T 21

REPORT OF THE COMMISSION ON DRUG SAFETY. COMMISSION ON DRUG SAFETY. WASHINGTON, D. C., FEDERATION OF AMERICAN SOCIETIES FOR EXPERIMENTAL BIOLOGY, 1964. 228 P. QV 500 C734R 1964

REPORT. BAHAMA INTERNATIONAL CONFERENCE ON BURNS. WEST END, GRAND BAHAMA, 1963. PHILA., DORRANCE, 1964. 239 P. WC 734 B151R 1963

RESEARCH IN INFANT BEHAVIOR, A CROSS-INDEXED BIBLIOGRAPHY. BRACKBILL, YVONNE, ED. BALTIMORE, WILLIAMS AND WILKINS, 1964. 281 P. ZWS 105 B797R 1964

•A 20

FEINGOLD, S. NORMAN. SCHOLARSHIPS, FELLOWSHIPS AND LOANS. CAMBRIDGE, MASS., BELLMAN, 1955- 2 V.

LIBRARY HAS V. 3, 1955. V. 4, 1962. REF LB 2338 F299S 1962

FENN, WALLACE OSGOOD. HISTORY OF THE AMERICAN PHYSIOLOGICAL SOCIETY, THE THIRD QUARTER CENTURY, 1937-1962. WASHINGTON, THE SOCIETY, 1963. 182 P. QT 1 F334H 196

Fig. 3 *Specimen entries from the Selected Acquisitions List (the Subject Index is in the same format), the Title Index and the Author Index of the Annual Catalogue.*

These methods, which were naturally very expensive to develop (the serials project cost about $20,000), are inexpensive to run after development. In line with the Public Health Service's belief in the desirability of communicating research results, and because the purposes of the research demand it, the Library has publicized these methods in professional journals. An application for training predoctoral library students here in machine methods through a one-year internship has been approved by the Public Health Service. As a result, a number of medical and university libraries around the country have begun to use or modify some of the methods developed here, as well as to develop their own systems.

As mentioned elsewhere, libraries have used computers mostly for record-keeping operations, especially the traditional library records of acquisition (to show which books and journals have been acquired, how much money has been spent, how much is still available, which journals need to be bound, what items that should have been received have not been obtained), indexing (either the book catalogue or the great *Index Medicus* and the whole MEDLARS programme), and accounting for their whereabouts (circulation routines). Smaller programmes of Selective Dissemination of Information have been tried in various libraries, including the author's (Fig. 4). These match up the subjects in which a reader indicates an interest with the subjects found in incoming works and then lists for him those books and articles (or summaries of them) which reach a certain level of agreement with his interests.

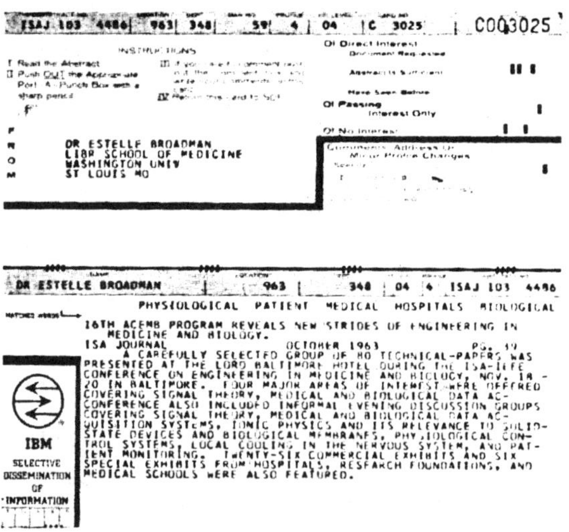

ISAJ 103 4486 | 963 | 348 | 59 | 4 | 04 | C 3025 | C003025

INSTRUCTIONS

I Read the Abstract

II Push OUT the Appropriate Port. A Punch Box with a sharp pencil

IV Return this card to SCI

Of Direct Interest

Document Requested

Abstract Is Sufficient

Have Seen Before

Of Passing Interest Only

Of No Interest

Comments, Address Or Minor Profile Changes

FROM

DR ESTELLE BROADMAN
LIBR SCHOOL OF MEDICINE
WASHINGTON UNIV
ST LOUIS MO

DR ESTELLE BROADMAN | 963 | 348 | 04 | 4 | ISAJ 103 4496

MATCHED WORDS → PHYSIOLOGICAL PATIENT MEDICAL HOSPITALS BIOLOGICAL

16TH ACEMB PROGRAM REVEALS NEW STRIDES OF ENGINEERING IN MEDICINE AND BIOLOGY.
ISA JOURNAL OCTOBER 1963 PG. 39
A CAREFULLY SELECTED GROUP OF 80 TECHNICAL-PAPERS WAS PRESENTED AT THE LORD BALTIMORE HOTEL DURING THE ISA-IEFE CONFERENCE ON ENGINEERING IN MEDICINE AND BIOLOGY, NOV. 18 - 20 IN BALTIMORE. FOUR MAJOR AREAS OF INTEREST WERE OFFERED COVERING SIGNAL THEORY, MEDICAL AND BIOLOGICAL DATA AC- CONFERENCE ALSO INCLUDED INFORMAL EVENING DISCUSSION GROUPS COVERING SIGNAL THEORY, MEDICAL AND BIOLOGICAL DATA AC- QUISITION SYSTEMS, IONIC PHYSICS AND ITS RELEVANCE TO SOLID- STATE DEVICES AND BIOLOGICAL MEMBRANES, PHYSIOLOGICAL CON- TROL SYSTEMS, LOCAL COOLING IN THE NERVOUS SYSTEM, AND PAT- IENT MONITORING. TWENTY-SIX COMMERCIAL EXHIBITS AND SIX SPECIAL EXHIBITS FROM HOSPITALS, RESEARCH FOUNDATIONS, AND MEDICAL SCHOOLS WERE ALSO FEATURED.

IBM
SELECTIVE DISSEMINATION OF INFORMATION

Fig. 4 *Traditional Selective Dissemination of Information Notification Card.*

The greater and more interesting, if more difficult, problem of using computers for the automatic extraction and transmission of scientific data has, however, been only partially successful. Some problems in this aspect of the field have to do with the automatic translation of documents from one language to another—say Japanese into English. Another problem, for which a solution is devoutly to be wished, is the automatic extraction of abstracts from the texts of scientific works. Much has been done on this phase of computer work, but libraries have not been able to use it as a regular work-a-day tool. Even the method of making sure that the user obtains the texts of the items presented to him through the computer needs further study. Automatic production of microfilm copies, or display of the entire text on television-like screens, is likewise under study. The possibility of procuring input to the computer as a by-product of the setting of type for printing is another promising development.

In these problems, of course, medical libraries are not working in a world of their own. The National Library of Agriculture, for example, has begun work on automating a Pest Control Center, which may well be the basis for other specialized information services. The Library of Congress has had a team working on automation of its work for several years now, and hope for the speedy application of computers to some phases of their work is now high; this would benefit medical libraries also. The medical libraries of Columbia, Harvard, and Yale Universities have been working co-operatively on joint computer storage of their catalogues. This is an exciting era for libraries and librarians.

REFERENCES

BILLINGS, J. S. (1876). A Century of American Medicine, 1776-1876. Literature and Institutions. Amer. J. Med. Sci., 72, 439-480.

MOORE, EVELYN A., AND BRODMAN, ESTELLE (1965). Communications to the Editor. Bull. Med. Lib. Assoc., 53, 99-101.

——————————————AND COHEN, GERALDINE S. (1965). Mechanization of Library Procedures in the Medium-sized Medical Library: III. Acquisitions and Cataloging. *Ibid*, 53, 305-328.

PIZER, IRWIN H., ANDERSON, ISABELLE T, AND BRODMAN, ESTELLE (1964). Mechanization of Library Procedures in the Medium-Sized Medical Library: II. Circulation Records. *Ibid.*, 52, 370-385.

————————, FRANZ, DONALD R., AND BRODMAN, ESTELLE (1963). Mechanization of Library Procedures in the Medium-sized Medical Library: I. The Serial Record. *Ibid.*, 51, 313-338.

The Permuterm Subject Index: An Autobiographical Review

BY EUGENE GARFIELD

Institute for Scientific Information
Philadelphia, PA 19106

The Permuterm Subject Index (PSI) section of the *Science Citation Index (SCI)* was designed more than ten years ago and has been published both quarterly and annually since 1966. There is, however, no 'primordial' citable paper about the *PSI*. It has been described and discussed from different standpoints in a number of papers[1,2], but none of them provides the formal description usually accorded a new bibliographic tool. This article is intended to provide such a reference point for future workers in information science.

The *PSI* was designed in 1964 at the Institute for Scientific Information (ISI) by myself and Irving Sher, my principal research collaborator at the time. In the subsequent development of the *PSI*, contributions were also made by others, including Arthur W. Elias, who was then in charge of production operations at ISI. In the early sixties we were too preoccupied with the task of convincing the library and information community of the value of citation indexing even to consider the idea of publishing a word index. But it was a logical development once we added the *Source Index* containing full titles.

The value of the *PSI* as a 'natural language' index is now well recognized and exploited by its users, but this was not the original reason for its development. The *PSI* was developed as one solution to a problem commonly faced by users of the *Citation Index* section of the *Science Citation Index (SCI)*. While the typical scientist-user could enter the *Citation Index* with a known author or paper, other users with a limited

Originally published in *Journal of the American Society for Information Science*, Volume 27 (September—October, 1976), pp. 288-291.

knowledge of the subject often lacked a starting point for their search. Before publication of the *PSI*, we told users whose unfamiliarity with subject matter left them doubtful about a starting point to consult an encyclopedia or the subject index of a book. If these failed, we told them to use another index, such as *Chemical Abstracts, Biological Abstracts, Physics Abstracts* or *Index Medicus*. Once the user identified a relevant older paper, it could be used to begin a search in the *Citation Index*. Users of the *SCI*—and librarians in particular needed some tool with which a starting point, or what used to be called a target reference, could be quickly and easily identified.

In those days the information community was preoccupied with Key-Word-in-Context (KWIC) indexes. The development of the KWIC index, which was subsequently vigorously marketed by IBM, undoubtedly had an enormous impact[3], [4], [5]. But I was never happy with the KWIC system for a number of reasons.

First, Sher and I felt that the KWIC index was highly uneconomical for a printed index. KWIC's use of space is prodigious, and it can be extremely time-consuming to use in searches involving more than one term.

Another aspect of the KWIC system (as used for example by *Chemical Titles*) that disturbed us was its indiscriminate use of stop-lists to eliminate presumably non-significant title words. In our view, it caused considerable loss of information on many subjects of interest to some users, if not to all. Consider the effect of deleting terms like METHOD and BEHAVIOR. In order to retain much of this information, but still prevent the useless entries generated by "terms" like THE and WHICH, we developed the concept of the semi-stop list, to be used in addition to a full-stop list.

The full-stop list for the *PSI*, which contains words that are completely suppressed, was and is quite small The semi-stop words such as METHOD, BEHAVIOR, CAUSE, REPORT and TECHNIQUE are suppressed as primary terms (main entries), but not as secondary or co-terms (subentries). In addition, certain frequently used two-word phrases, which have been identified through statistical analysis of word frequencies, are kept together and treated as a single term rather than being allowed to permute separately. Such phrases as GUINEA-PIG, NEW-YORK, ESCHERICHIA-COLI and BIRTH-CONTROL appear in the *PSI* as hyphenated terms, thus reducing look-up time in many types of searches. This is done by computer in the *PSI*, while in indexes like *Chemical Titles*, it is done by a manual process called "slash and dash."

Finally, the KWIC format was rejected because a number of studies had demonstrated that users of scientific indexes generally specify two or three terms when they use coordinate indexes. We reasoned that the optimum system would precoordinate any two terms, no matter how far apart in the title.

Over ten years of *PSI* experience has confirmed that "specificity" *per se* does not guarantee efficiency of a word as a search term. If used frequently enough, a seemingly highly specific term like DNA becomes as inefficient as more general terms that are used less frequently. The converse also holds; consider the term CREATIVITY. It is general, but because of the comparatively low frequency with which it occurs in the scientific literature, it is an efficient search term. Therefore, pairing—together with precoordination—becomes essential for high-usage terms, and merely convenient for low-usage terms. Triple coordination—and even higher-level coupling—may also be desirable if two terms occur together with a third frequently enough. But the threshold must be correlated with cost of processing and printing, not only with economies in users' time. The ideal system would handle three or more terms, but this proved too costly. We therefore settled on two terms, although recently precoordination of three terms has been built into the five-year cumulative 1965-1969 *PSI*, and an improved three-term precoordination routine will be achieved in the five-year cumulative, *PSI* for 1970-74, to be published by ISI in 1977.

The choice of name for the *Permuterm Subject Index* was quite deliberate. Ohlman suggested the term *permuted* from *cyclic permutation* used in mathematics[6]. It was in that sense appropriate to KWIC indexes. *Permuterm*, however, is a complete permutation of all title words to produce all possible pairs, including, of course, the inversion of every pair. As I and others have noted before, KWIC indexes are more appropriately called *rotated indexes*[7, 8]. For example, ISI's *Rotaform Index* section of the *Index Chemicus* is rotated formula index. The *Chemical Substructure Index* (*CSI*) is also a cyclic or rotated index. Using the Wisewesser Line Notation, the *CSI* rotates the line notation to create a main entry for every substantive constituent in each notation.

For each title in the *PSI* with n title words, $n(n\text{-}1)$ word-pairs are created by permutation. After applying the full-stop list and semi-stop list, this usually produces about 40 word-pairs for the typical seven-word title. It is by no means unusual for the *PSI* to contain over 100 word-pairs for titles with 11 or more words.

In the *PSI*, every significant word in the title is permuted [not merely rotated, as in a KWIC index (7)] by computer to produce all possible pairs of terms. Every word is potentially both a primary term and a co-term. On the printed page, each permuted word-pair is arranged alphabetically by primary term. All co-terms occurring with a particular primary term are indented as subentries and listed in alphabetical order under the primary term. Dashed lines lead from the co-term to the author, whose name can be used to locate in the *Source Index* section of the *SCI* the complete bibliographic data, including the title for the article.

As part of ISI's quality-control precoordination and spelling-variance unification procedures, every incoming term—that is, every word in every title—is passed against the established *PSI* vocabulary. In this computer comparison, wrong and variant spellings are corrected and coordination tests for accepted word-pairs are applied. Terms which are truly new are selected for human review and added to the vocabulary. Naturally, many author- or ISI-produced errors are identified and corrected in this process.

From the earliest days Sher and I were aware of the enormous potential of the *PSI* vocabulary for scientific lexicography. Besides allowing very specific searches on terms that would never have appeared in thesaurus-controlled indexing systems, the use of actual title-words reflects terminological innovation long before anyone but specialists in the affected field are aware of the changes. Every year nearly two-thirds of the words *added* as primary terms to the *PSI* vocabulary are "new" in the sense that they occurred only once or not at all in titles processed the previous year[9]. This does not, of course, mean that two-thirds of each year's vocabulary is "new."

The cumulated vocabulary of the *PSI* comprises an author-generated word-index to all the significant articles of science and technology—including letters, technical notes, and proceedings of meetings. It is a pity that the *PSI* vocabulary has not yet been used by lexicographers to identify and define new scientific terms and usages[10]. A dictionary based on the *PSI*, which could be updated quarterly, would be the first current dictionary of new scientific terms based on primordial sources.

From the outset, we were aware of the shortcomings of title-word indexes: the lack of resolution of obvious (and not-so-obvious) synonyms and the unavoidable fact that morphological variations of the same primary terms, *e.g.*, CLASSIFY and CLASSIFICATION, appear separately in the index. Even the plural of a noun may be separated from its singular, *e.g.* SUGAR and SUGARS. In Ohlman's permutation index to the proceedings of the ICSI 1958 conference, this problem was alleviated somewhat by restricting sorting of the first six characters of each term. However, use of this procedure is impractical for an index as large as the *PSI*[3].

Such problems were of minor importance as long as the *PSI* was regarded merely as a supplement to the *Citation Index*. We found that many scientists preferred a title-word index because it enabled them to retrieve a work by a word or phrase remembered from its title, or by subject words they knew to be relevant.

It was inevitable that librarians and others would begin pressuring us to make the *PSI* a search tool in its own right. Our response began with provision of cross-references and eventually led to certain standardizations, especially in the case of spelling variations. Today the so-called source-data edit procedures at ISI are quite systematic and comprehensive[11], and the *PSI* does stand on its own as both a current and retrospective subject index.

As early as 1969, I reported at Amsterdam on ISI's efforts to develop automatic procedures for hyphenating word-pairs into phrases, a process we called "precoordination"[12] to produce bound terms like BIRTH CONTROL. Such terms would be hyphenated automatically, provided they occurred with sufficient frequency. It was remarkable to discover that punctuation could be ignored if a given word-pair occurred above a certain very low threshold, about two or three times. One would not find too many titles in which the terms BIRTH and CONTROL were separated by a comma, such as "Season of birth, control of disease, and WHO statistics." Linguistic analysts have agonized over the problem of differentiating such items, but it is rarely a real problem.

Besides increasing the specificity and thus the informational value of the *PSI,* the main objective of precoordination is to reduce the number of permutations required. This did not prove to be as easy as we had first imagined. We have since found that precoordination is best performed by source-data edits, which requires constant monitoring of term-pair frequencies.

An important objective of permuted index display should be to minimize post-coordination by the user. For example, while BIRTH-CONTROL provides one level of precoordination, the resulting term is of such high frequency that one ought to be able to precoordinate BIRTH-CONTROL at a second level, with terms indicating drugs, devices, methods, etc., so as to narrow the focus of retrieval to less than ten articles for most searches. Obviously, the value of precoordination increases five-fold for a five-year cumulation, in which certain terms might occur dozens or even hundreds of times.

In closing this belated report on *PSI,* we should not overlook the application of the *Permuterm* concept in controlled or manual indexing systems. We first used *Permuterm* in a controlled indexing situation during the production of *Current Contents/Chemical Sciences.* Since then, we have used the method in producing the yearly index of the *Journal of the Electrochemical Society,* and some industrial organizations have used our *Permuterm* programs to generate their own indexes. Further, our on-line searching experience has demonstrated that *PSI* can be (and now is) used to facilitate searches of other data bases, such as MEDLINE, precisely because it displays term pairs that one might not think of or cannot find in thesauri such as MeSH. Otherwise, *Permuterm* indexing has had little application outside ISI.

A proper evaluation of *PSI* by the information community has yet to be published. Meanwhile, we can only report that *PSI* has been steadily gaining increasing acceptance among *SCI* subscribers. Most users today know how to optimize their use of the *SCI* with the most appropriate word index available for the time period covered in the search, whether for the period prior to 1965, when *PSI* first became available, or thereafter. Since 80 percent of *SCI* subscribers now also subscribe to *PSI*, it seems reasonable after more than ten years' development, to incorporate *PSI* into the *SCI* system. Thus in the future no user of the *SCI* will lack its complement, the *PSI*.

REFERENCES

1. WEINSTOCK, M. 1971. "Citation Indexes." Encyclopedia of Library and Information Science, 5 Vols. New York: Marcel Dekker, 1971; 5: 16-40.
2. GARFIELD, E. 1971. "Automation of ISI Services: Science Citation Index (*SCI*), Per-Muterm Subject Index (*PSI*), and *ASCA*." International Association of Agricultural Librarians and Documentalists, IVth World Congress, Paris, 20-25 April 1970. Paris: Institut National De La Recherche Agronomique, 1971; p. 107-112.
3. CITRON, J.; HART, L.; OHLMAN, H. 1959. "A Permutation Index to the Preprints of the International Conference of Scientific Information." Reprint no. SP-44, revised edition. Santa Monica, CA: System Development Corp. 1959, December 15; 37 pp.
4. "Keyword-in-Context Index for Technical Literature." Report RC 127, New York: IBM Corp., advanced system development division, 1959. Also published in: American Documentation. 1959; 11: 288-295.
5. STEVENS, M. E. 1965. "Automatic Indexing: A State-of-the-Art report." National Bureau of Standards Monograph 91. Washington, DC: Government Printing Office. 1965, March 30.
6. OHLMAN, H. Personal Communication, 1975, November.
7. GARFIELD, E. 1972. "Indexing Terminology and Permuted Indexes." Journal of Documentation. 1972; 28 (4): 344-345.
8. HEUMANN, K. et al. 1954. The Chemical Biological Coordination Center of the National Academy of Sciences. Washington, DC: National Research Council. 1954; p. 18.
9. WEINSTOCK M.; FENICHEL, C, ; WILLIAMS, M.V.V. 1970. "System Design Implications of the Title Words of Scientific Journal Articles in the Permuterm Subject Index." The Social Impact of Information Retrieval: The information bazaar, seventh annual national colloquium on information retrieval. May 8-9, 1970. Philadelphia, PA: The College of Physicians of Philadelphia, 1970; 181-200.
10. GARFIELD, E. 1969. "Permuterm Subject Index, the Primordial Dictionary of Science." Current contents. 1969 June 3; 22: 22.
11. FENICHEL, C. 1971. "Editing the Permuterm Subject Index." Proceedings of the American Society for Information Science, 34th annual meeting. Denver, CO. 7-11 November 1971; 349-353.
12. GARFIELD, E. 1970. "Citation Indexing, Historio-Bibliography, and the Sociology of Science." Proceedings of the third international congress of medical librarianship, Amsterdam, 5-9 May 1969. Amsterdam, The Netherlands: Excerpta Medica. 1970; p. 187-204.

The Development of a Library Minicomputer System: The Minnesota Experience

By Glenn Brudvig, *Director*
Bio-Medical Library
University of Minnesota

ABSTRACT

The University of Minnesota Bio-Medical Library received a grant from the National Library of Medicine in June 1972 to develop a low cost, stand alone, library controlled computer system which could be afforded by medium and large medical libraries. The system which is being developed is used solely for library operations with an integrated software system for handling all library processing. The system has been designed so that it can be easily replicated for other libraries. The project, therefore, has involved the development of a complete, integrated library data management system which would handle book ordering, serials check-in, binding, accounting, cataloging, catalog card production, circulation, and reference retrieval. The project is not yet operational but is nearing completion. The cataloging and acquisitions portion of the system will be implemented first, followed by serials, with circulation last.

Background

To provide a background for the development of the project, I would like to briefly describe the Bio-Medical Library and some of the computer applications which proceeded the development of the minicomputer system.

The Bio-Medical Library serves a user clientele of approximately 6,500 students, faculty, researchers and health practitioners. It has a collection of 240,000 volumes and subscribes to about 3,300 current serials. Its annual book acquisitions, however, is small compared to non-medical libraries, about 3,000 titles are normally added each year.

The minicomputer system is based on automated procedures which have

This project was supported by NIH grant LM-01507, awarded by the National Library of Medicine.

Originally published in *Automated Activities in Health Sciences Libraries*, Volume 1, Issue 2 (1975), pp. 13-17.

been in operation in the Bio-Medical Library for over seven years. The first automated system, serials control, went into operation in January 1968. This system, soon to be replaced, handles all aspects of serials control in a batch processing operation using a CDC 3300 computer. It produces a monthly check-in list of predicted journals, a monthly list of all journal holdings, cumulative daily supplements of new arrivals, a bindery ready list, binding instruction slips, and special lists of various kinds.

In July 1969 a second automated system went into operation for acquisitions, again using batch processing and a CDC 3300 computer. The acquisitions system produces periodic lists of all materials in process, including titles requested but not ordered, ordered but not received, received but waiting cataloging, and cataloged but the cards are not yet filed in the catalog. It prints purchase orders and handles all accounting operations.

In 1970 procedures for handling the payment history records for serials records were added to the system so that accounting records for both books and journals could be handled through one operation. These batch procedures have operated very successfully, with few problems, full staff acceptance, economy, and improvement of public services. The minicomputer system will incorporate these procedures for acquisitions, serials, and accounting and will expand the system to circulation, cataloging, and reference retrieval.

The batch systems which have been in operation do not have a direct relationship to the software design of the minicomputer system since a complete new design has been necessary to achieve an integrated system for operation on the minicomputer. The significance of these batch operations to the development of the minicomputer system has been in providing a background of experience for the library staff, and some of the systems people who worked on them, so that staff members could make meaningful contributions to the development of the new system. The transition to the mini system, therefore, will be relatively easy in terms of staff acceptance and involvement; the staff has developed an appreciation of the capability of the computer and an understanding of its potential and its limitations.

Although none of the software used in the present batch operations will be used in the minicomputer system, as much of the data as possible will be captured for the new system. Some of the data in the existing systems will have to be re-entered, other portions edited, but much of the information will be transferred directly into the new system, such as bibliographic data, vendor name and address files, payment history records, serials holding statements, and binding instructions. Some additional information will need to be added to the records to bring them up to full MARC standards.

Staff

After we received the funds from the National Library of Medicine to develop the system, the first task was to recruit staff. Audrey Grosch, who was directly involved in the design of the existing acquisitions and serials system, was already on the staff as was Carl Sandberg, Senior Applications Programmer, who had assisted in programming the batch systems. Eugene Lourey was with the University Library Systems Division when the minicomputer project was conceived and returned from other employment to help develop the system. He was instrumental in recruiting Bob Denney who brought to the project a wide range of experience in systems design. One additional Senior Applications Programmer, May May Johnson, was recruited to the staff to provide a total of four full time systems people for the project, plus the Library staff members who have been involved in various degrees in the project.

The project staff, therefore, had a good working knowledge of the Bio-Medical Library operations, a total familiarity with the present computer batch systems, and a wide range of experience in systems design. All of the people on the project are part of the Library staff.

Space

Space was made available in the Library for the minicomputer system by converting a former conference room into the computer room. No remodelling costs were involved other than to provide additional wiring and telephone outlets. The area was already air-conditioned.

Equipment

After the staff was recruited, the selection of equipment became the first priority. Specifications were prepared and sent out to 40 computer firms and custom engineering companies. Seven firms answered our bid and a Digital Equipment Corporation PDP 11/40 system was selected. The first equipment components were delivered in April 1973 with the second portion in May and June 1973. The first CRT terminal was received in December 1973, but the communication equipment needed to connect it to the computer was not installed until March 1974. We had considerable delays in getting equipment which slowed down the project by several months. Vendors had difficulty meeting delivery schedules because of heavy orders for minicomputers and components, but lately delivery schedules have improved considerably.

The hardware is described by Bob Denney in his paper, but I want to describe the distribution of terminals in the Library. There will be five CRT terminals wired directly to the computer; one in acquisitions, one in serials, one in cataloging, one in the circulation area, and one at the reference desk. In addition there will be one extra terminal which will be used with an acoustic coupler so that regular telephones can be used to access the system. This terminal will be used where necessary in the Library or to demonstrate the system. There will also be three slow speed printers, one in cataloging to produce catalog cards and cataloging worksheets, one in serials and acquisitions to produce purchase orders, claims, and accounting records, and one in the circulation department to produce circulation notices and records.

Cost Factors

In regards to the cost benefits of the minicomputer system, we have no cost figures for manual operations to compare it with, only the costs of the present batch systems. Costs for computer time for our present batch serials system averages $400 per month for 3,300 current titles, and the acquisitions and accounting operations averages about $500 a month. We also have costs for keypunch rental, punched cards and paper. The total costs for automated procedures at present, therefore, come to about $12,000 to $13,000 per year.

The annual costs for the minicomputer system will only be for maintenance since the system has been purchased. The maintenance costs will be approximately $9,000 per year for the system, which is less than we are paying for our present batch processing operations. The new on-line system will eliminate the need for keypunch rental, punch cards, and much of the paper now used for the various lists which are regularly produced.

The total costs of the equipment which we have, or will purchase, will come to approximately $160,000. This includes a Digital Equipment Corporation PDP 11/40 system with 64K core, six CRT terminals, three slow speed printers, one high speed printer, two tape drives, and two light pen readers for the circulation portion of the system.

Implementation Schedule

The initial grant which we received did not include provisions for a full circulation system. After the project got well underway, the need to develop a full circulation capability to have a complete integrated system became very apparent. The Library therefore applied for supplemental funding and received an additional $59,000 in February 1975 to develop a full, on-line circulation system.

The conversion of records has begun for the circulation system and also to support reference retrieval functions, acquisitions, and cataloging. We are converting full bibliographic data for all monographs from 1960 to date and selected titles before 1960, for a total of approximately 22,000 titles. We are using the shelf list to create the initial record, but will need to go to the main entry in the card catalog to get the full and complete bibliographic information. The main entry, brief title, call no., date, and Library of Congress number are entered onto a CRT screen from shelf list cards. This file will then be matched against a MARC tape file to capture full MARC data for as many titles as possible, which we estimate will be about 4,000—5,000 titles. Titles for which MARC data is available will be edited to match our records. The conversion of records is moving slowly at present because of the need to use the system for software development. However, during the summer we expect to make a full scale conversion effort so that all records will be converted by the time our current grant period ends in September 1975.

We have recently received funding for two additional years to continue the project. During the next two years, after the system is in operation, we will continue to improve the systems operating characteristics and adapt software so that it can operate on smaller, less expensive hardware. We plan to design interfaces with other computer systems, such as MEDLINE or other minicomputers, so that the system can switch information requests to other computer systems. We also plan to expand the subject search capability and to develop management information functions to provide information for more effective management of the Library's collections and programs. An important part of the continuing development of the system is to develop guidelines and instructional materials so that other libraries wishing to use the system would know what would be required in terms of funds, space and staff training. We also plan to replicate the system in at least one other medical library.

Problems

One of the problems which we have had, which has already been mentioned, was the delays in getting equipment. Another problem, and one which we did not fully appreciate when we developed the proposal, was the large amount of time which would be required to evaluate equipment for the minicomputer system, particularly the CRT terminals, printers, and the light pen readers. We have still not made a final decision on light pen readers and have had to accept a CRT terminal which is not ideal for the Library, but is the best that is now available on the market.

Another problem in the project, which I believe is typical for all developmental efforts such as this, is that the complexity of library problems was greater than we anticipated, even though we had a number of years experience in working with automated systems. We are using full MARC records in the system and this in turn introduced a number of complexities which required more time to work out than we initially anticipated.

One problem which we have not had, however, and one which concerns many library administrators, is staff acceptance. As I mentioned, the staff is very knowledgeable of library automation activities and has contributed to the development of the project, and we do not expect any problems as we switch over to a full on-line system. The automated processes which we have in operation have had two effects on staff. First, they have decreased the amount of clerical and professional time involved in acquisitions and serials and second, they have increased the para-professional staff. In other words, our clerical people have moved to higher level positions and have taken over some of the work previously handled by professional librarians. We expect much of the same to happen as we expand the system to other operations in the Library. However, most of our staff savings will be in catalog card production and in the management of circulation records. Any staff time which may be released will be reinvested in other areas of the Library, particularly to improve our public services. The end result of the on-line system will be a higher level of library service and an improved ability of the Library to perform increased services, or handle increased amounts of materials, without a corresponding increase in staff.

Present and Future Benefits

The operation of the minicomputer system will be described by Doris Owen in the following paper. We expect the system to reduce the costs of technical processing and circulation, but this is not the only or even the major benefit or purpose of the system. Our ultimate objective is to provide better service and improved access to the Library's resources. The conversion of catalog records back to 1960, and some before, will create a partial on-line bibliographic data base for the Library which will be kept up to date with new acquisitions. Eventually we hope to have all bibliographic records into the system and replace the card catalog, but this is still in the future. Until such time as we can replace the catalog, we will continue to produce catalog cards. The problem of providing terminals for patron use is one that we have not yet seriously investigated.

The on-line bibliographic records can be searched in a variety of ways for reference retrieval or technical processing, by author, title, subject, date, series, language, call no., Library of Congress no., type of material, etc., and in various combinations. The capability of the reference librarians to locate materials in the collection will thereby be much improved.

The system will have the potential to maintain a full management information system for the Library which we intend to develop within the next two years. Records on all library transactions can easily be collected by the system and a variety of data can be assembled, such as circulation of materials by subject or by type of user, so that we will know which users are putting heavy pressures on the collection and which are not, which portions of the collection are being used heavily, what titles should be duplicated and which should either be placed in storage or withdrawn. Information can be collected to relate circulation and use of materials to the cost of purchasing materials and servicing the collection. We hope to be able to determine the costs for providing services to different kinds of users or for different subject areas. The data thus collected will help justify and defend budget requests and allocations.

One of the most promising aspects of the minicomputer system is its potential for linking systems together so that one library would be able to gain access to the records of others and vice versa. This subject will be covered by Gene Lourey, but I want to give an example of how such a system would work. If a reference librarian or user was searching the bibliographic data files for a journal title and did not find it, the system could automatically search the journal file of a sister library, or to another library in the network, to see if it held the title wanted, and so on in a round robin search of linked systems. If the title was found, the system could be used to switch interlibrary loan requests from one library to another.

As I mentioned, during the next two years we hope to replicate the system in at least one other medical library and test the potential of linked systems. In addition, we are also planning to replicate the system in the main University Library, and possibly in the St. Paul Campus Library. When these systems are developed, the bibliographic records of each library will be accessible to each of the others in the system providing in effect a union catalog as far as a user is concerned.

The minicomputer has the potential to enable a library to be part of a network yet control and manage its own resources and services according to its needs and constraints.

The minicomputer system which we are developing is based on the premise that equipment and software should be available as a package in the not too distant future so that a library could purchase a complete system and avoid expensive developmental costs. The system is being developed so that it can be easily tailored or tuned to the particular needs of an individual library. Print formats such as purchase orders or catalog cards, data elements, and operating procedures can be easily changed to fit individual library requirements without changing the system software. The equipment can be run by non-technical people with equipment and software maintained by contracts with software and equipment companies. A library, therefore, would not have to have expensive software people on its staff to run the system.

We feel that there is tremendous potential for use of small computers and software dedicated specifically to libraries. Whether we will have solved all of the problems still remains to be seen, but at least we feel we are moving in the direction of providing low cost computer capability to libraries, or to groups of libraries.

REFERENCES

For other papers dealing with the Minnesota Experience: A minicomputer system at the University of Minnesota Bio-medical Library see...Automated Activities in Health Sciences Libraries Vol. 1, Issue 2, 1975.

GROSCH, A.N.: Approaches to Library Automation: Past, present, and future library computer systems design. pp. 8-12.

OWEN, D.L.: The Use of an On-Line System for Library Processing Operations: a Librarian's Point of View. pp. 18-23.

DENNY, B.: Systems Design and Hardware Consideration for an Integrate Library System. pp. 24-29.

LOUREY, E.: The Use of the Minicomputer in Library Networks. pp. 30-34.

JOHNSON, M. M.: Software Description for an On-Line Integrated Library System. pp. 35-43.

UPHAM, L. N.: MARC Formats in the University of Minnesota Mini-computer Project. pp. 44-53.

LOOKING FORWARD:

POSSIBLE DEVELOPMENTS IN THE PUBLICATION OF MEDICAL LITERATURE*

EILEEN R. CUNNINGHAM

Librarian, Vanderbilt University School of Medicine

IT HAS become increasingly evident that the publication of scientific literature presents certain difficult problems, and the various proposals for their alleviation which are constantly appearing indicate that scientists are dissatisfied with existing conditions. The problems which exist and the suggestions for their solution have been primarily concerned with three major factors: (1) the increasing quantity of material available for publication; (2) the increasing difficulties and complexities involved in obtaining and publishing abstracts of scientific literature; (3) the enormous, steadily increasing, number of journals, and the difficulty of supplying even a small proportion of these journals to investigators.

The amount of scientific data which should be published is constantly increasing, with a consequent overtaxing of the facilities available for publication. In order to cope with this situation the journals have been forced to request the elimination of charts, tables, and experimental protocols wherever possible, and editorial policies have been to urge authors to condense their papers to the utmost degree. This has meant that much material of value to investigators is unobtainable, and yet it is quite correct that these detailed findings are not of sufficient general interest to warrant publication. Another source of dissatisfaction is the fact that the time required for the publication of the average scientific paper is steadily increasing and investigators everywhere are complaining of this delay and are demanding more rapid publication.

We have then a paradoxical situation: the necessity for rendering more data available for scientists and increasing the rapidity of publication, but at the same time decreasing the number of pages published by the journals. In order to meet this situation the organization of central depositories for manuscripts and the utilization of modern photographic methods † for the reproduction of unpublished material have been proposed.

* Read at the Annual Meeting of the Medical Library Association, St. Paul, Minnesota, June 23, 1936.

† Many interesting articles regarding the latest developments in the field of microphotography as applied to libraries are to be found in the *Library Journal, 60,* 1935, and *61,* 1936.

Originally published in *Bulletin of the Medical Library Association,* Volume 25 (September, 1936), pp. 100-108. Reprinted by permission.

Dr. Seidell (9) of the National Health Institute and Dr. M. B. Visscher (12) were among the first to advocate the application of such methods to reforms in the publication of scientific literature. Their first articles were discussed in my paper given before the Second International Congress of Libraries and Bibliography (3). Dr. Seidell (11) reported in 1935 that further progress had been made in regard to the perfecting of mechanical devices for making film-strip copies of scientific publications. These devices have been put into practical application by Dr. Draeger of the U. S. Navy Medical Department, who wished to provide himself with a film library for use on shipboard and at distant navy posts, and who perfected a special camera for this work.

The problem of over-crowded publications has been, for some time, acute in the field of chemistry. The Office International de Chimie, organized several years ago, has attempted to enlist the aid of the International Institute of Intellectual Co-operation of the League of Nations in this problem, and it has been suggested that a comprehensive international guide to documentation be prepared.

Dr. Seidell (10) has discussed in detail the address given by Mr. Watson Davis before the Chemical Society of Washington, in which Mr. Davis presented a very comprehensive scheme for the reorganization of scientific publications. He suggested a central, co-operative, non-profit organization which he called the Scientific Information Institute (S. I. I.) for the double purpose of publishing current original material and the furnishing of bibliographies and photographic copies of current and previously published documents. Photographic reproduction would be substituted for all except papers of general interest, and journals would be practically reduced to review and abstract publications. Such a plan would of course completely revolutionize present systems of publication, and would be dependent upon the perfecting of the details of satisfactory and economical processes for photographic reproduction and the projection of filmed material so that it can be easily read.

At the ninety-sixth meeting of the American Association for the Advancement of Science the section on the Dissemination of Science (1) discussed further developments of Mr. Davis' plan and reported that efforts were being made to establish at once the Scientific Information Institute (S. I. I.). The report indicated that the first part of the program, *i.e.*, reproduction of papers which cannot secure prompt and complete publication and the reproduction of " out of print " papers, is capable of immediate realization. It is assumed that editors of journals would submit to the S. I. I. manuscripts which they cannot publish promptly or completely. The sponsoring journal would publish an abstract informing readers that the complete paper can be had from the S. I. I. in the form of photographic prints until reading projectors for films are more generally available. The bibliographic service will require much further planning and investigation before it can be realized. Details are obtainable from Science Service, Washington, D. C.

In my paper last year (3) I pointed out that, in order to make a central scientific organization for the publication of literature effective, it would seem advisable to have this organization's work carried out in co-operation with reliable journals and not by any attempt to supplant them, and that, as a result, more investigative findings would be rendered available to scientists interested in some particular subject, while the journals would not be over-taxed by details unnecessary for the majority of their readers. From a study of the latest available reports, it seems that Mr. Davis and his co-workers have come to somewhat similar conclusions, at least as a starting point for their plan for central organization.

A brief report of a somewhat similar plan was recently published by Dr. Polissar (8). In this plan, the unabridged manuscript would be deposited in typed form in twenty-five key libraries to be photographed and distributed to investigators desiring the unpublished details.

One of the most radical suggestions was that presented by the Association of Scientific Institutions of the Mining Industry in the U. S. S. R. (5) before the 1934 meeting of the International Geological Congress. They proposed that reprints be made of all papers, and that these reprints be handled by a central bibliographic institution for each subdivision of science in every country. They advocated that private individuals or companies publishing scientific periodicals introduce a twofold method of publication: separata and complete volumes. Scientists could then pay for only those articles actually needed. If such a plan were ever carried out, journals, as they now exist, would have to suspend publication.

Turning to the question of obtaining adequate and prompt abstracts of current literature, it is evident that present methods render the publication of this type of material expensive, cumbersome, and slow. It is also evident that there is a lack of co-ordination, resulting in the publication of abstracts of the same article in several publications while some articles are overlooked entirely.

Dr. Paul Lamson recently published a discussion of *Biological Abstracts* (6), in which he suggested the possibility of simplifying methods of obtaining abstracts for this publication. The plan outlined was that the co-operation of the editors of all biological journals be enlisted in an agreement that no paper would be accepted for publication unless accompanied by an author's abstract, and that this abstract would be mailed to the abstracting center as soon as the number of the journal was ready for publication. In this way an enormous amount of time would be saved for voluntary abstractors, and of expense for the publication. The advantages of such a plan are obvious; and while at first it might be difficult to get editors to insist upon authors' furnishing abstracts, there is no question but that abstracts would be furnished if this were necessary to obtain publication. The Wistar Institute has, for many years, applied this principle with great success to its own journals and bibliographic service. It is also quite obvious that this method could be extended to foreign journals as well, if their editors became convinced of the advisability of such a plan. This would very much decrease the difficulty of abstracting foreign articles, as it is much easier to translate an abstract than to abstract an article in a foreign language, with a possible misinterpretation of the author's meaning. Obviously, if this scheme ever received world-wide recognition, automatically a complete bibliographic record of all publications in medicine would be obtained.

A survey of medical journals (3, 4), indicates that again a somewhat paradoxical situation exists; for, in spite of the complaints outlined above in regard to the difficulty of obtaining prompt publication of investigative results, the number of journals is continually increasing. Approximately 2,221 medical journals were being published in 1935 (3). The multiplicity and high cost of these publications preclude the possibility of even the largest and richest libraries providing all of them for their readers. This results in a handicap to a rapid dissemination of knowledge of the work produced in different parts of the world, which is so essential if wasted time and effort on the part of the investigator are to be avoided. It is also obvious that many journals are publishing material which is of ephemeral value, or which does not contribute new data to investigative results already published.

The large amount of reprinted material being published seems both wasteful and unnecessary. In order to determine just exactly how many such publications exist in the United States, and their usefulness, a questionnaire was sent to all medical libraries by the Committee on Serial Publications of the Medical Library Association (7). It was found that 85 are being fairly regularly issued at the present time. While some librarians were loath to say that such publications were not useful, it became evident from the replies received that they were not used extensively in their present form. Naturally, a small library where many journals are not available is glad to have access to the articles in the reprint form. The questionnaire showed that there is evidently a tendency to place large libraries on the mailing lists to receive such publications, rather than small libraries. If the needs of the investigator were being considered, then these publications should be sent out primarily to libraries on the basis of their limited size and isolation from large library centers.

From the view-point of the institution which issues series of reprints regularly, two objectives are served: advertisement of work going on in the institution, and the obtaining of a permanent record of achievement for the institution. From the standpoint of advertisement, a sound reputation depends on the merit of the original work rather than on its widespread distribution in duplicate. On the other hand, undoubtedly it is of advantage to the institution to retain a permanent record of all published work. Such a record can be obtained from a few bound volumes of separate reprints deposited in the necessary offices or library of the institution. Lists of titles could be issued from time to time, if desired, for general distribution. Such a method would be far less expensive than reprinting the material again, or distributing great numbers of volumes of reprints.

Some of the difficulties which are at present being complained of in regard to the publication of scientific literature and some remedies which have been suggested for their alleviation have been briefly reviewed. If proposals such as those which have been discussed above, particularly the establishing of depositories for unpublished manuscripts and the utilization of photographic methods for the dissemination of scientific data, are placed in operation, it becomes of interest to determine what effect such procedures may have on the present system of the publication of medical literature, and if this system may be modified to the advantage of physicians and scientists throughout the country without initiating such radical changes that the publication of reliable printed journals would be jeopardized.

In clinical medicine, the number of journals has been enormously increased by the publications of state and other local societies. Much of the material contained in these journals does not add new data to investigative results already published in the general clinical journals. The chief purpose they serve is to afford the local physician an opportunity to report cases and to publish data of local interest. Is it possible to preserve this local means of self-expression and yet reduce the total number of publications?

If one divided the United States into ten zones arbitrarily by population, and established within each zone a medical society, one would have a sufficiently large group of physicians to support the society, but not so large that the organization would be cumbersome. It might be assumed that each of these organizations would publish a journal which would cover medicine and surgery in a general sense, and which would be issued at reasonably frequent intervals—say every two weeks (24 issues). This should give adequate opportunity for the publication of important contributions arising from a given zone. An editorial section could be maintained for the discussion of local problems, but it would be assumed that such journals would have no abstract sections except for papers from their own zone not of sufficient importance to publish in full. With proper editorial supervision, each regional journal would easily become the equivalent of from five to ten journals of the type at present published by the city, county, and state associations.

It would seem desirable to have some co-ordinating organization which might operate as the medical branch of the proposed " S. I. I.," or merely work in co-operation with it, to cover the clinical subjects. This co-ordinating clinical organization should publish a journal, preferably in several sections. This journal should contain: (*a*) review articles of general clinical interest, prepared on request by specialists in the subject to be covered; (*b*) author abstracts of all articles appearing in the ten regional journals; (*c*) a comprehensive abstract service covering all clinical material in the world, obtained as far as possible by authors' abstracts under the plan outlined above. The central organization would also be supposed to function as a depository for experimental data too detailed to publish in the journals, and for manuscripts of which only abstracts were published. This material could be furnished on request by the methods outlined in the discussion of the Davis plan.

The financial support would come in large part from the memberships of physicians in the regional societies; say for example $15 per year. This is undoubtedly higher than the membership the average physician is paying to his local society at present, but in return he would receive his regional journal, and in addition the journal published by the co-ordinating institution, which would give him a complete survey of everything being done in his own region and the other regions in the United States, as well as abstracts of world literature and reviews of achievements in various clinical fields. In addition he would receive information regarding unpublished material which he could obtain at reasonable prices, by photographic methods, if needed for his particular work. It is obvious then that the practitioner working in places in which there are no library centers could, for his membership fee, have the means at hand of keeping in touch with medical progress throughout the world, at a minimum expenditure of time and money.

The close interrelationship between medical centers and the practice of medicine which could be obtained by such means would be very valuable. One of the great weaknesses of our present system is the ease with which the practicing physician becomes dissociated from centers of intellectual activity. Much is to be gained by physicians' maintaining an interest in, and familiarity with, all of the educational facilities available in their section of the country. This familiarity should encourage them to seek postgraduate instruction, to obtain material from medical libraries more extensively, and the whole program of medical progress would become more closely interlocked.

What effect would such an organization have upon specific journals? It is difficult to foresee the answer to such a question, but it seems fairly certain that those journals really essential to general clinical medicine would continue to be published. It seems likely that those not essential would cease publication.

Many specialized journals now published in the United States maintain an abstract section.* In many instances the same articles are abstracted in several journals. This duplication is necessary at the present time in order to reach different groups of people, owing to the fact that not all the individuals involved subscribe to the same journals. The abstracts which would be published in the proposed central, clinical, abstracting journal

* The report of the Medical Library Association's Committee on Indexing Medical Literature indicates that approximately 45 American journals publish abstract sections at present.

would take the place of these abstract sections and relieve the specialized journals of an expensive and difficult task. The abstracts would reach a larger group than under the present system and save a considerable sum of money and time for the editorial staffs of the specialized journals. This increased saving in money, time, and space could be used by the journals to increase facilities for the publication of original investigative results and to lower the cost of the journals.†

It might seem wise to develop and maintain under the management of the central organization one or more journals in each specialty with separate but reasonable subscription rates. Such journals would furnish authors' abstracts to the central abstracting journal, and would deposit experimental details and manuscripts of value that they were unable to publish, issuing notice to this effect in the journal so that the specialists interested would know they were available on request, at slight expense, through the central organization.

There are great numbers of small medical organizations which undoubtedly offer to their members opportunity for an exchange of experience and development of ideas, and the individuals who particularly benefit from these organizations would question the effect that such a plan as has been suggested might have on their particular society. There does not seem to be any reason why an organization such as that outlined above might not fit into the present scheme of things to the advantage of smaller organizations. Any given county, state, or municipal society might affiliate itself with the zone organization without ceasing to have local meetings. It is, however, clear that in the majority of instances the papers read before these smaller organizations often consist of case reports which require only brief mention: this they could receive through the zone journal; and, if the editors thought the material of sufficient value, the paper could be deposited in the central organization for photographic distribution to those desiring it. The papers contributing data of investigative value or historical interest would be published in the zone journal. Such a method would give the practicing physician in smaller communities better opportunities for keeping in contact with medical literature, and this should more than compensate for the lack of opportunity for a few individuals to have published in full papers which do not contribute something fundamentally new.

It might be assumed that the proposals just discussed advocate such radical procedures that their accomplishment must be considered impossible. They do not, however, seem so difficult of achievement if one assumes that they would be initiated by, and developed in co-operation with, agencies which are already available. It is conceivable that the present organization

† The members of the Medical Library Association's Committee on Indexing Medical Literature under the Chairmanship of Miss Eleanor Fair, have come to the conclusion that a very real need for a clinical abstract journal exists; see the report of this Committee in the *Bulletin of the Medical Library Association, 25:* 33–38, (Sept.) 1936.

which is effectively publishing *Biological Abstracts* might join with governmental and other agencies in the centralization, extension and co-ordination of abstracting services for pre-clinical literature. Likewise, the movement toward establishing regional societies and publications might be developed from, and through, existing state and sectional societies in co-operation with the American Medical Association. The highly efficient and excellent character of the work already carried on by the American Medical Association would guarantee proper scientific standards for these publications. Indeed, a step toward the concept outlined above has already been taken by this Association in establishing and publishing their own *Journal* and such journals as the *Archives of Neurology and Psychiatry* and the *Archives of Pathology,* as well as other excellent journals covering special subjects, issued at reasonable subscription rates. Certain journals already in existence might well serve as starting points for regional journals. The *New England Journal of Medicine* already serves as the official publication for a large group of local affiliated societies. The *Southern Medical Journal,* in co-operation with the *Southern Surgeon,* could easily form the nucleus for a journal which could become the official publication for a regional group of societies.

In conclusion, certain facts seem apparent:

1. A reduction in the total number of medical journals is desirable. The amalgamation of local society publications into larger regional publications would be of value in this regard.

2. The elimination of serials containing reprinted material would be advisable.

3. The publication of a comprehensive abstract journal covering clinical material is needed. Material for such a publication should be obtained as far as possible by author's abstracts. Abstract sections in specialized clinical journals, with their consequent reduplication, could be eliminated.

4. Some co-ordinating institution should function as the publishing center for the clinical abstract journal and as a depository for manuscript data too detailed for inclusion in the clinical journals.

5. New developments in the photographic reproduction of literature will undoubtedly influence future methods of publication. It would seem wise for those interested in the publication of medical literature carefully to study and control their use. The immediate value of such methods seems to be in the reproduction of old and rare books and out-of-print material. In the production of current literature, photographic methods, at present, should be used to supplement printed publications rather than to supplant them.

If the future publication of medical literature continues to follow closely the pattern of the past, the next generation of investigators will have to surmount greater and greater difficulties. Dr. Mansfield Clark (2) in a recent whimsical address before the American Association of Bacteriologists depicts the plight of a scientific student in attempting to keep up with the literature in 1933. "He must feel like Alice in Wonderland," says Dr. Clark, "while the Red Queen cried 'Faster, faster. Here it takes all the running you can do to keep in the same place. If you want to get somewhere else, you must run at least twice as fast as that!'" At present there is no let-up in sight for the harassed investigator; most of us will be forced to agree with Dr. Clark that "scientific literature at the close of the first third of the 20th century is still growing like an infant in its second week after birth."

No one can foresee the nature of the mature development of this literature and its publication. It is quite possible that it will evolve on entirely different lines from those we have been discussing. The problem is a very serious one; it challenges the best mental efforts that those concerned have to offer; its solution will require the utmost of intellectual co-operation and endeavor. It will require the setting aside of individual jealousies and prejudices if the goal is to be achieved. The way may be long and beset with difficulties; but eventually it will be achieved.

Bibliography

1. American Association for the Advancement of Science: Report of Dissemination of Science Session, *Science,* N. S. *82:* 74, 1935.
2. Clark, W. Mansfield: Evolution toward a mature scientific literature, *Jour. Bacteriol., 27:* 1–18, 1934.
3. Cunningham, Eileen R.: The present status of the publication of literature in the medical and biological sciences, *Bull. Med. Lib. Assn., 24:* 64–81, 1935; and *Transactions of the Second International Congress of Libraries and Bibliography,* Madrid, Spain, May 20–30, 1935.
4. Cunningham, Eileen R.: Notes on medical libraries and certain developments in the publication of medical literature, *Phi Chi Quarterly, 31:* 542–550, 1934.
5. Goldman, Marcus: Reform in the system of scientific publication, *Science,* N. S. *80:* 380–381, 1934.
6. Lamson, Paul D.: Biological abstracts—a discussion, *Science,* N. S. *74:* 486–487, 1931.
7. Medical Library Association: Report of the Committee on Serial Publications for the year 1935–1936, *Bull. Med. Lib. Assn., 25:* 38–51, (Sept.) 1936.
8. Polissar, Milton J.: A new outlet for unabridged scientific papers, *Science,* N. S. *81:* 229, 1935.
9. Seidell, Atherton: The photomicrographic reproduction of documents, *Science,* N. S. *80:* 184–185, 1934.
10. Seidell, Atherton: Reforms in chemical publication (documentation). *Science,* N. S. *80:* 70–72, 1934.
11. Seidell, Atherton: Film-strip copies of scientific publications, *Science,* N. S. *81:* 174–176, 1935.
12. Visscher, M. B.: Reform in the system of scientific publication, *Science,* N. S. *80:* 245–246, 1934.

Building Precepts and Library Programs*

By Vern M. Pings, Ph.D., *Medical Librarian*

Medical Library
Wayne State University
Detroit, Michigan

ABSTRACT

The quality of a library's design can often be determined by the amount of preplanning done before it was built. The paper discusses three components of a library: the users, staff, and materials. Before any design is contemplated for new or additional space, a philosophy or purpose of the library must be determined. Some questions that need to be asked about users are used as an illustration to show the kinds of information that is needed before a librarian can begin to write a program. Only after such information has been gathered can textbook formulas be applied. The librarian will have to synthesize general purposes and facts into a functional program which the architect can use as a basis for design. A common way to demonstrate how space should be utilized is through diagrams. The determination of why one building is better than another for a specific environment is not a matter of guess work or applying formulas, but a matter of intellectual work.

EVERY health science librarian should be using at least part of his work week stewing about what needs to be done to improve the utilization of his library space. This stewing should be devoted to thinking constructively, not just complaining that he does not have enough space. Librarians should be thinking of space utilization in at least one of the following three ways:

(1) The present library should be abandoned and a new one constructed, but not necessarily a larger copy of the existing one.
(2) The present library should be renovated either by utilizing existing space more efficiently or adding more space for library functions.
(3) If you should be one of the lucky few who has just had a new library built, you should be actively thinking about, if not planning, future renovations.

*Presented as part of a "Clinic on Medical Library Buildings" at the Sixty-sixth Annual Meeting of the Medical Library Association, Miami, Florida, June 11, 1967.

Originally published in *Bulletin of the Medical Library Association*, Volume 56 (January, 1968), pp. 24-31. Reprinted by permission.

Why should I argue that all librarians should be thinking about space utilization? Not, let me repeat, *not* because the Medical Library Assistance Act of 1965 has money available to build or renovate. Librarians have the responsibility to society to support an important institution in the total communication process of health care. You must be convinced in your heart (or some equally autonomically controlled organ) that as a librarian you are making a contribution to the health care of individual citizens. With such a conviction, you will be able to see the library as a dynamic unit requiring special space utilization.

The Components of a Library

Architecturally a library is a relatively simple building. Even with the possible future use of a lot of electronic equipment, the library is still a simple structure. We have really only three components.

(1) The people who come to the building, or use some other device, to get access to information.
(2) The staff who works in the building whose function it is to see to it that people actually do have access to information.
(3) The equipment which people and staff must have to make it a library and not an airport terminal, e.g., books, journals (and if you must, the undefinable "multi-media material"), chairs desks, etc.

Since libraries are at least 5,000 or 6,000 years old, these three components, users, staff, and books should not present an architectural problem to society. Why should good library design be so difficult to accomplish? Three tomes have been published recently (or are about to be published) which are supposed to tell us how to design and build libraries (1). Metcalf, for example, is filled with formulas telling us how to space pillars, how many books you can store per square foot, and dozens of other tidbits. These formulas are vital after, and only after, the decision has been made what kind of library ought to be constructed. Formulas by themselves cannot build airplanes, bridges, or libraries. Before we start designing library space we have to be able to answer Robert Walkington's question, "Why have a library?" This is not a facetious question. As I interpret Walkington's question, why this particular library instead of another shape or size? Why this arrangement instead of another?

The Program

I should like to put these questions into another context. The publications I've mentioned emphasize that a librarian must write, let me stress, write a program before an architect is given the task of actually designing library space. But what is a program?

(1) It is a written document not just for the architect to read, but the faculty, the dean, the hospital administration, and anyone else you can get to evaluate it.
(2) The most important part of this document is a discourse on the philosophy or the specific purpose of the library.
(3) It is filled with as many objective facts and figures as can be gathered about users, staff, and materials as they relate to the lucidly written philosophy of the library.
(4) Equipped with a philosophy, facts, figures, the librarian then puts these disparate parts into some kind of order. This does not mean that the librarian designs buildings; that is the architect's job. But the librarian must provide the architect with relationships of function of units, or else you are apt to find the card catalog is on the fourth floor and the circulation desk in the basement with no exit except through a fire window.
(5) Finally, the program must argue that the architect has the responsibility to design an esthetic structure.

Far too many libraries now being designed are without programs, or are composed of programs made from formulas indiscriminately lifted from various publications. Why? My oversimplified answer is that as a profession we have failed to develop a strong philosophy of librarianship on which each of us can depend for support in our daily work as well as in the specialized interest of library buildings. To quote Shores from a recent issue of the *Journal of Library History:*

> Despite the late Pierce Butler's pointed observation that librarians "... belong to a profession which has never learned to think seriously about itself in general terms, a profession whose recruits are taught merely efficient routines in a growing concern ...," there is cumulative evidence in our professional literature of concern with ultimates. Not that we have changed our image very much yet; but ... here and there some of us have begun to brave the stares at conventions of the pragmatists. The word "philosophy" is not yet a respectable subject; but it is working its way tangentially into the professional blood stream under "types of libraries" and "kinds of work". . . .
>
> But if philosophy of librarianship is not boldly proclaimed by our literature, there are many significant professional beliefs tucked away in corners of practical articles, how-to manuals, (and) perennial surveys.... The problem is "how" to expose our philosophies of librarianship? Hopefully, philosophy was made one of the three major alternate titles of the *Journal*. From the beginning, the philosophy

of librarianship was established as a major editorial objective. But after a year and a half of one volume, plus two issues, no major essay, despite general and personal invitation, has been submitted to the editors[2].

According to Shores we have not been taught how to think seriously about librarianship in general terms. How do you go about developing a philosophy? I wish there were simple answers. Any philosophy or system of generalizations is difficult to write so that it makes sense and is not just a list of clichés. In spite of this, I shall try to give some sample questions about users for which you must find meaningful answers before you can begin to write a program and assist an architect and your faculty or staff to design an aesthetically functional library. Remember, users are only one component of the library. Questions have to be asked about staff and books in an equally sincere and searching manner.

The User

Before you begin, you must have in mind the length of time the space you are renovating or building is to function as a library. The formulas in textbooks suggest twenty years. I feel that if you can plan space for ten years you are a major prophet.

The first question to ask is who are the primary users: How do you find out how many bodies they represent? When Noah wanted information, he sent a dove from the ark, "And the dove came in to him in the evening; and lo, in her mouth was an olive leaf pluckt off[3]." Noah waited seven more days and landed. Librarians may start with an olive leaf which is a rumor that his institution is planning to expand within the next five to twenty years. What does this expansion mean interpreted into the number of medical students, interns, residents, nurses, and other health care personnel? Are the present schools and departments going to expand their enrollments? Are new schools and departments going to be created? These are obvious questions. The librarian cannot wait for the olive leaf. He should be sending out ravens and doves at very frequent intervals. He must have a communication channel which keeps him informed. This communication channel does not mean an occasional chat with a dean or a vice president or the reading of an annual report. Unfortunately, too few librarians have the status to be part of their institution's executive committees where total institutional planning takes place. An alternative is to have at least one, if not several, committees working on library problems. The membership of the library committees must be made up of individuals who are already on committees working on other buildings, regional planning, publications, curriculum, and other issues vital to the institution. Only such informed individuals can give you, or tell you from whom you can get, the information you need to contribute a philosophical foundation. Of course, such committees, be they executive or *ad hoc*, can only function if the librarian can match their imagination and can synthesize their collective thinking.

This brings me to another problem about users. Every good medical school and teaching hospital in the country is now in the process of examining its curricula, if for no other reason than to answer the Coggeshall and the Millis reports[4]. The position paper published in 1966 by the American Nurses' Association has, in effect, announced that about 60 percent of its profession is no longer really professional nurses since they have no baccalaureate degree. You cannot just look at the curriculum published in your institution's bulletin. You must be aware of changes in all the programs requiring library service. For example, I recently learned of a new nursing program to start in Detroit this summer in a 150 bed hospital. The program is designed to attract graduate nurses to the hospital so that quality health care can be maintained. The hospital has a three-fourth's time graduate librarian working with a collection that is above average for a hospital of its size. The library has ten effective user work spaces (there are more chairs). This program, approved by the Board of Trustees, is, among other things, to do the following:

(1) Raise the salaries of nurses by about 20 percent.
(2) To earn this salary each nurse will be assigned the full care of six patients, and she will be given as much work time as she needs to spend in the library to study about her patients. Imagine the competition between the physicians and nurses for the ten seats and the materials in the library if this program works!
(3) The third part of the program is that the hospital will pay the tuition for anyone who works toward a baccalaureate or advanced degree. How are the three collegiate nursing schools of the area going to give these students library service?

If my point is not clear, let me announce it more emphatically. The Director of Nurses may have an excellent program, but she made an assumption common with many administrators—she just assumed library service would be available. I have two questions: If the Director of Nurses had been sufficiently aware, are there librarians who could have explained to her what her program means in terms of library, people, space, money, and service? Two, if this imaginative program fails, could it be because the diagnostic and therapeutic instrument, the library, just was not available?

Many other questions need to be asked and answered about users before you begin writing your program. Where do they live in relationship to where they study and work? What other library services and study areas are available, and how do they relate to the library space you are designing? But these examples should give you enough insight into the intellectual as well as leg work that must be undertaken before you can begin to apply formulas.

The Formulas

Assuming you have all the information about your users that you can acquire, then you, as a librarian, should be able to make sensible estimates of the amount and kind of material you need to add each year to your library by asking searching, meaningful questions which can produce the information to define general selection and discard policies.

Armed with numbers of people and amounts of material to be added, and the number and kind of staff you need to provide user service and process your acquisitions, you can now go to the textbooks and apply the formulas to determine how much space you need. Even if you failed eighth grade arithmetic, it is not a horrendous job of multiplying, adding, and dividing.

Space Relationships

The next step, however, in preparing your program is not a simple one. You have to know what services are to be given, where they are to be given, and how they can be given to the users with the most efficient use of staff. Whatever the librarian of the future will deliver, within the next ten years his major function will still be delivering documents and references to documents. The librarian, then, must provide the architect with some idea of the space relationship calculated through the use of formulas. This does not mean, as I said earlier, that the librarian designs the library, but the architectural cliché "form follows function" can be used as a rule for the librarian who has synthesized the needs and functions of his library.

From my observations, there are two ways to show priorities of space relationships to an architect. A prose description may be satisfactory if you write well and your architect can visualize your prose into space relationships. However, for the librarian to describe space relationships well, he must be able to think dimensionally. It is often easier to translate this thinking into diagrams than to try to write it out completely. A diagram properly explained with an appropriate text can make the efforts of your study more meaningful, not only to the architect, but to yourself. There are three kinds of diagrams often used; (1) the free form, (2) the circle, and (3) the square. The following three figures are examples to demonstrate how librarians have tested their intellectual work into space relationships.

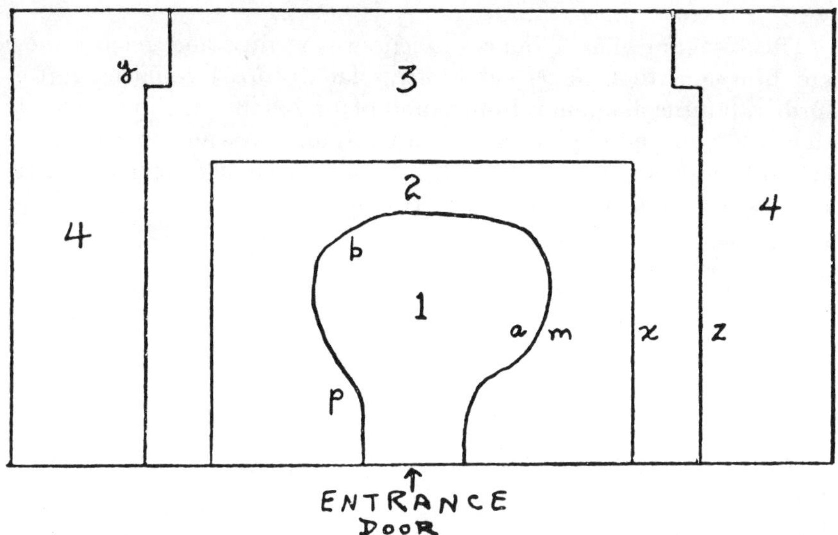

Accessibility Priorites are shown by the numerals 1, 2, 3, and 4. The entrance door gives immediate access to Priority 1 areas. All the areas in Priority 1 are necessarily near each other, e.g., area a and area b. This is not true in the case of Priority 4, e.g., areas y and z. Proximity is possible across Priority lines, e.g., areas a and m, or even areas a and x. Thus, it is possible to have a Priority 4 area like Cataloging staff at z reasonably close to a Priority 1 area like the Public Catalog at a. The diagram shows everything on a single horizontal plane. Possibilities for achieving efficient space relationships are increased by bringing areas into vertical proximity by a wise use of stairs and elevators.

FIG. 1—Accessibility Priorities for the Francis A. Countway Library (Source: Metcalf, *Op. cit.*, p. 381.)

This priority diagram has probably been seen by more medical librarians than any other. It was prepared by Esterquest for the Countway Library. The technique here is to assign accessibility priorities by numbers. Functional areas such as reference collections, the public catalog, etc., are labeled by letters. Although Esterquest has undoubtedly written one of the best medical library programs and prepared an excellent space relationship system for the architect, it didn't seem to get translated into the Countway Library. Nevertheless, the Countway Library is an aesthetic wonder and has the "feel" of a grand library. I am convinced that without Ralph's hard work, which went into the development of his program, giving him the ability to communicate intelligently with designers, Harvard might still have built an aesthetic wonder, but a monstrous library.

Figure 2: The Circle.

This diagram has grouped functions together and related these groupings into first and second priority relationships. I would discuss this further, but the diagram is from a draft of a program which was recently shown to two library planning consultants and presented to two faculty committees. The concept of the library is now so changed that an entirely new priority system is under development.

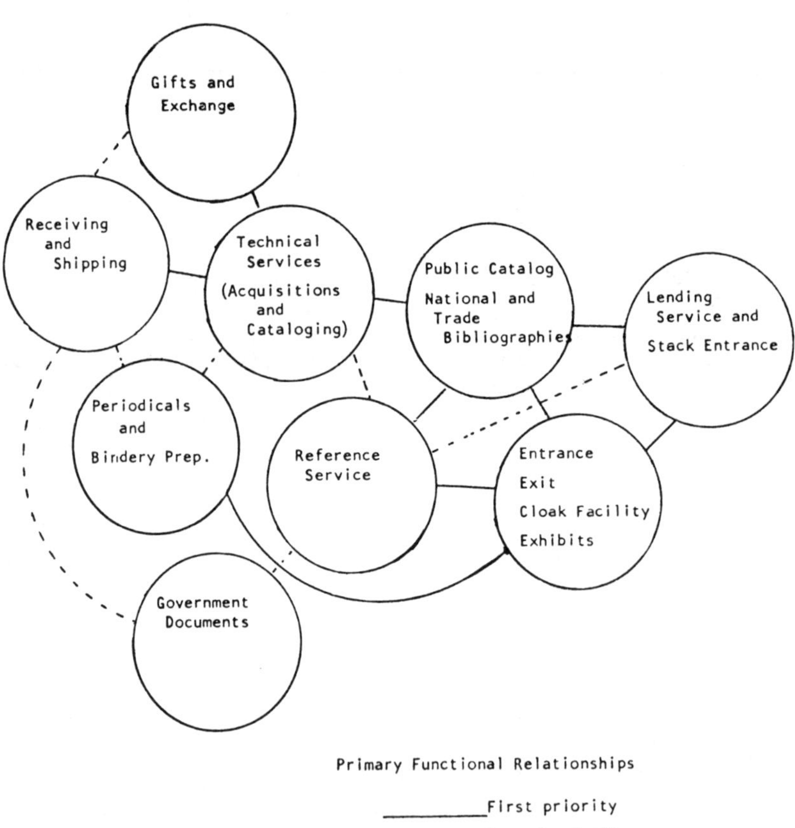

FIG. 2—Primary Functional Relationships of the Wayne State University Library Building Program.
(Source: Draft of Wayne State University General Library Building Program, March 1967.)

Figure 3: The Square.

The diagram, one of several used in the Wayne State University Medical Library Program, tried to show five things.

(1) Areas which must be contiguous are connected by solid lines.
(2) Those areas which are connected by dashes would be convenient to be contiguous, but need not be so if suitable direct access is available through passageways.
(3) The areas whose proximity would be convenient, but have lower priorities than the other two types of areas, are indicated by dotted lines.
(4) The broken line indicates that the areas can be located vertically to one another with suitable access to each other.
(5) The arrows try to show the relative movement between areas; some areas require movement of people or materials in both directions, while in others the flow is mainly in one direction.

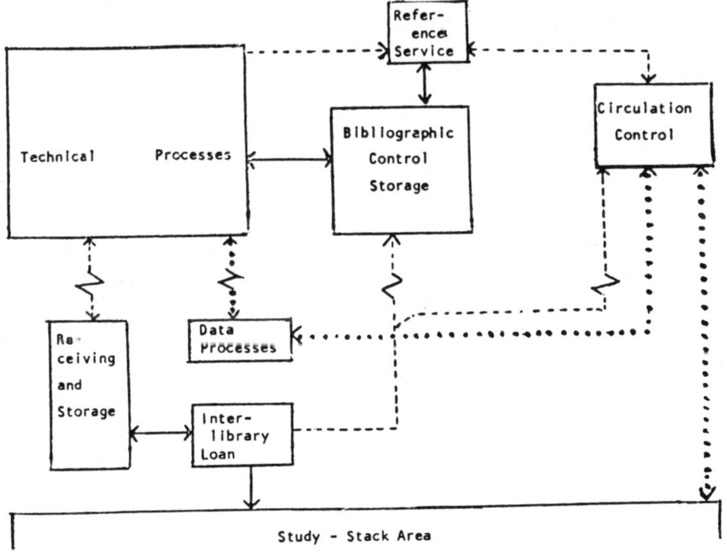

Space relationship of technical services and interlibrary loan service to other areas

————	those spaces which must be contiguous.
-----------	those spaces which it would be convenient to have contiguous, but allowing for suitable halls or aisles, can be separated.
....	those spaces which, while related, have less priority to be contiguous than other spaces. Direct passage space must be planned to this area.
——/__	a broken line indicates the space relationship may be either vertical or horizontal.

FIG. 3—Space Relationships of Technical and Interlibrary Loan Services (Source: A Program for Wayne State University Medical Library, January 1965.)

Figure 4: The Architect's Interpretation.

This is the fourth schematic of the first floor prepared by Wayne's architect trying to rationalize the philosophy and the priority diagrams given in the program. A fifth one is now in process to be reviewed once more by a gaggle of librarians, faculty, and administrators. My reason for stressing that six schematics or more may be necessary is that, no matter how good the program, the final building requires compromises. Without the exercise of preparing an intellectually sound program, the librarian finds himself at the mercy of an architect or a library committee.

VERN M. PINGS

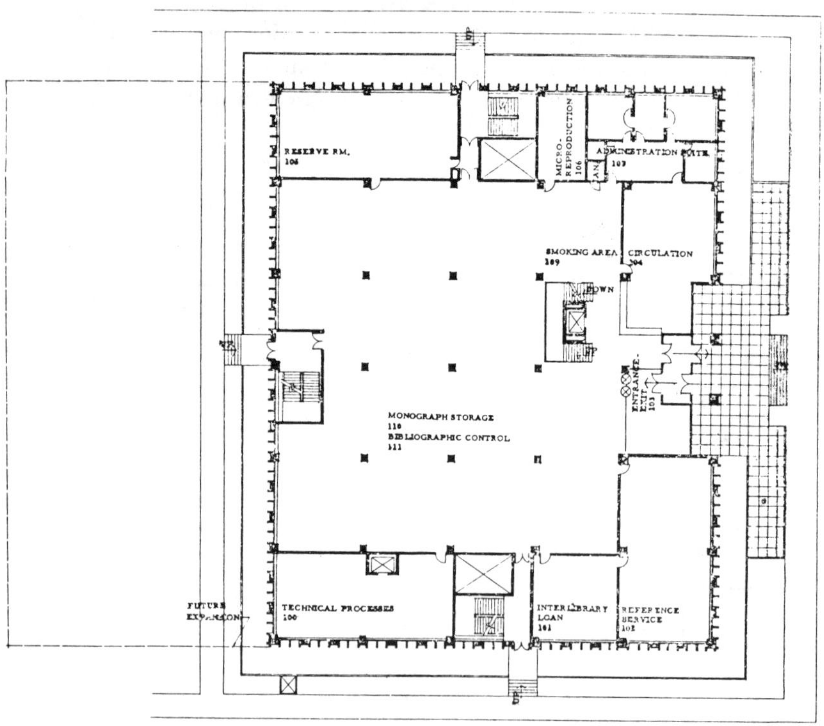

FIG. 4—First floor plan of the Vera Parshall Shiffman Medical Library (Source: O'Dell, Hewlett and Luckenback, Inc., Vera Shiffman Medical Library, August 1966.)

Summary

(1) The quality of the design of a library can often be determined by the quality of the original program written by the librarian.

(2) A good program depends upon a philosophy of library service which is developed from a knowledge of who the users are, how they work and study, and above all, the general philosophy and purposes of the parent institution.

(3) Only a librarian, let me repeat, only a librarian, can do the necessary synthesizing of the general principles and facts to prepare a functional program. He needs the help of his users and administrators, but it is ultimately the librarian who must be and remain the expert.

(4) Understanding and rationalizing why one building plan is better than another for a specific environment is not a matter of guess work and applying formulas but a lot of hard head and leg work.

Although not discussed in the paper, there is a point that must be added. If you are unsure of yourself in specifics or generalities, be not ashamed to ask for help from library planning and library building consultants, but be sure you find one who is capable of helping you solve problems, not just criticize the work you have done. All of us can be sidewalk critics, but few of us can teach or show others how to solve problems.

Acknowledgment

Although Robert Walkington, Construction Program Officer, Facilities and Resources Division, Extramural Programs, National Library of Medicine, cannot be held responsible for the content of this paper, he was my mentor, not only in writing the paper, but during the past year. I am grateful, therefore, for his specific help as well as the sincere effort he has demonstrated to insure that our nation will have the best possible medical libraries.

REFERENCES

1. Metcalf, K. D. Planning Academic and Research Library Buildings. New York, McGraw-Hill, 1965; Guidelines for medical school libraries. J. Med. Educ. 40: Part I, Jan. 1965; The health sciences library; its role in education for the health professions. J. Med. Educ. 42: no. 8, Pt. 2, Aug. 1967.
2. Shores, L. Epitome. J. Libr. Hist. 2: 92-93, Apr. 1967.
3. Gen. 8: 10.
4. Coggeshall, L. T. Planning For Medical Progress Through Education. Evanston, Ill. Association of American Colleges, Apr. 1965; American Medical Association. Council on Medical Education. Ad Hoc Committee on Education for Family Practice. Meeting the Challenge of Family Practice. Chicago, Sept. 1966.

Medical Librarianship, A Mid-Century Survey: A Symposium

Medical Library Architecture in the Past Fifty Years*

BY ALDERSON FRY, *Librarian*

Medical Center Library
West Virginia University

AND SCOTT ADAMS, *Librarian*

National Institutes of Health

SINCE the start of the BULLETIN in 1911 there have been 18 articles and five fairly important news notes published related to library planning and/or architecture. The news notes, chronologically, mention the new University of Michigan General Library (1); the second one gives the first floor plan of the Yale Medical Library (2); the third is a picture of the Oregon Medical School Library (3); the fourth reports an enlargement of the School of Medicine Library, University of Southern California (4); and the fifth one announces the completion of the Fulton County Medical Society of Georgia Library (5), probably the first (1942) air-conditioned medical library.

Of the eighteen articles, only four have to do with planning, and the remainder are mostly descriptive of individual libraries. Up until 1950, eleven times as much attention was given to the cost of German periodicals as to library plans and planning. (For reasons amounting to little more than prejudice the senior author refuses to gather together the numerous references to the difficulties pertaining to establishing a building for the Surgeon-Generals-Armed-Forces-National-Library of Medicine, with one exception, noted later.)

Although it wasn't until 1925 that an article on library planning appeared, Gilchrist, (6), Librarian of the University of Rochester, made a very fine contribution. Obviously the problem is not knowledge, but functional knowledge. Had this article been heeded, and the advice and information followed, then this history would have been quite different—and the entire course of medical education in this country would have been different also.

* Read at 56th Annual Meeting of the Medical Library Association, New York, New York, May 6–10, 1957.

Originally published in *Bulletin of the Medical Library Association,* Volume 45 (October, 1957), pp. 471-479. Reprinted by permission.

In 1925 he wrote: "It is not unkind to the architect to say that the librarian should know best how much space now and later should be provided for the staff." That states it gently enough, but the fact is yet to successfully penetrate some planners.

And he was more optimistic then, we think, than he should have been in concluding that architects are "generally considerate, helpful, and eager for the suggestions which a librarian may give them in making the library useful as well as ornamental. . ." (p. 1) A very important conclusion he made, that should have been taken to heart by all planners of libraries, was that "If the growth of the collection is diagrammed over a period it will probably be found that the increase is not arithmetical but geometrical—that every year the total added is greater than before." (p.2) Experience probably taught him that "No one but the librarian is likely to stick out for an adequate provision for stack space, or to insist on a plan which will make future additions to the stack possible without entirely reconstructing the building." (p.3)

He also recognized another problem. "The amount of space to be devoted to the staff is still more difficult to calculate with precision," and, "The most common mistake in planning workrooms is in estimating the working space merely as desk space." (p.4)

It was another ten years, 1945, before another planning article appeared. This one, by Robert Stecher (7) and one two years later (8) are excellent contributions toward the lighting problem.

Miss Lora-Frances Davis (9), in "Instructions for a Medical School Library Planning Survey," resulting from her survey for the new Florida Medical School, makes a good start toward studying background conditions. It is useful, but only introductory, and her complete survey should be made available.

Fourteen of the articles are descriptions of nine different libraries. The first library described, in 1917, by A. S. Warthin, is an excellent review of the situation and the history of the Medical Library of the University of Michigan. The library occupied the entire fourth floor of the north stack and a part of the same floor of the south stack. It is interesting to note that the Homeopathic Library was above it on the fifth floor.

Another article, in the same issue, by W. W. Bishop (11) described the Main Library without mentioning the location of the medical library. He gives the first floor plan of a library to appear in the BULLETIN, but it is for the Main Library.

By some strange coincidence the last article with a plan, covered by this survey, (which is in the BULLETIN for October 1956) by David Kronick (12) is about the University of Michigan's new Medical Library, and contains excellent descriptions and this sage advice: "I know of no way of anticipating the space requirements for work room short of estimating the maximum space requirements and then doubling them." (p.427).

Four articles are on the New York Academy of Medicine. The first, in 1922, briefly details the building history of the library since 1847 (13), and includes the essential services the library performs, indicating that it was, in 1922, the third largest medical library in the world. The building at 17 West 43rd Street was the fifth building the Academy occupied, thus a different building every 15 years, each outgrown.

Dr. Malloch (14) gives a description of the new (and present) building. Seemingly all sorts of provisions were made for adding stacks, floor onto floor, but no figure is given as to expansion, but merely, "There is ample room for expansion for some years to come, as we could house 250,000 volumes with the present shelving, and the books and bound periodicals have been arranged on the shelves so that new accessions can be added as they come in." (p. 11–12).

The following year Dr. Williams, welcoming the MLA Convention thirty years ago said, "The original plan for the new building provided for a stack centrally located in the building, and which was a fixed unit. Fortunately the plan was modified so that the present building is constructed in three parts—the stacks so constructed that it is possible to almost double its size upwards and make it half as large again to the east which would house ultimately about 600,000 books." (p.5)

The last article on the Academy, by Miss Janet Doe, (16) depicts the situation as of 1952.

The only other article to appear before World War II was by Miss Marguerite Campbell (17). It is a description and history of the Biology and Medical, or Billings Library at Chicago, indicating that the two units are separate, but in charge of one librarian. Size is about 60,000 volumes.

Increased interest, or increased space in the BULLETIN, led to the publication of a number of articles after World War II. The first by Miss Louise Darling (18) is not a discussion of general problems, but of those specific to UCLA. No floor plans are given, and some changes were made after this article was written.

The above article appeared in 1950. In 1953 Fry (19) reported on the new Health Sciences Library at the University of Washington in detail, including the architects. In that same year Miss Heck (20) described the new library at Oklahoma, and in October there was an article by Miss Eldridge (21) on the Dental Library at the University of California. In 1954 Miss Dorothy Cramer (22) gave a specialized but interesting report on the NIH Library, including methods as well as a description of the physical plant.

Also in 1954, John Oley (23) gave a specialized description of the Armed Forces Medical Library's building program—and it will be nice to get that problem off the agenda of the Association.

One problem may have growing importance for the future, that of the historical collection. Miss Gertrude Annan (24) discusses this problem in another publication than the BULLETIN. She says: "Fundamental changes in our attitude toward both history and book-collecting have in the past twenty-five years widely affected historical collections." She details the earlier disregard for housing historical material, which changed about thirty years ago. "Before any of the large eastern libraries took the step, the Lane Medical Library in San Francisco led the way by assigning its top floor to its well known historical collection of material earlier than 1850. In 1933 the New York Academy of Medicine added to its building space for a Rare Book and History of Medicine Department." (p.68).

The steps seemed logical at least if belated. First the assignment of a separate floor, then the addition of a wing, then a complete division, as when the Army Medical Library sent to Cleveland in 1942 its material printed before 1801. In 1940 the Yale Library planned a separate but equal wing. The destruction of valuable old material has been so rapid that soon air-conditioning will be a must just for the preservation of material if nothing else.

RESULTS OF THE SURVEY

Space is the word this report starts with, and the word it ends with is space. In the past fifty years there have been examples of intelligent planning in relationships, lighting, flow patterns, and other things, and there have been mistakes, but about eighty per cent of the troubles subsum under a single word—Space. The rest of this report simply amplifies this thesis.

As to architecture: W. Poole, speaking at an ALA meeting in 1883 said, "The architect is the natural enemy of the Librarian." Then he was right, but it is less true today. Too often medical library buildings, in some cases right up to the Forties, were more for the glorification of the architect and the University than for the use of the librarian and the patron. Today the chances of reasonable cooperation are far better.

Little can be said about the external form of medical libraries of the past fifty years. Frequently they have followed the current fashion and the demands of surrounding buildings, which fashion was usually a Bastard Collegiate Gothic. Ceilings were too high, but they had no forced circulation then. Fenestration was usually overdone, but they had expensive electricity and no fluorescent tubes. Foyers were too large, stairways too sweeping, marble too prominent, and Veblen's "Theory of the Leisure Class" too much in evidence.

Today external style in libraries occasionally shows the same lack of daring. We think little can be done about it, for while librarians should fight for the internals of the machine, when it comes to exterior design he will be met with the knowing sneer of superior knowledge, soi disant, on the part of the architect and possibly the planning committee.

An excellent book written a while back is "Space, Time, and Architecture." That is the problem here, in a way. Space is needed, time is the enemy, and architecture could solve the problem. It may be that the architect, when he talks in terms of economy of line, too frequently translates it into economy of space. But we must leave that problem, for most of this paper is on the internal, rather than the external problems of the past fifty years.

To find out what librarians think of planning which was done for them in the past, whether by architect or faculty committee, we recently circulated a questionnaire. Forty-five schools replied, twelve county and similar libraries replied, and a few others. For lack of time we will consider only the schools.

But before going on, I wish to thank all who took the considerable amount of time needed to answer an awkwardly worded questionnaire, to ask all who haven't to please return the questionnaire so this may be a comprehensive and ultimately an historical study. I want also to pay tribute to the amazing ingenuity displayed by librarians in adapting sometimes very poor plans and structures to intelligent function.

Of the libraries replying on schools, 45 of them, they range in age from 1834 to 1957. Eleven per cent were built before 1900, nine per cent in the Tens, thirty per cent in the Twenties, thirteen per cent in the Thirties, and thirty-five per cent since World War II. Only seven of these libraries occupy a building separate from the school they serve.

(Figures given from now on apply only to those giving replies that could be used, which frequently does not include all 45 libraries.)

Comparing the holdings of books and periodicals we find that thirty-five per cent of the library holdings are in books, or one-third. There is little difference whether the library was built fifty years ago or recently, except for a slight tendency for there to be more periodicals than books in the newer libraries.

The total holdings of these libraries range from 16,000 to 210,000 volumes, with concentration in the 28,000 to 70,000 volumes. We asked for capacity and holdings. An interesting figure developed. Nine libraries report their capacity and their holdings as exactly equal, 18 libraries report their holdings as less than their capacity, and 12 libraries report their holdings as in excess of their capacity. As a matter of fact, the total holdings of the libraries reporting are so much in excess of their capacity that, if the new University of Michigan Medical is eliminated, all the libraries in the country that report unfilled shelves could barely shelve the holdings of the libraries that have exceeded their capacity. In other words, there are 300,000 volumes of medical material in our libraries that seemingly are not on the shelves of the libraries owning them.

The average space of the eleven libraries built during the Twenties was 6,532 square feet. The eleven libraries built since 1947 have an average of 13,918 square feet. Therefore the average space of the newer libraries is a bit more than twice the average of thirty years ago. These statistics are offered as encouragement to librarians who want to double their Dean's estimates.

Ignorance of this growth rate can lead to tragic consequences: Two libraries built since 1949 indicate they are out of space. A picture that emerges shows that libraries are frequently planned for twenty years use, they run out of space in about ten years, scrounge around for space another six years, and are considering a new library four years before the twenty years are up.

Fremont Rider's calculations showed that research libraries in this country in the past have doubled every sixteen years. While there are a number of reasons why this rate will not necessarily obtain in the future, it is worth looking at the records of some medical libraries and trying to discover what has been happening.

These figures, taken from the American Library Directory, covering a few of the libraries that are in this report, need to be qualified. Reorganizations, different methods of counting and reporting holdings, and other factors have affected them, but this is what we find:

Library	1914	1927	1935	1942	1951
A		3,500	11,464	15,162	22,500
B		11,000	21,500	28,750	41,875
C	7,316	23,604	68,775	91,870	115,763
D		3,485	10,000	16,617	21,891
E		6,902	19,895	30,870	47,220
F	8,478	13,230	28,000	32,000	62,000
G		5,000	8,977	12,732	17,846
H		8,595	21,500	32,551	48,805

Charted, these figures roughly approximate a geometric growth with a slope of $x = 5y/3$, or put another way, these libraries have tended in the past to double in size every twelve years—at least from 1927 to date.

There you have a considerable explanation of why medical library architecture in the last fifty years has led to so much temporizing, adding stacks, finding storage space, working out unwanted discarding routines, and asking for new libraries long before the one in use has been worn out. The stack space is just not big enough in nearly all medical libraries. Space for other uses is frequently inadequate, but stack space easily heads the list.

The same is true of future plans. Medical library architects should do very well. The reports show that eighty-eight per cent of the libraries are planning significant alterations; twenty-seven per cent are adding stacks, and thirty-one want new libraries very soon. And if previous patterns are followed, twenty per cent of these new libraries will be out of space within nine years.

An effort was made to find out who planned the libraries that needed changes soonest. It would seem that the poorest choice for successful planning is an architect alone, but two of the worst examples, in terms of anticipating needs, indicate the planning was done by "Lord only knows," and a blank in the questionnaire.

Next poorest for planning is the combination of an architect and the main university library authorities; next is the architect, a committee, and the business administrator; and best is the librarian working with any of these combinations and a consultant.

The evidence is insufficient, but the poorest person, it would seem, to determine the size of the library is the business administrator and the best is the librarian, the administration, and a building committee.

The question on what was planned and what was achieved was a failure, for we hoped to discover why libraries plan better than they achieve, why so frequently the size is not what was planned for, or certain services are not in the final building. This was not answered. The answers did range from "Like Topsie, we just growed," to "I got what I wanted." Nearly all who answered were very kindly toward those who built the library a long time ago.

The common report on the basic plan was that it was adequate as conceived, but now inadequate, and where the basic plan is considered inadequate, it was usually planned by the architect alone. One person reported the basic plan, "called for one person, goal achieved." Another said "Planned for a junior college, achieved just that." There were cases where promises by the architect and/or the administration were not carried out, but only one report of a failure to achieve goals because of a cut in appropriation.

The relations of the architect with authorities over the past fifty years have ranged from "very pleasant," "architect cooperated fully," "cooperative," to "non-existent" and "uncooperative." This part of the study was not too significant because many of the librarians were not around when their structure was planned.

As to making present and future plans, the relationship between the architect and the librarian does seem to have improved somewhat. Sixteen reported the relationship good, eight reported it as non-existent, and the other five range between.

The section on lighting was very simple. No library built before 1947 had adequate lighting (one had gone through candles, gas, bulbs, and fluorescent), and ten of the libraries built since 1947 reported the lighting as adequate, with three giving qualified answers. Twenty-seven libraries reported there had been changes in their lighting, eighteen of the changes to fluorescent, the remainder indicating they had put in more lights, sometimes bulbs, or simply indicating a change had been made.

Only ten libraries could furnish plans or published articles on the library; only three were known to have planned from an original prospectus or study; and two of these were available.

One third of the libraries are working toward expanding their stacks, from "in preliminary stages" to "being constructed." One fifth of the libraries are getting more floor space, one-fifth are getting more workroom space, and plans for either new libraries or major changes in older ones were indicated by more than one-third of the libraries, ranging from "in confusion" and "wishful thinking" to waiting for a final decision from the authorities.

An indication of future needs for shelving was asked for. Twenty-eight libraries answered, wanting space for from 20,000 to 500,000 volumes, with a total of 3,690,000 volumes wished for. This was from libraries with a present capacity of 1,928,400 volumes. Forty-four per cent of the libraries want more seating space, twenty-five per cent want larger charging areas, up to "ten times as much," and next most important after shelves was need for workroom space, wanted by thirty-nine per cent of the libraries. The answers were such that they cannot be added, but would seem to indicate a need for at least two to three times as much workroom space as libraries presently have.

On the last question about opinions from the dean, etc., further discussion, and notes, varied answers were given. One library indicated the figure for shelving space was calculated on the public library figure, which was twenty-five per cent too high. Many notes were added indicating that answering the questions was quite difficult, and one librarian wrote she had answered as best she could, but the person to consult was the former librarian, who was now dead.

In the last fifty years the external form of the library has followed the dictates of surrounding architecture or current styles of the time, there has been a gradual growth in the size of libraries in terms of square feet, material has grown at the geometrical rather than an arithmetical rate, libraries are coming downstairs and nearer the entrance, and while there is of course intelligent and unintelligent planning, the overwhelming need is simply for more and more square feet. Given sufficient room, librarians seem to be highly adaptive organisms, and can do very well if there is sufficient room for the growth of their holdings, their patrons (I started to say their seats), their services, and their personalities. Just give them space.

REFERENCES

1. Bishop, W. W. in Minutes of the 19th Annual Meeting held at Detroit, June 12, and Ann Arbor, Michigan, June 13, 1916. Bulletin 6: 16, 1916.
2. Miscellaneous Notes. Bulletin 28: 161, 1940.
3. Main floor plan University of Oregon Medical School Library. Bulletin 29: 122, 1940.
4. Bulletin 33: 103, 1945.
5. Miscellaneous News. Bulletin 30: 134, 1942.
6. Gilchrist, D. B. Some fundamentals in library planning. Bulletin 15: 1–8, 1925.
7. Stecher, R. M. Let there be light—at least enough for reading in libraries. Bulletin 33: 220–230, 1945.
8. Stecher, R. M. Why light in the library or comments on illumination. Bulletin 35: 137–145, 1947.

9. DAVIS, LORA-F. Instructions for a medical school library planning survey. BULLETIN 41: 273–276, 1953.
10. WARTHIN, A. S. The medical library of the University of Michigan. BULLETIN 4: 46–53, 1917.
11. BISHOP, W. W. The University of Michigan's new library building. BULLETIN 6: 53–57, 1917.
12. KRONICK, D. A. The University of Michigan's new medical library. BULLETIN 44: 424–427, 1956.
13. The New York Academy of Medicine and its new building project. BULLETIN 12: 19–21, 1922.
14. MALLOCH, A. The library of the New York Academy of Medicine. BULLETIN 17: 8–17, 1927.
15. WILLIAMS, L. R. Address of welcome. BULLETIN 17: 5–6, 1928.
16. DOE, J. The Library of the New York Academy of Medicine. Bull. N. Y. Acad. Med. 28: 197–203, 1952.
17. CAMPBELL, M. E. The biology-medical library of the University of Chicago. BULLETIN 18: 23–25, 1929.
18. DARLING, L. Planning the biomedical library building at U.C.L.A. BULLETIN 38: 246–252, 1950.
19. FRY, A. Plan and equipment of Health Sciences Library, University of Washington, Seattle. BULLETIN 41: 24–31, 1953.
20. HECK, L. B. New library at the University of Oklahoma School of Medicine. BULLETIN 41: 238–243, 1953.
21. ELDREDGE, A. The dental library in the organization of a new medical center library. BULLETIN 41: 393–395, 1953.
22. CRAMER, D. M. & FOX, F. K. The National Institutes of Health Library. BULLETIN 42: 176–182, 1954.
23. OLEY, J. A. Basic elements in the planning of a new building for the Armed Forces Medical Library. BULLETIN 42: 454–457, 1954.
24. ANNAN, G. L. Recent trends in medical historical libraries of the United States. Libri 5: 67–74, 1954.

Random Thoughts about Medical Library Planning*

By Alderson Fry, *Librarian*

Medical Center Library
West Virginia University
Morgantown, West Virginia

ABSTRACT

There seems to be enough material about library planning, but since mistakes, obvious ones, are made, maybe it is information without meaning. Sources of planning material are discussed, and some new libraries are considered. The necessity of discarding is urged, and methods of bringing it about are suggested.

When I accepted this assignment to bring up to date the 1957 paper on fifty years of medical library architecture (1), I did not know William Beatty would publish his excellent study, "Recently Built Medical School Libraries in the United States," summarizing his findings on twenty libraries built since 1955 (2). Two other ideas, when explored, had also been covered, enough to make another paper needless in the two fields. So, this paper is an olla podrida or, as I titled a paper last year, "Some Random Thoughts While Thinking about Library Planning."

But first, some philosophy of sorts. While in the Orient six months ago, I visited about twenty-five or thirty libraries. Outside of Japan, they are mostly pretty bad as concerns space and contents—the space was not built into the library from the beginning, and the storage of unneeded material has taken up too much of that limited space.

In one library (and I tried not to be a critic) the plan was poor, by any standards. But most surprising, the librarian and the committee that planned it had collected an excellent file of material on planning and were aware of much of its contents. I was surprised, though I prob-

* Presented at the Sixty-third Annual Meeting of the Medical Library Association, San Francisco, California, June 4, 1964.

Originally published in *Bulletin of the Medical Library Association,* Volume 51 (October, 1963), pp. 501-506. Reprinted by permission.

ably should not have been, cynic that I am. Anyhow, I thought about it and realized that here was a fairly common mistake. The information was available, certainly enough of it to be useful, but the meaning was not in it. Question: What is wrong with articles on library planning that they fail to communicate?

Information, shall we say, is not *meaning*, but a technical term related to degree of ordering, the method of presenting organized material, or the content presented. Meaning is a more difficult matter, not necessarily related to information, but a larger term, something super-added. The desire to sacrifice what we know to what we think creates more of a hippogriff than a working library. The information is there, but some planners cling to their memories and fantasies as if they were the spring-board to achievement.

Somehow we must put meaning into our information about planning. Maybe we are publishing our articles in the wrong places. Maybe we should find another word for "flexibility," because it is sometimes used to avoid planning in detail. Maybe there are too many people—or too few—between the plan and the building. But something is wrong somewhere. There is lots of information on how to plan a good library, but there is too little meaning in that information or too little old-fashioned preaching about it.

Help, I think, is on the way. There is more talk, or writing, about the meaning of the library. Ralph Esterquest points out in a recent article that the library will be with us for quite a while (3). He suggests what makes a good library, but here again is the problem of getting knowledge to work.

Quite useful reading, also, is the chapter on libraries in *Bricks and Mortarboards,* published this year by the Educational Facilities Laboratories (4). Some of the examples, I thought, were extreme, but the sermon is well delivered. Another excellent study is a German publication on the public library building (5). It should help expand the imagination and implant information. There is another publication by EFL, "The School Library" (6). Mention should also be made of Scott Adams' paper, "Medical Library Resources and Their Development" (7).

I would like to retract a statement I made some time ago that you should not visit many other libraries before planning your own, because such visits might lead to a bastard product and some confusion. I now think seeing other libraries is a good idea, particularly if you can spend long enough time in them to find what is right and what is wrong with them. But the selection of libraries should be judicious.

For instance, I think there is little to be learned from the National Library of Medicine about planning a health sciences library. There is too much disparity in size and function. (I must interject here I also think we make the mistake of sending visitors from abroad, who might plan a library, to the big ones we are so justly proud of. They should be sent to the libraries just a bit larger than the ones they might achieve. One visitor I had from Africa last year said he wanted to plan for an NLM library, starting with a room of about 10,000 square feet, to be gradually expanded into a national library.)

This is also true of the New York Academy of Medicine Library and, because it is no example of anything, of the College of Physicians Library at Columbia, probably the most outgrown library in the country right now.

Personally, I would add the new Francis A. Countway Library to this list. It is too big to be relevant, and it has some ideas that I hope will not be accepted elsewhere. "The Program for a New Library to Serve the Harvard Medical Center," March 1961, is a model of program writing, may be read by all with profit and edification, and can be reasonably copied if you must write a program, though it is too long for most. But I do object to that tremendous vault, 75 feet high, that sits in the middle of the library. This hole is 42 x 49 feet in size, occupying 13,706 square feet, and therefore is bigger than about one-third the medical libraries in this country. And, since Harvard paid about thirty dollars per square foot, it would cost $410,000. I am sure Harvard has good and sufficient reasons for this type of architecture that seems so out of place with today's air conditioning, but before anyone uses that idea he should take a long, thoughtful look at it.

The new Harvard library has some excellent ideas, though. I particularly liked the idea of placing the light transformers in their own room where they can hum away at all times. This library has done away with the main-reading-room concept, thus truly achieving a juxtaposition of student and book, and, remarkable for so large a library, separated the old books and periodicals from the new.

A large library that can be recommended is the new John Crerar Library. It is tasteful, well designed, illustrative of many new ideas, and built with remarkable economy. Few of us will be planning million-volume libraries, but, just in case, look at this one.

There are two more separate buildings that can be usefully studied. The Health Sciences Library of the University of Maryland in Baltimore can be visited with profit. On four floors, with 70,500 square feet of space, it has been well designed by Mrs. Marion Robinson. It is neat, with good lines, and if it has faults they are the use of valuable space on the main floor front for staff and the existence of a few too many separate rooms.

Relevant to the problems most of us have is the new Medical College of Georgia Library in Augusta. Planned by the Librarian, Sadie Hill Rainsford, it is one of the most beautiful in decor of the medical libraries around right now. It was finished last year. It has two floors and no basement, occupying 28,300 square feet—cost $600,000, including the modern furniture—and is a pleasure to see. Particularly notable is the complete use of nonwooden furniture. I am sorry to say I think the floor plan can be faulted. The reference tools are on the first floor, with the catalog and charging desk, and the books and periodicals are on the second floor. And the history room occupies space beyond its importance.

Since this paper is compounded of some facts and some prejudices, I shall not consider any libraries, segregated or integrated, of less than about 28,000 square feet, because today's medical or health sciences library in the United States should not be smaller than that.

And while expressing prejudices, I shall give you as a good example of the integrated library one that is part of a medical center, my own library in Morgantown. It has about 30,000 square feet, is air-conditioned and well lighted, holds about 350 students and 140,000 volumes, has 16 study rooms, and is very easy to explain to the new patron. The charging desk and work area are to the right of the entrance, a reading room and the new periodicals are to the left, and there is a "Calling Dr. Kildare Room" for those on call. The reference tools are together, and the most used books and the last twenty years of periodicals are on the main floor, with the remainder on the up or down floors of the storage area, which is near the center of the main room and is central core-stack construction. The reading rooms are broken up into three areas, and there are eight different types of chairs, both for decor and choice of seating. Visitors are invited.

Now that the information and meaning of library-planning material has been considered and some examples of planning described, I want to take up a third point, that of discarding, which I think is important. I said many of the libraries in the Orient have used much of their limited space for what seems to me to be unneeded material. That situation is true of our own libraries also. Here again, we have the information that should lead us to discard, but it does not seem to have any meaning for us or does not mean enough to lead us to take action.

Ralph Esterquest in his *Strengthening Medical Library Resources in New York State* makes the strong recommendation, with a plan for implementing it, that New York State build no more great storage libraries, but rely on those already in the state (8). He points out that new libraries can depend on the big ones for little-used material, and they should.

But he overlooks, I think, one point. He suggests a good working library size of from 70,000 to 90,000 volumes. By the time a library hits about 80,000 volumes, unless it is a fairly old library, it has generated a good head of steam and will very quickly go past that point. A library that size will be taking about 1,000 to 1,200 periodicals, acquiring about 3,000 books a year, and, if it is a fairly new library, still filling in some backlog. So at 6,000 to 7,000 volumes a year it very rapidly crosses the 100,000 volumes size and is still going strong. Very soon there is a new library to be built, or a strong discard program must be initiated. Here I wish to repeat some material I gave last year in Chicago, which, insofar as I now know, does not seem likely to be published.

Most of the rest of this talk is devoted (and you may consider that word either in the sense of the minister or the agent provocateur) to an attack on the idea that most of us must keep building bigger and bigger libraries, or at least putting more and more books in them. We must be concerned (1) with adding to that huge mass of books we have back in the bowels, or megacolon, of the library or (2) with getting rid of this matter altogether. This latter action will result in saving money, running more efficient libraries, and, unfortunately for some of you, building fewer libraries. Natually I think it will be fortunate for the rest of society.

Some of my attitude is easy to illustrate. Thank God for that accretive hi-fi set, the engaging TV, the amiability of the car, and the blessings of medicine in eliminating a great deal of only marginal health, thus making available energy for something besides reading. They are breaking the stranglehold of the writer-publisher-critic guild, which would have us believe reading is man's highest pursuit. As Peter Dooley said, "Readin' ain't thinking." And Oscar Wilde said, "Work is the curse of the drinking class." Well, print is the curse of the thinking class.

But let us suppose that some reading does lead to some thinking. It is perfectly clear that no one person, not even any 5,000 persons, could read, or would want to read, or should read, all the books that have ever been printed, acquired, cataloged, and shelved. What, then, is worth reading—and hence worth giving expensive storage space?

Some people have thought about this problem. Our great Harvey Cushing has written: "Too often libraries are but the graveyards of forgotten books, whose oblivion is disturbed only by the exigencies of time, which has necessitated their transfer for lack of space from the smaller cemetery to the larger." And Marian Patterson, Academy of Medicine, Toronto, wrote, ". . . we do not want our libraries to be regarded as tombs for tomes and ourselves as members of the royalty in the solitude of the crypt."

But aren't we, as librarians, mummified in a printed desert of paper trash in which only a few oases break the useless landscape? Patricia Knapp's dissertation, *College Teaching and the College Library*, is the latest and one of the best studies of the use of library books (9). She studied Knox College, whose library held 79,144 volumes and was a good library. More than 90 percent of the loans were for course purposes. Two-thirds of the loans were from the reserve collection. And, most important, everything was taken care of by 5,000 titles. Only about one-sixteenth of the collection was oasis. Of the rest, if I may quote from one of the books that probably was used, "boundless and bare / The lone and level sands stretch far away."

I don't know that a hundred such studies would force the librarian to stop accumulating and saving so much. But they ought to be made, if only to show that our dinosaur libraries are becoming so unwieldly that, like the stegosaurus, we have had to add a second brain—the computer—to take care of the tremendous size. Possibly we, like the stegosaurus and the other dinosaurs, are witlessly plodding toward tar pits made of our own books.

As we plod along, we are aware enough that storage is one of the library planner's biggest problems. We speak of the need for flexibility, and we seek to avoid the central core stacks or a large undigestible mass of stacks. But both our brains have missed the point. It is not the stacks that are indigestible, but the books that go on them. The gin-drinker's liver, if you remember, is treated by getting rid of the gin, not by doing away with or enlarging the liver itself. In other words, there is nothing wrong with our stacks except the way we treat them. (Libraries have the colic, because we are bucolic about books.)

Very well then, let us make an heuristic rule. Twenty percent of the median sized college library holdings are useful. The rest are for storage, if not for discard.

Now let us work to find out how nearly right this rule is and find a proper sliding scale for it, such as a percentage indicating that as a library gets bigger the percentage of active usefulness gets smaller. With such a scale, library planning would be simplified. And you would have the possibility of learning another, most valuable figure: what percentage should be discarded.

To get myself off the hook, please remember I am not talking about discarding all books, but merely the worst 10 or 20 or 30 percent. The moment you mention this subject, people react by saying, "You want to throw out Shakespeare!" They use the top 10 percent as a shelter under which to hide the bottom 20 percent. They are not only unable to see the trees because of the forest, they are unable to see the forest because of the woodpulp.

The reef on which library planning is wrecking is that big, undigestible mass of volumes in storage. There is a sick book title that goes "Around the Block in 80 days with the Cerebral Palsy Marching Band." Well, librarians are moving at about that pace toward a solution, and if there is to be a modern trend in library planning and administration, it must be toward a solution at a faster rate.

For example, it seems that all plans presented, year after year, call for bigger and bigger areas. Such plans are invariably accompanied by the selfcontradictory illusion that while libraries get bigger and bigger, the book and the reader are getting closer and closer together. You know when you blow up a balloon that you are at the uninflated start in contact with a relatively large part of its surface. But as the balloon gets bigger and bigger, as you blow harder and harder, you are less and less in contact. And sooner or later, there's going to be a blow-up.

Now one answer to successful planning would be to have all the money you could possibly use, like Harvard. But this won't bring the reader and the useful book together when the needed book is one among hundreds of thousands of relatively worthless, if not completely worthless, books. Space might seem to be the answer, but in this context space is a function of money, so space just defers the problem.

I wrote a while back that 90 percent of the problems of successful library planning can be summed up in one word: "Space." Well, 30 percent of these problems may be solved by the application of one word: "DISCARD!"

Of course all this has been said before. The introduction to a medical book in my library starts off: "There is nothing in this book that has not been said at least 500 times before—but nobody seems to listen." I understand what he means. In library planning there is no Bellman to insist that what he tells us three times is true.

The architect cannot solve the problem. It is not his business. The college president or your dean cannot solve it, because he is caught in a competitive situation and a need for grants. The students cannot solve it—they are in the position of "vexation without representation." Accountants, though they might be horror-struck by a cost-function analysis of those old books, cannot solve the problem and would not listen to our unscientific, unproven, and probably unprovable lofty generalities.

In short, though the librarian may be caught in a status-symbol bind and a Parkinsonian web, he is the only man who can solve the problem. I hasten to add that he has help.

Perhaps the answer lies in the already existing regional plan. Perhaps it lies in greater use of microfilm, something quite feasible since the introduction of the reader-printer. But using microfilm for worthless material is not a solution.

Perhaps the answer is to be found in such libraries as the Butler Library, the Lamont Library at Harvard, and the Heritage Library. Certainly the Princeton plan, with a central library and about a dozen libraries at other places, has a great deal to be said for it. But, I must say, none of these are really discard programs.

Maybe the teaching machine will help. Programming them calls for a very careful assessment of useful knowledge, and minds trained on that kind of diet could very well learn to reject the trash—something that is not being done now.

But the one answer we have available right now, at no added expense to speak of, is a workable and working discard program. So, let me make a Modest Proposal, or Proposals.

We all know we are cowards about discarding, fearing, if nothing else, the finger of scorn, so let us try to devise some working rules. One would be that circulation, exclusive of Reserve, must at least equal the holdings, or vice versa.

Also, set up a traveling fund out of the money saved by discarding, by not building new libraries, and by not buying in the first place to be used to send the sometime, or summer, scholar to a large storage library to continue his work. Very few on the staff, really, are doing any way-out-yonder research. How many lockable carrels, so eagerly gobbled up by the faculty when first made available, are ever used?

I have other suggestions. Since the retiring librarian is a knowledgeable person, hire him, since no one can jump him for what he throws away, to do your discarding.

Select three or four thousand books in a given subject field for possible discard. Invite the faculty and graduate students in that field to come help themselves. Then as they leave the library take the books they have selected away from them. Now you have the books judged best by competent persons (who might otherwise say, "Keep them all"). Return these to the shelves for keeping, and burn those that were left behind, that no one wanted. And I do mean burn, or sometime the weight of libraries will gradually sink this entire continent gently beneath the Atlantic and Pacific oceans.

Another method of arriving at what to discard would be to gather at a sort of summer camp, where there are no libraries and no bibliographies, all those concerned with certain disciplines, then ask them to list all the books they could remember by author and title. Put these in a composite list and discard all books not listed. That would get rid of 98 percent of your holdings.

The administration could make the library pay five dollars back into the general fund for every book more than fifty years old it keeps. Discards made before a book is twenty-five years old would be good for a five dollar credit.

Or (and this isn't a bad idea at all), if the library operates with departmental funds, after a book is, say twenty-five years old, give those in charge of the departmental fund the privilege of either discarding the book or paying the main library out of departmental funds five dollars for every book that is kept beyond that period. That will force a judgment on lots of worthless books.

Recently there has been developed paper that will last longer than fifty years. Maybe that is going in the wrong direction. Maybe we need a paper that, regardless of how it is kept, falls suddenly into dust at the end of fifty years. Then we would make a reevaluation of our books and keep only a few of them.

What does this have to do with library trends or recent developments? In an anonymous article recently there is the statement that:

> on the average, some 4,000 technical articles (enough to fill seven sets of the Encyclopaedia Britannica) and 50 new books are published *daily* in the United States alone: the world's store of knowledge has increased by better than 80 per cent in the last four years, and will probably be trebled in five years; that's even faster than the population explosion.
>
> The American Institute of Biological Sciences reports that technical writing in the United States costs some 10 billion per annum. This includes military weapons manuals, however, the cost of which is put at 2.8 billion and accounts for six per cent of the total military expenditures. More than 90,000 people are currently at work in this country on full-time editing, writing and publishing of scientific and technical material. By 1970 the number, it is expected, will be 160,000 people (10).

I question the above, but the situation is bad enough. A more sensible view is presented by John C. Green (11). I think this can safely be said: Ten years from now at our regular meeting, if the trend continues, you will be told that the average health sciences library should have about 60,000 square feet and hold 180,000 to 200,000 volumes. So, in summary of this discard sermon, we must solve this problem of overgrown libraries by screwing our courage to the chucking point. If the librarian will only get concerned enuf, worried enuf, he might get mad enuf to blow his stack.

One last word on the problem of information and the meaning of information. Despite the publications on library planning, some libraries are still being planned that could have been, in the view of a panel of experts, improved on in a meaningful way. Possibly a consultant, or consultants, is the answer. Certainly calling in a consultant would give fairly cheap insurance against a bad mistake or two, and if the library costs more than half a million dollars, probably there should be two independent consultants. If you follow trends, there is a trend in that direction, dictated by the growing size and growing complexity of our library plans.

REFERENCES

1. Fry, Alderson, and Adams, Scott. Medical library architecture in the past fifty years. Bulletin 45: 471–479, Oct. 1957.
2. Beatty, William K. Recently built medical school libraries in the United States. J. Med. Educ. 38: 725–729, Sept. 1963.
3. Esterquest, Ralph T. Improving the quality of the medical school library. J. Med. Educ. 39: 451–458, May 1964.
4. Educational Facilities Laboratories. Bricks and Mortarboards. New York, The Laboratories, 1964.
5. Mevissen, Werner. Büchereibau. Public Library Building. Essen, E. Heyer, 1958.
6. Ellsworth, Ralph E., and Wagener, Hobart D. The School Library. Edited by Ruth Weinstock. New York, Educational Facilities Laboratories, 1963.
7. Adams, Scott. Medical library resources and their development. J. Med. Educ. 38: 20–27, Jan. 1963.
8. Esterquest, Ralph T. Strengthening Medical Library Resources in New York State. Albany, New York State Library, 1963.
9. Knapp, Patricia. College Teaching and the College Library. Chicago, American Library Association, 1959. (ACRL Monograph, No. 23.)
10. Quality, quantity, and the scientific press. The Sciences 2: 2, June 15, 1962.
11. Green, John C. The information explosion—real or imaginary? Science 144: 646–648, May 8, 1964.

The Medical Library Center of New York: An Experiment in Cooperative Acquisition and Storage of Medical Library Materials*

BY ERICH MEYERHOFF, *Director*

The Medical Library Center of New York
New York, New York

IN 1951 the director and planner of the Midwest Inter-Library Center surveyed the history of storage libraries and outlined the program for the newly established regional, cooperative facility for the universities of the Midwest (1). The Midwest Inter-Library Center received wide and deserved acclaim throughout the library world for its imaginative planning and its elegant execution and development. Indeed, a recent review of "The State of the Library Art" concludes: "It may be certainly said that no single activity has contributed as much overall to the impulse given cooperative planning as this one. Whether it be judged successful or not, its importance in guiding the thinking of modern libraries towards the future has been considerable" (2).

The Medical Library Center of New York bears a heavy debt, not only to the Midwest Inter-Library Center, but to the New England Deposit Library and the Hampshire Interlibrary Center. They demonstrated the economic advantages of integrated, cooperative housing and cooperative acquisition of library materials. They provided administrative methods for these activities. However, they supported general academic library programs while the Medical Library Center of New York serves a specialized subject area, medicine and its allied disciplines.

Cooperation among libraries in the New York metropolitan area has traveled a rocky road. It may suffice to say that the meetings and deliberations of the heads of the large research libraries and the college and special libraries which began in 1948 ended in failure. Nearly ten years later

* Presented at a meeting of the Medical Society Libraries Group, Medical Library Association, Chicago, Illinois, June 6, 1962.

Originally published in *Bulletin of the Medical Library Association,* Volume 53 (July, 1965), pp. 374-383. Reprinted by permission.

the Council of Higher Educational Institutions in New York City obtained a grant from the Avalon Foundation and employed Mr. Warren James Haas, now Assistant Director of the Libraries of Columbia University, as a full-time consultant to investigate the needs for cooperative action among the libraries of the institutions of higher education in the City of New York and to develop a set of recommendations. Mr. Haas developed a plan (3) which was coordinated with the recommendations of the Committee on Reference and Research Library Resources of the Commissioner of Education of the State of New York (4). These plans called for regional cooperative libraries aided by State funds. So far these plans have failed to obtain the approval of the New York State Legislature. Most recently, Ralph T. Esterquest, the Librarian of the Harvard Medical Library, was retained by James E. Allen, Jr., Commissioner of Education of the State of New York, to survey the adequacy of medical library resources and develop a plan for the improvement of medical library service in the State of New York (5). Esterquest's interesting plan also required extensive state aid, and the plan has not been carried out either in toto or in part.

The plans for cooperation among medical libraries, initiated in 1958, proceeded slowly but steadily. After the medical librarians in the New York area had indicated a definite interest in cooperative planning, steps were taken by the Director of the New York Academy of Medicine, Dr. Howard Reid Craig, to interest the deans of the medical schools of the city and the chief administrative officers of medical research institutions to organize an agency which would obtain funds and develop a program.

On November 20, 1959, the Medical Library Center of New York was incorporated. The medical schools of Columbia, Cornell, New York University, Yeshiva, and New York Medical College, as well as the Rockefeller Institute, the Memorial Sloan-Kettering Cancer Center, the New York Academy of Medicine, and the Department of Health of New York City, became associated with the Center. The Board of Trustees consists of the deans of the medical schools and chief administrative officers of the other institutions mentioned. The purposes of the Center are given in the Charter as follows:

1. To provide additional stack facilities and book storage for the medical libraries of the medical colleges and research institutions in the City of New York as well as for the libraries of other medical and scientific institutions which the trustees may deem eligible to participate in the maintenance and use of such facilities.
2. In furtherance of the services and activities of such libraries:
   a) To maintain a union list of current medical literature available in the New York area;
   b) To develop uniform systems of cataloguing;
   c) To facilitate the acquisition and sharing of medical books and periodicals and medical library equipment; and

d) To provide facilities for research and experiment in the field of medical library practice and administration.

During the next year financial support was obtained from the Avalon Foundation, the Commonwealth Fund, the John and Mary R. Markle Foundation, the James Foundation, and the Health Research Council of the City of New York. The John A. Hartford Foundation gave a grant of $127,000 for the establishment of the Union Catalog of Medical Periodicals and organizational expenses of the Medical Library Center. In May of 1961 a director for the Center was appointed, and on December 15, 1961, an eight-story garage building of 160,000 square feet, located in the immediate vicinity of the New York Academy of Medicine, was purchased for the total of $950,000. Shortly thereafter the architectural firm of Steinmann, Cain, and White was selected to prepare preliminary drawings for the conversion of the sixth and seventh floors of the building for library purposes. The alterations and the equipment for the Center are estimated to cost an additional $509,000. The space will be ready for occupancy in February of 1964. The initial capacity will be 39,000 running feet of shelving for 300,000 volumes.

Program of the Medical Library Center of New York

The program of the Center is related to the general framework within which it operates: (1) It is a library for other libraries, and its services, therefore, benefit individual users only indirectly. (2) Its scope is a specific subject area. (3) Its associated institutions and organizations are located within a relatively small geographic area.

The functions of the Center may be divided into six major categories:

1. *A joint housing facility of less-used library materials in medicine and its related disciplines.*

The determination of what is little used is left to the librarians of each of the affiliated libraries on the assumption that the librarian, who must provide for the literature needs of his clientele, is most qualified to make this judgment. The categories which the Center will accept for deposit, however, are carefully defined, and among these are:

(*a*) clinical and basic science serials;
(*b*) serials in related disciplines, such as nursing, optometry, medical technology, pharmacy, veterinary medicine, parasitology, mycology, biochemistry, physics, even sociology, as long as they are actually in the collection of a participating library;
(*c*) text books and monographs;
(*d*) dissertations and theses in medicine and its allied disciplines;
(*e*) international, national, regional, and local government publications in the field of health;

(*f*) institutional publications such as catalogs of schools of medicine, nursing, etc., and annual reports of hospitals; and

(*g*) catalogs of dealers of rare books and second hand books, principally covering medicine and related sciences.

The Center controls the input of materials and interprets whether materials offered are in scope. It can, therefore, insure to a large extent that it will house less-used materials and eliminate trivia. The librarians of the participating libraries themselves plan to make this a useful collection. This is indicated by the type of journals which they intend to give to the Center; for example, early issues of the Scandinavian *Acta*, the *American Journal of Roentgenology*, the German *Ergebnisse*, etc.

A library may place materials in the Center in three ways: It may make a free gift and relinquish ownership. It may retain title to its materials but may demand their return only upon the dissolution of the Center (this applies primarily to institutions unable to give up ownership because of legal or statutory restrictions). It may rent storage space at the Center and retain full control of its materials.

2. *A cooperative central acquisitions program of less-used currently published serials and of reference works.*

The Center will acquire medical, biochemical, pharmaceutical, veterinary, and dental journals, which are listed in pertinent abstracting and indexing journals such as *Index Medicus*, which are not currently received by any of the participating libraries, and which are judged to be of sufficient importance by the librarians of the participating institutions. It will also acquire reference works, mainly in languages other than English, whose use can be shared through a central information service.

3. *An information service to interpret the collection at the Center.*

4. *Dissemination of materials held by the Center.*

The Center follows the National Library of Medicine in providing, wherever possible, electrostatic copies of the articles requested. It will also have a daily messenger service which will pick up and deliver materials from the associated libraries. Requests for books and journals will be received by telephone and by mail, and during the hours when the Center is not staffed an automatic recording device, installed in the telephone, will take incoming requests.

5. *A Union Catalog of Medical Periodicals for the New York metropolitan area.*

As previously mentioned this program has been separately funded by a grant from the John A. Hartford Foundation. Mrs. Jacqueline W. Felter assumed the direction of this project in September of 1961. The Catalog will list holdings, not only of the libraries associated with the Center, but of all pertinent collections in the New York metropolitan area. The

Union Catalog will provide current information from its card files, and it will also publish a union catalog in book form, which will be distributed to its contributors and will be available to other libraries.

Microfilming of the files of the libraries of the member institutions has begun. These films allow us to make Xerox copies, which constitute the working file of the Catalog. These will be integrated, and at present an investigation is under way on the use of punched cards with print-out possibilities.

The Union Catalog will indicate duplication of materials; it will reveal fragmentary files of journals, now scattered in several locations, which may be united to form files which are complete; and it will enable us to determine important journals which are not presently received in this area.

6. *A program of research to find cooperative solutions to help libraries to deal with the problems of storing, disseminating, and interpreting information.*

Such a program should serve the practical needs of the Center but need not be limited to applied problems. A study of serial entries used by the participating libraries which would lead to recommendations for uniform cataloging entries for serials has been suggested. The basic data will come from the Union Catalog of Medical Periodicals. Since the Union Catalog will provide uniform entries and will probably be organized on punched cards, it may be possible to supply a participating library with a new and revised card catalog.

One of the by-products of the microfilming of serial catalogs has been the actual reproduction of an entire serial card catalog for a member library which needs a duplicate at a distance from its main catalog.

Perhaps the most important function of the Union Catalog may be in finding materials cited on the MEDLARS computer tapes of the National Library of Medicine.

Financing

No final figures are available on the cost of this undertaking, but the present plan will hold the cost to the participating institutions to a minimum. Since the Medical Library Center will use only the space it actually needs for efficient operation, a major portion of our building will continue to be rented and produce income. This income will cover nearly two-thirds of the operating expenses of the Center. Of course, as more space is needed, rental income will decline.

It is difficult to arrive at an equitable way to share operating expenses, and some arbitrariness can hardly be avoided. It was realized that actual use of the materials at the Center would be of little help in establishing sharing ratios, because the need for less-used material is completely random. The Trustees decided that for the present the expected operating deficit would be shared equally by the participating institutions. Although these institutions differ in their overall budget, their share of the Center's operating costs is still a very small portion of their total budget. It is unlikely that this situation can be maintained, however, when other institutions with smaller resources become members of the Center.

REFERENCES

1. Esterquest, Ralph T. The storage library and beyond. Libri 1: 239–252, 1951.
2. Orne, Jerrold. Storage warehouses. In: Shaw, Ralph, ed. The State of the Library Art. New Brunswick, N. J., Graduate School of Library Service, Rutgers–The State University, 1960, v. 3, pt. 3, p. 27.
3. Council of Higher Educational Institutions in New York City. Cooperation in Library Service for Higher Education. New York, 1960.
4. Commissioner's Committee on Reference and Research Library Resources. Report. University of the State of New York, State Education Department, New York State Library, December 1961.
5. Esterquest, Ralph T. Strengthening Medical Library Resources in New York State. Albany, N. Y., The University of the State of New York, State Education Department, New York State Library, 1963.

VII
HISTORY OF MEDICINE AND THE LIBRARY

Introduction

Every discovery, however important and apparently epoch-making, is but the natural and inevitable outcome of a vast mass of work, involving many failures, by a host of different observers[1].

Why should we be interested in history? To us and we hope to other medical librarians, it is because we like it. This is reason enough. Further than that, medicine is blessed with a rich heritage, and a knowledge of the developments of modern medicine from primitive beliefs should be a great source of cultural satisfaction.

Besides the cultural aspects, there are several more reasons for the study of medical history. As many have pointed out, today's medicine is the outgrowth of yesterday's, and many of the principles guiding present-day physicians owe their origin to past discoveries.

Another reason for studying medical history is the possibility of rediscovering in the older literature important concepts about disease that may be applicable to present-day medicine. Often, too, medical investigators unaware of past endeavors may claim priority in the discovery of a concept or therapeutic measure only to hear from their history-studying confreres that what they considered to be new and original had been better described many years before.

Study of the history of medicine will lead the reader to the classic descriptions of diseases and other important discoveries relating to the entire field of medicine. How much better to read descriptions in their original setting or in a translation of an original paper than to read from a secondary source! The reading of original descriptions can also be thrilling and provides accuracy, whereas a partially quoted or paraphrased secondary source may be inaccurate.

History, like other disciplines, has a mission. It not only teaches us about things of the past but also suggests, if only by implication, the things to come. The greatest advances in medicine have occurred in the last 100 years, and the task is not finished. Not only must physicians continue the conquest of diseases that still cripple our civilization but also they must consider as part of their task the large overall problem of arriving at man's understanding of man. The mission of the medical librarian is to aid physicians as much as possible in this respect.

The writings included in this chapter selectively share the thoughts, activities, and contributions of authors who have been, or are, involved in the history of medicine.

The *Fabrica* by Andreas Vesalius was a revolutionary book that had a decisive influence on the development of scientific thought. This book, published in 1543, one of the greatest of all books in the history of medicine, ushered the study of anatomy into the modern age. It also paved the way for William Harvey and his 1628 epochal contribution, the concept of unidirectional circulation of the blood in the body, published in *De Motu Cordis*. Dr. Max Fisch, author of the classic article selected for this chapter, discusses well both Vesalius and his great book. The *Fabrica* is a major treasure of any medical library that owns it.

Dr. Francis Packard narrates the life and works of William Macmichael, who was both a physician and a librarian. Packard reviews in some detail Macmichael's *The Gold Headed Cane*, which was first published in 1827. With this book, Macmichael reawakened interest in the history and in the achievements of the illustrious men who had been associated with the Royal College of Physicians. The book is an autobiography of the adventures of the famous gold headed cane as it passed through the hands of Radcliffe, Mead, Askew, William and David Pitcairn, and Baillie and then retired to the library of the Royal College of Physicians of London.

In "On the Reading of Medical Classics," its author, Dr. Owsei Temkin, argues the virtues to those involved in medicine of a close companionship with the great works of the past.

Dr. David Kronick offers good advice to the librarian who is collecting historical medical books. He also shares interesting comments on some of the great works in medicine.

Gertrude Annan, one of the most knowledgeable individuals on rare medical books in our time, comments on collecting for the history of medicine. Drawing on a background rich with personal experiences, she contributes excellent suggestions for persons in this area of librarianship. Miss Annan's practical and helpful list of "Do's and Dont's for Rare Books" is also reprinted.

Henry Schuman, in his day a great friend to librarians and libraries, details his personal involvements with the Lawrence Reynolds Collection. This remarkable collection pertaining to the history of the medical sciences took Dr. Reynolds, with the collaboration of Schuman, about 40 years to form. He annotates the "highlights" in the collection and describes his personal relationship with its collector. Today the collection resides in a great Alabama university medical library.

Another great friend to medical librarians was Murray Gottlieb of the Old Hickory Bookshop, New York City. His friendship, advice, and encouragement enriched the lives of those who knew him. Mr. Gottlieb, with pleasure and personal commitment, was a matchmaker, placing important medical books that came into his hands with the appropriate library or collection. In "This Business of Rare Books," he shares much of himself and his experience, values, and philosophy.

In "Physicians and Books," Dr. William Bean reminds us of the importance of books and libraries to persons charged with responsibilities for health care and lives ("they built our great tradition").

Dr. Peter Olch brings this chapter to a close with his delightful comments on the oral history movement, a description of efforts for oral history in the life sciences, and personal views.

With much regret, we are not able to include Myrl Ebert's article "The Rise and Development of the American Medical Periodical, 1797-1850" (Bull Med Libr Assoc 40:243-276, 1952) because of its length. This excellent historical essay is a classic and deserves recognition. It is must reading for anyone interested in the history of medicine.

REFERENCE

1. Starling: Cited by MORTON LT: A Medical Bibliography (Garrison and Morton): An Annotated Check-List of Texts Illustrating the History of Medicine. Third edition. Philadelphia. JB Lippincott Company, 1970, p v.

Vesalius and His Book

By MAX H. FISCH

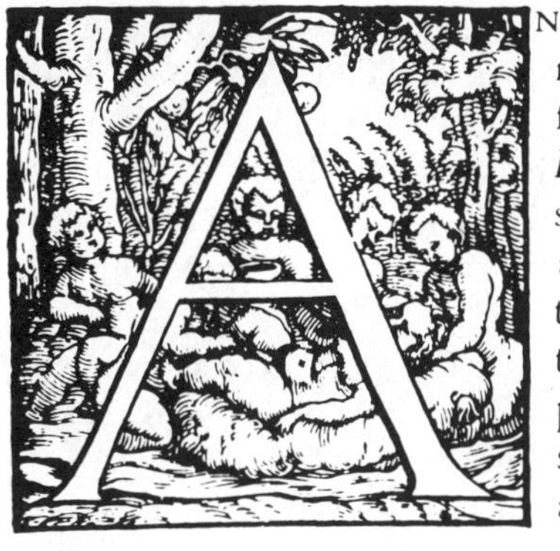

NDREAS VESALIUS has long been recognized by historians of medicine as the founder of modern anatomy; and his *Fabrica*, whether in the first or in the second edition, is the chief treasure of any medical library that owns it. But in the larger history of science and of culture Vesalius has not yet been given his place as the embodiment of the renaissance spirit in the field of medicine; and though the artistic merits of the *Fabrica* have been sufficiently admired, its unique position in the development of the printed book as a medium for the communication of descriptive science has not yet been generally appreciated.

Among the familiar notes of the renaissance are two in unstable equilibrium and frequent conflict: the passion for exploration, discovery, manifold experience; and the cult of antiquity. Both were strongly developed in Vesalius from childhood, assuming the special forms of a passion for dissection of animals on the one hand, and a reverence for the Greek medical tradition on the other. The conflict between the two did not emerge until he reached maturity, for he had the renaissance knack of persuading himself that each was a corollary of the other.

Vesalius was the fifth of a line in which the medical profession had passed from father to son. The first had written a commentary on a part of Avicenna's Canon of Medicine, and had had copies made for himself of all the medical texts then in use, which were handed down in the family. The second had been professor of medicine, astronomy and mathematics in the University of Louvain, and later city physician of Brussels; and had established the family fortune. The third had been physician to the Emperor Maximilian, and had written commentaries on

Originally published in *Bulletin of the Medical Library Association,* Volume 31 (July, 1943), pp. 208-221. Reprinted by permission.

the work of the Arab physician Rhasis, and on the Aphorisms of Hippocrates. The fourth, Vesalius's father, was apothecary to Margaret of Austria and later to the Emperor Charles V. Vesalius himself in turn became physician to Charles V, and later to his son Philip II of Spain, the two dominant figures in sixteenth century European politics.[6, 7]

Vesalius's mother was Elizabeth Crabbe, and the family home in Brussels was on land that had belonged to her father, Jacob Crabbe, who was probably of English origin. Behind the house there stretched a vacant and partly wooded area, called Gallows Hill, at the farther end of which condemned criminals were executed and their bodies left exposed.[7] There the boy Vesalius could observe from day to day the crude dissection performed on these bodies by time, the elements, and birds of prey; and could gather the bones he was later to describe so carefully in the *Fabrica.* Quite early he began himself to dissect rats, moles and dormice, with now and then a cat or a dog.

His father was away from home most of the time, accompanying the Emperor on his journeys and campaigns; but his mother seems equally to have cherished the medical tradition and vocation of the family into which she had married. It was she who preserved the books that had come down from Vesalius's forebears, and especially those which they had written themselves. She must often have turned their pages with the son who was to follow in their footsteps. She lived to add his book to the others; indeed it was she who procured the imperial *privilegium* for the *Fabrica* and sent it from Brussels to Oporinus at Basel.

Certainly in Vesalius's youth there was no conflict between tradition and experiment in his own mind. Was not his a family after the pattern of the ancient family of the Asclepiads, in which, as Galen put it, the boys learned dissection at home along with reading and writing? And was it not from just such families that a rebirth of medicine must come?

After the usual schooling in Latin, Greek and the liberal arts at Brussels and Louvain, Vesalius went to Paris in 1533 to study medicine. His chief teachers were the anatomists Jacques Dubois and Guinterius of Andernach. Fernel, a deeper man than either of these, and a deeper man than Vesalius became, seems not to have touched him; perhaps because he did not teach anatomy. But what Dubois and Guinter really taught him was not anatomy but Galen. The occasional dissections by a barber-surgeon in their courses were aimed at the elucidation of Galen, and were largely confined to the viscera. "Except for eight muscles of the abdomen, disgracefully mangled and in the wrong order, no one . . . ever demonstrated to me any single muscle, or any single bone, much less the network of nerves, veins and arteries." The *fabric* of the human body was a continent reserved for his own exploration. When his fellow-students, and through them his teachers, learned that he had practised dissection from boyhood, they encouraged him, at the third dissection he attended, to take the knife himself; and he readily performed a more thorough and skilful dissection than the barber-surgeons could provide. This was followed by others quite beyond their range. As at Brussels, but now with a band of fellow-students to help him, he also collected bones at the cemetery of the Innocents; and at Montfaucon, where the bodies of the hanged were exposed and their bones lay in heaps, they fought off the dogs to secure the specimens they wanted.

While Vesalius was at Paris, Guinter compiled from Galen a small textbook of anatomy, without illustrations. In the first edition (1536) he spoke of Vesalius as "a youth of great promise, with a remarkable knowledge of medicine and of Greek and Latin, and great dexterity in dissection." It was by the help of Vesalius, he said, that he had finally traced the spermatic arteries to their origin. In a later edition (1539) he acknowledged that he had been assisted throughout by two able dissectors, Vesalius and Michael Servetus. "With the aid of these two, who attended my lectures on Galen, I have examined in the bodies themselves all the muscles, veins, arteries and nerves of the limbs and of the other external parts." But even this was an understatement, if we may judge by Vesalius's later *apologia pro vita sua* in his China Root Epistle of 1546:

> I reverence him on many counts, and in my published writings I have honored him as my teacher; but I wish there may be inflicted on my body, one for one, as many strokes as I have ever seen him attempt to make incisions in the bodies of men or beasts, except at the dinner table. Nor do I think he will take offense if I say of him, as of not a few others, that he is largely indebted to me for whatever he knows of anatomy apart from what is in the books of Galen, which are common property.

On the outbreak of the third Franco-German war in 1536, Vesalius returned to the University of Louvain. With the help of his friend Gemma Frisius (the teacher of Mercator), he smuggled in from the gallows outside the city walls a skeleton which they had found still held together by the ligaments and still possessing the origins and insertions of the muscles. Under the sponsorship of Jean of Armentières, professor of medicine, he set up this sketeton beside the dissection table, and "somewhat more accurately than at Paris expounded the whole fabric of the human body in the course of dissecting."

In February, 1537, as if to balance this innovation by a token of respect for tradition, Vesalius published a paraphrase of the ninth book of the *Almansor* of Rhasis, "On the cure of diseases from head to feet," a favorite compendium of general therapeutics, largely Hippocratic and Galenic. He had been encouraged to undertake this paraphrase by his teachers at Paris, and probably thought of it as a companion text to Guinter's Galenic *Institutiones Anatomicae*. to which, as we have seen, he had also lent his hand. His paraphrase was not based on the Arabic original, but on previous translations. He had by him also his grandfather's commentary on Rhasis, and doubtless intended his first publication as a tribute of filial piety to his medical forebears, and a mark of his coming-of-age in the family succession. Indeed he projected a paraphrase of the entire ten books of the *Almansor*, which he later completed but destroyed when he gave up teaching and entered the emperor's service.

The prefatory epistle to Nicolaus Florenas, physician to Charles V, was dated at Brussels, February 1, 1537, a month after Vesalius's twenty-second birthday; and the book was published at Louvain before the end of February. The next fixed date in his life is December 5 of the same year, when he received the degree of doctor of medicine at Padua, after some months of clinical study at Venice. We do not know when or by what route he went from Brussels to Venice; but from the fact that a second edition of his Paraphrase of Rhasis was published by Ruprecht Winter at Basel in March, 1537, I infer that he went by way of Basel; and from the far superior accuracy of the Basel edition I infer that he did not see the proofs of the Louvain edition, but went directly from Brussels to Basel and was there for a month or more seeing the second edition through the press.

Winter had three partners: Platter and Lasius, who had published Guinter's *Institutiones Anatomicae*; and Oporinus, who was later to publish Vesalius's *Fabrica*, *Epitome*, and China Root Epistle. Vesalius formed intimate friendships with these and other Basel printers.[6] In 1539 he had his Epistle on Bloodletting published by Winter, and in 1543 he stood godfather for Winter's son Hans. The earliest recollection of Platter's son Felix, himself an eminent physician, was seeing Vesalius in his father's home. In 1555 Johann Herwagen the elder sought his aid in securing the imperial *privilegium* for a book he wished to print, and an appointment as imperial notary for a nephew he wished to advance. When Henricpetri printed an edition of Rhasis in 1544, he included Vesalius's Paraphrase; and it was largely through Vesalius's personal application to the emperor that Henricpetri was knighted in 1556. But above all it was Oporinus who attracted Vesalius by his classical scholarship, by the mastery of medical terminology he had acquired under Paracelsus, by his meticulous proofreading, and by his *Gemütlichkeit*.

These friendships with Basel printers were Vesalius's tribute of gratitude, I think, for their having opened up to him the possibilities of the printed book with illustrations. Basel was now the chief publishing center of Europe; and it was especially pre-eminent in woodcut ornamentation and illustration, largely as a result of Holbein's collaboration with Froben and other printers there. It is no accident that the finest illustrated medical books of the century—Fuchs's *De Historia Stirpium* (1542), the most beautiful of all herbals, and Vesalius's *Fabrica* (1543), the most beautiful of all anatomy books—were printed at Basel.

It is not improbable that the dream of the *Fabrica* began to take shape at Basel in March, 1537. Certainly one of the first things Vesalius did after reaching Venice was to seek out an artist to help him prepare anatomical drawings for woodcut reproduction. Perhaps it was by applying to Titian that he was put in touch with Titian's pupil and his own fellow-countryman, Jan Stephan van Calcar.

Their collaboration began not later than December 6, 1537, when Vesalius assumed the chair of anatomy at Padua. Elaborate preparations had been made. A skeleton had been articulated and was set up beside the dissection table, as at Louvain, so that his audience might have constantly before them the basic framework of the body. Three cadavers

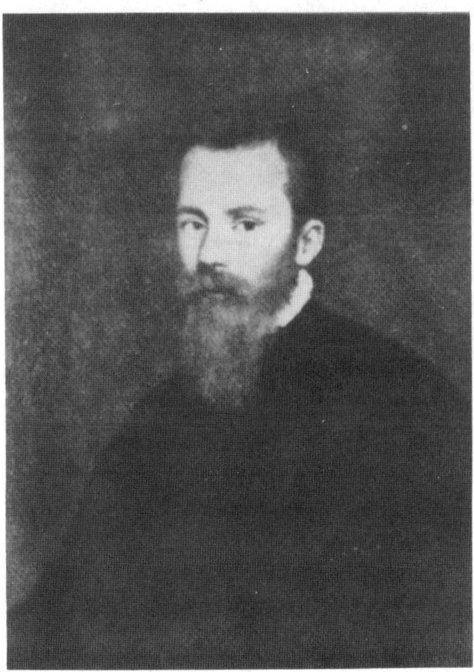

FIG. 1. Portrait of Vesalius by Calcar[2]

were provided, and the alternate dissection of them continued for three weeks. The first fruits of the collaboration of Calcar were the six Anatomical Tables which Vesalius dedicated to Narcissus Vertunus, chief physician to Charles V, under date of April 1, 1538, from Padua. The drawings for the three skeletal tables were made from Vesalius's skeleton by Calcar, and the wood engravings for all six tables were probably made at Venice under Calcar's direction. The sixth bears the colophon: "Printed at Venice by B. Vitale at the expense of Jan Stephan van Calcar. For sale at the shop of D. Bernardo. 1538."

Vesalius used as his anatomy textbook Guinter's Galenic *Institutiones Anatomicae*, but found in the course of his dissections that it needed extensive revision. He incorporated his revisions in a new edition which he published shortly after the Tables, with a dedicatory epistle to Jean of Armentières, professor of medicine at Louvain, under date of May 5, 1538. Thus within the first five months of his professorship he had published a textbook incorporating the results of his first-hand observations, and a set of tables in partial illustration of the textbook. But the text and illustrations were still essentially Galenic, and his revisions were conceived as corrections not of Galen but of Guinter. He preserved his renaissance bivalence by using his own observations, and even the Tables, to restore the original sense of Galen.

Nearly two years later, on January 1, 1539, in the concluding sentences of his Epistle on Bloodletting, addressed to Nicolaus Florenas, physician to Charles V, he reported his further progress in the work of providing adequate anatomic illustrations. Two new tables of the nerves, later used in the *Fabrica*, were ready; but those for the muscles and for the internal organs were still to be done. He had tried to conduct the dissections of the year in such a way that these could be made, but the throng that attended the course (often as many as five hundred) had made it impossible. He was being urged from all sides, and particularly by Marcantonio Genua, the professor of philosophy, who had become "as it were a second father" to him, to hasten the completion of the great work to which he had set his hand. And "if I have bodies enough to work with, and Jan Stephan, the outstanding painter of our age, continues to play his part, I shall not evade the task."

About this time the Giunta press at Venice projected an edition of Galen in Latin, asked Vesalius to revise the best existing versions of the *De nervorum dissectione*, the *De venarum arteriarumque dissectione*, and the *De anatomicis administrationibus*, and supplied him with a collection of variant readings of the Greek text for the purpose. When the Giunta edition appeared in 1541, the editor said in his preface that after

Vesalius had "corrected in many places" the translation by Antonio Fortolo of the first two tracts, it was only with the greatest difficulty that he was persuaded to revise the translation by his former teacher Guinter of Galen's great work on anatomic procedure. In the end, however, he had done this so thoroughly that as now printed it was "almost a new treatise."

In preparing his Paraphrase of Rhasis and in revising Guinter's *Institutiones,* Vesalius had innocently used his own observations to restore the sense of what he took to be corrupted passages. But now, as a result of examining the Greek texts of Galen more carefully, and checking Galen's statements by his own dissections, he was driven to the conclusion that Galen's anatomy was essentially that of the anthropoid apes, conjecturally but often erroneously extended to man. As he later put it in the *Fabrica:*

> It is quite clear to us, from the revival of the art of dissection, from a painstaking perusal of the works of Galen, and from a restoration of them

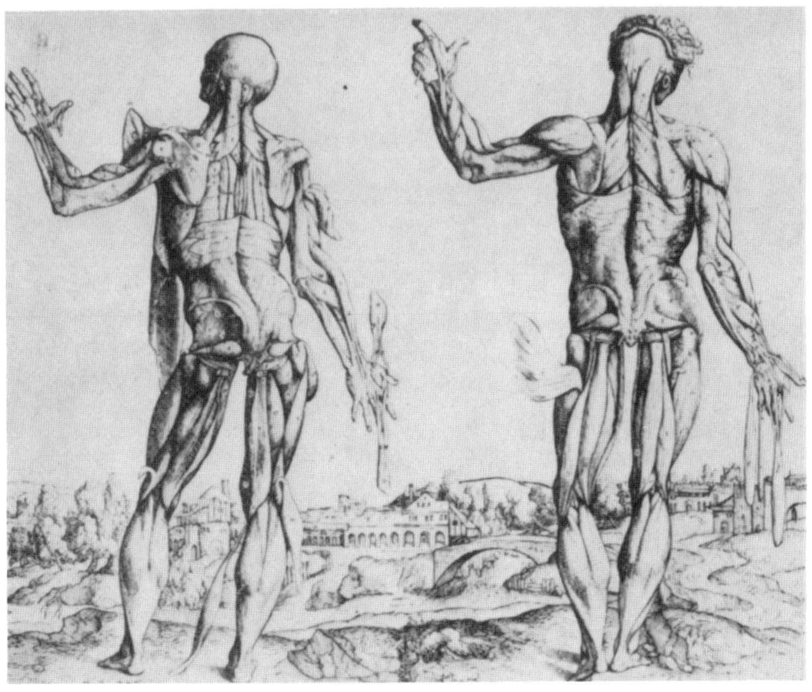

FIGURE 2. Muscle Tables XI and X from the *Fabrica*

in several places, of which we have no reason to be ashamed, that Galen himself never dissected a human body lately dead.

After making this discovery, Vesalius gave up reading his own observations into Galen; and when they were at variance with what he found there, he frankly presented them as corrections of Galen. The results of this change in his method of teaching were reported in the *Fabrica:*

> The medical profession are wont to be upset when *in more than two hundred instances,* in the conduct of the single course of anatomy I now exhibit in the schools, they see that Galen failed to give a true description of the interrelation, use and function of the parts of man. They scowl from time to time, and examine every inch of the dissection in their determination to defend him. Yet they too, drawn by the love of truth, gradually abandon that attitude and, growing less emphatic, begin to put faith in their own not ineffectual sight and powers of reason rather than in the writings of Galen.

So strong, however, was Vesalius's reverence for antiquity that,

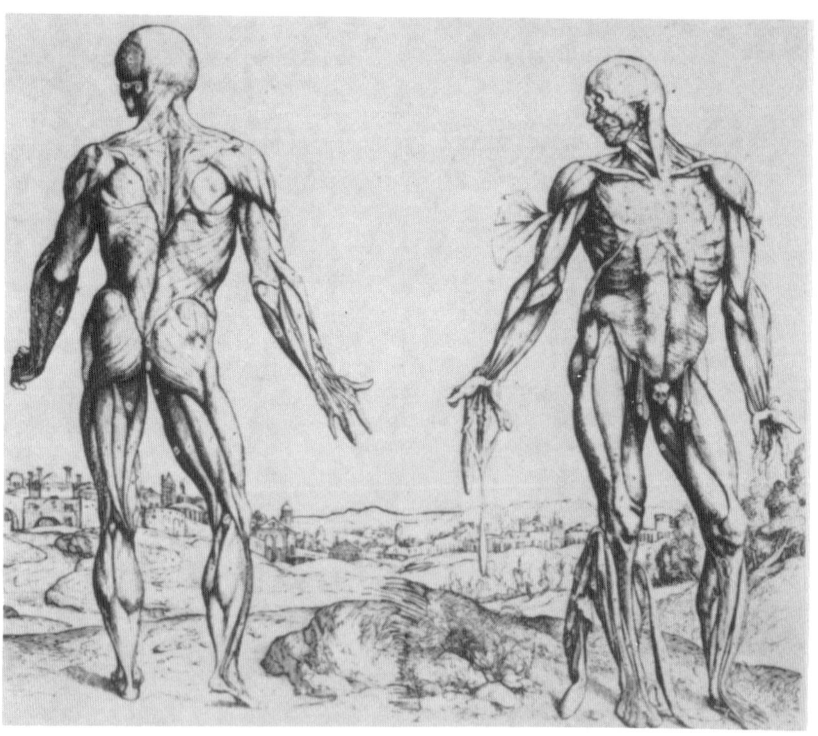

FIG. 3. Muscle Tables IX and IV from the *Fabrica*

now that Galen had failed him, he imagined for himself a pre-Galenic anatomy based on dissection of the human body. "Deceived by his monkeys," he says, "Galen often wrongly controverts the ancient doctors who had trained themselves by dissecting human corpses." And much as Bacon later lamented the loss of the writings of the pre-Socratic natural philosophers, Vesalius regretted that the pre-Galenic "writings of Eudemus, Herophilus, Marinus, Andreas, Lycus, and other princes of anatomy have not been preserved to us." There was no disrespect for Galen in this, for Galen himself had looked back on a golden age in which anatomy flourished because the Asclepiads learned dissection in boyhood. Thus it was still possible for Vesalius to preserve his reverence for antiquity and to regard his reformation of anatomy as a renaissance.

If Vesalius had had any lingering doubt, it was now, however, obvious that further revisions of Guinter's text, supplemented by further fugitive sheets like his own Anatomical Tables, would not suffice. Since the works of those pre-Galenic anatomists who dissected the human body had not survived, what was needed now was an entirely fresh exposition of "the fabric of the *human* body," based throughout on dissection and first-hand observation, and incorporating in the text itself a complete series of illustrations, carefully drawn from the object itself in the course of dissection.

By 1540, when Vesalius was twenty-five, the plan of the *Fabrica* had been laid out, several of the plates were ready, and Calcar had drawn the programmatic frontispiece.[1] Dissection-scene engravings were not new in anatomy texts, as appears from those in Mondino's *Anathomia* and in Berengario da Carpi's *Isagogae Breves*. In these, however, the professor reads the lesson out of a book from an elevated desk, while at a table below the barber-surgeon dissects the cadaver and the demonstrator beside him supervises the process and points with a wand to the parts as they are referred to in the text being read. In the frontispiece of the *Fabrica,* Vesalius himself stands at the table and unites into one the three rôles of lecturer, demonstrator and prosector. The barber-surgeons are reduced to keeping his instruments sharp below the table, and a skeleton sits above in the position formerly occupied by the professor. Moreover, Vesalius lectures from the cadaver and skeleton, not from a book.

In its calculated contrast at every point with the traditional dissection scene of the Mondino and Carpi manuals, the *Fabrica* frontispiece is the manifesto of an educational reform. But so much is Vesalius the medical man of the renaissance that he conceives even this reform as a rebirth. Medicine had flourished from Hippocrates to Galen because doctors of every school were masters of all three branches of the art—dietetics, pharmacy, and surgery.

> But after the ruin spread by the Goths, when all the sciences that had previously flourished and been properly practised went to the dogs, the more fashionable doctors . . . began to be ashamed of working with their hands, and delegated to slaves the manual attentions they judged needful for their patients. . . . Methods of cooking, and all the preparation of food for the sick, they left to nurses; compounding of drugs to apothecaries; surgery to barbers. . . .
>
> This deplorable dismemberment of the art of healing introduced into our schools the detestable procedure now in vogue, that one man should carry out the dissection of the human body, and another give the description of the parts. The lecturers are perched up aloft in a pulpit like jackdaws, and arrogantly prate about things they have never tried, but have committed to memory from the books of others, or placed in written form before their eyes. The dissectors are so ignorant of languages that they are unable to explain their dissections to the onlookers, and merely botch what they are supposed to exhibit in accordance with the instructions of the physician, who never applies his hand to the dissection, but contemptuously steers the ship out of the manual, as the saying goes. Thus everything is wrongly taught, days are wasted in absurd questions, and in the confusion less is offered to the onlooker than a butcher in his stall could teach a doctor. . . .

The educational reform proclaimed in the *Fabrica* frontispiece was therefore a means to, and an integral part of, a needed reform of medicine itself. The art of healing had suffered dispersion, and its severed parts had atrophied and decayed. It must be born again, whole and entire. And only a teacher who did his own dissecting could train doctors who would not abstain from surgery as from the plague, lest they be slandered as barbers by the mandarins of the profession. It need scarcely be added that Vesalius was applying to medicine the renaissance humanist's ideal of totality, and reading it back, in the renaissance fashion, into the rounded Greeks who not only saw but lived life steadily and lived it whole. When the humanist disdained to be but a fragment of a man, could the doctor content himself with being but a fraction of a physician?

The hoped-for reform proved abortive, and the progress of medicine came by increase rather than by decrease of specialization, and by the rise of sciences undreamed of by Vesalius. Though the ideal of totality was not thereby discredited, it was postponed perforce to some heaven of omniscience and omnicompetence. Vesalius's permanent contribution to medicine was the founding of the basic science of human anatomy on the dissection of human bodies. And his permanent contribution to education was not his attempted reform of anatomy teaching, but the perfecting of the printed book as a medium for the spread of scientific knowledge. This was the task that filled the years from 1540 through 1542, and the six months or more that Vesalius spent at Basel seeing the *Fabrica* through the press in 1543. This was the crowning achievement not only of Vesalius, but of Calcar and his associated artists and engravers, and of Oporinus the printer; yet above all of Vesalius, for there was scarcely any detail of preparation or execution which he did not personally plan and supervise. The teaching reform could plausibly be regarded as a return to the Greeks, but the book was a new creation, beyond the dream of any earlier age. Even the Basel printers with whom, as we believe, Vesalius first canvassed its possibilities in the spring of 1537, can scarcely have imagined anything which the fulfilment did not surpass.

The art of writing had from time immemorial made possible the permanent recording of the spoken word, and its indefinite multiplication by copying, so that an unlimited number of people in different times and places could read the same words. But what was physically possible was neither economically nor psychologically possible; for copies made by hand and one at a time were prohibitively expensive, and all texts suffered cumulative corruption by the errors of copyists. The art of printing from type had recently reduced the economic limitation by mass production methods, and nearly eliminated the psychological limitation by enabling the author to insure the accuracy of thousands of identical copies by correcting one proof. The arts of drawing and painting, of wood and stone carving, had from time immemorial made possible the permanent recording of visual impressions; but copies of these recordings made one at a time were even more expensive than copies of the written word; and exact copies of the original were not merely psychologically improbable, but physically impossible. The art of printing from wood engravings, however, had now virtually eliminated all obstacles except those inherent in the wood itself as a medium for recording the original visual impression.

These arts of printing from type and from wood engravings were closely associated from the beginning, and needed only the rise of a descriptive science like human anatomy to induce their fusion into a single art of communication. The anatomy lecture could be recorded, and the lecturer could control the record more completely than he could control his own tongue. The visual impression of the body under dissection could be recorded and revised under his scrutiny until a proof was run off which satisfied him. The two records could be reconciled with each other and with the physical fact, and woven together into a

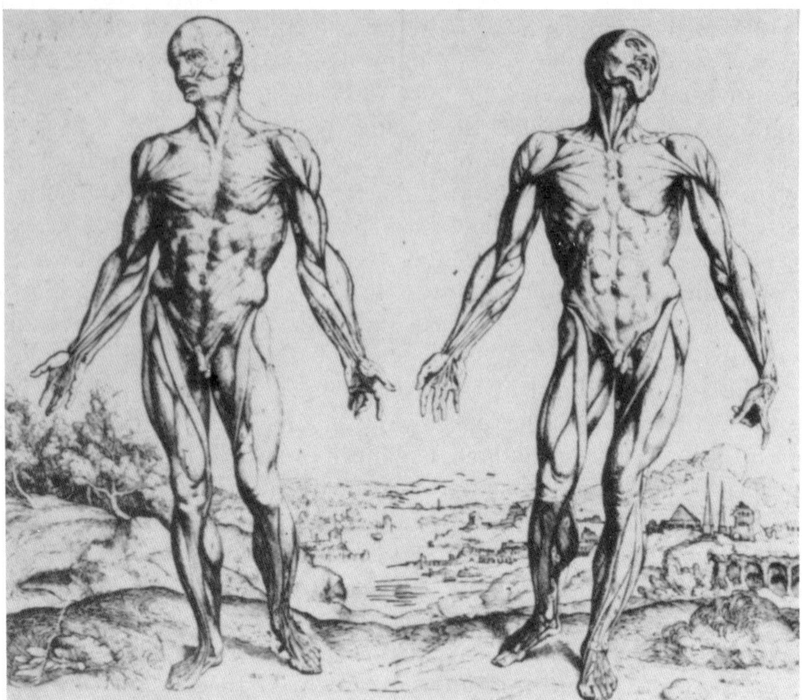

FIG. 4. Muscle Tables III and I from the *Fabrica*

single record. And by an elaborate system of cross references between printed text and printed picture, an integral effect could be achieved not unlike that of the simultaneous address to the eye and the ear in the dissection-room.

The illustrated book was of course no substitute for attendance on, and practice of, actual dissection. The picture could not really *be* the body; like the verbal description, it was only *about* the body. It was a highly selective report, a rendering, a translation, with conventions of its own, analogous to those of language itself. Yet for purposes of communication there were certain advantages arising out of this very limitation. Most of these are so obvious as to need no comment, but some attention to two in particular is essential to a full appreciation of Vesalius's achievement in the *Fabrica*.

Whereas multiple meanings with a penumbra of suggestiveness, or even entire absence of objective meaning, may be positive virtues in

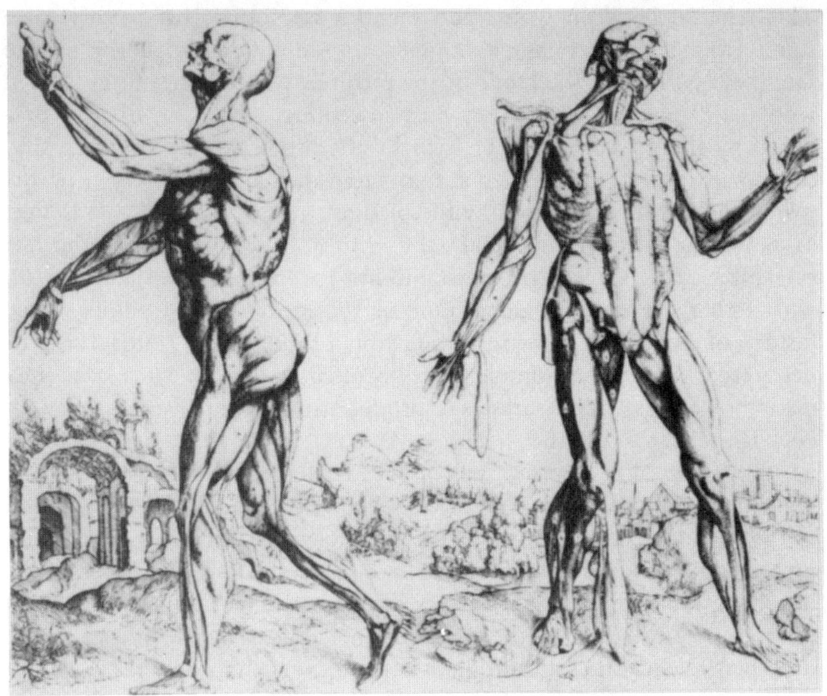

FIG. 5. Muscle Tables II and V from the *Fabrica*

imaginative literature and poetry, the ideal of science must be a single, precise and unambiguous meaning for every statement. But a descriptive, non-mathematical science, even with the help of a technical vocabulary, cannot altogether eliminate ambiguity from its verbal statements, and cannot always insure that the verbal statement alone will have a meaning at all. These hazards are reduced in the physical presence of the object described. In the case of anatomy, the visual experience of following the dissector's knife or the demonstrator's wand provides a running interpretation of the lecturer's words, both giving them meaning and restricting the range of their possible meanings. But pictures can be made to serve both these purposes even more effectively, for the reason that the picture is itself a statement, while the incision and the pointing are not. Moreover, the picture says something which not only cannot be said by operations, gestures and pointings, but cannot be said by words; so that it does not merely fix the meanings of the words as a facing translation into another language might, but makes a contribution all its own to a total meaning which the words could not convey alone. This relation between words and pictures is mutual; for pictures also suffer from ambiguity, and though words cannot say what the picture can, they can restrict the range of the picture's possible meanings. When words and pictures seem to say the same thing, that is an illusion produced by the interpretation of each by the other, so that together they convey an integral meaning not analyzable into a part conveyed by the words and another conveyed by the pictures, just as the integrated effect of binocular vision is not analyzable into a part conveyed by the left eye and a part conveyed by the right, and is certainly not identical with what either eye conveys alone. One of the great turning points in the history of education was the production of the first printed book of descriptive science so completely illustrated and with such a perfect mating of words and pictures as to produce this binocular effect throughout. The *Fabrica* was that book.[3]

But there was another potential advantage of the picture, also dependent on the fact that it was not the body; and in its exploitation of this second advantage the *Fabrica* was not merely the first of its kind, but remains unique. It was always a dead body that lay inert on the dissecting table, or at best was suspended for the vertical position. Even for the practical ends of the surgeon-to-be, this was a handicap in the days before anaesthesia; for the bodies on which he operated would seldom be inert. And from the point of view of the general physician, as from that of the renaissance humanist, the purpose of dissecting dead bodies was of course to know the fabric not of the dead body but of the living man. No doubt a teacher like Vesalius could and did appeal to the imagination of his students to make the translation; but it was not within his power to make it for them, or even to assure himself that they had made it. And as the dissection proceeded over a period of three weeks, the progressive decay of the body would overpower the senses of sight and smell, and inhibit any such effort of translation on the part of even the most hardened student.

By the help of Calcar and his assistants, however, this translation from the dead to the living body was made in the plates of the *Fabrica.* The muscle figures, for instance, were all animated, and the muscles exhibited in the state of contraction required to produce the movement in progress, and the position of the moment.[4] To enhance the illusion, the artists took or drew a renaissance panorama, divided it into sections, and superimposed the figures upon them.[5]

Even the skeletal figures seem miraculously alive. The spirit of the

Lord had set the prophet of old in the valley of dry bones and asked, "Son of man, can these bones live?" There was an earthquake, and the bones came together, bone to bone; and lo, there were sinews upon them, and flesh came up, and skin covered them above; and the breath came into them, and they lived, and stood up upon their feet. So wherever Vesalius taught, he articulated a skeleton, set it up above or beside the corpse that lay on the table, and invited his students to take the muddy vesture of decay which he anatomized before them, reknit its parts, made clean and sweet again, project it in imagination onto those dry bones, and breathe again into its nostrils the breath of life. But it must have been a rare student, even in the renaissance, for whom the miracle came to pass at the master's word. What the word could not evoke, the craft of artist, engraver and printer enacted in the *Fabrica.*

REFERENCES

1. CRUMMER, LE ROY. An original drawing of the title-page of Vesalius' *Fabrica.* Annals of Medical History. *2*: 20-30, 1930.
2. FEYFER, F. M. G. de. Een portret van Andreas Vesalius. Nederlandsch Tijdschrift voor Geneeskunde. *1*: 60-73, 1932.
3. IVINS, W. M. The woodcuts to Vesalius. Bulletin of the Metropolitan Museum of Art. *31:* 139-142, 1936.
4. SPENCER, W. G. Vesalius: his delineation of the framework of the human body in the *Fabrica* and *Epitome.* British Journal of Surgery. *10:* 383-402, 1923.
5. SPIELMANN, M. H. The iconography of Andreas Vesalius. London, John Bale, sons & Danielsson, 1925.
6. ROTH, MORITZ. Andreas Vesalius Bruxellensis. Berlin, Georg Reimer, 1892.
7. WAUTERS, ALPHONSE. Quelques mots sur André Vesale, ses ascendants, sa famille et sa demeure à Bruxelles. Mémoires couronnés et autres mémoires publiés par l'Academie Royale des sciences, des lettres et des beaux-arts de Belgique. *55:* 1897, 48 pp.

THE GOLD HEADED CANE AND ITS AUTHOR, WILLIAM MACMICHAEL.

By FRANCIS R. PACKARD, M. D.

I have chosen for my theme this evening the life and works of one who was both a physician and a librarian and who has preserved in two books, which his modesty caused him to publish anonymously, the most delightful record of the lives of some of the great English masters of medicine. To these books we are indebted for the perpetuation of some of the choicest stories which have become professional classics and for the preservation of lifelike portraits of some of the great men whose names adorn the medical annals of Great Britain. But for the labor of love of Dr. Macmichael these records would have been totally lost or buried in oblivion in scattered places, inaccessible save to the laborious searcher.

William Macmichael, the author of the Gold Headed Cane, was born at Bridgenorth, in Shropshire, in 1784, and after receiving his education at the grammar school of that town, entered as a student at Christ Church, Oxford, where, after receiving his degree of Master of Arts in 1807, he graduated as a Doctor of Medicine in 1816. In 1811, he was elected to the Radcliffe Travelling Fellowship which owed its foundation to the generosity of Dr. Radcliffe, about whom he writes so delightfully in his chef d'oeuvre. These fellowships were founded with the purpose of giving their holders the opportunity of travelling in foreign lands, and Dr. Macmichael passed several years journeying in Russia, Turkey, Greece and Palestine. That he was an observing and interested traveller is manifested in a little work which he published in London in 1819, entitled "A Journey from Moscow to Constantinople, in the years 1817 and 1818." He was, for a short time, physician to Lord Londonderry while the latter was ambassador to Vienna. He settled in London in the practice of medicine in 1818, and was elected a fellow of the College of Physicians of London in the same year. At the outset of his career as a practicing physician, he had the good fortune to secure the friendship of Sir Henry Halford, to whom the College was indebted for the gift of the Gold Headed

Originally published in *Bulletin of the Medical Library Association,* Volume 4 (July, 1914), pp. 1-11. Reprinted by permission.

Cane, which had descended to Sir Henry from the distinguished line of bearers about whom Macmichael centered its autobiography. Sir Henry Halford's influence in professional and social circles in London was immense. His name was really Henry Vaughan. His father was a physician in Leicester, who devoted his entire income to the education of his seven sons, all of whom proved themselves worthy of the parental self-denial by the eminent positions which they subsequently obtained in the professions which they respectively adopted. Sir Henry after graduating from Oxford, secured an advantageous social position for himself by his marriage to the daughter of Lord St. John of Bletsoe. He inherited a large property on the death of Lady Denbigh, the widow of his mother's cousin, Sir Charles Halford, Bart., and by an act of Parliament in 1809, changed his name from Vaughan to Halford. In the subsequent year he was made a baronet. He attended in a professional capacity George III, George IV and Queen Victoria, and after the death of Matthew Baillie, he had the largest and most fashionable practice in London.

Halford was the president of the College of Physicians of London from 1820 until his death in 1844, and it was during his presidency that the College was removed from Warwick Lane to Pall Mall East. Those who envied his position attributed his success to his courtly manners and he was nicknamed "the eel-backed baronet." The story is told how he galloped from the death bed of George IV out to Bushy Park in order that he might have the honor of being the first to inform William IV of the glad event. He was present at the opening of the coffin of Charles I, in 1813 and published an account of the proceedings on that occasion. J. F. Clarke, in his autobiography, accuses him, amongst other things, of retaining possession of part of the fourth cervical vertebra of the king through which the axe passed, and displaying it at his dinner table as an interesting curio.

Halford, in the words of Dr. Munk, "at the height of his success, and when his duties at Court were the most onerous, found it necessary to have in reserve some physician, on whom he could implicitly rely, to act as his representative and substitute when such was needed. His choice fell on Dr. Macmichael, who, through Sir Henry's influence, was appointed in rapid succession Physician Extraordinary to the King in 1829, Librarian to the King in 1830, in place of a very eminent physician, Dr. Gooch, recently deceased; and finally, in 1831, Physician in Ordinary to the King."

Halford had been obliged to resign his position as physician to the Middlesex Hospital owing to the pressure of other duties as early as 1800, but it was probably also due to his influence that twenty-two years later Macmichael was appointed to the same position. Macmichael was very active in the affairs of the College of Physicians, served among its officers on several occasions, and read a number of communications before it. He wrote various articles on contagion and infection, none of them possessing any great value. In spite of his powerful backing and the important positions he held, Dr. Macmichael lacked the ambition or did not possess the aptitude to acquire a large practice. In 1837, at the age of fifty-seven, Dr. Macmichael suffered an attack of paralysis which obliged him to retire from professïonal life and he died two years later at his residence in Maida Vale. Sir Thomas Watson, the famous London physician, was one of Dr. Macmichael's friends who knew him many years. In 1878 Sir Thomas Watson wrote of him as follows, to Munk, 1. (Footnote 1, Roll call of the Royal College of Physicians, article on Macmichael) "Dr. Macmichael was fond of society, and qualified alike to enjoy and embellish it. Having travelled long and seen many cities and the manners of many men, he possessed a large stock of general information, was fertile in various and amusing anecdote, and was wont to mix, with a certain natural ease and grace, in lively and interesting discourse, without making his own share in it unduly prominent. His cheerfulness, equanimity of temper, and kindness of heart, endeared him to a large circle of devoted friends, of whom a very few only, at the time of this writing, survive to commemorate his engaging qualities and to regret his loss."

Under Sir Henry Halford's presidency, the College of Physicians underwent a great awakening. It acquired, largely through his individual efforts, a splendid new home and he also originated the evening meetings which were henceforth held in the Hall. These were held once a month during the first six months of the year, at nine o'clock in the evening. Tea and coffee were provided. The meetings were attended not only by physicians but by many persons of prominence in the various walks of life. The papers presented at them were, therefore, as a general rule, adapted to a mixed audience. They were not read by their authors, but by the Registrar of the College, except in the instance of the President, who was permitted to read such communications as he might wish to make himself. A great part of Sir Henry's Halford's success in these innovations was due to the active part taken by Macmichael in seconding his efforts, in this as in every other way by which he could show his gratitude and aid his friend and benefactor. In nothing could he have succeeded better in awakening renewed interest in the venerable College than by directing attention to its past history and to the achievements of the illustrious men who had been connected with it. It was probably this desire which led Macmichael to utilize his erudite knowledge of the subject in the compilation of the fascinating book to which he gave the name of "The Gold Headed Cane."

The new College was opened on the 25th of June, 1825. According to its veracious autobiography on the previous day, the Cane was deposited in a corner closet of the new building, "with the observation that I was no longer to be carried about." The Gold Headed Cane now occupies a glass case in the Library of the College, where it may have the consolation of feeling that it is gazed on by many visitors who have read its history and been stimulated by it to wish a close view of the author.

The Cane was carried successively by Radcliffe, Mead, Askew, Pitcairn and Baillie, and bears their various arms engraved upon its head. It was presented to Sir Henry Halford by Dr. Baillie's widow, and he in turn placed it in the College.

Dr. Macmichael's happy inspiration to write its autobiography was carried into effect at the time when the enthusiasm of the Fellows at the acquisition of their splendid new hall was at its height. The first edition was published in 1827, and a second edition in the succeeding year.

The third edition, edited by Dr. William Munk, was published by Longmans, Green & Co., in 1884, forty-five years after Macmichael's death. Dr. Munk was Harveian Librarian of the College of Physicians, and speaking in that capacity for the Cane, he brought the latter's recollections down through the presidency of the College by Dr. Thomas Mayo to the latter's death in 1871. He also added some interesting footnotes to the matter contained in the two previous editions. Munk's continuation is written in very good imitation of the easy narrative style of Macmichael and is a valuable contribution to English medical biography. His edition, however, lacks the quaint illustrations which ornamented the others and added to their charm.

The Cane in ancient days was regarded as an essential part of the equipment of every physician. Dr. Munk in the third edition of the Gold Headed Cane adverts to this fact and also explains the origin of the custom. The cane usually carried by physicians had for its head a knob, of gold, silver or ivory, which was hollow, and perforated so that it served to contain aromatic preparations which could be inhaled as a preventive of contagion. The favorite preparation for this purpose was the "vinegar of the four thieves," or Marseilles Vinegar, an aromatic vinegar which, according to the confession of four thieves who had robbed the plague stricken in Marseilles, had prevented them from contracting the disease while pursuing their nefarious occupation.

The Gold Headed Cane was adorned by a cross bar for a top instead of a knob, a fact which Munk explains by the statement that Radcliffe, its first owner was a rule unto himself, and very possibly preferred a handle of that kind for his cane as a distinction from that used by the majority of physicians.

The Cane begins its autobiography by narrating some of its experiences while carried by John Radcliffe (1650-1714), who was physician to King William III. The account of the physician's visits to his royal patient is told with a delightful verve and there is no reason to doubt the veracity of the portrait drawn of that great but most unattractive personage.

Radcliffe accumulated a fortune of which he left a large portion to Oxford University and much to charity. Shortly before his death, Radcliffe gave the Cane to Richard Mead (1673-1754), who succeeded to most of Radcliffe's practice and occupied his late residence. The account of the adventures of the Cane while in the hands of Mead is one of the best parts of the book. It opens with a description of a consultation between Mead, Sir Hans Sloane and Dr. Cheyne on the case of Bishop Burnet. George Cheyne (1671-1743) was a man of immense bulk, at one time weighing thirty stone, which by observing a diet of milk and vegetables, he succeeded in reducing to less than half that weight. He was very witty and many stories and repartees are attributed to him. Sir Hans Sloane (1660-1753) is now chiefly remembered as the founder of the British Museum. 1. (Footnote 1. In the first edition of the Gold Headed Cane, Macmichael states that Sir Hans Sloane "had shortly before been created a baronet by his Majesty George the First, being the first physician upon whom an hereditary title of honor had been conferred." Dr. Munk in the third edition corrects this statement in a footnote stating that Sir Edward Greaves, M. D., was created a baronet by King Charles the First at Oxford, May 4, 1716.) At his death he desired the nation should benefit by the wonderful collections which he had made, and directed that although they had cost him £50,000 they should be offered to the Government for the sum of £20,000. Parliament voted the necessary funds and thus the British Museum came into existence.

Mead was an erudite scholar and an observing and skillful physician. He wrote a treatise in Latin on smallpox and measles to which he subjoined a translation into the same language of Rhazes' commentary on smallpox. He was a strong advocate of inoculation for smallpox. Lady Mary Wortley Montague had witnessed the beneficial results of inoculation as practiced by the Turks during her residence at Constantinople, and on her return to England in 1722 determined to introduce it to her fellow countrymen. Whilst professional and public opinion was yet weighing its efficiency, Caroline, Princess of Wales, nearly lost one of her children by an attack of smallpox. She was desirous of having her other children inoculated, and obtained from King George the First pardons for six condemned criminals on condition of their submitting to be inoculated. Five of the felons contracted the disease; the sixth who concealed having previously had the smallpox was not infected. At Mead's suggestion, a seventh criminal, a girl of eighteen, was subjected to the experiment by the Chinese method, which consisted of introducing into the nostrils a tent soaked with the matter taken from ripe pustules. The girl contracted the disease and recovered.

The Cane relates an oft repeated story which shows Mead's powers of observation leading to an innovation in practice of permanent value. It was frequently observed that in cases of persons with dropsy, when tapped and the effusion suddenly drawn off, the patient swooned and often died with great suddeness. Mead determined to replace the pressure of the fluid thus suddenly withdrawn by external means and devised the expedient of placing a broad bandage around the abdomen which was gradually tightened as the fluid was removed. The Cane relates that it was frequently present and saw this method used, "more especially in the case of Dame Mary Page, wife of Sir Gregory Page, Bart., who was afflicted with this disease. *** In sixty-seven months she was tapped sixty-six times, and had two hundred and forty gallons of water taken away, without ever once fearing the operation." These details are carefully recorded on a monument to this lady in Bunhill Fields cemetery. In Mead's time political feeling was at fever heat. Although he was an ardent Whig, he numbered the Tories Garth, Arbuthnot and Freind among his intimate associates. When the latter was imprisoned because of his supposed implication in the Atterbury plot for the restoration of the Stuarts, Mead visited him in the Tower, and secured his release in the following remarkable manner. Sir Robert Walpole was taken ill and sent for Mead. The latter availed himself of the occasion to plead Freind's cause. The latter was a member of Parliament and his chief offense seems to have lain in some intemperate speeches. Mead extenuated these, spoke of Freind's public services as a physician to the British army in the Spanish expedition and in Flanders, of his erudition and his scientific attainments, and finally refused to prescribe for the Prime Minister unless he liberated him, which he accordingly did. The evening following there was a great assembly of guests at Mead's house all anxious to congratulate Freind. As the latter was leaving, Mead drew him aside and presented him with a bag containing all the fees which he had collected from Freind's patients during his imprisonment. 1. (Footnote 1. In the two first editions the amount was stated to have been 5,000 guineas, but Dr. Munk in the third edition points out in a footnote that as Freind was only imprisoned for three months this is hardly credible. He thinks the sum might have been five hundred guineas, increased to five thousand by an error in transcription.) Freind reciprocated Mead's friendship by writing a "History of Physick from the Time of Galen to the Beginning of the Sixteenth Century—chiefly with Regard to Practice—In a Discourse written to Dr. Mead."

This work was begun during his imprisonment, and shows much sound learning and original research. Mead used to love to gather his friends at stated periods in his wonderful library. The Cane describes the talk at several of these meetings in a delightful way. Thus at one of them Mead discourses on the careers of Linacre and Caius and Freind displays his learning in a brief review of the great anatomical discoveries of the seventeenth century. The conversation then deals with Harvey and with many of the benefactions by which he manifested his great interest in the College of Physicians. The fortunes and misfortunes of the College are followed most delightfully. The great fire of London destroyed its home and many of its most interesting treasures. Only 112 books were saved of the already large collection which it contained. After the fire of 1666, the College moved to new premises in Warwick Lane where was built the hall which it occupied until 1825. Among the interesting consulations which the Gold Headed Cane heard whilst in the hands of Dr. Mead was that upon Sir Isaac Newton. Cheselden was the surgeon who was in attendance upon Sir Isaac who suffered from a stone in the bladder, and the Cane states that "It was my lot often to be in company with the eminent surgeon whose name I have now mentioned; for the public seemed universally to have adopted the sentiment of the popular poet of the day:

'I'll try what Mead and Cheselden advise.'

Pope.' "

The Cane gives a beautiful account of the great philosopher's closing days; and then relates how Sir Hans Sloane was elected his successor as president of the Royal Society of Great Britain, being the first medical man to be chosen president of that Institution. Mead died in 1754, in his 81st year, and the Gold Headed Cane passed into the hands of Dr. Anthony Askew (1722-1774).

The Cane's new possessor had travelled widely, not only throughout Europe but through the East, and was as ardent a bibliophile as its late owner. As the Cane says, "Our house in Queen Square was crammed full of books. We could dispense with no more. Our passages were full; even our very garrets overflowed; and the wags of the day used to say that the half of the Square itself would have done so, before the book appetite of Dr. Askew would have been satiated." *** "As a collector of books Dr. Askew was the first who brought bibliomania into fashion; and no one exhibited his various treasures better than himself. The eager delight with which he produced his rare editions, his large paper-copies, his glistening gems and covetable tomes, would have raised him high in the estimation of the Roxburgh Club. Some, indeed, were of such great rarity, that he would not suffer them to be touched, but would show them to his visitors through the glass cases of the cabinets of his library, or, standing on a ladder, would himself read aloud different portions of these inestimable volumes."

In the chapter on Askew there is a very interesting account of the Heberdens, the elder of whom was Askew's contemporary. William Heberden (1710-1801) lectured on Materia Medica at Cambridge for a number of years before settling in London, and the Gold Headed Cane tells of his celebrated essay on Mithridatium and Theriaca, published in 1745, which once and for all time disposed of the claims of those two much vaunted antidotes to any value in the treatment of poisons, although at the time he wrote they were still included in the English dispensatory. He was a profound Greek and Latin scholar and furnished out of his own means, which were large, the money necessary to the publication of a number of classical works. He published from a Harleian manuscript in the British Museum, Conyers Middleton's "Appendix to his Dissertations on the servile condition of Physicians among the Ancients," and afforded on the other hand a curious proof of his piety and generosity by paying to the widow of Conyers Middleton the money which she had been offered by a publisher for a manuscript left her by her husband on the "Inefficacy of Prayer," which Heberden judged unedifying, and burnt after purchasing. No less an authority than Samuel Johnson spoke of him as "Ultimus Romanorum, the last of our learned physicians." He was the first to describe the disease angina pectoris

His son, William (1767-1845), was as piously inclined as his father, and also inherited his classical tastes. He likewise achieved great success in his profession. He was appointed physician to George the Third and was in the heyday of fortune when in 1812, his wife died leaving him a widower with nine children. He retired to a country village in Buckinghamshire and devoted his entire time to the education and care of his children with the sole exception of visits to his royal patient, at such times as his professional assistance was required. He lived thus for fourteen years solacing himself by translating and publishing some of the Greek and Latin classics and writing a little treatise on education. In 1826, he returned to London, largely actuated by the design of aiding one of his sons who had entered upon the study of medicine. Two years later this lad met his death as the result of a wound received while dissecting. The deaths of another son and a daughter led Heberden to devote himself to religion and the study of the scriptures. He subsequently wrote several theological works, as well as a small work on the diseases of children.

From Askew the Gold Headed Cane passed to Dr. William Pitcairn (1711-1791), a brother of Major Pitcairn of the British Army, remembered by all Americans as one of the officers slain at Bunker Hill. Pitcairn had the leading practice of his time in London, but the account of the Cane's career during it possession by him is chiefly interesting because of the other notabilities to whom it introduces us, among them Dr. Richard Warren (1731-1797), and George Edwards (1694-1773) the Librarian of the College of Physicians and one of the most distinguished of English ornithologists. Edwards had for a patron Sir Hans Sloane and the Cane's account of the latter's closing years and the manner in which he secured for the English nation the benefit of his enormous collection, the nucleus of the British Museum, is excellent.

From Dr. William Pitcairn the Cane passed to Dr. David Pitcairn (1749-1809) his nephew. The latter was a Fellow of the Royal Society and to its meetings the Cane frequently accompanied him, being thereby led into a most interesting account of the origin and history of that learned body. Pitcairn was the first to point out the frequency with which valvular heart disease is associated with rheumatism. One of the most prominent of Dr. Pitcairn's contemporaries was Sir George Baker (1722-1809) who also served a number of terms as president of the College of Physicians. Baker was an excellent classical scholar, especially skilled in writing vers d'esprit in Latin. The Cane gives his Latin epitaph on a Mrs. Vanbuchtel, the story of whose corpse is a medical classic. The lady died at the age of forty and at her husband's desire Mr. Cruikshank, under the supervision of Dr. Hunter, injected into her arteries spirits of turpentine, coloured by vermilion. Mr. Vanbuchtel kept the body thus preserved in his house during his life. When he died his son presented it to the College of Surgeons, where it is still to be seen in a mahogany case. Sir George Baker rendered a great service to his native country of Devon by his discovery that the so-called "endemial colic" of Devonshire was really a form of lead poisoning due to the use of lead in the vessels used in the manufacture of Devonshire cider. The disease was entirely eradicated by the use of differently constructed vessels.

From Dr. David Pitcairn the Cane passed into the hands of Dr. Matthew Baille (1761-1823). Baille's mother was Dorothea Hunter, sister of William and John Hunter. His sister Joanna won fame as a poetess, receiving high encomiums as a daughter of the Muses, from Sir Walter Scott. Matthew came to London at the age eighteen and lived with his Uncle William Hunter. The latter not only gave him every possible aid in his studies, but at his death bequeathed him his house and collections, with the provision that the latter should ultimately go to the University of Glasgow. William Hunter also left Baillie the family homestead at Long Calderwood. The latter, Baillie most honourably turned over to William Hunter's brother John, to whom it rightfully should have been left, but whom William had deprived of it because of their historic quarrel. In 1795 Baillie published his famous work on morbid anatomy, the first English work on that important subject. It was dedicated to his friend Dr. David Pitcairn, and was notable not only for the extent of the observations which it contained, but also for the excellent illustrations with which it was embellished. "Baillie was considerably below the middle size, with a countenance rather plain than prepossessing, a Scotch dialect, and blunt manners." In spite of his personal disadvantages, he acquired a very large practice and under the pressure of work his natural irritability greatly increased. The Cane tells how "After listening, with torture, to a prosing account from a lady, who ailed so little that she was going to the opera that evening, he had happily escaped from the room, when he was urgently requested to step upstairs again; it was to ask him whether on her return from the opera, she might eat some oysters: 'Yes, Ma'am,' said Baillie, 'shells and all.' "

Baillie possessed the collecting zeal of his uncles, the Hunters. He presented his anatomical preparations, most of which had been made by his own hands, to the College of Physicians in 1819. Four years later he died, his health failing gradually but to such an extent as to cause his retirement from the duties of his profession several year's before his death.

With Baillie's death the autobiography of the Gold Headed Cane as compiled by Macmichael ended. When, in 1884, Dr. Munk, the learned chronicler of the College of Physicians of London brought forth the third edition of the little book, he added a number of pages written in the Macmichael style and adding much information to the previously garnered store. Thus he gives us little sketches of Sir Henry Halford, who had presented the Cane to the College, and under whose auspices the new hall of the College was opened in 1825; Dr. Macmichael, the originator of this unique autobiography; and Drs. John Aryton Paris and Thomas Mayo, who were respectively presidents of the College in succession to Sir Henry Halford.

In 1830, Macmichael published "Lives of British Physicians," of which another edition was published by Thomas Legg in 1846. Macmichael himself contributed himself to it the lives of Linacre, Caius, Harvey, Sir Thomas Browne, Sydenham and Radcliffe. The biographies of twelve other English medical worthies were contributed by Dr. Bisset Hawkins, Dr. Parry, Dr. Southey, Dr. Munk, and Mr. Clarke. The book is a small volume containing portraits of some of the more famous subjects. It was dedicated to Sir Henry Halford. Although not so happy in its conception and execution as the Gold Headed Cane, this little work is a most valuable contribution to English medical literature. The lives are well written, accurate, and contain information much of which is derived from sources inaccessible to the general reader.

If in this hurried review I have been able to awaken interest in Macmichael's charming little medical classic, if, perchance its perusal might stimulate some medical librarian or literary physician to undertake a similar labor in a new direction, how happy would be the result.

On the Reading of Medical Classics*

By Owsei Temkin†

In his *Areopagitica* John Milton wrote[1]:

> For Books are not absolutely dead things, but do contain a potencie of life in them to be as active as that soule was whose progenie they are; nay they do preserve as in a violl the purest efficacie and extraction of that living intellect that bred them.

To modern medical library practice, these well-known words constitute something of an embarrassment. The huge increase in the production of books and the speed with which contents become obsolete have forced libraries to handle their books as subject to aging and even to death. Active life is limited to about twenty years, when they are "cut off" and retired as elderly to less accessible areas. Those which pass through the process of aging are resuscitated in the historical collection.

In past times, scientific progress was slow compared to ours; important new discoveries were made at lengthy intervals, and the conservatism of many universities prolonged the lives of authoritative works. In 1644, when the *Areopagitica* was published, not only Hippocrates and Galen, but many other ancient authors and even Avicenna were still printed and studied as sources of medical knowledge and science. The final break with the ancient past, its relegation to history, belongs to the mid-nineteenth century. Even then the content of medical books could count on a lengthy period of acceptance. For instance, in 1866, Austin Flint's *A Treatise on the Principles and Practice of Medicine* was still oriented toward the Paris school and showed little regard for contemporary German achievements which, among other things, had produced cellular pathology.

It was formerly, therefore, relatively safe to entrust new scientific discoveries to books, as did Vesalius, Harvey, Auenbrugger and Jenner. Not only was the danger of concomitant discovery by others smaller; a book could also count on readers with sufficient leisure to peruse it. The feeling of urgency to acquaint the world with one's discoveries and to learn

*This essay is dedicated to my old friend, Samuel X Radbill, M.D., a lover and reader of medical classics.

†419 Alabama Road, Towson, Maryland 21204.

Originally published in *Transactions & Studies of the College of Physicians of Philadelphia*, Volume 42 (July, 1974), pp. 113-120. Reprinted by permission.

what others had discovered as quickly as possible may not have been as strong as it is today; the less developed means of communication may not have fostered the fear of missing the latest contribution; the way of life of a less industrialized society may not yet have bred the feeling that time was of the essence and the concomitant unrest that overtakes us if we are expected to follow arguments in discursive books not packed with information. Whatever the causes may have been—and they are hard to assess—the compulsion to obtain the most recent information did not manifest itself as strongly as it does today.

By Jenner's time, medical journals were already well established and had replaced the epistolary commerce by which scholars of the seventeenth century used to let their colleagues and friends know of their novel thoughts and discoveries. The frequently appearing issues of a journal brought information more quickly than a book, but journals too are now being overtaken by the torrent of scientific events, for rarely can a contributor count on having his article published within less than a year's time. Journals become volumes which also crowd the shelves, and their contents too become obsolete, though the continuity of a journal, and hence the frequent need to go back to an older article, delays the process of aging.

Nor has the progress of technological science that has created some of the difficulties for our libraries by-passed the libraries themselves. From places where books and journals are deposited and catalogued, libraries are turning into information centers, places where ingenious mechanical processes retrieve information, not only saving the reader's time but also making the coverage more extensive. Audio-visual devices offer information on selected topics in concentrated form; they also relieve the viewer of the need to read. There is a constant endeavor to save space by the use of micro-cards and microfilms, and the ideal goal would be reached if the volumes of books and journals could altogether be replaced by less space-consuming material. Indeed, some types of books are already facing doom[2].

This discourse on the problems of our libraries, by one so little competent for it, is intended to illustrate the intellectual situation in which we find ourselves. We need ever more information; we have to make room for it in our brains, no less than in our libraries, and we also have to rid ourselves of what is no longer valid and had best be forgotten, lest it do harm. Yet we realize that we cannot destroy all the informative books and journals without obliterating the traces of our civilization and of our own medical activities. In course of time, all books (and for simplicity's sake the term is here to include journals as well) assume some degree of historical value. From giving medical information to us they change to giving information about us. Thus they reached the heaven of the historical collection. Not all elderly books are saved, however; many of them leave the purgatory of the distant shelves only to disappear for ever in such hell as fire, pulping, or other tortures provide.

The great need for increased information, without which our economic, political, and administrative life could not function and without which science and medicine would stagnate, tends to encourage a cult of information that overlooks the fact that even knowledge needs more than information. It needs an integration of data into a comprehensible context, and what makes things comprehensible depends very much on the assumptions and rules we acknowledge when information reaches us. Information must be expressed and it must be organized, both of which can be done well or badly. Even the most purely informative book containing nothing but statistical material can be good or bad, depending on the way it handles that material[3]. Moreover, the material may be correct but irrelevant, i.e., either not pertinent to the theme of the book or related to matters to which we are not willing to assign much value. Or the book is worthless because the material it contains, even if correct, is a mere rehash of earlier publications.

Obvious as these remarks may be, they remind us that every book contains something that is not just informative and that interferes with the prearranged march from young and "active" to "elderly" and then to "old." Some books are judged so worthless that they are not even admitted to the home of the elderly. (Paradoxically, they may then become valuable as rarities.) On the other extreme stand those books that are deemed "timeless," the classics, with which we are now concerned.

What is essential for making a medical book, or article, a classic? Examples from non-medical literature are helpful in the search for an answer. For religious persons, the Bible is "the book," because it reveals divine truth, and even others will admit that it has much wisdom to impart. Wisdom is more than knowledge, or all who know much would also be wise, which unfortunately is far from being the case. Few will be insensitive to the moving power of prophetic speech, to the feeling of human grandeur and vulnerability conveyed by a Greek tragedy, or to the beauty of Shakespearian sonnets. Few will escape meeting in real life such fictitious characters as Don Quixote, Hamlet, Pickwick or Babbitt.

But long ago, Claude Bernard pointed out the difference between personal contributions in the arts and the sciences. Science, being cumulative, a discovery if confirmed is assimilated into later work, without leaving traces of its origin. Not so in the arts, where Plato's philosophy, Shakespeare's plays, and Dickens's characters do not become dissolved in the works of later authors. As Claude Bernard[4] put it: "The past keeps all its worth in the creations of art and letters; each individuality remains changeless in time and cannot be mistaken for another."

Medical classics probably would not exist if they were to be read for their substantive content only. I doubt that a modern neurologist will learn much about epilepsy from Hippocrates's *On the Sacred Disease*, that Fracastoro's *Syphilis sive De morbo gallico* has much to teach about the clinical manifestations of syphilis as seen today, or that Virchow's *Cellular Pathology* contains much that a modern textbook of pathology has missed. To be sure, *On the Sacred Disease* is the first monograph on epilepsy and *Cellular Pathology* the first work basing human pathology on the life of the cell. To be "the first" may make a book very interesting from a historical point of view, and I am the last to discourage historical interest. Nevertheless, a historically important book is not necessarily a classic.

Because medical classics, I believe, are not read primarily for the sake of their substantive content, they are not widely read altogether outside of required class work, with which I am not concerned here. How much they are read voluntarily is hard to gauge. The multitude of reprints (facsimiles, paperbacks, anthologies) points in one direction; my personal impression, I regret to say, points in another. However that may be, it will hardly be claimed that medical men are given to avid reading of medical classics. If this evaluation of the state of affairs is correct, there should be no hesitation on the part of many physicians to proclaim the reading of medical classics a waste of precious time. Yet I do not believe that such a proclamation would find a large number of subscribers. Unless the hesitation is attributed to fear of being held lacking in cultural polish, we must look for a motive strong enough to prevent disrespect. In spite of the absence of perceptible immediate usefulness, there must be a belief, or at least a suspicion, that reading such books or articles carries its reward in itself and is, perhaps, indirectly useful.

Since this is not written to promote the classics among the heathen, telling them why they have to read them, the analysis had best begin with an incontrovertible fact: There are those who derive enjoyment from such reading, and there are others who do not. The number of persons incapable of finding a single book that they would be willing to accept as a classic is probably very small. But education and reading habits may stand in the way of accepting many an established classic. There is nothing here to single out medical works from others. The *Oedipus Rex* of Sophocles is an established classic and may have an overwhelming effect at first reading. Some readers, however, if honest, will admit with more or less diffidence that the play leaves them cold. That may be a final judgment, or it may yield to admiring enjoyment on repeated reading. Set off from average books, even from good books, classics require an attention all their own.

Not all of them are necessarily well written in the literary sense of the word. The author's intent, his line of thought, his placing of values need careful scrutiny. A superficial perusal may be misleading and a bar to enjoyment. It may conceal our having brought the author down to our level of understanding, instead of working ourselves up to his. The recognized classics have stimulated a huge amount of interpretative writing—none more than the Bible—and new points are constantly discovered. Interpretation, i.e., assimilation of a work by our minds, is an act that a few master intuitively, but most of us have to acquire. In bygone days, education included a painstaking, and often painful, study of languages, especially Latin, and taught the pupil to cope with what was difficult and strange. With the decline of the thorough study of languages, dead or alive, this educational help can no longer be counted on.

There is no contradiction in the contention that enjoyment of books is often coupled with work; in music and the visual arts too full enjoyment has to be earned. Better perhaps: the work done on a classic, and crowned by understanding it, can be enjoyable.

De gustibus non est disputandum said a scholastic adage—no arguing about tastes! Only a questionnaire could supply an answer to what readers actually do enjoy in medical classics; nevertheless, a few points suggest themselves. The enjoyment may act as a mental stimulus, refreshing the intellect, increasing the eagerness to go about one's own task and overcome the obstacles in its way. Depending on the content of the book in question, the gain can be more specific. Harvey's *De motu cordis* is a model for the development of a revolutionary scientific idea of great significance, incompatible with generally accepted doctrine. It can be read with a single-minded concentration on its thesis, that the blood circulates, and on Harvey's arguments, his methods, his diction, only in as far as they prove that thesis. But such an approach bereaves us of the pleasure of meeting the Harvey who was not just the discoverer of the circulation. Harvey had his predecessors; sooner or later somebody else would have given us this discovery. Sociologists have familiarized us with the idea that discoveries usually are made independently by several persons around the same time. But that is only true as far as "the discovery" is concerned. In reading *De motu cordis* we also learn the particulars of Harvey's approach to the discovery, what it meant to him, and the mental images he associated with it. We meet a particular mind, William Harvey's, trying to be as convincing as he knew how.

Claude Bernard was not the inventor of experimental medicine, yet a similar case can be made for his *Introduction to the Study of Experimental Medicine,* which gave it a philosophical exposition unmatched for breadth, lucidity of style, and persuasiveness stemming not only from logical coherence but also from the harmony between theory and the illuminating examples from his own research. There is much to criticize in Bernard's book, to mention only the lack of appreciation of the statistical method. But rarely, if ever, will medical classics represent the last word about a subject. "That living intellect that bred them," to use Milton's words, is the main thing. To meet that intellect is a privilege; it speaks to us and compels us to listen attentively to its every word.

As long as the reading of classics is felt to be a chore, it is a barren enterprise and had better be dropped, for it does neither the reader nor the books any good. It makes us rebellious and brings them into disrepute, heightening the barrier to a potential source of productive joy. The barrier need not be constitutional. Indifference or even hostility in early years may be dispelled by the discovery later in life of a book that strikes us as above the ordinary. We find sympathy where we thought to stand alone, we find a keenness of observation that puts us to shame, a clear grasp of ideas behind primitive techniques, or an attitude towards medical duties that we cannot but admire. Instead of a chance discovery, a rational approach can also lead to classical works. At some time in our life we realize that the basic concepts of medicine, which appeared so familiar, are more puzzling than complicated problems of molecular biology. Then we shall ask when and under what circumstances this concept was introduced and how it developed. That is the historical path. But even without tracing the steps through the past, we may interview the men who forged these concepts.

Our very familiarity with these concepts has prevented us from seeing the inherent assumptions. And so we rightly turn to authors who made the assumptions stand out, because they were not yet conventionalized. We know more about "inborn errors of metabolism" and of "chemical individuality" than Archibald Garrod could possibly have known. But the ideas were his, and this accounts for the fact that interest in his book is very great today, much greater than it was during his lifetime[5].

Whatever the occasion for a meeting with medical classics may be, the meeting becomes one between master and pupil. Not all of us have had the benefit of being taught by great medical teachers *viva voce*. The classics teach silently; they are teachers who will not answer every question, but who will help us to ask the right questions and to find the way by which we ourselves may work out the answers.

Yet reading such works is not without danger, for the light they shed may be dazzling. We may forget that in reality matters were not always as clear and unequivocal as the mind of the master makes them appear in his presentation. The logic of Henle's *On Miasms and Contagions* makes it hard to understand how his contemporaries could fail to accept the microorganismic theory of infectious diseases. Only by immersing ourselves in the literature of the day do we realize how confusing the situation was.

Another, though minor, danger threatens even those who do not turn to the classics for historical understanding. Classics have to be read carefully, because we expect their authors to have used their words carefully. Such reading, however, should not lead to contempt of what may be ephemeral yet important for doing "what lies clearly at hand." The words are Carlyle's, they are cited by Osler[6] and I quote them to obviate the misunderstanding that there is bound to be antagonism between works of information and classics.

This is reminiscent of Osler's advice to a budding medical man[7]: "Let the old men read new books; you read the journals and the old books." Among the old books, Osler here specifically included the ancient Greeks, Sydenham, and Laennec, many, if not all, of whom would be considered classics. His subsequent remark, "as a teacher you can never get *orientiert* without a knowledge of the Fathers, ancient and modern," indicates that the young man was a teacher, present or prospective. Altogether, it would seem that when speaking about the reading of medical classics, Osler exercised his role of medical educator. His activity in the United States belonged to the early period of medical reform; it ended about five years before the Flexner Report was issued, and when the Johns Hopkins School of Medicine was still a new venture, barely twelve years old. The fight for better preparation of prospective medical students, for the academic character of medical schools, for a thorough scientific training of the physician and for his unremitting contact with scientific progress, formed the background of much of Osler's thought about "Books and Men," if we may use the title of this essay as denoting the theme dominant or touched upon in many others. Osler was pressing for good medical libraries and for good reading habits, in which he wisely included non-medical works.

Many of Osler's desiderata have been fulfilled, though not always quite as he had envisaged them. The humanistic side of the education of physicians has not kept pace with their scientific training; on the other hand, medicine has moved closer to public health and to the social sciences. But the provision of good medical libraries is as little a matter of debate today as is the provision of good laboratories. If, in Osler's days, not enough important medical literature was housed, the question now is one of providing proper housing for the medical literature that is pouring out like a torrent.

With this question we are back where we started, only that our specific problem now is: Where do medical classics stand in this changed world? Do they belong with the active, informative books, or do they belong in the historical collection? Or should Osler's wish[8] be heeded that there be "in each library a select company of the immortals set apart for special adoration"? It would be simple to send all classics to the historical collection—if classics only had to be old and clearly separable from current life. And a chapel dedicated to the immortals could combine the practical with the decorative—if only the selection of the immortals were a matter of easy agreement.

As long as potential readers can find the books, their physical placement is a matter that concerns the librarian more than us, who ask whether classics have to be old and how a decision can be reached whether a book is immortal.

Books that have been read for many generations are said to have passed the test of time, a test which is unreliable for classics. One of the collections of Osler's essays from which I quoted carries the subtitle, "and Other Papers That Have Stood the Test of Time." Indeed, many of the essays are still read in Anglo-Saxon countries; I wonder how well they are known in other parts, even of our own Western civilization. Classics are bound to their respective civilizations. And there are essays by Osler that did not appeal to my students, required to read them. Indeed, I must admit that "A Way of Life," breathing, as it does, the optimistic spirit of 1913, does not easily fit into our benighted world. Characteristic as it may be for Osler's view of life, its prescriptions may be unconvincing and its prescriptive style sound harsh to young ears today[9].

Osler too was time-bound, and reading him and holding him up as an ideal should not become a substitute for emulating him. Where the humanities are concerned, it seems to me that what Galen said of Hippocrates could also be said of Osler: Most physicians admire him but do nothing to emulate him[10]. Emulating Osler means actually reading books (beside the informative ones) and forming one's own judgment about them, even at the peril of disagreement with the master.

My argument is not directed against the established classics as such, and the value of lists of "great books" for the schoolroom need not be denied, particularly if there is a competent teacher to select, to advise and to comment. But there is a difference between books that should be read because our civilization has been formed by them and the advocacy of reading classics for their intrinsic value.

It is customary to refer to all ancient Greek and Roman authors as "classical," and in the historical sense this appellation is justifiable. But their intrinsic value may not warrant it. Galen's *Ars medica,* the *Microtegni* of the Middle Ages, is a great medical book that helped to form the outlook of medical men for hundreds of years; nevertheless, I would hesitate to offer it to a physician as a classic. One generation may well need a vacation from such classics as another may restore; "timelessness" and "immortality" should not be interpreted so rigidly as to deaden response and bar newcomers.

The opposite extreme to mere traditionalism is the devaluation of all classics by the cheapening of the very word. It is good that reprints, paper backs, and anthologies put so many books within easy reach, thereby purging them of possible snob value. But the cheapening that derives from promiscuously naming all kinds of books "classics" is not good. It weakens our sensibility and creates disrespect for greatness. It is in line with the carelessness that calls any theoretical thought "philosophy," and misnames any knowledge "wisdom." As a result of such leveling we have no words left for real philosophy, real wisdom, and real classics—all of which are rare. Where everything is made to look like gold, real gold will not look different from anything else.

If the test of time cannot be relied on and everyday parlance is treacherous, on what shall we rely? On ourselves, I would suggest. If, upon reading a book (or an article) carefully and thoughtfully, having assured ourselves that enthusiasm has not made us read into it more than it demonstrably contains, nor left out parts because we cannot understand them, if then we judge the work to be exemplary of its kind, to set a standard, we shall have judged it a classic. Exemplary can refer to presentation, novelty of experience or interpretation, breadth of concept, coherence and consistency of thought, fullness and keenness of observation, ingenuity in experimentation, nobility of deed, or any other value that makes this work stand out even among good ones and tells us: This is the way to think, to write, or to act.

We shall have judged it a classic because, for us, individually, it has fulfilled the demands that can be made of a classic. If the book already stands in the alcove of the immortals, we shall have confirmed the judgment of those before us. In the case of elderly books or of active ones, others will or will not share our judgment, and the book will or will not gain the general approval we think it deserves. Official classification is the concern of educators, literary critics, bibliographers, and librarians. Classification becomes meaningless if classics are not read and either reconfirmed or suspended. And their being read depends on our capability, active or potential, to recognize their worth.

Two serious objections may be raised. To base the reading of classics on subjective experience makes greatness relative, and only the absolute, it may be said, is binding. There is, perhaps, no better reply to this objection than the following words of Jacob Burckhardt, the author of *The Civilization of the Renaissance*[11]:

We take our departure from our dwarfishness, our confusion, and distraction, Greatness is what *we* are *not*. To the beetle in the grass, being nothing but a beetle, even a hazel-bush (provided it takes any notice of it) may already loom very large. And yet we feel that the concept [of greatness] is indispensable and that we must not allow it to be taken away from us. Only it will remain relative; we cannot hope to reach an absolute concept.

Eschewing a systematic discussion and admitting all kinds of dangers, Burckhardt insisted that the feeling for greatness, though relative, is yet inescapable. Thereby he saved this concept from being lost in a discursive debate over its essence. This seems important in our time, when greatness is often attributed unreflectingly, sometimes even irrationally, or its existence denied altogether because it does not easily fit into a statistical world of quantities.

The second objection questions whether upholding the standard of the classics is not tantamount to perfectionism. Will it not induce us to hide our own light under a bushel? I agree that perfectionism is sterile when it becomes an excuse for never finishing a piece of work. But to quote a "classical" author, Propertius[12]: *in magnis et voluisse sat est,* "in mighty enterprises it is enough even to have willed success." There is nothing wrong with trying to do one's best, and our libraries amply prove that our times do not suffer from a surplus of bushels.

Like all classics, medical classics too lead a pitiful existence if, like gods on Olympus, they are separated from us. In libraries they must not be shelved out of sight, even though their choice may demand a constant exchange of opinion within the medical community. For us as individuals they must be like the Roman *lares* and *penates*, gods of the household.

REFERENCES

1. MILTON, JOHN. 1959. Complete Prose Works. Vol. 2. New Haven: Yale University Press. P. 492.
2. BENJAMIN, C. G. 1974. Soaring Prices and Sinking Sales of Science Monographs. Science 183: 282-284.
3. By definition every book has a literary aspect, however small a role that aspect may play.
4. BERNARD, CLAUDE. 1949. An Introduction to the Study of Experimental Medicine. Trans. by Henry Copley Greene. Reprinted by Henry Schuman. P. 43.
5. CHILDS, BARTON. 1970. Sir Archibald Garrod's Conception of Chemical Individuality: A modern appreciation. The New England Journal of Medicine 282: 71-77.
6. "Our main business is not to see what lies dimly at a distance, but to do what lies clearly at hand." OSLER, WILLIAM. 1958. A Way of Life. In A *Way of Life and Other Selected Writings of Sir William Osler.* Reprinted New York: Dover Publications P. 240.
7. OSLER, WILLIAM. 1963. Internal Medicine as a Vocation. Aequanimitas and other papers that have stood the test of time. New York: W. W. Norton. P. 84.
8. "Books and Men," in a way of life (cited above, note 6). P. 38.
9. My experience goes back many years, and generations of students are notoriously apt to change their opinions. DR. JAMES A. KNIGHT's experience seems to be different from mine;

see his essay on "The Relevance of Osler for Today's Humanity-Oriented Medical Student." In *Humanism in Medicine.* 1973. John P. McGovern and Chester R. Burns, eds. Springfield, Illinois: Charles C. Thomas. P. 95.

10. Galen. Quod Optimus Medicus Sit Quoque Philosophus, ch. 1.
11. Burkchardt, Jacob. 1941. Weltgeschichtliche Betrachtungen. Werner Kaegi, ed. Bern: Hallwag. P. 314. Italics in the text. Burkchardt was not displaying false modesty; he referred to the encounter with what makes us feel small.
12. Propertius. Elegies 2. 10.6 H. E. Butler's Trans. Loeb Classical Library. P. 91 (slightly modified).

Collecting Historical Medical Books

There are many differences between the private book collector and one who collects books for institutions like libraries. The private collector, for the most part, collects to satisfy the needs of his own scholarship, or to satisfy his own whims and predilections. The institutional collector has largely custodial responsibility for the books he collects, and the whims and predilections are not necessarily his own but those of the institution he serves. He is, therefore, sometimes faced with the problem of justifying or rationalizing his activities, in distinction to the private collector who needs, if he doesn't have sufficient strength of character that is, to justify his activities only to his wife. These rationalizations or justifications, sometimes dignified with the term policies, are difficult to evolve even for the everyday research and information needs of the library's clientele, but there are more or less tangible guides which can lead to somewhat workable solutions to this problem. When, however, the librarian concerns himself with those books which have the misfortune of being labeled "historical," or what is even worse "rare," he finds himself in an even greater dilemma.

In the first place the same kind of utilitarian arguments that are made for current research books do not seem quite as acceptable for historical books. There is a whole series of conventions built up around "rare books" which put them in a class by themselves. Arguments on the basis of utility seem somehow to detract from the sense of devotion that antiquarian booksellers sometimes think should be involved in any transaction involving "rare books." It appears that they regard themselves more as matchmakers than salesmen. "I never try to sell anyone a book," one bookdealer has been quoted as saying, "I simply bring the book and its prospective owner together and let him fall in love with it." I almost said "fall in love with each other," because you get the impression from some dealers that there really is a reciprocal relationship in some way involved, and that the book is for the owner as much as the owner is for the book. There is a method in this madness, of course, because by bringing this notion of romantic love into the transaction, consideration of price no longer partakes of the nature of a commercial exchange but becomes a form of love token. In a sense the higher the price paid for the book, the greater is the gift that is bestowed on the beloved.

None of this should detract from the essential service performed by the book dealers both for the private and the institutional collector. Most of the great medical book collections in the country could not have been built without their help. However, while some of these romantic notions may titillate the private collec-

Originally published in *Bulletin of the Cleveland Medical Library,* Volume 9 (October, 1962), pp. 67-76. Reprinted by permission.

tor, they place the institutional collector in a rather unfavorable light. In the first place, since he generally ends up as a custodian of collections which have been donated by individuals who have presumably enjoyed this romantic attachment with their books, he is somewhat in the same position as the employee of an oriental institution involving collections of a rather different kind. This notion is enhanced by the slander which is sometimes circulated about librarians, that a librarian who reads is as bad as a bartender who drinks.

It is certainly true of the Cleveland Medical Library and probably true of a great many other public collections, that its "rare book" or historical collections are largely the result of gifts or donations which accrue to the library not on the basis of any pre-arranged policy but rather from the random benefactions of its friends and well-wishers. The result is that collections of this kind sometimes are not really collections at all, in the sense that they are orderly and reasoned gathering together of books for some specific purpose, but rather accumulations. This does not gainsay that these collections may consist almost entirely of desirable and worthwhile books, as is the case with the collection of the Cleveland Medical Library. One of the reasons that collections assume the character of randomness they sometimes seem to have, is that they are often based on a notion of rarity rather than on such utilitarian notions as providing an adequate basis for scholarship in some field, or demonstrating an orderly progression and evolution of ideas, or providing a tangible physical contact with some of our intellectual ancestors.

Librarians sometimes try to get away from the esoteric qualities associated with rare books by calling them "special collections." This permits them to include within the confines of such collections, such things as manuscripts and other archival materials. The term "rare book" does, however, still have some usefulness. It can, I suppose with equal justice, be applied to a book that is rare in the sense that it contains a rare contribution to intellectual, aesthetic, or social history. The emphasis we usually find unfortunately is on the kind of rarity which can be easily applied to buttons or to street car transfers which have been as avidly collected as books. This is the emphasis that is sometimes apparent when a library counts its treasures in "incunabula," the early books printed before 1500. The Cleveland Medical Library does have in its collection a representative sampling of medical incunabula, but none to compare with the holdings of the Boston Medical Library (674), the National Library of Medicine (532) or the College of Physicians of Philadelphia (412). The holdings of the Cleveland Medical Library are more on the order of the Library of the Royal College of Surgeons of England (56).

Most of the incunabula in the Cleveland Collection are a part of a special group of books known as the Nicolaus Pol Collection, since they were all part of the library of a physician by this name who flourished in the last part of the 15th and the early part of the 16th centuries. He inscribed his books in a bold hand "Nicolaus Pol Doctor 1494." They are interesting as a group since they represent the kinds of books a learned physician was acquiring in the first half century after the introduction of printing. This collection has been described in detail by Max Fisch in a book published for the Library in 1947[1] on the occasion of the Library's 50th anniversary, so there is no need to say much about it here. It represents only a very small part (40) of a library estimated to have contained more than 1300 books of which, however, only 500 seem to be known. The titles are representative of some of the characteristic medical texts of the period, heavily weighted as they are with Arabic writers like Albucasis, Avenzohar, and Rhasis, but including also some of Pol's closer contemporaries like the physician Ugo Benzi, sometimes called the "prince of philosophers" although I seem to recall that there are other claimants to this title.

In the opinion of some scholars it would be most wasteful for a research library to spend a great deal of its funds on acquisitions in this field. From the point of view of intellectual history, or the history of medicine, many scholars are convinced that the incunabula represent one of the least important parts of our medical literature. The great science historian, George Sarton,[2] certainly felt this way. He analyzed the bibliography of scientific and medical incunabula which Klebs[3] published in 1938 and came to the conclusion that taken by and large 15th century book printing, like book printing today, represented the publisher's or the printer's estimate of what he thought was a good economic risk. Of the 657 titles listed in the Klebs bibliography over half (377) were written in the second half of the 15th century. Sarton is convinced that most of these were written by mediocre writers. In short he regarded the collection of incunabula as a form of "veneration of relics." Other students of medical incunabula are not in complete agreement. To Osler they had interest primarily because they documented one of the great human inventions—the invention of printing. He also valued them for aesthetic reasons, because they are among some of the most beautiful books which have ever been produced. Other students have valued them for their role in preserving a large part of our classical heritage and for their importance in the study of the history of ideas. In a sense it is just as important for a research library to preserve the bad books as the good books, because the student of intellectual history is interested in erroneous ideas just as the physician is interested in any pathological conditions in gathering the history of his patient.

Incunabula have been treasured for many reasons but it is incontestable that rarity is an important one. Rarity has a basic appeal to human values which has little to do with the importance or intrinsic value of the artifact collected. It is useless to deny its power and much of the zest of collecting doubtlessly would be lost without it. The kind of rarity that leads people to become concerned about the surviving number of whooping cranes is even more important when applied to books, because books, at least in a biological sense, do not really reproduce themselves. Some of the objects which are collected because of their rarity may seem strange to some people. Rarity is not an absolute quality, it is more like the quality of beauty which exists to some extent in the eyes of the beholder. It is because of the strange predilections of some collectors that some objects survive at all in the world today.

Over-emphasis, however, on antiquity as a motivation in book collecting may lead to a neglect of some of the real classics in the history of science and medicine. For instance the anomaly has been pointed out, which leads us to cherish with loving care in a beautifully restored leather binding a medieval book on the beauty of women, spuriously attributed to Aristotle, while a first edition of one of the world's truly great classics like Darwin's *Origin of Species* languishes dog-eared and unnoticed in the stacks. It is undeniable that some of these later-day classics may be rather undistinguished in appearance, as is true of many 19th century books, but this does not detract from the fact that they are monuments of our intellectual history. One of our distinguished medical librarians has suggested that instead of rare book rooms in medical libraries we should have collections devoted to "milestones" or "monuments" of medical history. A book would be added to this kind of collection because of the nature of its contribution and not because of its age or rarity. This would provide us with some assurance that the important books of our own era would not all be worn out but that some of them would be preserved for future generations. A library historian has pointed out that sometimes our impressions of the intellectual preoccupations of our ancestors are based not so much on the books that they read as upon those that survived. This accounts, he says, for the fact that some historians think that theological literature was an abiding interest of this country's early settlers. It may be difficult, for this reason, to understand why book collectors place so much emphasis on copies in which the pages have not been cut. They do of couse represent copies in a more perfect state of preservation, one might almost say virginal, but this brings us back to the romantic basis of collecting we were trying to avoid. To the uninitiated, however, they may represent books which were unable to entice their owners to open them.

There are other standards applied in book collecting that are even more difficult to understand, especially by students of medical history whose interest is primarily that of gathering working texts. Not too long ago I visited a friend in the Midwest who is in charge of a University Library special collection. This library had recently acquired a distinguished history of science collection, and my friend regaled me with an account of some of the treasures it contained. Did I, he asked, have a Semmelweis in my library collection? My first reaction was that this was a species of Alpine flora, and that while we had some strange things in our collection, the only flowers we had were those in our herbals, and an occasional pressed flower that wandered in inadvertently in a gift collection. Before I disgraced myself however, I recollected that he was referring to the author of the famous book on puerperal fever. It seemed that as a result of acquiring the collection they now had three Semmelweises (a veritable garland) while our library had not even one. My friend wishing to remedy this imbalance offered, if my memory does not fail me, to sell one of the Semmelweises for three thousand dollars. When I demurred that this would leave my book budget at that time with something less than a negative balance, he said he could let me have one of the other copies for three hundred dollars. When not too unnaturally I inquired what the difference was between the two copies, he said that the second unfortunately was perforated, that is marked with a library stamp. I am sorry to say that we still don't have a Semmelweis, either perforated or unperforated, at least in a first edition. But completeness is a bane of the collector because this leaves him with nothing to collect. We do have a fine copy of Oliver Wendell Holmes, *Puerperal fever as a private pestilence,* published some five years before the Semmelweis. Although this does not detract from the importance of the other book, it does point up the fact that it is dangerous to insist on any kind of priorities in medical history, or any other field for that matter without liberally hedging the claim with qualifications.

Both the Semmelweis and Holmes books would qualify for any special medical collection both on the grounds of rarity and of significance. In fact it seems fairly clear that rarity and significance are each a function of the other. Books generally do not become rare, or known to be rare, unless they are sought after. One way to identify the significant books in the history of medicine would be to try to list those ideas or developments which historians have judged to be the most important in the development of medicine—in other words those ideas which were considered seminal or germinal. This is an interesting kind of intellectual exercise, but I doubt if any two people would come up with exactly the same list of names, and that one would have a tendency to be either too generous or too selective. I suppose that literally the only seminal contribution would be that of Leeuwenhoek, who saw the spermatozoa for the first time in his primitive microscopes, and the only really germinal idea — but you have anticipated me here, I am sure.

This kind of collecting may be more difficult because it is based on historical judgment rather than some arbitrary or accidental standard of rarity. It is also easier because one of the functions which rarity serves as a basis for collecting is that it tends to eliminate the number of objects in the class that are available to collect. This is especially true today when because of the increased interest in recent years in the history of science and medicine, many important books have practically disappeared from the market. A good example of what has happened to the trade in medical rare books in recent years is Harvey's great book on the circulation. It has been called the most important book in the history of medicine, but it is not an example of the highest standards in the bookmaking arts. It was most unattractively printed and most of the copies appeared on poor paper. It was for a long time a mystery why Harvey sent his little book to Frankfurt to be printed by an almost unknown publisher. One theory was that this was the quickest way to get it into the continental book trade through the fairs, and also that it was cheaper and more efficient to produce it that way. Harvey had expressed his new ideas about the circulation of the blood in lectures some ten years before the publication of the book, so speed could not have been of importance to him. An article published by the Bibliographical Society in *The Library* some twenty years ago helped to solve the puzzle. Harvey made his choice of publishers, it seems, through the influence of his friend Robert Fludd, an English physician who had had some of his books published on the continent by a publisher in the well-known DeBry family. Fitzer, who published Harvey's book, was originally an Englishman who had married one of the DeBry daughters and took over the family business but apparently not their skill in publishing or printing. A few copies of this important book were printed on good thick paper.

In a census of copies of Harvey's book made in 1940 some 46 copies were located—most of them in England but several in great libraries on the continent and in this country. It is interesting to note that Osler had his hands on as many as four copies at one time or another. He bought three of them in 1906: one ended up in his own library now at McGill, another he presented to Dr. Walter James who in turn gave it to the New York Academy of Medicine, and the third he presented to the Johns Hopkins Medical School Library. He bought a fourth in 1912 and presented it to the Royal Society of Medicine in London. He bid on another copy at the Pearson sale at Southeby's in 1916 but his bid of £40 was under the £48 bid by Maggs Bros. who bought it for a New York dealer. Osler probably did more than any single individual to influence the collecting of medical and scientific books in this country and in England. It has been noted that before Osler began to collect early medical books, a copy of a first edition Harvey was for years exhibited in a show case of an English bookseller for £5. Of another famous medical book, the *De Fabrica* of Vesalius, it is said that because of Osler's interest in the book, no medical library could afford to be without a copy, but few could afford it.

The Cleveland Medical Library, unfortunately, does not have a copy of the first edition of Vesalius, but we do have a fine copy of the handsome second folio printed just a few years later, still close enough in time to its author to provide us with the sense of contact which we spoke about earlier. This may be tinged a little with the romantic notions of book collecting we seem to be trying to avoid, but it is nevertheless real. It is not necessary to prove this to any librarian who has, for instance, found for a reader a copy of the original publication of

Dupuytren's fracture and has seen the almost visible evidence of the physical presence of the author in the reader's reaction. In looking for a single quality to characterize several of these books we have in our special collection, the first edition of Auenbrugger, Laennec, Beaumont, the quality that makes them important is, I think, that they all still have about them the excitement of new discoveries. This feeling is embodied so well in a line of Malpighi. It is a headline to one of the letters he wrote to Borelli on the capillary circulation which were printed in 1661. The line has a quality of breathless awe and excitement: "I see with my own eyes a certain great thing." The line had a certain biblical quality about it, as I remembered it. In trying to verify the line I checked first in Fulton's history of physiology[5] where I found it given as: "I see with my eyes a work trusty and great" which does not have nearly the flavor of the first so I was much relieved when I finally found it cited in Foster's book on the history of physiology.[6]

Malpighi's little book is quite rare and much sought after, but frequently some of the most exciting and productive ideas have been published in a form which is not as inviting to the book collector such as the Dupuytren we mentioned above. This has been particularly true ever since the development of the scientific journal from its early beginning in the later half of the 17th century until today when almost everything of any new significance in medical thought appears first in a periodical. In the last decades of the 17th century the *Philosophical Transactions,* one of the earliest of the learned periodicals, was publishing the curious observations Leeuwenhoek was making in Holland. At the end of the 18th century the Royal Society which had taken over formal responsibility for the *Transactions* may have helped to create an item for collectors when it turned down Edward Jenner's paper on the cowpox which he published separately as a 75 page pamphlet in 1798. By the last half of the 19th century all of the important contributions were being printed in journals, some of them on paper which has already deteriorated to the point where they cannot be handled. Robert Koch's classical paper on the etiology of tuberculosis was published in 1882 in the *Berliner Klinische Wochenschrift,* and many of Ehrlich's contributions appeared in the *Deutsche Medizinische Wochenschrift,* and the *Zeitschrift für klinische Medizin.* Pasteur's important papers appeared in the transactions of various scientific societies. Joseph Lister published his first paper on antiseptic surgery in 1867 in the pages of the English medical journal *Lancet.* Some of these papers of course are collected in the form of reprints and highly prized. This was brought home to me recently when I saw a reprint of Einstein's first published paper on relativity being offered by a dealer for the same price as a first edition of Newton's *Principia,* but for the most part many of the important contributions to medical science in the 19th and 20th centuries exist only in the form of journal articles which are in many cases in a very poor state of preservation.

Because our library has a fine journal collection, including one of the few complete sets of the *Philosophical Transactions* of the Royal Society of London beginning with the first volume which appeared in 1665, the Cleveland Medical Library is rich in this kind of material. Most of it was collected not to augment our historical collections but in the course of carrying out the primary role of the Library, which is that of supplying the sources needed by its members in their daily activities in practice, teaching and research. The Library will and must carry on this primary function, but the question may be asked whether it should take any strong overt steps to increase what might be called its historical collections. There is a fine, in fact almost a non-existent, line between materials collected for current research purposes and materials collected for purposes of historical research. It might be argued that a research library if it did a good job with the former would have no problems with the latter. This would be true, for instance, if it had existed and had purchased a copy out of its current book funds of the *De Motu Cordis* when it first appeared. The fact remains, that these judgments are much easier to make in retrospect than they are in prospect.

One axiom that is frequently quoted to guide libraries in building their collections, both for current and historical research needs, is that they should build on their strength. That is, since no library can hope to collect exhaustively in all fields, it should attempt to make those areas in which it is already strong as definitive as possible. The Cleveland Medical Library already has several areas which could be developed in this way. First there is the Marshall Herbal collection, a collection of some three hundred items, including the rare *Herbarius* published by Peter Schoeffer in Mainz in 1484 and a complete copy of the *Grant Herbier* published in Paris in 1500 of which only one other copy (an incomplete one) has been recorded. The Cole collection on syphilology and venereology provides a great deal of the source material on the history of these subjects. Thanks to the generous benefactions of two of its good friends the Library has excellent collections in two subject areas which provide a basis for historical collections. Dr. Henry John's collection of books on diabetes mellitus, including some early dissertations on the subject, has been added to the existing materials in the Library's collection on this subject. Dr. Robert M. Stecher has from time to time added to the Library's holdings in the field of rheumatology and arthritis with the result that this area is beginning to grow in greater depth. Dr. Stecher has also brought together for the Library what is tantamount to a definitive collection of the original papers of the father of psychoanalysis, Sigmund Freud. This has recently been significantly augmented by his gift to the Library of a collection of early psychoanalytical journals which contain many of Freud's original papers. In addition the Library is in possession of a fine collection of many of the important classics in the history of medicine as well as many of the secondary works of importance. Many of these are in the collection of Dr. Edward H. Cushing, an eclectic collection in subject matter but not in quality, since it contains such treasured items as a first edition Auenbrugger, a Laennec, a Beaumont and many other fine editions.

Thus it is largely through the efforts of private collectors that the Library has been able to build its resources in the history of medicine. The Library will probably have to continue to augment its historical collections largely by this means. In the first place in order to collect effectively in any subject field, a great deal of study is required, and no matter how much scholarship the Library's staff is able to muster, it will never be sufficient to do justice to all the diverse fields which its collection covers. The other reason is an economic one. With the great demands that contemporary scientific publication makes on its resources, the fewer are the funds available for historical books. I hope that the Library will always be able to squeeze enough out of its budget for an occasional indulgence in an irresistible book. It is for this reason that such funds as the D. Kirk Spitler Memorial Fund are so valuable to the Library. This Fund was established a year or so ago in memory of one of our past presidents. The income from this Fund, for instance, made it possible for us to acquire recently a handsome and important book: the *Bibel der Natur* (Leipzig, 1752) of Johann Swammerdam (1637-1680), the famous Dutch biologist and microscopist, which was first published long after his death by Boerhaave in 1737.

There is an area of collecting perhaps even more important than any we have discussed, and furthermore one that requires more of an expenditure of energy and time, than it does money, though it's not often certain which of these commodities are in the shortest supply. If it isn't axiomatic that history like charity begins at home, it should be. If we don't take an interest in our own local history there will be few others who will do so. The great sweep and progression of medical history can sometimes be as effectively demonstrated on a small stage as it can be on a large one. The materials which provide the basis for this history are more than rare; they are usually unique, in the form of letters, manuscript memoirs, notes and records—records of all kinds. Many of these unfortunately are lost forever unless active efforts are made to gather them into archives.

Books can be enjoyed and they can be utilized in many ways. They represent one of the most important resources any community can gather unto itself. The community's regard for and devotion to learning will be measured in some respect by the degree to which it devotes its energies to building its libraries, just as its regard for beauty is reflected in its art museums and its musical institutions. Books have been and they can be collected as artifacts. There is no reason why they should not be. They are frequently just as beautiful demonstrations of the craftsman's art involved in making books, as the vase is of the art of the potter. But their primary importance is what they embody in the form of realized experiences, insights and informed opinion. If a Library collects with these purposes in mind, it need not worry too much about such concepts as "rare books."

DAVID A. KRONICK, PH.D.

Cleveland, Ohio

REFERENCES

1. Fisch, M. H. *Nicolaus Pol Doctor 1494.* New York, Cleveland Medical Library Association, 1947.

2. Sarton, G. The scientific literature transmitted through the incunabula. *Osiris,* 1938, **5**:41-245.

3. Klebs, A. C. *Incunabula scientifica et medica.* Bruges, St. Catherine Pr., 1938.

4. Weil, F. William Fitzer, the publisher of Harvey's de Motu Cordis, 1628. *The Library,* 1943/44, **24**:142-64.

5. Fulton, J. F. *Selected readings in the history of physiology.* Springfield, Ill., Thomas, 1930, p. 65.

6. Foster, M. *Lectures on the history of physiology.* London, Cambridge, 1901.

Collecting for the History of Medicine*

By Gertrude L. Annan, *Librarian*

New York Academy of Medicine
New York, New York

ABSTRACT

Value of books depends on their place in the collection, and it is not suggested that the librarian become an expert in the prices of rare books. The dealer should be trusted as an adviser. The same is true about disposal of rare books.

An account is given of earlier practice at the New York Academy of Medicine Library in the acquisition of rare books, and some notable items are listed. The importance of pamphlets, reprints, and annual reports is discussed.

Building a collection of the institution's own records is commended, and various examples given of how an unbalanced or inappropriate collection loses its value. Good examples of special subject collections are quoted.

Care and preservation of rare material are discussed.

FEW medical libraries planning a historical collection begin without some resources. There are usually at least a few volumes or small groups of material which point in specific directions to guide the librarian in adding to or in weeding from the shelves. Weeding and building the collection must of course be based on the same principles.

A major point to remember is that the value of any item in any collection does not depend upon its market value. It is the value of the particular text within the particular collection. Nothing should be added to or discarded from a collection because it is expensive or not expensive. The item itself, the text in the collection, is the only concern in passing judgment. A knowledge of prices and values is useful for a librarian to have, particularly when buying early materials or collectors' items of later periods, and in judging the disposal of duplicates. Unfortunately, there is no easy way to learn the values of these historical materials. It is a life's work, and takes many years of reading sale catalogs, following book auction prices, and realizing the fluctuations in the antiquarian book market, because this, as in all commodities, follows supply and demand.

*Based on a lecture given at the Institute sponsored by the Committee on Continuing Education, Medical Library Association, in Denver, Colorado, on June 5, 1968.

Originally published in *Bulletin of the Medical Library Association,* Volume 58 (July, 1970), pp. 330-335. Reprinted by permission.

The librarian, however, can be comforted by the fact that he is not expected to be an expert in the prices of rare books. He is not a dealer nor should he assume that prerogative. The Antiquarian Booksellers Association of America issues a directory of members which includes also brief general information about books and values. This emphasizes that dealers are appraisers, that it is their business to be concerned with the ever changing picture of prices in the rare book market. This was rightly stressed at a meeting of ALA's Rare Book Section in 1967. Here the librarian was advised that he should not appraise except in certain cases, for example, when there is a donor who gives a few items and wishes evaluation for income tax purposes. If they are not very valuable and the librarian feels capable of appraising them, this may be done. If the gift is an expensive book, or a collection, then the librarian should feel free to tell the donor that he should have a professional appraisal. Some donors will offer to pay for this; others expect the library to cover the expense, often 10 percent of the value. As the Internal Revenue Service is much more strict than formerly, a professional appraisal is a protection for both donor and library. This same advice serves to help the librarian receiving demands for appraisals from those unfamiliar with the many problems appraising may cause. A firm rule, gently stated, should meet with understanding. Such a rule should cover all requests, including those frequent demands for assigning the costs of secondhand books without any examination of copies. Librarians can say with authority that they are not dealers, no matter how many years they have spent in historical collections. Librarians with such expertise are the most adamant in refusing.

The same general attitude may be assumed toward disposal of duplicates or other unwanted volumes. Practical advice given at ALA's meeting of the Rare Book Section was quoted in *Antiquarian Bookman:*

> The usual method for the disposition of special collections is the tried and true one of establishing a relationship with a number of booksellers who know the collections in the library; are likely to want the type of duplicates which may show up in it and in turn likely to be able to offer, at the time or later, something wanted or needed by the library. Except for the simple and obvious requirements of notations or receipt and credit memoranda, the arrangement seems always to be an informal, if not unofficial one based on the indispensable factor of mutual trust between librarian and bookseller. And it seems to work with all parties benefiting.

I cannot emphasize too strongly this point of view. Some medical libraries send priced lists of duplicates to libraries and patrons. Financially, this is impractical. The staff must spend in staff time an equivalent of whatever profits accrue. Perhaps more important, however, is the danger of upsetting library-dealer relationships. Every librarian with a historical collection knows the dependence upon a friendly dealer in building a collection. When librarians appraise duplicates, price them low for the benefit of their own clientele and their colleagues in other libraries, they are appreciated by those who benefit. It can hardly fail, though, to make difficulties for dealers. More than once items worth about $75 have been listed at the very low price of $5. The physician who orders one of these after it has been sold may try to get another copy from a dealer who expects to get the market value. The prospective buyer will probably not consider that the price of the duplicate was particularly small, but rather claim the dealer is a pirate. Examples of this are many. One man, outraged because a dealer priced an important contribution at the then market price of $250, has never been convinced that the library's $40 was in error, rather than the dealer's. Confidence in a dealer's integrity may be unwittingly destroyed. Furthermore, a dealer should not be asked to offer special prices or reductions to those who are not regular customers. A client of long standing may hope for special privileges and consideration, not a stranger. It is unrealistic to demand from a book dealer what one would not expect other business men, such as antique dealers, to offer. Librarians, then, wishing to please their clientele with underpriced material should state very explicitly at the top of the list of duplicates that these prices do not reflect the market value but are priced below it for the benefit of friends and colleagues. Otherwise, the librarian would do well to have a professional appraiser engaged. This would protect dealers and prevent knowledgeable collectors from snapping up bargains with the intention of selling them at a profit.

Although the librarian cannot suddenly overnight become an expert in book values, he can learn about the different types of material and what makes them rare. It is seldom that there is only one factor. Today a book is not as a rule valuable for age alone, scarcity alone, size alone, beauty or typography alone, provenance alone, or type of publication alone. The one single factor of great importance is that of contribution to knowledge. This should be emphasized, because twenty years ago the most important factor was age, and librarians collected chiefly the classics of medicine, early editions, manuscripts, sixteenth century publications, and early Americana.

At the New York Academy of Medicine Library in the thirties and forties the money available for the purchase of rare books was so very little that it was impossible to add to our incunabula, medieval manuscripts, or the most costly of the sixteenth century items. The few hundred dollars regularly available were spent with care, consideration, and no little anxiety, on important texts of the seventeenth to nineteenth centuries, the very material which has since then risen so spectacularly in price. There was no prevision that this would be so. Poverty of funds dictated that the early classics other libraries were adding were far too costly. There are many examples of low-cost purchases. An eighteenth century Italian book concerning a hospital which treated patients with mental illnesses, acquired for $8.00, was offered not long ago for $275. The value of Carpue's small piece on plastic surgery of 1816 has soared unbelievably since 1929 when the Academy's copy, described even then as scarce, was bought for ten shillings. Editions of Hippocrates and Galen, or fifteenth and sixteenth century texts, have not risen in value as astronomically. Some are very little higher, a few even lower. Important contributions, however, have steadily increased. Even the *Wall Street Journal* published an article on the subject. Libraries do not buy for investment, but there is satisfaction in knowing that scientific texts have gone up in value as some literary and ecclesiastical volumes declined. A collection of 112 editions of the *Vicar of Wakefield* was presented to the Academy, because Goldsmith studied medicine. The donor was proud of the first edition obtained for $4,000. Kept in the vault for some years, it was finally removed when it was apparent that tastes had changed so much that its price had sunk to $400.

Although the librarian need not try to become an expert in market prices, he should turn his attention to a consideration of the types of publication which may have value in a historical collection. The first and most needed lesson is to learn that the large handsome volume may well be of much less value, intrinsically and financially, than a small unattractive piece. The first edition of Harvey, beyond question the most costly of all printed medical books, is in reality a poorly printed pamphlet on poor quality paper. Many years spent in working with early material have taught that the librarian should and must learn that above all the small fragile piece must be of concern. The New York Academy of Medicine Library was extraordinarily fortunate in having a man of remarkable foresight in the nineteenth century who saved thousands of pamphlets, chiefly in bound volumes, that his contemporaries were discarding as worthless. He knew instinctively what the historian of the future would want saved for his needs. One of our most valuable Americana, Samuel Bard's thirty-three-page tract on diphtheria, 1771, Dr. Samuel Purple literally retrieved from an ashcan. Early nineteenth century murder trials containing medical testimony by leading physicians of the day are in some cases unique survivors. One of our most knowledgeable medical bookmen, seeing the many bound volumes containing these pamphlets, estimated that if put up for sale they would bring at least six million dollars. Often today, when pamphlets are offered at very high prices in sales catalogs, the staff checks to see if our copies are safely in the locked precincts of the Rare Book Department. Last year Ashbel Smith's early Texas medical imprint,

An Account of the Yellow Fever, Galveston, 1839, was offered for $1,500. Our copy was immediately rescued from the pamphlet file in the main collection, where an unscrupulous reader might be tempted to take it away in a convenient pocket. The very next day after that incident, Goodspeed's *The Month* described an early eighteenth century Boston pamphlet on inoculation for sale at $1,600. Our holdings of those early smallpox pieces are most distinguished, and as this particular one was not present, an immediate telephone call ordered it. Unfortunately it was sold. At the time there were no funds for such a purchase, but its importance to our already fine holdings would surely be of sufficient persuasion to attract funds from some of our Friends. These two incidents are cited to emphasize how valuable pamphlet material may be and how little today age is a factor. Twenty years ago the inoculation pamphlet would have been very costly, the Smith, not at all.

Other material often slighted by librarians are annual reports and annual school catalogs. Those who have little historical insight often discard potential treasures. A member of the Library Committee of the Academy advised that instead of careful weeding of hospital reports we should discard them all. The previous day another Committee member, an astute bookman, telephoned to say that he had been going through similar material at a local dealer's, found some interesting reports he was sending to us, and he would buy for his own library any we did not need. There were many early reports of the Institute of Living in Hartford, Connecticut, only one of which we lacked. The Menninger Foundation, *Short Title Catalogue of the Rare & Historical Collection*, Topeka, 1967, has a splendid listing of hospital reports, pp. 48-63, which should assist any librarian in demonstrating the value of retaining them. With these as with other desiderata, judgment must be determined on the importance of the material to the library and its users. A report that lists donors to an unfamiliar small hospital may be discarded without concern, but reports containing information which will be of obvious use to the historian should receive careful consideration.

Nor should the lowly reprint be scorned, even if the original journal article is in the collection. Reprints of outstanding contributions to science, especially those signed by the authors, are collectors' items of great cost. Librarians must look at reprints, not as trash to be thrown out without question, but rather as potential rarities. The staff of the Academy library are well aware that out-of-date, unwanted textbooks, particularly duplicates, may be discarded without further questioning, but pamphlet material, small pieces, must have authoritative judgment passed upon them. A duplicate pamphlet, Philadelphia, 1837, Jean Baptiste Bouillaud, *New Researches on Acute Articular Rheumatism*, was sent for decision.

Fortuitously, the previous day it had been noticed for sale in a catalog at $75, so that, obviously, its fate was not the wastebasket. Librarians cannot be expected to be knowledgeable about such items, but must be aware of general principles, and must at least question the importance of a text. The reprint of Oliver Wendell Holmes' paper on puerperal fever is hardly a handsome publication, but is many times more valuable than a copy of the journal from which it was reprinted. Claude Bernard, Lister, Roentgen, all the giants of medicine are collected in reprint form. Twentieth century giants are no less important. A library exhibit, "Yesterday's Throwaways, Today's Treasures," brought together astonishingly valuable pieces, surprising to librarians and collectors alike.

Alert to these considerations, the librarian faced with building a collection must begin by having a written plan, the product of consultation with bookmen, collectors, dealers, even more than with historians, unless the latter are bookmen as well as historians. The historians are enormously helpful in determining policies, but their own specialized interests may on occasion prevent objective planning. The collection must be planned for the future as well as the present, and one must consider the holdings already available, and the possibility of adding collections being built by those close to the library, but since it is obvious that too broad an acquisitions policy prevents rather than stimulates wise collecting, the librarian cannot please every historian by collecting in his field. The physician who is shocked to find the library does not have anything about the materia medica of Madagascar may insist that such a collection be inaugurated. Such a collection might be most appropriate, but decision should be reached only after extensive efforts to determine how it fits into the present collection, where other collections are, who are experts in the field to advise, what dealers can help. In some fields expertise is far more important than available funds. Money is necessary for most collecting, but time and expertise are far more necessary. Here the dealer can be expert consultant, a friend in need as well as a bookseller. Librarians without contacts with dealers should acquire a directory of the members of the Antiquarian Booksellers Association of America from their Center at 630 Fifth Avenue, New York, and make an effort to meet and know any geographically convenient one who may cover medicine and science. The librarian, the bookman, the historian, the dealer all have vital roles to play.

Changes in the study of the history of medicine in these twenty years have been as great as those in collecting. When Dr. Richard Shryock was Director of the Institute of the History of Medicine at Johns Hopkins University, he reported that those applying to study there were from other disciplines rather than medicine. A major reason was that at the time there were few opportunities for full-time historians of medicine. Today the situation is in reverse, with chairs not filled because there are not enough trained applicants. On the other hand, in the training of rare book librarians, for the first time there are opportunities to learn that expertise outside in-service learning. The establishment of a Rare Book Section of the Association of College and Research Libraries, and the pioneering at the Lilly Library in training rare book librarians are major and exciting and badly needed steps toward supporting and providing the expertise so necessary. The same may be said of advancement in the care and processing of archives. When the Academy started its archival program, there were no guidelines or sources of information and advice. Today the Society of American Archivists has annual meetings of great practical value and publishes an important journal. This supplements Theodore R. Schellenberg's *The Management of Archives*, New York, 1965. Oral history, too, has grown up in this same period. Librarians must concern themselves with the records of their own institutions, and encourage administration to insist upon saving and preserving them. Gilbert Clausman, Librarian of the New York University Medical Center established a model program, and others in the New York metropolitan area have been alerted to the importance of establishing and maintaining these services in accordance with the size and age of the facility. Some hospitals have lost all records of their distinguished history. Others are more fortunate in early administrators who realized the value to the institution for information and in public relations as well as the history of medicine.

Establishing the institution's own records is surely the first step in building a historical collection. Then decisions must be made regarding the scope of the collection. This depends upon the goals, upon the teaching needs, upon the special interests of the institution. The greatest danger is to be too ambitious in scope. Lee Ash has said in a survey he made of a library in Canada (quoted on the cover of an issue of the *Antiquarian Bookman*): "A good collection is expensive; a poor collection is extravagant and wasteful." An examination of several collections may show this, so we may first look at some of the collections given over the years to the New York Academy of Medicine. The Streeter Collection, purchased by a group of Fellows of the Academy in 1928, is a particularly good example. It was brought together by a physician who bought whatever appealed to him without any special plan or design, and without any expertise, without knowledge of condition of copies, of editions, of importance of texts. Some of these volumes are highlights of the library today, such as the superlative illuminated English manuscript of Guy de Chauliac. But as a collection it can only be called extravagant and wasteful, or more properly it may be said that it was not a collection, but a group of books which have been scattered through the Academy's library. A few years later, Dr. Margaret Barclay Wilson presented her collection on foods and cookery, some 4,000 items relating to the subject. This is not as extravagant and wasteful, for it has a basic idea and brings together volumes and information belonging together. Unfortunately, she, too, was not advised about condition of copies, or selection of editions or texts, but added whatever came her way, so that there is great unevenness, with excellent holdings by one author, but no important edition by such a figure as Brillat-Savarin. On the other hand, it was wasteful to have this collection given to a medical library where it is seldom that readers wish to know what an Italian kitchen of the sixteenth century looked like, how poultry was carved in the seventeenth century, or how elegantly an eighteenth century table could be decorated. This is surely out of scope in a medical library, except for texts on nutrition and diet. It is especially sad to see a collection brought together with such love and interest little used and not being added to as such a collection might be in a more appropriate home.

Several collections received in the last decade are worthy of examination as models to follow. Rufus Cole, Director of the Hospital of Rockefeller Institute, interested in the development of scientific research, collected the writings of Francesco Redi, an eminent Italian experimental physiologist of the seventeenth century. From this one author his efforts were extended to assembling the writings of Redi's colleagues. Redi was a member of the Accademia del Cimento, that first great scientific society whose writings reflected the ferment, the exciting and varied experiments of the scientists of the period. Here are the works of Bellini, Borelli, Steno, Kircher, Malpighi, Magalotti, and others, all in one place for the historian of experimental science in that century, a superb concept for a collection. Fenwick Beekman's John Hunter collection is of equal importance, uniting not only the many contributions of that great surgeon, but also the work of his contemporaries. Another small group of material Dr. Beekman collected may be called unique, and is surely fascinating, if not a little macabre. It relates to the resurrectionists, that notorious pair, Burke and Hare, who robbed graveyards for the benefit of surgeons wishing bodies for dissection. One volume contains pictures in color of "Daft Jamie" and other victims, many ballads, a woodcut of the scene of the execution, and a letter written by William Burke, addressed to the keeper of the "Lock up House," on the night before the hanging. Again, the historian has in one place a treasure of information.

A totally different kind of collection came to the Academy, one that required little in money, but much in thought, perseverance, enthusiasm, even dedication. Michael Davis for over fifty years was intimately involved with medico-socio-economic movements of the period which led to Medicare. He saved correspondence, published and unpublished reports, legislation, pamphlets, books, a mine of pertinent information that anyone wishing to report on these events in the history of health care and economics must consult. This collection can serve as a classic example of what may be accomplished by one man deeply concerned in his work.

Most large collections are the result of amalgamation of a number of these personal collections, and the librarian must work toward coordinating them, supplementing, not allowing them to stagnate. A dynamic program should be encouraged, and the various collections placed within a general scheme so that progress may be made in developing the collection as a whole, rather than separate goals pointing in many directions. With large collections this is difficult, but planning should be started early. Sir William Osler's collection, remarkably varied in scope, was carefully structured. This was possible only because of his varied interests and wide reading in the history of medicine. Also, he had the good fortune of pioneering at a time when it was possible to haunt bookstores for great bargains. His careful planning, however, is still pertinent to the librarian.

Acquiring material is only the first step for the librarian; it must be cataloged, it must be cared for. Too many libraries, overburdened with many activities, have put aside for the future the care and cataloging of their gifts and purchases. This discourages donors who prefer to give to institutions which obviously cherish their gifts and make them available. Often it has been difficult to persuade donors to send manuscripts and other archival material to the appropriate library because previous gifts have not been unpacked and cataloged. Since the Academy library has always made every effort to process such material it has been the reluctant recipient of many items more properly offered elsewhere. Librarians wishing to encourage donations should emphasize their willingness to care for them.

Preservation is a most important problem today. Fortunately, there is now information available, although it is not always a simple matter to find an expert. Yet expertise in this field is all important. Much damage has been done by amateur mending, by accepting a salesman's words about laminators or supplies, by lack of interest, by assuming every large library must know what procedures should be correct. Librarians should at least learn what not to do, should feel a grave responsibility to keep up with the literature on the subject, should not order supplies and equipment without consulting the enormously useful publication of Talas, Division of Technical Library Service, *Tools & Supplies for Bookbinding; Book Repair; Book Conservation*, New York, 1967 and Supplement, 1968. The series of pamphlets issued by the Barrow Laboratory: Permanent Durable Book Paper, The Virginia State Library, Richmond, should be at hand. Articles by Frazer Poole, Preservation Officer, Library of Congress, Paul Banks, Conservator of the Newberry Library, and Hannah B. Friedman,

Collections Preservation Coordinator at the New York Public Library, appear in the literature. Workshops by such an expert as Carolyn Horton are of great importance for all staff members.

There are of course differing opinions and methods, and each librarian must use judgment. A rare book librarian who recommended that materials in a library should be divided for preservation procedures, the sheep from the goats, should surely pause at the awesome responsibility of these decisions. They should not be left to the whim of a staff member. Experience has taught that unless one knows that a Roentgen reprint is of great value it is apt to be treated as any other reprint, and tragic errors have been made by unknowledgeable treatment, with stiff hinges cutting through fragile title-pages. The advice—at least do no harm—should be a command for all types of material, old, new, fragile, ugly, and handsome.

Any collection is brought together for the future as well as the present. It is a heritage from one generation to another, or from many centuries to another. It may be of staggering financial worth or it may in its initial stages be modestly collected as those of Samuel Smith Purple and Michael Davis. Time, interest, knowledge of a subject, enthusiasm, and determination bring rich rewards to library and librarian.

DO'S AND DON'TS FOR RARE BOOKS

By GERTRUDE ANNAN

DO remember that the value of any book in any collection has nothing in the world to do with its price on the market. Librarians are not in the book business. It is the value of the text to your collection that should concern you.

DO trust your antiquarian book dealer who can be of enormous service to you, and remember that the price you pay covers that service as well as the cost of the volume. The dealer's years of experience, means of getting material, subject knowledge, interest in your collection, is of great value, and the time you may spend checking on the price of a book can be more costly than the price quoted.

DON'T think that because an item is a pamphlet or a broadside, or even on occasion a lowly reprint, or of insignificant appearance, that it is therefore valueless. Many collector's items are of just such material. Ephemera of yesterday are scarce and valuable today precisely because they were ephemera and not saved for the future.

DON'T unwittingly buy a defective copy. Stop worrying about what the dealer charges for a book and start worrying about the condition of a copy. It is your responsibility to check to see that the copy is complete before paying for it, not several years later when you accidentally discover it.

DON'T compete with other libraries in collecting, cooperate instead. No librarian should buy a book in order to swell statistics, to brag of holdings or to get ahead of another collection. Competition and useless duplication among libraries is wasteful and expensive.

DON'T take anyone's word for anything in historical research. All historians are fallible, even as you and I. Go to the source. Many historians have passed on to posterity the errors of their predecessors. Let us not do so if we can avoid it.

DON'T let uncaring hands mark, stamp, cut, hinge title-pages or other leaves. If expert attention is not available, wrap carefully and preserve rather than mutilate further.

DON'T think of a book as rare, as costly, as a museum piece. *Do* think of it as a contribution to knowledge, a product of man's thought and ingenuity, a piece in the long story of historical development.

Originally published in *Bulletin of the Medical Library Association,* Volume 48 (January, 1960), pp. 104-105. Reprinted by permission.

DO read booksellers' catalogs regularly—day time or bed time reading for enjoyment, information and profit.

DO enjoy the enchantment of the past; the charming, the beautiful, the fragile, sometimes the pathetic or funny, but always fascinating record of an earlier day.

A Dream Come True: The Lawrence Reynolds Collection*

BY HENRY SCHUMAN
New York, New York

AN EVENT of the greatest significance for the cultural and scientific life of the University of Alabama Medical Center, of the University itself, of the city of Birmingham, of the South in general, is in the making. I refer, of course, to the gift by Dr. Lawrence Reynolds of his remarkable collection of books, manuscripts, and autographs pertaining to the history of the medical sciences, formed over a period of forty years, much of it—I cannot refrain from boasting—with my collaboration.

One could comment on the Reynolds treasures for a solid week—the duration of an old-fashioned filibuster. In this paper I can but leap from peak to peak and highlight for you some of the more dramatic gems.

But first I want to say a few things about Dr. Reynolds, whose cultural benefaction to this area will be felt as long as books remain a concern of civilized men. Is it not natural to wonder, to ask, what manner of man is Dr. Reynolds? I offer in justification of my hardihood in essaying to give you a brief portrait of a most difficult subject the fact that my relationship with him goes back 27 years to 1932.

It was early in that year that I turned professional bookseller, spurred by the Great Depression of 1929 which deepened progressively, undeterred by the pronouncements of two American leaders of that period, one the President of our country, Herbert Hoover, the other the economist, Roger Babson. Both had made the public statement the previous year that 1931 would be the biggest year in America's economic history. In my own experience this prediction fell so comically short that by the end of 1931 my wife and I accepted the inevitability of a standstill in our business and decided to venture into the unknown terrain of what we liked to think of as a profession—bookselling. I had for some years been something of a collector of literary works, yielding to my sentiment for a few of my favorite contemporary authors, among them Stephen Crane, Dreiser, Anderson, Shaw, and Galsworthy. The first editions

* (Based on a talk given before the Alabama Society of Medical History, March 6, 1957.)

Originally published in *Bulletin of the Medical Library Association,* Volume 47 (July, 1959), pp. 235-252. Reprinted by permission.

of these authors were part of our general library of about 3,000 volumes which constituted our initial stock in trade.

A few Detroit collectors found us almost at once. They happened to be mostly doctors interested in literature. One of them, my good friend, Dr. Richard McKean, whose interests spanned both literature and the history of medicine, said he would bring in a bookish friend of his before long, a doctor concerned principally with the literature of medical history. This friend did indeed visit our shop shortly afterward and made inquiry about "a Laennec." That was the beginning. I hadn't the slightest idea who Laennec was, nor of the subject of the history of medicine, but in two years I had become a specialist in this field, by grace of the enthusiam and patience of the seeker of the Laennec—Dr. Lawrence Reynolds. I found the subject so engrossing, so fresh and novel a vista from which to view the history of civilization, that I pursued it to the exclusion of my old interests and made medical and scientific literature the sole basis of our rare book business.

I found the first edition of Laennec (1819) for Dr. Reynolds, and much else since, although he had been gathering books from his early years, his natural collecting instinct warmed by his father's gift of four medical historical works when he went off to Johns Hopkins. And at Hopkins he could hardly miss the atmosphere favorable to the study of the history of medicine, an atmosphere created by John Shaw Billings who gave a course of lectures on the subject in 1876, again in 1891, and in 1893, and, with the opening of The Johns Hopkins Medical School, was made Lecturer in the History and Literature of Medicine, a position he held till 1905. Further inspiration was provided by the founding, in 1890, of the Johns Hopkins Hospital Historical Club by Osler, Welch, Kelly, and others.*

Dr. Reynolds himself has recently touched on his book-collecting activity in an article for the new publication, *De historia medicinae*, official organ of the Alabama Society of Medical History:

> "I finished the Johns Hopkins Medical School in 1916, and entered the Hospital as a resident in the Department of Radiology. During this time World War I had begun and I enlisted in the services of the United States Armed Forces. After service of two years in the Army overseas, I came back to Baltimore to finish my residency training, and very shortly thereafter I was invited to come to the Peter Bent Brigham Hospital in Boston for an interview concerning my taking charge of the X-Ray Department there. Here, I met Doctor Cushing and he and I became friends. Being the great scholar and bibliographer that he was, Doctor Cushing further stimulated my interest in books. It was while at that institution, drawing a very modest

* GEORGE ROSEN. Victor Robinson: A Romantic Medical Writer. (First Annual Victor Robinson Lecture in History of Medicine, Temple University School of Medicine, Sept. 23, 1958)

salary as Chief of the Department of Radiology, that I purchased the first edition of Vesalius' book on anatomy. Doctor Cushing was at that time writing his great book—*The Biography of Sir William Osler*—and it was my privilege to read some of the pages of this book in manuscript form. During my association with Doctor Cushing, my library grew in the acquisition of some choice editions; as the years went by and my earning ability increased, my interest in book collecting became an obsession. Being a bachelor I could indulge in this hobby to a greater degree than some of those who had the care of families. As Doctor Sosman so aptly said in his address at the time of the dedication of the gift of my library to the University of Alabama Medical Center, 'My collection of books became my vicarious children.' What to do with these 'children' gave me serious concern as to how they might be properly 'clothed, housed,' and made available to those seriously interested in the advancement of knowledge and medicine."

The problem of "what to do with these children" was one that was to occupy Dr. Reynolds' thoughts over many years. Over lunch, from time to time, or in the course of a visit to our shop, he would raise this question, seeking advice, but it was not anything about which he could come to an easy resolution. His sensitiveness made him keenly aware of his many allegiances—to the various institutions with which he had had fruitful associations and to Detroit where his name became so notable over a long professional career which continues to this day. But about his basic sentiment, his natural inclination, there could be no doubt. It was his native region, Alabama, for which he had never lost his profound feeling, and his alma mater, the University of Alabama, that he hoped could become the dwelling place for his great collection. All credit is due this forward-looking University for creating the desirable conditions, including a separate building, which made the gift to it of the Reynolds Collection natural and inevitable. Dr. Reynolds' wrote:

"Most of my family, both sisters and brothers, nieces and nephews, have been students of the University of Alabama throughout these many years. My father and two of my older brothers who studied medicine were graduates of the University of Alabama Medical College when it was in Mobile, Alabama. I, having been an undergraduate of the University of Alabama, decided that my collection of books should go to the University of Alabama Medical Center. I discussed it with a number of friends whose opinions I valued, and they agreed with me. So, there today it is. . . ."

Some time in 1957, before the completion of the Reynolds Library building, I visited Dr. Reynolds in his office at Harper Hospital. He was looking forward to its completion and dedication with an emotion he could not conceal. And as we discussed his library, its future in its new habitat, he said, reminiscently, "A dream come true."

But I have not yet touched upon the question: What manner of man is Dr.

Reynolds? The fact, as I have mentioned, that I have known him as bookseller and friend since 1932 does not make the task of answering that question any easier. In Dr. Reynolds you have a man at once simple and complex, innocent and sophisticated, articulate and reticent, warm and reserved.

The bare facts of his life I know very well. His inherited medical leanings stem from a whole cluster of Alabama medical forebears—grandfather, father, brothers. He was born in Skipperville, near Ozark, in 1889, and was educated at the Ozark High School, the University of Alabama, and Johns Hopkins Medical School. During World War I he served as a Captain in the Medical Corps, with overseas service in France. He began his teaching career by serving as Instructor in Roentgenology both at Johns Hopkins and at Harvard. Licensed to practice both in Alabama and Michigan, he went into private practice in Detroit in 1922, and has continued his teaching career there at Wayne University College of Medicine as Professor of Radiology, 1945–52, and as Clinical Professor of Radiology since 1953. Dr. Reynolds, also, has been Chief of Staff at Harper Hospital, Detroit, since 1948. As Editor, since 1930, of the *American Journal of Roentgenology*, he is known to radiologists and librarians the world over. Member of some 20 professional and learned societies, he has been an active participant in their affairs, at present serving as President of the American College of Radiology. He has received many awards: A citation in the form of a plaque from the Fifth International Congress of Radiology, Chicago, 1937; the Gold Medal Award, December 1956, of the Radiological Society of North America; honorary degrees from the University of Alabama and Wayne University and from numerous foreign societies; and an award from the Michigan State Medical Society, "In deep appreciation and grateful recognition of distinguished service rendered by him to medicine and medical education." But Dr. Reynolds' concern has not been solely with medicine. He is a member of the Board of Governors of the William L. Clements Library (of Americana) of the University of Michigan, and he is Past President of the Detroit Public Library Commission. It was in connection with his long service as Library Commissioner that he was awarded, by Mayor Cobo, the "Citation for Meritorious Service" of Detroit. Here is a man who has achieved high rank as practitioner, as teacher, as community servant, as scholar and collector.

But what else? We must now assess the less tangible ingredients that go into the making of character, of personality. There was, for example, his extraordinary boyhood experience, from age twelve to sixteen, as "sight and guide" to his blind father. Coming out of the Civil War with disturbed vision, his father entered medical school, though in his last year he had to hire someone to read to him. Warned by an eminent ophthalmologist that to persist in his medical career was to run the risk of total blindness, he became a successful and well loved physician, though completely blind. His son, Lawrence, never knew his father when he was not blind. Indeed he looks back upon the four years of his boyhood spent in reading those books his father loved as a source of great inspiration and in turn the son grew to love the same books when he reached maturity. Notable among these was Osler's famous *Practice* which together they read again and again; this experience accounted in large part for the son's abiding affection for Osler.

There are people who feel that to discuss "personalities" is to be "nosy," that it smacks of gossip (well it may!) and isn't exactly "refined." But about those people who have somehow come to occupy the center of the stage, it is natural that we want to know everything, whether what has propelled them has been the buying and selling of junk (*Born Yesterday*) or the gazing at the heavens, as with Galileo. The late Professor George Sarton, the beloved historian of science, always said, as he does in his recent posthumous work, *Six Wings—Men of Science in the Renaissance:*

"I am . . . a humanist, a man deeply interested in the humanities of science, and above all, in the personalities of scientific investigators. It is very strange, by the way, that this kind of humanism is less common in science than in other fields. People interested in art are curious to know all they can concerning the artists, the creators of beauty; is not that natural enough? And is it less natural for a scientist to want to know about the lives, as well as the works, of his predecessors? Unfortunately, some scientists are merely technicians who want to master the facts, theories, and tricks of their branch of science and have no time or curiosity for anything else. That is not enough."

Emphatically it was never enough for Dr. Reynolds, whose intellectual and personal curiosity brought him to the charming mania of book collecting.

In the history of the mania of the collecting of medical books by physicians, the aphorism, "Physician, heal thyself," was seemingly given little heed, for the roster in the history of medicine of those notable figures who were, so to speak, slaves to books is long and impressive. I cite a few: The sixteenth-century physician-naturalist, Conrad Gesner, one of the earliest of medical bibliographers, the Swiss poet-physician von Haller, Richard Mead and Anthony Askew (both in McMichael's *Gold-Headed Cane*), Sir Hans Sloane (his collection formed the core of the British Museum), William Hunter, Lettsom, Paget, D'Arcy Power, Osler, Cushing, Fulton, and Waller. And in America the tradition is by no means as thin as foreign commentators on American culture like to think. In the library of the New York Academy of Medicine are to be found three fat volumes containing some 20 sale catalogues of medical book collections, sold at auction between about 1860 and 1890, formed by many distinguished American physicians. To name a few, Réné la Roche, the yellow fever man, Frank Hastings Hamilton, William A. Hammond, Surgeon-General of the U. S. Army, 1862–64, George M. Beard, the pioneer neurologist, Isaac Hays, one of the founders of the *American Journal of the Medical Sciences* and pioneer American ophthalmologist, and there is the Southerner, J. C. Nott of Mobile, founder of the Medical College of Alabama, whose collection was sold in New York on December 4, 1872.

Collectors buy rare books, build collections, for different reasons, some of them naturally overlapping. With Dr. Reynolds, I have always felt that in the acquisition of a first or rare edition embodying an idea or discovery, he was offering his admiration, respect, and homage to the author for his achievement, while the book itself became a viable symbol of that achievement which one could see, touch, read and draw therefrom ever fresh inspiration. But there is more, I feel, to Dr. Reynold's collecting of important works in medicine than the esthetic impulse, the love of a book for its own sake, or the desire to pay homage to an author for his achievement; there is the pedagogic or, if you will, the missionary impulse.

According to the French entomologist, Fabre, "History celebrates the Battlefields whereon we met our deaths, but scorns to speak of the plowed fields whereby we thrive; it knows the names of the king's bastards, but cannot tell us the origin of wheat. That is the way of human folly." One need hardly belabor the parable. Dr. Reynolds is acutely aware of this folly as it occurs in the medical profession. He sees it as nothing short of deplorable that the average physician is ignorant of the origin of his own specialty, to say nothing of the origin of medicine as a whole. He sees, as do many education theorists concerned with the humanities, a society run by what Lewis Mumford calls "fragmentary men." Dr. Reynolds feels the necessity of medical history in the curriculum in the Oslerian sense, of a "living need." I borrow the following quotation from Theodor Puschmann, from the remarkable Garrison Lecture given last year by Dr. Poynter, Librarian of the Wellcome Historical Medical Library:

> "When the history of medicine and of the sciences is seen as a part of the general history of culture and is thus presented, when the teacher follows its relation to the other arts and sciences, and, vice versa, calls attention to the influence of the latter on natural science and medicine, when he considers at once political events and social conditions, and gives to the whole the characteristic aura of the age, his lectures will complement and broaden the education of the students in every way."

Then Dr. Poynter added:

> "But whatever may be provided for the undergraduate, the postgraduate student and the medical teacher should at least be well grounded in the history of his own specialty. . . ."

At the beginning of Descartes' classic of science, *Discours de la méthode*, 1637 (there is a beautiful copy of this edition in the Reynolds Collection), he considers the reading of historical books to be much the same as traveling in

* VON LEYDEN, W. Antiquity and authority: a paradox in the Renaissance theory of history. J. Hist. Ideas. 19: 473–492, Oct. 1958.

foreign countries, which he believes enlarges the view and enables one to form sound judgments.* Dr. Reynolds is in every sense the traveler.

HIGHLIGHTS IN THE REYNOLDS COLLECTION

Andreas Vesalius. The *Fabrica,* that monumental and epochal work, is represented by the first edition of 1543, the more beautiful one of 1555, as well as the now unobtainable *Compendium* published by the Italian engraver, Thomas Geminus, in London in 1545, which was among the most important anatomical works in England of the sixteenth century. The title page is the first copper engraving of artistic merit to be produced in England.

Ambroise Paré, the greatest of the army surgeons before Larrey, began his life as a humble barber-surgeon and ended as the greatest surgical authority in Europe, and the best beloved man in France. He was not trained in the schools; he was not as great a scientist as Vesalius. He was a practical clinician, who went through the world with his eyes open, and brought to bear upon his task hard common sense, impatience with vapid tradition, and enormous experience, gained during a remarkable, adventurous, romantic, and brilliantly useful career. He was with the army in time of war; he practiced in Paris during the intervals of peace. As Paget, his biographer, says, "he was a man who heartily disliked change, self-will, skepticism, controversy, politics, and foreigners." Paré's early works were in the vernacular, and so popular that, like school books, they were "thumbed" away and few copies remain—one of the reasons why they have become prized possessions in the hands of collectors. Among Dr. Reynolds' books there are about ten original editions of Paré's works, including the little duodecimes issued between 1545 and 1575 which are among the "Koh-i-noors" of rare books.

William Beaumont. The story of Beaumont, the pioneer physiologist of the United States, and of Alexis St. Martin, the subject of his experiments, has often been told—how, in Osler's words, "the man and the opportunity had met" and a book resulted from Beaumont's indefatigable efforts. To quote Osler again, "To the medical bibliographer there are few more treasured Americana than the brown-backed, poorly printed octavo volume of 280 pages with the imprint 'Plattsburgh, Printed by F. P. Allen, 1833.' " This famous first edition of Beaumont's *Experiments and Observations on the Gastric Juice, and the Physiology of Digestion* is represented, as are most of the editions which followed as well as the earliest *Journal* appearances.

Nicholas Culpeper. He was an extraordinarily popular writer in his day and his books, in general, are among the most common today on the rare-book market, save one, the first American edition of his *English Physician,* which has the remarkable distinction of having been the first medical book to be published in the United States, at Boston in 1708. This edition is of the utmost rarity, and only four copies of it are on record, including Dr. Reynolds' copy.

This is the reason why this peculiar character is included in his collection. Culpeper was a special favorite of Dr. Cushing, who had 65 editions of the *English Physician*—but not this edition.

Rudyard Kipling, in *Rewards and Fairies,* has devoted a poem, "A Doctor of Medicine," to Culpeper, and when presenting a copy of his book to Sir William Osler, he wrote in the accompanying letter, "Nicholas, who could write even if he couldn't cure for nuts—says at the beginning of his Herbal, 'I knew well enough the whole world and everything in it was formed of a composition of contrary elements, and in such a harmony as must needs show the wisdom and power of a great God.' " And he was indeed a religious fellow of sorts, and when the end came he said to his wife, "My dearest girl, live as I have done, then thou wilt die as I do. For now I speak it, when it is no time to dissemble in the presence of God and his angels, I *did* by all persons as I would they should do by me. I was always just in my practice; I never gave a patient two medicines when one would serve the turn. Farewell, my dearest, I am spent." Thus he died.

Medical Americana. But this Culpeper rarity is only the starting point for an extensive group of medical Americana. In this category is to be found a run of the earliest medical American publications—the early eighteenth century inoculation tracts by the Mathers and Boylston. Dr. Reynolds is especially proud of his acquisition a few years ago of one of the most elusive items in all military medical literature, the *Confederate States Medical and Surgical Journal* of 1864–65, published in Richmond, Virginia. This set had been in the possession of Dr. Hunter Holmes McGuire of Richmond, a leading Virginia surgeon active in the Confederacy, and sometime medical director of Lee's army. Dr. McGuire presented this set with autograph inscription to his Irish colleague, Dr. George Foy of Dublin, in 1892. For full particulars about this important item, I refer you to the excellent account of it by Eleanor B. Lanier of the University of Alabama Medical Center Library in the February 1959 issue of *De historia medicinae.*

Early Spanish Medicine. Because of his sentiment for Spain, Dr. Reynolds has brought into his collection a group of the earliest significant medical books of the sixteenth century originating in that country. Two of the items are most outstanding. The first is the Spanish text for midwives, which is considered to be the second one on the subject in any modern language, Damian Carbón's *Libro del arte de las comadres o madrinas y del regimiento de las preñadas y paridas y de los niños,* printed at Mallorca in December 1541. Only three copies besides this one are extant in American libraries. Dedicated to a nobleman on the occasion of his lady's first pregnancy, the work discusses the anatomy and physiology of the organs of generation, male and female; the signs and hygiene of pregnancy; miscarriage and its causes; birth, its mechanism and difficulties; the extraction of the after-birth, and puerperal fever. Of particular interest is the chapter on lactation. Carbón comes out against the use of cradles and against singing babies to sleep.

An equally interesting companion piece to the Carbón work is the first anatomy in the Spanish language, the *Libro de la Anothomia del Hombre* by Bernardino Montaña de Monserrate, Valladolid, 1551. As Saunders and O'Malley have written, Montaña de Monserrate was the first in Spain to recognize, even as an afterthought, the superiority of the Vesalian illustrations. His text shows the same important stirrings which were to bring forth much fruit in all Europe but which were to be choked in the bud in the case of his native Spain. If we are to judge by its rarity, his small volume must have proved highly popular, and we are reminded that the first edition of his English counterpart, Vicary, was apparently used to extinction.

Medical Incunabula. There is a group of choice medical incunabula, including the first edition of Celsus, 1478, and the second edition of 1481; Arnold of Villanova's book on wine, the first on this subject, 1479; the beautiful anatomy of Johannes de Ketham of 1500; Maimonides' medical Aphorisms of 1489; the *Almansoris* of Rhazes, printed in 1483; several editions of Giovanni Michele Savonarola, who was the grandfather of Girelamo Savonarola, the great Florentine preacher and religious reformer, whose education he supervised.

Oliver Wendell Holmes, the great doctor, wit, author and, Boston Brahmin, who will always be affectionately remembered as "The Autocrat of the Breakfast Table," is a great favorite with Dr. Reynolds. It is difficult to realize today the measure of popularity enjoyed by Holmes, of whom Osler has said that he was "the most successful combination the world has ever seen of physician and man of letters." His poems and epigrams still live on the lips of English-speaking people everywhere, and his contributions to science are part of medical history, and the fine run assembled by Dr. Reynolds well shows Holmes in his double role in the world of medicine and of literature.

In 1843, at the age of 34, Oliver Wendell Holmes wrote a paper, *On the Contagiousness of Puerperal Fever*, which is a milepost in the history of medicine and in the attitude of physicians toward infection. The paper was written for the Boston Society for Medical Improvement and published in a journal which ceased to exist after the first year, the *New England Quarterly Journal of Medicine and Surgery*. Because of its small circulation and the storm of controversy aroused, Holmes republished the paper in 1855. It is a masterpiece of medical literature which every physician should know. According to Eleanor Tilton, Dr. Holmes' biographer, a few offprints of the original paper were struck for Dr. Holmes' personal use—in too small a quantity as he later realized—one of which Dr. Reynolds is proud to have been able to acquire for his collection. And speaking of puerperal fever, it is not surprising to come upon a splendid copy of Semmelweis' immortal work on this subject: *Die Aetiolgie, der Begriff und die Prophylaxis des Kindbettfiebers*, 1861. This makes a perfect companion piece to the Holmes work. Holmes had the correct concept of the nature of puerperal fever, but was unable to reveal its etiology and prophylaxis. This scientific discovery was the work of the emotional young Hungarian assistant in obstetrics, Ignaz Philipp Semmelweis (1818–65), whose tortured professional life led him to a lunatic's death in an asylum, one of medicine's great martyrs.

It was about 1860 that Holmes invented the "American Stereoscope," as it was called, which coincided with his interest in photography; it was a hand stereoscope. He described and discussed his invention in an essay entitled *The Stereoscope and the Stereograph*; the original manuscript of 31½ pages is among Dr. Reynolds's prized possessions.

William Harvey. There is a fine run, not only *De Motu Cordis* of 1628, but other important editions as well. Quoting Sir Geoffrey Keynes, Harvey's bibliographer, "Harvey's *De Motu Cordis* is justly considered to be one of the most fruitful and important books ever published. Harvey's treatise is, in fact, more important as a demonstration of scientific method in biological research than as an annunciation of the fact of the circulation of the blood. From this beginning has flowed all subsequent biological knowledge in an ever widening stream." This, Harvey's first and greatest work, usually known by its short title, *De Motu Cordis*, was printed in 1628 at Frankfort-on-the-Main. Most copies of the book are printed on thin paper of inferior quality and are very unattractive objects, though they are the most sought after of medical classics.

John Aubrey (1626–97), a noted antiquary—a kind of immature Boswell, the DNB calls him—details a gossipy morsel about Harvey in his work, *Aubrey's Lives*. This book is a rich source of private scandal about his seventeenth century learned contemporaries. He tells us that Harvey came to London in July 1646, and lived with his brother. It would not be like Aubrey to fail to inform us that he kept a pretty young girl to wait on him, and, in quite the spirit of scandal, says he no doubt made of her for warmth. He took care of this young woman in his will, which may or may not be a piece of corroborative evidence of Aubrey's story. As with so many great discoverers, Harvey was estimated a madman by many of his contemporaries and lost much of his practice following his announcement of doctrine respecting the circulation of the blood.

Robert Boyle Collection, a most comprehensive collection of the works of this Irish genius. Marie Boas, in her recent book, *Robert Boyle and Seventeenth-Century Chemistry*, has given the most up-to-date interpretation of Boyle's importance as a scientist: "Foremost among the theoretical chemists of the age, one of the few highly-skilled chemists who made contributions to natural philosophy as well, was Robert Boyle. . . . His public reputation has always been greater as a physicist than as a chemist. . . . But he thought of himself as primarily a chemist and his influence on chemistry was enormous. . . . Our greatest difficulty in estimating Boyle's importance lies, it is reasonable to suppose, in our own confused picture of the developments of chemistry during his lifetime. We know, roughly, the things the chemists did, but not why they did them." Boyle was the true precursor of the modern chemist. He was the first to distinguish definitely a mixture from a compound; with him originated the definition of an "element" as a hitherto undecomposed constituent of a compound; he introduced the use of vegetable color-tests of acidity and alkalinity. He actually prepared hydrogen. Boyle's voluminous writings procured him an immense reputation, both at home and abroad. He was a "decorous bachelor, but prolific as the father of many children of the mind," as Fulton charmingly put it in an address on Boyle.

Anesthesia was a native American discovery—and a fine dramatic tale it is—involving a four-ring controversy over priority of discovery. The Reynolds Collection contains a splendid group of works, including the famous Ether volumes of the *Boston Medical and Surgical Journal* and an extraordinary run of rarities by the Scotsman, Sir James Y. Simpson, who was responsible for introducing chloroform as an anesthetic in England in 1847. About him there is the story involving his contemporary, Walter Scott, who suggested as a motto for Simpson's heraldic emblem when knighted: "Does your Mother know you're out."

A recent acquisition is a somewhat spectacular collection of ten rare items by Sir James Y. Simpson and three additional ones closely connected with him. The whole group in its composition provides insight into the four aspects of Simpson's historic personality—that of anesthetist, of gynecologist and obstetrician, of teacher, and of writer.

The collection once belonged to one of Simpson's pupils, and most of them carry an autograph inscription by Simpson or by their original owner, all dated 1847 and 1848. This owner was Dr. Thomas Cunningham, of Belfast, Ireland, a medical graduate of the University of Edinburgh in 1849, who practiced for a number of years in the neighborhood of that city, but returned to Belfast in 1858, where he died a year later. Particularly choice items are: the very rare first edition of Simpson's *Anaesthetic and Other Therapeutic Properties of Chloroform*, 1847, which is a follow-up of his original report on chloroform of that year; *Remarks on the Superinduction of Anaesthesia in Natural and Morbid Parturition*, Edinburgh, 1847, his second important publication on chloroform anesthesia; the first edition of Simpson's *Answer to the Religious Objections Advanced Against the Employment of Anaesthetic Agents in Midwifery and Surgery*, which followed shortly after the preceding item in the same year; and *Remarks on the Alleged Fatal Case of Chloroform-Inhalation*, 1848, giving the detailed facts of this case. There are the memorable address, *Remarks on the Conduct and Duties of Young Physicians*, second edition, Edinburgh, 1848; and *Report of the Edinburgh Royal Maternity Hospital from 1844 to 1846*, published 1848, which includes a summary analysis of the obstetric practice of that institution. Then follows Simpson's *Observations Regarding the Influence of Galvanism upon the Action of the Uterus during Labour*, 1846; *Case of Delivery, without Operative Aid, through a Pelvis Extremely Deformed by Malacosteon*, 1847; and *On the Duration of Labour as a Cause of Mortality and Danger to the Mother and Infant*, 1848.

Included in this collection is Thomas Cunningham's manuscript notebook on the Midwifery Practice at the Edinburgh Maternity Hospital, containing 50 reports of cases he managed and proof of the early administration of chloroform in obstetrics at the hospital. The collection is rounded out by two items about Cunningham.

Here also are two other anesthesia classics of great rarity, both by another Englishman, the pioneer John Snow, the first professional anesthetist: his paper *On the Inhalation of the Vapour of Ether in Surgical Operations* of 1847, which contains an account of his regulating inhaler, the first to control the amount of ether vapor received by the patient; and his book, *On Chloroform and Other Anaesthetics*, London, 1858, which put the administration of chloroform and ether on a scientific basis. The 1847 paper is evidence of the link of scientific communication existing between Britain and America; Snow had sent this copy to Isaac Hays, "Editor of American Journal of Science," and one of the earliest American ophthalmologists.

There are even more exceptional items: Two reports on the successful application of Mesmerism for surgical anesthesia in an obscure American Midwestern mesmeric periodical, *The Saint Louis Magnet*, 1845–1847 (all published), of which the *Missouri Imprints Survey* (no. 462) locates only the Harvard University copy. These two reports precede any American publications on ether anesthesia, and perhaps may be regarded as the first pronouncements on the subject printed in this country.

Perhaps the earliest German publication on chloroform anesthesia is that by Aloys Martin and Ludwig Binswanger, *Das Chloroform in seinen Wirkungen auf Menschen und Thiere*, Leipzig, 1848. This slender volume is dedicated to James Y. Simpson. And what is probably the first Italian publication dealing with ether anesthesia is G. B. Poggi's *Dell' etere sopente nelle operazioni della chirurgia*, 1847, in which credit for the discovery of the narcotic properties of sulfuric ether is given to Charles Jackson, information which is unknown to all authorities on the subject.

Daniel Drake Collection. These are works by and about Drake, originally gathered together by myself, for myself. Eventually a dealer must stop behaving like a collector; the Drake group is now one of the outstanding features of the Reynolds Library.

Daniel Drake (1785–1852) was the most eminent early nineteenth-century physician of the Central West. His parents both came from New Jersey from a long line of obscure farmers. They made the dangerous trip down to the Ohio and into Kentucky. It was on the Drakes' barge that they met a man who in the middle of this wilderness wore the powdered hair and gold-headed cane of the medical man, Dr. William Goforth, to whom Dan Drake became apprenticed. For all his foibles, Goforth was a good doctor. He had been well educated in New York before he hit the frontier, and was the pioneer vaccinator in the West. A year after Waterhouse received the cow-pox serum from England, Goforth managed to put his hands on some which he lost no time in trying out on his apprentice, Daniel Drake, who thus became the first person to be vaccinated west of the Alleghenies.

There is justice in the appelation of Drake as the Benjamin Franklin of the West. He was constantly improving his own education and he had great ambitions for Cincinnati as a center of arts and sciences and did much to promote his goal. For himself he deeply desired intellectual fame, but his high idealism suffered frequent frustration and involved him in many quarrels with colleagues. A formidable controversialist he must have been. Referring to one of his backbiting opponents he wrote: "To give a full-length portrait of this *gentleman* would be a labor similar to that of dragon-making in the romances of the 16th century. It would be to combine all that is cunning and contemptible in the moral world. As it relates to his intrigues in the medical college, he is like his household idol, *cash,* the root of all evil, like a general infection of the body everywhere present, corrupt and corrupting." There is a story about his meeting an opponent head-on in the street. "I do not propose to step aside for a fool," said his antagonist. "*I* will," replied Drake and stepped aside.

I have tarried on Drake terrain a bit because of Dr. Reynolds' intense regard for Drake, heightened by the fact that his grandfather, Dr. John Reynolds, had his medical diploma from the University of Cincinnati.

Sir William Osler. Here is a fascinating group of 60 holograph letters that Osler wrote to his Canadian boyhood friend who stayed "home"—"Ned" Milburn. The letters cover the years 1865–1919, the year of Osler's death. Cushing in his biography of Osler, speaks of this friendship which originated in Osler's boarding-school days at Barrie, a town on the western arm of Lake Simcoe. It is Dr. Reynolds' plan to edit these letters for publication.

Louis Pasteur. There are two stunning groups of Pasteur manuscript material, all unpublished. One deals with the silk worm, the other comprises about 20 scientific letters on rabies to a colleague, Louis Thuillier, and to Emile Roux. These letters are extraordinary for their scientific interest, written as they were in the period when Pasteur was polishing his treatment of *rouget*—pork disease—and when he was continuing his labors on rabies. In one of his moving letters to Thuillier, Pasteur promises not to publish anything on *rouget* or rabies before the former's return from Egypt where Thuillier had gone early in 1883 and where he was to die of cholera in September of the same year. Editing these letters, also, is another project on Dr. Reynolds' agenda.

Electricity, Magnetism, and Radiology. This is one of the most extensive sections of the collection, naturally, because it falls into the sphere of Dr. Reynolds' own professional specialty. Dr. Reynolds himself arranged a splendid exhibit of his extensive collection of books on the subject for the Fifth International Congress of Radiology, Chicago, 1937, and prepared a printed annotated catalogue. The catalogue opens with a Pliny *Natural History* in the beautiful edition from Jensen's famous press, Venice, 1472. This is included because Pliny calls attention to the magnetic properties of amber when rubbed.

There is a copy of the translation of the famous letter of *Petrus Peregrinus* (Pierre de Maricourt) to his friend, Sigerus de Foucaucourt in Picardy, written in August 1269, which is the earliest work on the magnet. The letter is divided into 13 chapters and forms the most original, extensive, and important treatise on the subject prior to Gilbert's *De Magnete.* A manuscript version of this famous letter will be mentioned a little later.

There is, of course, a copy of the first edition of William Gilbert's *De Magnete*, London, 1600, a remarkable work in the history of scientific discovery, in which Gilbert shows that a freely suspended magnet is controlled by the earth and not, as supposed, by extraterrestrial influence. Gilbert also proves that other bodies besides amber possess the property of attracting, after being rubbed. It is in this book that he first uses the word "electrisis." Gilbert was physician to Queen Elizabeth and James I, and one of the founders of experimental science. According to Mr. Bern Dibner (*Ten Founding Fathers of the Electrical Science*), it was the first forward step in the field of electricity since the time of Thales.

The Benjamin Franklin material includes the first edition of Franklin's first basic paper on electricity, *Experiments and Observations on Electricity, made at Philadelphia in America*, published at London in 1751. There is Hans Christian Oersted's fabulously elusive four-page paper, published in 1820, in which he announced his discovery of the magnetic effect of electric current. The comprehensive coverage of the history of radiology is rich with an extensive run of Röntgen holograph letters and pamphlets and early X-ray books and pamphlets.

Of *Early Scientific Manuscripts*, there is an impressive group from among which the following may be highlighted:

ALBERTUS MAGNUS. *Liber physicorum sive auditus physici.* (French, c. 1350.) 92 leaves on vellum. This well preserved manuscript contains the full text—in eight books—of a great early interpretation of an Aristotelian scientific work. One of the most interesting features—a positive guide in dating the manuscript—is a partially legible note on the inside of the back cover, dated 1350, which would imply that the manuscript was written about that time. Other notes of ownership have been partially erased, leaving only an indication that by the fifteenth century the volume was in possession of a person or institution in Florence. The first printed edition of the text appeared at Venice in 1488, with a commentary by Matteo Battiferri, an Italian physician.

The author of this interesting and highly valuable medieval scientific text was the teacher of Thomas Aquinas. In Osler's words (*Incunabula Medica*), "The great Dominican's long life was an uninterrupted triumph of fruitful accomplishment. Though, like other learned men of his generation, he was accused of magic, he accomplished a colossal task, and left a memory equalled only by one or two of his generation and surpassed only by his great pupil, Thomas Aquinas. He recognized the importance of the study of nature, even testing it by way of experiment. . . ."

BERNARDUS DE GORDONIO. *Tractatus de flobotomia. Tractatus de urinis. Tractatus de pulsibus. Tractatus de regimine sanitatis.* A remarkable manuscript in Latin on 24 vellum leaves, double columns, probably Italian, sometime in the first half of the fourteenth century, it is written in a much abbreviated cursive, about 76 lines to the page. There are four large initials, one at the beginning of each treatise, painted in blue and red with scroll-work ornament. All headings are written in red, paragraph marks and initial supplied in alternate red and blue, foliation supplied by an old hand. Bernard of Gordon, the author of the four texts, was born at Gordon in the French province of Rouergue in the thirteenth century. A celebrated physician, who at an early time recognized the importance of Arabic medical texts, he taught medicine at Montpellier from about 1285, dying there in 1320. He is considered now by some to be the greatest medieval physician after Arnoldus de Villanova. The faculty of Montpellier rivalled in fame the school of Salerno. Manuscripts of Bernardus' works are rare, and none are listed in De Ricci's *Census* as being in America. Bernard's works are known to us only in a few fifteenth and sixteenth century editions, all of them of great rarity. Sudhoff believed that these four tracts belong under one heading and were intended to be four parts of a major work on the conservation of human life. Throughout the work Bernard stresses the importance of studying the composition of blood, and blood in his opinion is the most important component of the human body. There are observations of leukemic blood and some believe that Bernard observed leukemia among Northern peoples, which would fit the theory that he was not French but of Scottish origin. Chronologically this is Bernard's last work, written when he was at the height of his career.

ARNOLDUS DE VILLANOVA. *Regimen sanitatis ad regem Aragonum;* JOHN OF TOLEDO. *Dietarium*; and three other medical tracts.

This outstanding illustrated medical manuscript in Latin on 41 vellum leaves, Italy, fourteenth century, is written in a Gothic book hand in double columns with numerous ornamental initials. It is illustrated by 26 colored drawings, including representations of people seated at dinner, an old man in bed discoursing with a woman seated at the foot, a table set with wine and food, various herbs and fruits. Arnoldus de Villanova (c. 1234–1311), Catalan physician, alchemist, astrologer, diplomat, social reformer, visionary, was one of the most extraordinary personalities of medieval times. He realized the value of natural science and suggested that it should be given more importance in education; he even had some slight understanding of the experimental point of view. He was a famous medical practitioner, who was consulted by various kings of Aragon and popes. A great many writings have been ascribed to him, most of them dealing with medical subjects. His commentary on the *Regimen Sanitatis* is not to be confused with the *Regimen* itself. This famous poem constitutes, one might say, the backbone of all practital medical literature up to the time of the Renaissance. It has been estimated chat there are almost three hundred editions of this poem which was supposedly written about the middle of the thirteenth century, so that it was already old in Arnold's time, who was its earliest known editor. The wise sayings this vade mecum of the layman contained clung in men's memories with the tenacity of proverbs. In fact, many of the popular maxims which constitute the hygienic knowledge of the average man even of today are derived, without his knowing it, from that poem, which crystallized into a definite form all the folklore it contained and impressed its own indelible stamp upon it before transmitting it to posterity.

John of Toledo, a Hispano-Jewish translator from Arabic into Latin, who was converted to Christianity, flourished in Toledo about 1135–53. His *Dietetics* was translated from the Sirr al-asrār, Secretum secretorum, and it is of great interest as a prototype of the famous Salernitan *Regimen sanitatis*, with which it is combined in this manuscript.

RHAZES. *Ninth Book of the Al-Manšuri.* Expounded and commented by Gerard de Solo and translated into Hebrew by the physician Tobiel ben Samuel de Leiria (of Portugal). A Hebrew medical illuminated manuscript, 206 leaves, vellum and paper, written in square (title and headings) and rabbinic (semi-square) Hebrew characters of the Portuguese, or Spanish, type, 24 lines to the page, early part of the fifteenth century. The beginning of the manuscript (title-page), the headings of the chapters, and occasionally other prominent places (about 30 pages throughout the manuscript) are illuminated with fine drawings in various colors. These illuminations consist mostly of fancifully intertwined arabesques and grotesque forms of fantastic animals or distorted human faces; at that early age the Jewish artist did not dare to draw normal figures of man or animal in a Hebrew book in order not to violate the second Commandment. Rhazes, abu Bekr Muhammed ibn Zakkariah (860–930 A.D.) was the leading figure in the field of medicine of his time. As a great clinician he ranks with Hippocrates, Areteus, and Sydenham, and he was one of the original portrayors of disease. He was a true follower of Hippocrates in the simplicity of his practice, and was the first to introduce chemical preparations, especially mercurial ointments, into the practice of medicine. The most outstanding work of Rhazes was his *Al-Mansuri*, consisting of ten parts (books) dealing with the various branches of medicine.

The Ninth Book of the Al-Mansuri, which deals with the problems of therapeutics, was one of the most popular textbooks for students and physicians of the Middle Ages. It was later revised by Vesalius, and it became the standard source of therapeutic knowledge until long after the Renaissance. Gerard de Solo, the expounder and commentator of the *Ninth Book* of Rhazes, was one of the most famous medical scholars of his time and a leading figure in the Western world of medicine. He was professor and later chancellor of the University of Montpellier from 1300–1320. It was his comments and additional medical information which made Rhazes' *Ninth Book* popular. The Jewish medieval physicians, who played an important part in the study and practice of medicine, soon realized the importance of this work and translated it into Hebrew for the use of Jewish physicians and students. Until the present manuscript was discovered, and now for the first time properly identified, two different Hebrew translations in manuscript form were known to exist. With the appearance of this new manuscript a new Hebrew version of this important work came to light. The translator of this new Hebrew version was the Portuguese physician Tobiel ben Samuel de Leiria. This Jewish physician and Hebrew translator was unknown to Steinschneider as well as to Friedenwald.

* * *

In 1895, Sir William Osler wrote a charming biographical sketch called *An Alabama Student* which became the title of one of his books of medical-literary essays now familiar to every medical man. The Alabama student about whom Osler was writing with such warmth and appreciation was Dr. J. Y. Bassett of Huntsville. In Bassett, Osler recognized what he called "a kindred with the great of old." Dr. Reynolds adores Osler, and were Osler alive today, he would inescapably be moved to reciprocate this warm regard, and would characteristically give expression to his feeling by writing a sketch he would call, with his usual aptness, "An Alabama Collector."

It is fitting that this splendid Collection should find such a beautiful residence at the University of Alabama. But it is not only the attractive physical housing that is important, it is the sympathetic receptivity for these cultural-historical materials that the Medical Center has already demonstrated in the building of one of the outstanding historical dental collections in this country. (Alabama, by the way, was the first state to pass a dental law, in 1841. This followed by only two years the establishment of the first dental collection, Baltimore, in 1839.) The value of such collections as these remind one of the versatile Rudolf Virchow when he wrote in his "Standpoints in Scientific Medicine"* "...we were convinced that the only genuine knowledge is historical knowledge, that justice toward others is the only counterweight to exaggerated self-esteem, and also that valuable lessons can be drawn from the study of error. We have not forgotten these things....

"He who has only once through his own efforts tried to trace back the long path trod by his predecessors, who has felt how clear and luminous his own knowledge becomes as he grows aware of the historical circumstances out of which it has arisen, and who discovers the basis of the errors through which even genuine investigators have been misled, he who has learned that a kernel of truth sticks in every error, will not place himself with those who despise historical studies...."

* Bull. Hist. Med. 30: 537–543, Nov.-Dec. 1956.

This Business of Rare Books*

By Murray Gottlieb

Old Hickory Bookshop
New York, N. Y.

THERE was a famous Philadelphia physician, Benjamin Rush, of whom Osler wrote to a correspondent: "I have collected a number of his works and read many of them. Years ago I made notes for a lecture which I gave on his life and work, but it was never published. . . . Should you ever come across collections of his pamphlets and minor works please remember my library, as I should be glad to buy them. . . ."

Among Dr. Rush's major works is *Diseases of the Mind*, published in 1812, and, incidentally, the first American book on the subject. In it the ancient and honorable profession of bookselling is immortalized by the following highly quotable observation: "The frequent and rapid transition of the mind from one subject to another. . . . It is said booksellers have sometimes become deranged from this cause. . . ." One of the subjects to which the bookseller's mind is constantly being diverted, in the midst of his myriad tasks, is to provide a satisfactory solution to that deathless question as to the precise nature of a "rare book." Discussions, dissertations, and disputations will doubtless be sempiternal. For my part, however, I am completely contented to accept (and I hope you will be, too) an interpretation so simple, so clear, and so sound, that the words "rare book" are stripped of any mystical and unwarrantedly awe-inspiring shroud with which they may be covered.

In 1951, Paul S. Dunkin, in an 85-page brochure entitled *How to Catalog a Rare Book*, wrote: "The rare book is a fascinating material object . . . a document in the history of civilization. If people wanted only to read it, a microfilm or reprint would do. The fact that the rare book is a material object must be the keynote of any useful approach. I have not attempted to define 'rare book.' It would take a good-sized treatise to do just that. Its rarity has been decided before the book reaches me. Any book which has value primarily as a physical object is a rare book. . . ."

* Read at the Regional Meeting, Medical Library Association, New York City, April 26, 1952.

Originally published in *Bulletin of the Medical Library Association,* Volume 41 (April, 1953), pp. 103-109. Reprinted by permission.

As all of you know, there are rare books and rare books. Sometimes the price tag is breath-taking, and the higher the price, the greater the publicity which attaches to it. Press and radio combine to herald the fact that the *Bay Psalm Book* fetches $151,000 at auction; that the Wilmerding sale in a New York auction gallery attracts American and European bidders who pay $569,000 for 2,387 lots, many of the items bringing thousands of dollars; that the Oliver Barrett Lincoln Collection inspires heated competition and more thousands of dollars; and, comparatively recently, the Rosenbach Company sells 73 volumes of Shakespeare folios and quartos to a Swiss banker for a sum purported to be in the neighborhood of two million dollars. That class of rare book is not within our province (imagine a medical librarian with two million dollars to spend!), but the publicity attendant upon such transactions is. It frightens away the uninitiated, as well as many of those who ought to know better. The inference is clear. Unless you have lots and lots of money, rare books are not for you.

Actually, for every volume that runs into four figures, there are literally thousands of rare books priced under $25.00, and as many under $10.00. Especially is this true of medical books, where a sales price of four figures, with one or two exceptions, would assuredly create a stir. Yet, for rare Americana, and rare English literature, in fact, for any literary rarity not in the medical fold, astronomical prices are not unusual, and not one murmur of dissent is heard if these prices fluctuate hundreds of dollars one way or the other, depending, sometimes, on whether or not this or that "genuine blank flyleaf" is present.

To return, however, to those old and rare medical books whose purchase can be envisaged even by those librarians with meager coffers. Gathering together a small library of rare medical books is possible without huge expenditures, and there are, moreover, ways of doing so without dipping into already slender appropriations. But more about that later on. First, you must decide whether or not rare medical books deserve shelf space at all.

How often have we been asked by visitors to our shop, looking for what they call an "old book" published a year or two ago, and seeing instead shelf on shelf of venerable and, to them, utterly unfamiliar volumes, bright and fresh centuries ago, but now bearing the bruises of time and undeserved neglect, "Do you mean to say," they ask, "that doctors actually buy this stuff?" When we were tyros at the game, we accepted such challenges eagerly and quoted lengthily from the writings of all the famous medico-bibliophiles. Though we ourselves learned a great deal from the ammunition we gathered so laboriously, our adversaries left not one whit closer to what Osler, in his essay "Books and Men" so eloquently described as "a third class of men in the profession, to whom books are dearer than to teachers or practitioners—a small, a silent band, but in reality the leaven of the whole lump. The profane call them bibliomaniacs, and, in truth, they are at times irresponsible and do not always know the difference between *meum* and *tuum*. Loving books partly for their contents, partly for the sake of the author, they keep alive the sentiment of historical continuity in the profession. We need more men of their class, particularly in this country, where every one carries in his pocket the tape-measure of utility."

Now, after many head-on clashes, and deeply wounded by the modern practitioner's unbelievable contempt for "the touch divine of noble natures gone," we are less inclined to dissipate our energies. The sceptics are shown the printed catalogue of the *Bibliotheca Osleriana*, and the Catalogue of the Cushing Collection. If these do not impress them, we merely shrug and walk away. There is a limit even to a bookseller's endurance and proselytizing.

When I received your gracious invitation, I immediately gathered around me many volumes and articles pertinent to the scheduled theme. I have sedulously read them all. They have revived half-forgotten thoughts, and recalled beautifully expressed and appropriate quotations on the subject of rare medical books. But none of them attempted to solve the problems of a librarian, who is weighing the pros and cons of adding such books to the library, and is, simultaneously, confronted with the dilemma of limited space, even more limited funds, and the formidable barrier of a library board antagonistic to affording shelf room to anything earlier than the next to the last edition of the latest text on pathological anatomy. Perhaps if each of you were endowed with a spacious library building and an inexhaustible budget, all friction would disappear, and the life of a librarian would be less harried and harassed.

Dr. Holmes once said: "Apart from any practical use to be derived from the older medical authors, is there not a true pleasure in reading the accounts of great discoverers in their own words?" Add to that Osler's fond wish that he "should like to see in each library a select company of the Immortals set apart for special adoration," and, further, Harvey Cushing's jocular warning in his address on "The Doctor and his Books" at the opening of the Allen Memorial Building of the Cleveland Medical Library Association, in 1926, "beware of books as an expensive habit. Some day when you have the endowment you deserve you will come to enlarge your collection of the early treatises . . . those of the 16th century should be gathered in when they turn up, even though, to use an expression of Osler's, you may have to 'bleed the Fellows' for the wherewithal. . . ." and you begin to understand why I felt uneasy about continuing along these lines. Holmes' original accounts of great discoverers, Osler's Immortals, and Cushing's early treatises were, to say the least, just a wee bit less expensive in their times. My concern at this juncture is not primarily the long-established, large, and book-rich medical libraries. Earlier, I said a small library of rare medical books could be built up with a minimal outlay, perhaps even without any money coming directly out of the library's budget. But first I had to try to convince you that rare books are not a luxury, but an essential part of an historical library.

Each of you, whether you approve of it or not, is a custodian of a library at least partly historical. To quote Dr. William Jerome Wilson of the Armed Forces Medical Library, "By mere existence for a considerable number of years, any library on any subject or subjects becomes at least partly historical, and the longer it lasts, the more historical it is. The reason is simple. Every subject that human beings study makes some progress from age to age, and the books that were of current practical interest a generation ago, may be of merely historical interest today. This process is sometimes fast, sometimes slow. The faster and farther knowledge advances, the more rapidly the books recording that knowledge becomes outmoded."[1]

Undoubtedly, many of the volumes acquired on publication date have, unheralded and surreptitiously, joined the ranks of rare books. A wise librarian would do well to note the fact, and, if practicable, gather them together on one shelf. Users might then accord the volumes better care, and perhaps greater esteem. That is one way of starting a rare-book section inexpensively. But another, that requires a sprinkling of imagination, a dash of research, and a pinch of initiative, is the collecting of American medical books of bygone years. Many of these are still to be had at modest prices, and will, I feel safe in predicting, increase in interest and value as time goes on. First or early editions of the works of such American medical giants as David Hosack, Godman, Samuel L. Mitchill, Physick, Dorsey, Eberle, the Becks, Chapman, Bartlett, Francis, and Samuel D. Gross, to name but a few, can be picked up under $10.00. Not all, of course, but sufficient to supply "the bait to set the trap," as Cushing says, "so that the young doctor will walk into it unawares. He will, in turn become your great supporter, learn the value of books, begin to make his own collection, which in turn will be deposited with you. Books," Dr. Cushing concludes, "are bibliotrophic, one attracting the other." We, ourselves, have sold enough books to enough doctors who have given their collections to favored libraries to know how right Dr. Cushing was.

My first suggestion is, read a good history of American medicine, and, though Packard's *History*[2] contains a wealth of material, personally we recommend Mumford's *Narrative of American Medicine*,[3] so enchantingly written, and withal so informative. Note down, as you read, the names of those early contributors to the American medical scene that are more likely to appeal to

[1] Wilson, William Jerome. Historical libraries—new style. Coll. and Res. Lib. 11: 54–63, 1950.

[2] Packard, Francis R. History of medicine in the United States. N. Y., Hoeber, 1931. 2v.

[3] Mumford, James Gregory. Narrative of medicine in America. Phila., Lippincott, 1903.

the needs and tastes of those who frequent your library. In the beginning limit yourself, if yours is a specialized library, to books relating to that specialty. Later, you can add non-American contributions to present a fuller survey of the classic works in your field. The more costly items you may be able to acquire through developing what the larger libraries call "Friends of the Rare Book Room." You might even approach lay people in your community for so noble a purpose. We know of a number of such donors, and one in particular, most generous in his contributions, who is helping a library build an enviable collection in a specialty on which one of his medical ancestors had written a book or two in the early part of the 19th century. A few discreet letters, or better still, visits to professional and lay people in your locality appealing for funds for such purposes may bring satisfying returns. It unquestionably is worth trying. At the same time, once you know specifically what you would like to add to your collection, contact with non-medical librarians, the local public library, or historical society library, or any others in your community, may result in locating such items on their shelves, and with a little diplomacy, finding their way onto your own.

There is another comparatively inexpensive and extremely important avenue of collecting. It embraces the ephemeral medical writings, generally in pamphlet form, bearing upon your immediate environs and especially upon the institution with which you are connected. Cultivate the librarian of your local historical society, if you have one, and enlist her aid in compiling a working bibliography. This undoubtedly will take some precious time away from ever-pressing work, but I am sure you will find it rewarding. You might even end up with all their medical duplicates! In the process, many of you will develop a respect for that fragile rarity, the pamphlet. Unbound, and containing anywhere from 10 to 100 pages, these fast-disappearing medical gems constitute a wealth of unexploited historical material no where else to be found. They are the delight of the historian and research worker, yet treated with deplorable disdain by altogether too many librarians We are dismayed, sometimes, when a pamphlet, ordered from our catalogue where it has been accurately described, is returned to us with some scathing remark about its lack of binding, or its lack of bulk, or both. It is usually identified in booksellers' catalogues by the word "wrappers."

In the pages of the BULLETIN of your Association, I have noted much emphasis laid upon medical incunabula and 16th century medical books. These fall into the category of rare medical books and, as you are well aware, they cost a lot of money. They are the rightful province of the large library. But in American medical books the small library can play a role in building up a collection of rarities. If, in the course of this self-imposed task, you inspire but one to join Osler's "small, silent band," the shades of all the great medical bibliophiles of the past will brighten for a moment in appreciation of a job well done.

I should like to spend a moment or two on the out-of-print book, which I place in a special category. Though kin to the rare book, the out-of-print book is still not primarily valuable as a physical object. It should not, therefore, be included in the rare-book classification, despite the fact that often the out-of-print book is as difficult to locate as the rare. The out-of-print book problem is an intricate one and full of pitfalls. The most cogent advice I can offer, is to make out a list of desiderata and send it to a bookseller in whom you have confidence. If he does not have the books in stock, he knows where he may be able to locate them quickly, or, failing that, tries the many means at his disposal. You will find this easier and more practical than doing the work yourself. Contrary to the belief of some librarians, this method is not more expensive. Actually, there is a significant savings in eliminating all the correspondence, record-keeping, check-writing, attendant upon multiple purchases. Usually, the asking price will be higher than the published price. However, this is not because the bookseller you have entrusted is trying to wax fat upon your list of desiderata; it is merely that old price-influencer, the law of supply and demand, up to its customary tricks. On the other hand, and this occurs frequently, the book may be offered to you at less than the published price because the supply is greater than the demand. Occasionally, there is no relationship between the published price and the asking price. The desired volume has quietly become a modern medical classic. Few know the market better than a bookseller, and he is, therefore, less likely to overpay. He can be of genuine assistance to you in solving your out-of-print book problem.

The bookseller is, you will agree, an integral part of "this business of rare books." Yet, he is seldom accorded the esteem he merits, and more often, is maligned. Particularly, is this true of the American dealer in rare medical books. Indeed, the highest-priced dealers of museum pieces and historical texts in non-medical literature are treated with great respect and showered with honors. But consider the case of the American medical bookseller. In the pages of your own BULLETIN an eminent director of a famous New England medical library accuses him of a booksellers' inflation and profits of 500%! Now, we do not deny that the prices of many rare medical books are higher than they were five or ten years ago, but so are those of food, clothing, and all other commodities, without exception. It is unkind, to put it mildly, to impute to the bookseller that terrible ordeal of modern times, inflation. We do not wish to labor the point, but our own costs of doing business have almost trebled in the same period. The problem of rising prices is not quite so easily explained; there is much more to it than that.

All librarians would, naturally, like to acquire as many rare books for as little outlay as possible, and frustrated by the comparatively higher prices, have overlooked, in my opinion, the main, impelling force in this directional movement. It is a matter of history, not booksellers' necromancy. Interest in rare medical books is more wide-spread and more intensified than before. More collectors and libraries have entered the book-buying arena, encouraging booksellers into greater activity to supply an earnest demand. However, owners of medical libraries, and even single volumes, are now no longer content with merely discarding them. Competitive offers are not only solicited—they are the order of the day. Rare medical books cost the bookseller ever so much more than formerly, and despite his activity, rare books, being what they are, turn up infrequently. Inevitably, prices had to rise—the law of supply and demand again. Frankly, and this is true of more than 99% of all booksellers, for the amount of energy, intellectual and physical, each one puts into the business, the pecuniary return is inconsiderable. As Alfred Goldsmith, that erudite and altogether charming bookseller, once pointed out: "Bookselling is a very pleasant way of making a very little money."

Fortunately, more and more collectors and librarians have come to appreciate the role of the bookseller. In his Rosenbach Lecture on "The Great Medical Bibliographers," Dr. Fulton had some heart-warming words to say in our behalf. Discover for yourselves how booksellers are regarded by that distinguished bibliophile, Dr. Erik Waller, of Sweden. I could mention many others, but I have elected instead to lean once more on Dr. Wilson of the Armed Forces Medical Library. His address on "Historical Libraries—New Style" shows a rare understanding of the rare bookdealer. Permit me this final quotation. "Enter at this point a third and quite important character. Some would call him the villain in the piece, but in that I do not concur. He provides an element of conflict, it is true, but he is no more of a villain than is the historian or the librarian. This third character is the rare book dealer. He has been absolutely indispensable in the building up of historical libraries to their present state of excellence. He has conducted his business usually on quite high ethical standards. He is also surprisingly generous in giving service. If you are a librarian in a recognized institution, or if you are an accredited private collector, he will send you a book or manuscript on approval, and if for any reason you do not want it, he will take it back. In his sales catalogues he gives descriptions of his wares, and if any volume that you buy has defects that were not mentioned, he will make an adjustment. Complaints are sometimes heard that the profits of the rare book dealer run from 100 to 300 per cent and occasionally higher. In reality this is not exorbitant. Turnover is slow in the rare book trade, there is no mass market, and there are some risks."[4]

It would be presumptuous of me to try to improve upon what Dr. Wilson has said, but I would like to point out that bookdealers do not enjoy being regarded with suspicion by librarians, and even though this attitude is slowly disappearing, it still manifests itself uncomfortably often. To an appreciable extent librarians singularly fortunate in acquiring rare books can credit their friendly and intimate relationship with bookdealers as a strong contributing factor. Actually, no bookdealer who wishes to remain in business can afford to be other than fair and ethical. He can become a most useful, unofficial part of the library's staff. In my opinion, he is worth cultivating.

[4] Wilson, William Jerome. *Op. cit.*, p. 57.

Physicians and Books *

By William B. Bean, M.D., *Professor of Medicine*
University of Iowa
Iowa City, Iowa

THE great Lord Bacon said "The images of men's wits and knowledges remain in books, exempted from the wrongs of time and capable of perpetual renovation. Neither are they fitly to be called images, because they generate still, and cast their seeds in the minds of others, provoking and causing infinite actions and opinions in succeeding ages. So that if the invention of the ship was thought so noble, which carrieth riches and commodities from place to place, how much more are letters to be magnified, which, as ships pass through the vast seas of time, and make ages so distant to participate of the wisdom, illuminations, and inventions, the one of the other?"

We are here today to celebrate the realization of an old dream, the culmination of a phase of our history in which the physician has continued to grapple with unwieldly knowledge by putting it into words, putting words into books, putting books into libraries and sometimes reading them. Slowly and painfully through the ages man has learned to concentrate and select facts, hoping thus to acquire knowledge and gain wisdom. Though this is necessary in all crafts, arts, and sciences, it is especially so for medicine if physicians are to improve the care and cure of the sick and troubled. You have heard and will hear more of the wise and noble men, past and present, whose skill and devotion, so often unnoticed by drowsy contemporaries, have brought forth and will continue to develop this monument to medical scholarship, medical humanities, and humaneness.

Our great theme today is books. Voices raised by the skeptic and the cynic cry disparagingly that facts and knowledge grow exponentially while men's wits grow in linear fashion if they grow at all. Knowledge, like the

* Presented at the dedication of the National Library of Medicine Building, Bethesda, Maryland, December 14–15, 1961.

Originally published in *Bulletin of the Medical Library Association,* Volume 50 (April, 1962), pp. 159-166. Reprinted by permission.

retreating galaxies, is exploding away from us. Those who clutch at it find it is receding at an ever accelerating pace. Others in perplexity wonder if the written word may characterize an ephemeral phase through which man has to travel in his worried passage through time as he moves towards a future of gigantic electronic machines. Are such paraphernalia for getting and marshalling knowledge—extrapolations of man's mental energy built in his mind's own image of itself—merely substantial means to an insubstantial end? Others, more bitter, carry gloom still further, suspecting that speech, our word symbols, may also be temporary, a chapter in our march to unknown heights or depths. Time, which the writer first, and then the printer, shackled, will now be chained by the low amperage engineer with his feedbacks, internuncial circuits, currents and tapes—finite containers for an infinitude of data. Will this lead to brilliant new syntheses of thought or a game of intellectual squat tag? Will the silk purses of inspiration and imagination come from the sow's ears of facts, and the birth of truth be forced by some law of mass action, with short circuits as inadvertent midwives?

Those of even more acrid and astringent mood further spread this pall through which they peer, half in horror, prophesying a time when all the raw data of existence are "programmed" into vast electronic gaboons, all-containing cuspidors, which in ancient manner feed back a mist of data for developing brains in characterless automatons according to the master blueprint of a gigantic stereotype.

But doom-mongers always thrive on misconstructions and misapprehensions. Their judgment is false, but whether through ignorance or obtuseness is uncertain. An antidote for such visions of dismay may be found in history, and even prehistory, the more hopefully to see the future.

Man emerged from chaos in fear, terror, and confusion. Ultimately he gained some mastery of his environment because he gained control of himself. From crude gestures and grunts came symbols as words arose and, with words, ideas. The fragile first records are all gone, written on wood, bark, and sand. Crude images and amulets suggest slow and painful progress. The first traces of an intelligible language growing out of the simplest symbols remain in the clay tablets of Babylon and in the papyrus scrolls of Egypt. The clay tablet, though it had good survival potential, was wonderfully awkward. Reading a book must have been like getting ready to tile a bathroom or build a brick wall.

Such early recording enabled one man to teach many; one generation could codify and record enough experience to be of value to the next. The emergence from Stone Age into the Copper or Bronze Age was closely related to the development of paper rolls, early forerunners of books. Though easier to handle than the earlier skins and parchment records, they were cumbersome to use and to store.

Books, words, language, and grammar grew in parallel lines. Grammar emerged from language and at first was not a skeleton on which speech, words and language developed. Its origins are as hard to understand as the complex origin of the intricate human body and the evolution of its myriad functions. Probably Homer would have been appalled at the very notion of grammar. To him grammar was innate, like air and breathing. Grammar came from the necessity for communication. Science came from the necessity for understanding. Language and grammar require books and libraries. Science requires language, grammar, books, libraries, and laboratories.

Rather than retrace the well known story of Hippocrates and the many books ascribed to him, let us see how collections of books first began to change the form and fabric of civilization and medicine as certain philosophers became scientists. The library at Alexandria developed hand in hand with the Museum. It was a single institution with two separate but interacting functions. Support for a vast program of building intellectual capital came from the Ptolemys. We cannot tell how scholars came to be accepted since at that time none really was able to explain or command Nature, despite incantations and horoscopes.

The Museum and Library were not public but reserved for only a few wise men. Here for the first time a museum, a hall of the Muses, became a laboratory for observation. This made possible early research and experiment by asking Nature for answers rather than listening passively, the immemorial eavesdropper technique. Now for the first time thought was directed beyond the musings of old men, the heroic urges of poets, and the residual mental output of philosophers. The charming daintiness of abstract thought had to confront messy reality. Wild horses of speculation began to feel the snaffle of stubborn facts. This never halted the mental chariot race of abstractions but kept it in an intelligible and strait curriculum.

As the world of learning grew, the library extended its functions. Magic was losing ground to the keen practicality of Greek and Alexandrian medicine. Astrology was merging into the beginnings of astronomy. Travel and trade along the far reaches of the Mediterranean were giving form to geography as it shook off the dust of geomancy and fable and began to escape from the fabulous mythology which far lands have always conjured up in man's mind. Philosophy, philology, and belles-lettres continued despite the intrusion of sciences into the hallowed shrines of literature. None of this could have happened without words, writing, paper, charts, and books, maps, and libraries.

With the Museum as laboratory the Library served multiple functions, just as our university libraries serve many divisions and departments, and this National Library of Medicine will serve them all. Trained librarians and "scientists" worked hand in hand. The library was a source of great pride for the Ptolemys. They developed the nasty little habit of requiring all travelers who reached Alexandria to surrender their books. The stranger then was given cheap papyrus copies. If the library already had the scroll, the original was returned. Happily, such forms of acquisition no longer prevail. Rulers and generals from Persia and later from Rome, as they became less compulsively destructive, sometimes preserved libraries more or less intact and took them home.

Thus in olden times it was realized that books represented power. They are man's memory—classic, scientific, and historic—the symbol and embodiment of the words and speech which elevate man above other animals.

No doubt the users of the great library of Alexandria were already fretting at the perennial nightmares of librarians; how to accommodate the needs of the general reader to those of special readers; how to control books so they can best serve most users. It was recognized very early that the functions of a library for the humanities and for the sciences differ. The astronomer will find out about the stars but he will not be able to see the heavens. The anatomist will find texts and illustrations but will not actually see the human body. But the treasures of the humanities and the classics, the very substance, are the books themselves. Physicians must use books in both contexts.

In Alexandria for the first time many scholars were assigned to library service. It must have been excellent. Because books were scrolls the mechanical part of the librarian's job was more awkward than that of a modern library, which at least has a recognizable unit with all kinds of opportunities for classification and storage—alphabet, subject, size, date, even color, or anything which can bring logic to the deposition and the disposition of books. Great bins had to be arranged to contain the overwhelming plenty of papyrus rolls. They all had to be classified, edited, identified, and put where they could be found. Librarians kept all this information in their heads. It is hard for us to imagine the chaos which simple problems of identification presented to those who shepherded the growing band of philologists, humanists, and scientists among the great bins and stalls which contained these early codifications of knowledge.

All books were hand written. This set a limitation on wide dissemination of knowledge, though papyrus scrolls greatly expanded the possibility of sharing information. The manual multiplication of papyrus scrolls gave only a faint preview of the colossal expansion and explosion in reading and writing which occurred with the invention of the printing press nearly two millennia later.

The parallel growth of the Library and Museum set the stage for the parallel development of the anatomy of the human body, and grammar, the anatomy of language. This could occur only where there was a large fund of empirical knowledge and observation.

The quantity of books may have a curious relationship with quality. Scholars have commented upon the melancholy fact that ancient literature began to decline as libraries began to grow. Perhaps there was a tendency for the rigor of criticism and thought to slacken. For the first fifteen hundred years of the Christian era ancient knowledge was copied. The interrogation of nature to gain new knowledge declined. For many reasons there was a great diastole of the intellect. Scientific inquiry went into eclipse.

Changes in the craft of bookmaking occurred slowly at first. In the third century the scroll began to give way to the codex or book. An enormous amount of work was needed in the change-over from scrolls to books of modern format with the great boon of convenient handling. A shortage of parchment led to the introduction of vellum. The first vellum was dried sheep tripe. Our vellum is fine-grained calf or lamb skin, or vegetable fibers used in imitation. Books were rare and some were beyond price. Still it was possible for the happy Benedict of Clusa to boast in 1028 A.D., just over nine centuries ago, "I have two large houses filled with books . . . , there is not in the whole world a book that I have not." No one today would dare hope to get all the books published the world over in any one week.

The great change came with the introduction of movable type in printing, the development of illustration, and later the advent and perhaps the corruption of medical periodicals. Printing with movable type was introduced into Europe during the second half of the fifteenth century, a major contribution of the Renaissance. It changed the character and scope of Western civilization. The rise of modern medicine parallels the expansion of bookmaking. A man born in 1453 A.D., the year Constantinople fell, if he lived for fifty years, could look back upon a lifetime in which maybe eight or nine million individual volumes had been printed; probably more than all the monks, all the scribes, all the writers of Christendom had been able to produce since the birth of Christ. No one dares to think how many times this number may be turned out now in any calendar year. If one adds journals to books, scientific and medical, printed in a current year, the "monstrous regiment" is vastly more than the total production of all manuscript writers before the age of printing.

Printing and bookmaking depend upon advances in technology. When books were made of sheepskin, a folio of about 200 pages required 25 sheep. In the days before printing the cost of hiring a scribe was small compared to the cost of 25 sheep. Thus, without the manufacture of paper which reached Europe in the twelfth century from Islam printing would have been but a modest advance. Likewise the development of satisfactory ink, lampblack boiled in linseed oil, was essential. Printing with fixed blocks and from movable type certainly came from China where printing paper money, playing cards, and religious charms had evolved. No one knows who first found that a mirror image of a letter of the alphabet could be produced in metal by casting with accurate metal molds. Decorations, color printing, relief printing, and intaglio printing developed slowly. Mass production of books had to wait until a little over a hundred and fifty years ago when it became possible to manufacture paper in continuous reels rather than making it by hand, sheet by sheet.

Illustrations of scientific articles and books has depended on the technology of the times. The first illustrations were from woodcuts; no other methods of reproducing drawings were known. They were black and white; color could be painted in later. Only when scientific principles of illustration were established could interpretive and imaginative work develop. The results of experiments could be presented in graphs, diagrams, or three dimensional drawings. Even hypotheses could be presented graphically. From the woodcut evolved etching, lithography, engraving on metal, and many other new techniques. Etching metal was introduced about the year 1500 although some engraving had been done on copper in Florence as early as 1477, but such engravings did not come into general use in illustrating books until the sixteenth century. They completely replaced wood blocks in the seventeenth century.

The advance of science has depended on the development of symbols in printing, especially simple line diagrams, just as the development of algebra depended on a set of symbols. As an example Christopher Wren, working with Robert Hooke, was one of the first to make exact drawings of things he had seen under the microscope. Robert Hooke developed this with great skill. It was only about a hundred years ago that Jacob Henle, the great anatomist, developed illustrations to indicate structure in three dimensions. Walter Roberts found out how to print a copy of an original drawing. Thus it became possible to magnify or reduce the scale.

Medical illustration and art are separate. The graphic artist produces his drawings and paintings as his best and most beautiful representation of what is going on in his mind. The scientist's major concern is to make accurate reproductions. Fortunately scientific books and illustrations can be technically superb. They may be valid art. There is no necessary conflict between the two. Vesalius and Calcar exemplify the divine conjunction of scientific discoverer and artist, putting a capstone on one phase of medical advance. Leonardo da Vinci exemplifies the combination of scientist and artist in one person.

But Leonardo must be reckoned a failure as a scientist, for he was oblivious to literary tradition. I follow Sarton here. Leonardo's culture was manual and oral; his formal schooling was meager and he probably never read a Latin book. His mirror writing, done for secrecy or out of some repugnance, was anecdotal—single statements without supporting data. He never wrote for publication, corrected no galley, and seemed to lack the ability to organize evidence or build up scientific proof. Even as an anatomist he was so taken with Galen's ideas that he not only "saw" pores in the heart's interventricular septum, but he drew them. Unaware of printing or engraving, his message had almost no audience, and in medicine, no influence. The seeds have ripened only in our time, too late except for us to marvel at lost opportunities. If a discoverer must convince he fell short, perhaps paralyzed by his own genius, shipwrecked by an overweight of knowledge and erudition. The scientific progeny of his gigantic intellect were largely stillborn.

In sharp contrast stands his slightly younger and I think less lavishly gifted contemporary, Albrecht Durer, who was practical, capable, and efficient, with a good eye for business. He was less deep but more fertile. He prepared and printed three books in the printing establishment he organized himself. Durer's anatomy, unlike the dissections of Leonardo, was surface anatomy. But he advertised, and carried his engravings to sell at fairs and markets, well aware that there was a large profit to be had when he could reproduce a drawing a hundred times instead of making it only once. His proprietary interest caused him to sign his pictures. But he wanted to influence people. Durer's impact was enormous. His instructions for the use of the compass and ruler and his book on the canons of proportion of the human body had important effects. The key to the difference between Durer and Leonardo is that we have got to understand and use books and illustrations in the literary tradition.

What lessons are there for us? Of course we must use books. This Library, this treasure of books, has been arranged with great care for the most efficient use, retrieval and recall with new electronic devices and especially designed equipment. In collaboration with the American Medical Association this Library prepares a huge monthly index to help ride herd on new medical information. We must be sure that the wisest experts advise in newer ways to store and recall knowledge. Their skill in designing new machines must control this proliferating repository of facts lest it become a mausoleum of mummified knowledge, data encysted in mile after mile of shelves, the tombs of tomes, melancholy memorials to a gigantic writer's cramp. I sometimes wonder if the secret bane in Pandora's box was not a printing press.

The spirit of Gesner, Klebs, Cushing, Osler, Billings, Fletcher, Garrison, Fulton, and other great medical bibliographers, bibliophiles, and librarians hovers about us here. They would marvel at this palace of learning, this shrine of medical scholarship. Perhaps they would warn us that literacy does not guarantee understanding, that mass production of books brings no assurance that all are good or that many will be used wisely, and that great electronic machines with instant and total recall will not substitute for the intellect though they may deaden it in a literary atrophy of disuse. We must have good and beautiful books, for the love of books has no substitute. They must teach us to face bravely our battle against the world's absurdities and irrationalities. We must not waste our hatred for things on persons, nor our strength for doing battle with the world in quarreling among ourselves. Books remind us of friendship. They lead us to equanimity and peace, at least peace of mind. They help us maintain our individuality without the austere and crushing loneliness of those who love only themselves. The wisdom we gain from books leads us to act as though we were building our ideas for eternity, mindful that the nature of life and death are so ordered that we and our works are fleeting and falling grains of sand in the hourglass of time. If we can avoid the apathy of those who claim to know that nothing matters and the sheer folly of those who know that they personally matter immensely, we shall have been worthy successors to that silent company of physicians, our medical forebears whose spirits watch over us here. Through the careful and scholarly making and the wise use of books and libraries they built our great tradition. By following them we must add to it as physicians wise and humble in the care, the comfort, and sometimes in the cure of our fellows in their sickness and in their sorrow.

A Dirty Mind Never Sleeps and Other Comments on the Oral History Movement*

By Peter D. Olch, M.D., *Deputy Chief*

History of Medicine Division, National Library of Medicine
Bethesda, Maryland

ABSTRACT

Oral history has become an increasingly popular technique for gathering information. Viewed by some as the last word in historiography and by others as the latest word in histrionics, it is in fact nothing more and nothing less than a technique with many worthwhile applications if handled with reason and proper preparation.

A brief historical review of the oral history movement is followed by a description of the current efforts in oral history in the life sciences. In conclusion the author expresses his personal views on the probable future of oral history.

It is imperative that I begin with an explanation of this title as I am acutely aware of the copyright laws and do not wish to offend the W. W. Norton publishing company or Mr. Max Wilk, the author of a delightful book entitled, *A Dirty Mind Never Sleeps*. In this humorous work, Max Wilk presents one facet and some of the fervor behind the oral history movement, though one hopes in a purely fictitious manner. For this reason I will quote several passages from Mr. Wilk's book[1].

> Because history is a half truth. How can it be anything else? It's a pile of facts and dates, mixed together with dollops of hypothesis and conjecture. Compounds of legends and old-wives' tales, what archeologists dig up, or what's washed ashore; tomb stones, carvings, and let us not forget, great lacings of

*Delivered at the History of Medicine dinner held during the Sixty-ninth Annual Meeting of the Medical Library Association, New Orleans, Louisiana, May 19, 1970.

The author was expressing his own views and not necessarily those of the National Library of Medicine or the Oral History Association.

Originally published in *Bulletin of the Medical Library Association*, Volume 59 (July, 1971), pp. 438-443. Reprinted by permission.

propaganda. (Of course the local monks were honest, but you can be damned sure they were not writing down and illuminating anything about Big Duke up in the castle that he might find irritating to himself and Big Duchess. Ah no, sire, those monks knew where *their* next pot of gold leaf was coming from.)

This is not to say history is fraud.

(Why am I carrying on like this about history? Flunked it regularly.)

But I'm beginning to understand why I flunked history.

Couldn't relate. Read texts and studied maps and charts. Nothing. No *essence*.

No sense of smell, and frustration, no boils and nightmares and bitching, sweat, the touch of skin, the drives—

Began to get some of it out of Shakespeare. But then began to question him, too.

For instance—what *else* did Julius Caesar say when Brutus let him have it?

Et tu Brute?

Brief, poignant, dramatically right. A great scene for an actor, obviously a crowd-pleaser at the Mermaid and the Globe.

But—was that all he could think of to say?

To have *been* there and seen and heard it—not like *See It Now*, with all the actors reading carefully scripted TV folksy-historic speeches in response to questions from Mike Wallace and Bill Leonard—no, I'm thinking and trying to *feel* Caesar.

. . . he probably staggers back with his hand on the hole in his toga, and gasps, "Why—you treacherous bum—after all I've done for you—*aach*—and you give me the shaft right here in front of the whole Senate—*whoo*, that hurts—like some plebeian you caught in the sack with your *uxor*—"

. . . bang, he hits the floor.

Senators all shaken up—

"Hey, he stabbed *Caesar*!"

". . . He's bleeding like a pig—"

". . . What a mess!"

"The old man's dying—"

"Who do you think'll get the Number One spot?" etc., etc.

That's my kind of history.

What do we really know about—say—Wilbur and Orville Wright, that day at Kitty Hawk? (Went and looked that one up. You can read Orville's diary with its eyewitness description, but it's easy to see he's holding back on all of the personal stuff.)

It's a chilly December day out on those windy dunes, and the boys have decided to go for broke. Orville lying flat on that rickety damned box kite with a motor, and it rolls along the bumpy ground, putt-putt-putt, and then all of a sudden, off she sails, seven crazy miles an hour, up up, and away!

. . . what do you think Wilbur said?

"Great Heavens, we are vindicated! All our labors—our deepest dreams and ambitions and hopes have come to glorious fruition—our gallant little craft has conquered the mysterious kingdom of the Air."

I'm trying to *think* Wilbur. Who wants to bet me he said something like "Sonofabitch—The damn thing works!"

And then—"Dammit, how come my brother *always* gets to be first?"

I'll never sell that version. Why?

My generation has no Shakespeare. But it does have Darryl F. Zanuck and *his* history lessons. We're brainwashed every night on the Late Show.

Play Associations.

Queen Elizabeth? Bette Davis.

Paul Gaugin? George Sanders. What did Henry V look like? Sir Laurence Olivier. John Brown—Raymond Massey. Henry VIII—Laughton. George M. Cohan—Cagney. Abe Lincoln? Why, let's see—Henry Fonda the Young and... Raymond Massey the Old!

—and the things they said. Paul Muni and Spencer Tracy, and the ever-popular Donald Ameche, all face-haired up, acting out a storm. "Ach, Sigmund, give opp zis madness of ze mind and come to bed—tonight all Vienna is laughing at you, but never mind, *liebchen,* I believe in you." "I tell you, Mr. Disraeli, England will never stand for your lunatic proposal to create a Suez Canal!" "... Son, y'see that hill over there? Well, mebbe I'm jest a-dremin' a dream, but someday there's goin' to be a city there, with wide streets and tall buildings, risin' right up to the skies, 'n I'm thinkin' folks'll call it...*Denver.*" "...Mummy, is that Queen Elizabeth in the box behind the black horse?" "*Shh,* yes child." "... But Mummy, she was such a *little* woman..." "... Rough Riders, we are here at the foot of San Juan Hill—now I want you to carry our beloved Stars and Stripes up to the top there—hit the line hard—bully-*charge*!"

That's history?

....

....

I'd like to tune in on the truth. What some of those Rough Riders were saying under their breath, while Teddy was giving them that Cuban pep talk (the canned bully beef was rotten and how their guts must have ached). And what about old George W. at Valley Forge? Stone me, ladies of the D.A.R., but did our country's Father really spend all his time giving out with those chin-up-men readings? Isn't it possible there was one nasty night when he blew his cool and yelled (through his wooden teeth, which didn't fit properly), "All ri, all ri—we *are* up the creek—but for God's sake will one of you stop bitching and go out and chop some firewood?"

Did Emile Zola ever have writer's block, and if so, how did he handle it? When Byron quarreled with Lady Caroline Lamb, were his epithets elegant, or merely earthy? ... and Napoleon—and I don't mean Charles Boyer with a spit curl and his hand fingering his navel, I mean the *man*—what was he really like? How did he behave, say, the night before the retreat from Moscow? Is it possible that he had a few shots of cognac (the good stuff, our of his private trunk, not the Army-issue slop), got slightly bombed, lapsed into maudlin self-pity, sang, and then groaned, "*Bon Dieu,* why didn't I listen to the little cabbage back at Malmaison? She always told me to stav out of Russia—after this she will be insufferable!"

... and the guard outside, on duty, freezing in the Russian night, listening to his Little Corporal belching and singing inside in the warm tent? I'd like to hear what *he* said.

I'd like to hear lot of things. What those Zealots up on the top of Masada said to each other when the Roman Legion showed up down below. How Michelangelo must have complained about the arthritis in his back as he lay there painting the Sistine Chapel ceiling, and what the Viking crew was discussing on the seventy-fourth night of their trip across the Atlantic. The dirty jokes that must have been passed around the court while Elizabeth played footsie with Essex, and dear Adolf's last words (after you, liebchen?) in the Berlin bunker. The arguments over whose wagon went where in the line the day before the opening of the Cherokee Strip, and G.B.S. arguing over scrip changes with one of his early managers, and the complaints of those poor lost kids on the Children's Crusade ...

Where's all that? *That's history—*

... gone, all gone.

While it was happening, nobody was collecting it. It didn't seem important enough, there were no cassette portable tape recorders, and even if there had been, everyone was too busy living it to be bothered.

... the sound of music?

It's the sound of people that matters. People talking—not for publication, or for an NBC News mike, but completely off the record, unconsciously, never suspecting anyone's listening....

It's exhausting to think about doing it.

But *that* would be history, courtesy of Sony and Minnesota Mining.

Though amusing, there is in fact a message here. Surreptitious recording *is* not a practice of the oral historian. but an important facet of the oral history movement is to "tell it like it is," to delve beneath the surface of the prepared and considered statement in order to obtain candid commentary. Such a goal is quite worthy, if coupled with a reasonable set of standards which will honor the respondents' desires for restrictions on access.

I would like to present a brief historical review of the movement, to discuss the present "state of the art," and to share my feeling about the future of oral history.

Dr. Louis M. Starr, the Director of the Columbia University Oral History Research Office, and one of the field's most enthusiastic supporters, traces the origin of the term "oral history" to a certain Bowery character named Joe Gould who set out on a life-long task of compiling what he called "an Oral History of Our Times." This was to consist of an endless series of chance remarks, fleeting bits of conversation as heard and overheard by this denizen of the Bowery, on every subject under the sun. (One finds an element of this in Wilk's chapter entitled "The Old Piano Roll of Life or Sock the Sixties to Me.") The biographer of Joe Gould finally concluded that this monumental Oral History was a figment of Gould's fertile imagination, but there was the term recorded for posterity. In 1948 when Allen Nevins established the first organization at Columbia to obtain systematically from the lips and papers of living Americans a fuller record of their participation in the political, economic, and cultural life of their time, he selected the name Oral History for the process and it has remained.

Whatever the origin of the term, two things are abundantly clear: (1) the term "oral history" is misleading; and (2) the technique is here to stay. While it is true that oral history begins with oral narration, usually in the presence of a tape recorder run by the interviewer, the end product is generally a typewritten transcript, edited, indexed, bound, and preserved—not as history, but as one man's views and interpretations of a series of events or individuals in his recent or distant past. The transcript is, therefore, a historical resource which we hope will be useful to historians. That it is here to stay is unquestionable, not, I fear, because of its proven value to scholars or historians, but because it utilizes a "gimmick" and anyone can learn to press the "ON" and "RECORD" buttons simultaneously.

From its inception in 1948, the Columbia program has created the largest collection of oral history transcripts. Dr. Starr and Elizabeth Mason, his assistant, have traveled throughout the country as consultants and advisors to most of the later programs to appear on the scene. In 1965 Columbia published a list of ninety-two oral history programs in the United States[2]. There probably are more than double that number now.

In 1966, James V. Mink, the Archivist of the University of California, Los Angeles, and his colleagues in the UCLA Oral History Program, put out a call nationally for all parties involved or interested in oral history to assemble at Lake Arrowhead, California, for the first National Colloquium on Oral History. Seventy-seven individuals gathered representing academe, industry, government, and religious institutions. Any doubts as to the existence of varied backgrounds, uses, or purposes of oral history were confirmed in the session on Objectives and Standards. Near chaos reigned as the arguments of the tape savers vs. tape erasers; transcript editors vs. verbatim transcribers; and concerned archivists and historians vs. those who owed allegiance to a technique rather than a discipline, split the cool mountain air in an ever rising crescendo. The obvious multiplicity of backgrounds and objectives represented in this group was to be responsible for the major problems faced by the group while at the same time greatly contributing to the charm, stimulation, and unique nature of the membership. The multiplicity of backgrounds, the lack of agreement on objectives and standards also quickly dampened the attempts of the UCLA contingent to form a national association on the last day of this meeting at Lake Arrowhead. However, there was no question that the groundwork and foundation had been laid. The assembled participants agreed they should form an Oral History Conference, an informal organization without constitution or bylaws, in order to have a confederation permitting oral historians to keep in contact with one another.

In the ensuing year the Steering Committee of the Oral History Conference published the proceedings of the Arrowhead meeting and the first of a series of newsletters. They began to develop a series of "Goals and Guidelines" for oral history programs and a bibliography of the literature on oral history. This Committee also prepared a constitution and the necessary Articles of Incorporation in the hope that a permanent organization would be one result of the second meeting scheduled for the fall of 1967 at Arden House in Harriman, N.Y.

The November meeting was again in a remote conference center where the natural beauty of the location, the cuisine, and wine list challenged the stimulating presentations by Henry Steele Commager, Luther H. Evans, Alfred Knopf, Cornelius Ryan, and others for top billing. Those of the 146 participants who were members of the Oral History Conference reviewed and modified the proposed constitution, approved the Articles of Incorporation, and selected a slate of officers, and the entire package was submitted to the full Conference membership by mail ballot. The prolonged labor pains of the Oral History Association (OHA) were about to end, as within a month the organization was voted into being.

In 1968 eighty-nine participants gathered in Lincoln, Nebraska, to hear a program featuring William Manchester, Walter Lord, and James Rhoads, the Archivist of the United States, and this past year, 165 gathered at Airlie House in Warrenton, Virginia, to hear Elie Abel, Barbara Tuchman, Frank Mankiewicz, Saul Benison, and Nathan Reingold. Lest you believe that the Association meetings are merely exposures to the interviewing experiences of leading authors and journalists, I hasten to add that the bulk of each program has included such topics as "Oral History and the Law," "The Art of Interviewing," "Oral History in the Classroom," "Interdisciplinary Views on Oral History," to name but a few. The membership of the Association at this time is approximately 400, including institutional and individual members.

As one who has attended all four of these meetings, I continue to marvel at the disparate make-up of the group, with respected and recognized scholars participating side by side with young, enthusiastic, bright-eyed (and frequently miniskirted) practitioners of oral history whose limitless enthusiasm and boundless inquisitiveness keep their animated discussions going until the wee small hours of the morning, when, as often as not, they are interrupted for a 2:00 A.M. swim! Seriously though, the group as a whole does share certain concerns for the practice of oral history. The two major points on which most would agree are (1) the need for adequate and serious preparation on the part of the interviewer, and (2) the importance of adhering to an ethical code whereby the respondent's request for confidentiality or restricted access is honored. The numerous points on which the group disagree are quite understandable, as each has his own definition of oral history. To the National Park Service it is "living history" or "interpretive oral history" such as a mountaineer in the Great Smokies describing his recipe for "white lightning" or an Indian in Arizona describing ceremonial dances. To the National Library of Medicine it is a technique to gather information to supplement the written word, generally a man's personal papers. To the Presidential Libraries it is a technique to elucidate further the life and career of past presidents, and to the Mormon Church it is a means for gathering genealogical data. With such diverse goals, the lack of unanimity is to be expected.

As for oral history in the life sciences, there are probably some twenty-five to fifty oral history programs (depending on how you define this term). These vary from a long term study of the development of biochemistry and molecular biology being planned by the American Academy of Arts and Sciences to a series of interviews with past presidents of a variety of professional societies.

At the NLM we currently have about 290 interview hours of oral istory materials including those in process. It is perhaps regrettable that we have not limited our area of subject coverage. I say regrettable in the sense that the limited man hours devoted to oral history could accomplish more if each individual interview was a building block toward the next interview. It is already becoming apparent that there is a need for a "clearing house" or central listing of who is doing what in oral history related to the life sciences. As the American Academy of Arts and Sciences is preparing to support a program on the development of biochemistry and molecular biology, it finds that the NLM has already interviewed a number of leading figures in this field. and the Salk Institute for Biological Studies, in La Jolla, California, has initiated an Archive of Contemporary Biology which includes the preservation of manuscript material as well as tape recorded interviews with a number of members of the same population within the scientific community.

Two steps have been taken to remedy this problem. The National Union Catalogue of Manuscript Collections, following a series of discussions between Mrs. Arlene Custer and representatives of the OHA, will now accept and publish listings of catalogued collections of oral history materials which either accompany manuscript collections or stand alone as collections of oral history transcripts. I feel that this is a most important development and over the long haul will make the scholarly community aware of those oral history collections of substance which can be important sources of historical information.

The OHA is developing a list of oral history programs which will include information on size, scope, and availability of collections which should be published within the year. It is hoped that this will be a complete list of oral history programs or activities throughout the country. The Association has also arranged for the revision and updating of a publication entitled *A Bibliography of Oral History*.

As I try to visualize what the immediate and distant future holds in store for the oral history movement, I am reminded of a comment made by a speaker at the National Academy of Sciences recently, namely, "A young lady's future seldom takes shape before she does." Nevertheless, as the oral history movement enters the decade of the seventies, it is characterized by enthusiasm tempered by an increasing awareness of the pitfalls of the technique. The loud voices which proclaimed the technique to be the salvation of historians in the face of disappearing holographic documents are now muted. The legion of recorder-bearing individuals rushing to the doors of prominent Americans are now walking and giving more attention to their preparation and showing a concern for overlapping interests with other programs, to say nothing of the ethical and legal considerations of importance to the oral historian. Increasing numbers of oral historians, or perhaps more accurately oral history practitioners, are taking pause and wondering whether they stand alone as "technicians" or whether in fact they are members of more ancient guilds such as historians, archivists, or journalists who have latched on to a "new" technique which transiently at least sets them apart from their brethren.

The "establishment historian" who scoffed at oral history a few short years ago has at least loosened his starched collar to admit publicly that oral history memoirs can often be a source of interesting anecdotal material and vivid expression. Some have even admitted that information otherwise unavailable has been gleaned from oral history materials.

I believe it is safe to say that oral history *as a technique* is beginning to gain a modest degree of respectability even among the hardcore doubters who will swear by the written word but immediately suspect the spoken word. The burden rests upon the the practitioners of oral history. If reasonable standards are followed and our products can withstand impartial review of content in the same sense as a published work, I foresee a long and useful life for oral history. The time has come, if you will, for oral historians to actively seek out critical and penetrating analyses of their products. This idea was vigorously put forth at the Fourth National Colloquium by Dr. Saul Benison and I heartily agree. It is not enough to keep a tally of how many individuals consult your collection or how many authors credit your oral history collection as a reference. It is time for oral history products to stand or fall on the merit of their content and not on the unique qualities of the technique.

In closing, I would like to quote from Allan Seager's preface to his book, *A Frieze of Girls: Memoirs as Fiction*[3]. Herein is a message to all who would make extravagant claims for oral history.

> I am old enough to know that time makes fiction out of our memories. Some people, some events it pulls front and center. It stores others in the attic until we find some use for them. It discreetly buries a few forever. Can anyone remember his life accurately, objectively the way a camera and a tape would have recorded it? I doubt it. We all have to have a self we can live with and the operation of memory is artistic—selecting, suppressing, bending, touching up, turning our actions inside out so that we can have not necessarily a likable, merely a plausible identity. In this sense we are always true to ourselves....

REFERENCES

1. WILK, MAX. A Dirty Mind Never Sleeps. New York, 1969. By permission of W. W. Norton & Company, Inc. Copyright (c) 1969 by Max Wilk.
2. Columbia University. Oral History Research Office. Oral History in the United States New York, 1965.
3. SEAGER, ALLAN. A Frieze of Girls: Memoirs as Fiction. New York: McGraw Hill, 1964.

VIII
BIOGRAPHICAL VIGNETTES

Scott Adams has had a long and distinguished career in medical librarianship and related fields. Mr. Adams was born in Agawam, MA. He attended Yale University, graduating in 1930. After working as a jobber for the wholesale distribution of books, he attended Columbia University School of Library Service, where he graduated with honors in 1940. He was soon associated as head of acquisitions at Teacher's College Library, Columbia University. Mr. Adams held a similar position with the Providence Public Library from 1942 to 1945.

In 1945, he became chief of the acquisitions department of the Army Medical Library. Here he designed the program of collecting important publications in medicine and related fields, especially those significant in furthering research. Aided by Gen. Joseph McNinch, who became the director of the Army Medical Library in 1946, Mr. Adams dedicated his employment to make this Armed Forces library more available to scholars and medical librarians. When Col. Frank B. Rogers became director of the Army Medical Library in 1948 and took a year's leave of absence to study at Columbia, Mr. Adams served as acting librarian. In 1949, he became librarian of the National Institutes of Health Library in Bethesda. From there, Mr. Adams went, in 1960, to the new National Library of Medicine as deputy director.

In 1970, Mr. Adams served as special assistant to the foreign secretary of the National Academy of Sciences, and in 1972, he was senior staff scientist in the Science Communications Division at George Washington University. He became a professor in the School of Education at the University of Louisville in 1973, his current position.

Of his many honors and offices, only a few are mentioned: president of the American Society of Information Science, 1954-1955; president of the Medical Library Association, 1967-1968; recipient of the Marcia Noyes award, 1969; and member of the International Advisory Committee on Documentation of Libraries and Archives to UNESCO, 1967-1970.

Gertrude L. Annan was born in Providence, RI, and attended Brown University, receiving a B.A. degree with a major in English literature. She began her library career at the John Carter Brown Library as a cataloger. One suspects that this important library of priceless books, maps, and prints relating to North and South America during the colonial period nurtured her love of rare books.

From 1929 to 1933, Miss Annan served as cataloger of the New York Academy of Medicine's Rare Book Library, and from 1933 until 1953, she headed the Rare Book Library. In 1953, Miss Annan was promoted to associate librarian, and on the retirement of Miss Janet Doe, she succeeded her as the librarian of this great library, holding this position until her own retirement in 1969.

A distinguished medical librarian, Miss Annan held all the important offices, including the presidency of the Medical Library Association. In 1968, she received the Marcia Noyes award for her many contributions to medical librarianship. Her publications substantially advanced medical librarianship, as did her editing, with Jacqueline Felter, of the third edition of the Association's *Handbook of Medical Library Practice*. It's a tribute to Miss Annan that she was chosen to deliver the first Janet Doe lecture.

James Francis Ballard, one of the most colorful members of medical librarianship, was the director of the Boston Medical Library. As Walter B. McDaniel, 2nd, said:

> The Director of the Boston Medical Library, Mr. James F. Ballard, died 15 May 1955, with, as they used to say, his boots on. A few months short of his 77th birthday, he still, because he wanted to, guided the destinies of the great library which he had served for 63 years[1].

Mr. Ballard was born at Saranac Lake, NY, and at the age of 14 (1892) entered the service of the Boston Medical Library at a minimal position. He pleased his superiors, and his title became second assistant librarian in 1900; then, in 1909, he was named assistant librarian. Since the librarian was by tradition a physician, the trustees found the solution to his further advancement—in 1928, Mr. Ballard was named director. Although self-educated, he accumulated a vast sum of knowledge, especially about rare medical books. It is interesting to note that Mr. Ballard was 20 and had been with the Boston Medical Library for 6 years when the group later to become the Medical Library Association came into being.

His first paper, "Some Problems in the Administration of a Medical Library," was presented to the Medical Library Association in 1914. From that time on, Mr. Ballard gave many talks and held countless offices in the Association. He was president from 1937 to 1939. He had much to do with improving the financial affairs of the Association. For several years, too, Mr. Ballard served as the unofficial parliamentarian. At the Association's

50th meeting, held in Denver, CO, in June 1951, he received a much deserved tribute, the Marcia Noyes award.

Perhaps Mr. Ballard will best be remembered for his classification scheme of the Boston Medical Library. He improved on an older scheme, and in 1921, the Standard Classification Committee of the Medical Library Association recommended that it be officially adopted. The classification was published in a third edition in 1946. In subsequent years, the rapidly changing character of medicine made for newer and more nearly complete systems. Mr. Ballard also was the compiler of the important *Catalogue of the Medieval and Renaissance Manuscripts and Incunabala in the Boston Medical Library* (1944).

After Mr. Ballard's death on May 15, 1955, a tribute was paid in his memory:

> Acknowledged as the Dean of Medical Librarians throughout the world, James F. Ballard, self-educated, compiled for the Boston Medical Library one of the country's outstanding collections of medical books and periodicals, and amassed, personally, a tremendous fund of knowledge of medical literature that he graciously shared with his confreres throughout the world and with the student, physician, or scientist who sought his services[2].

William Bennett Bean was born in Manila, the Philippines, on Nov. 8, 1909. He attended the University of Virginia in Charlottesville, receiving an A.B. degree in 1932 and an M.D. in 1935. He interned at the Johns Hopkins Hospital from 1935 to 1936 and was assistant resident physician at Boston City Hospital from 1936 to 1937 and also a teaching fellow in medicine at the Thorndike Memorial Laboratory at Harvard University. Dr. Bean served as senior medical resident at the Cincinnati General Hospital from 1937 to 1938 and held the title of assistant attending physician from 1941 to 1946. From 1942 to 1946, Dr. Bean served in the Medical Corps of the Army of the United States, achieving the rank of lieutenant colonel. He returned as assistant professor of medicine at the Medical College of Cincinnati (1946), advancing to the rank of associate professor in 1948. Dr. Bean then left this position to become professor of medicine and head of the Department of Internal Medicine at the University of Iowa College of Medicine, Iowa City. Dr. Bean was also physician-in-chief of the University Hospitals. He continued in these capacities until 1970, when he became Sir William Osler Professor of Medicine (a lifetime appointment). Since 1974, Dr. Bean has also served as the Harris Kempner Professor of Medical Humanities and professor of internal medicine (acting head of the Department of Dermatology) at the University of Texas Medical Branch, Galveston.

Dr. Bean has received many honors, including the John Horsley Memorial prize (1944) and the Groedel medal (1961). He was a special consultant to the surgeon general of the U.S. Army and was appointed by the President of the United States to the board of regents of the National Library of Medicine, serving two terms. Dr. Bean received the Gold Headed Cane award in 1964 from the University of California.

Dr. Bean belongs to many medical and allied organizations, including the American College of Chest Physicians, American Medical Writers Association, American Association for the Advancement of Science, American Association for the History of Medicine, College of Cardiology, American College of Sports Medicine (charter member), and American Osler Society (charter member and first president).

Among his many publications are several excellent books: *Sir William Osler, From His Bedside Teachings and Writings, Vascular Spiders and Related Lesions of the Skin, Aphorisms From Latham, and Rare Diseases and Lesions.*

William K. Beatty has been professor of medical bibliography at Northwestern University Medical School since 1962. He has been active as a writer and editor, serving as the author of a column in the *Bulletin of the Medical Library Association* since 1959, as book review editor of the *Journal of Medical Education* (1965-1970), and as a member of the editorial board for *Familiar Medical Quotations* (Little, Brown & Company, 1968). He has been coauthor, with Geoffrey Marks, of five books published by Charles Scribner's Sons: *The Medical Garden, Women in White: Their Role as Doctors Through the Ages, The Story of Medicine in America, The Precious Metals of Medicine,* and *Epidemics.* In addition, Mr. Beatty has been author or coauthor of 73 chapters and articles and of many book reviews.

The Medical Library Association awarded him the Ida and George Eliot prize in 1973 for his work as editor of *Vital Notes on Medical Periodicals.* The Special Libraries Association named him John Cotton Dana lecturer for 1968, and the University of Illinois College of Medicine invited him to give the D. J. Davis Lecture on Medical History in 1974.

Mr. Beatty has been active in library, medical history, and literary organizations and has served in a variety of offices: Association of Hospital and Institution Libraries (president, 1965-1966); Medical Library Association (board of directors, 1966-1969; chairman, Convention Program Committee, Louisville meeting, 1969; Nominating Committee, 1976-1977); Special Libraries Association (board of directors, 1964-1967; president, Illinois chapter, 1969-1970; chairman, Biological Sciences Division, 1963-1964; chairman, Hospital Division, 1960-1961; professional consultant); American Association for the History of Medicine (council, 1965-1968; chairman, Osler Medal Committee, 1965-1966); American Osler Society (founding member; board of governors, 1976-1979); Institute of Medicine of Chicago (editorial board, 1970 to present); Society of Medical History of Chicago (council, 1963-1971, 1973-1976); and Chicago Literary Club (corresponding secretary, 1971-1978; vice-president, 1978-1979).

Warren Phillip Bird was born in Rochester, NY, on Dec. 27, 1933. He attended Georgetown University, Washington, DC, from 1953 to 1956, when he received a B.S. degree in physics. He was a biophysicist at Columbia University in New York City from 1958 to 1964. From 1963 to 1964, Mr. Bird attended Columbia University in New York City, where he received an M.S. in library science in 1964. He then was appointed a library systems analyst (1964-1965).

From 1965 to 1968, Mr. Bird was chief of ibrary mechanization at Duke University Medical Center, Durham, NC. At that time, he was appointed associate director and assistant professor of medical literature. He has also served as visiting lecturer at the School of Library Science of the University of North Carolina at Chapel Hill. Mr. Bird is currently librarian at the Duke University Medical Center.

Mr. Bird holds memberships in the Medical Library Association, Special Libraries Association, North Carolina Library Association, American Society for Information Science, Institute of Electric and Electronic Engineers, BSA, and American Association for the Advancement of Science. He edited the Library Telecommunications Directory (1968-1969) and has contributed articles to the professional literature, especially on different aspects of library systems and automation.

John Shaw Billings was born in Cotton Township in Switzerland County in southeastern Indiana in 1838. He attended Miami University, Oxford, OH, at the early age of 14 and received an A.B. degree with honors 5 years later in 1857. Deciding on a medical career, he received an M.D. degree from the Medical College of Ohio in Cincinnati in 1860 and for a while served as demonstrator of anatomy.

With the advent of the Civil War, Dr. Billings decided on an Army career. He appeared before the local medical examining board and passed the examination at the top of the list. He received his commission, and after serving in the field, he was put in charge of an Army hospital. Because of his superior work, Dr. Billings was named executive officer of a Philadelphia hospital. His efficiency and good judgment in taking care of the thousands of wounded were noticed by his superiors. In April 1864, the surgeon general assigned Dr. Billings to be inspector of the Army hospitals. Working under the medical director of the Army of the Potomac, he gathered and consolidated statistics and, during battles, traveled from hospital to hospital, obtaining records and in some areas overseeing surgery.

In the summer of 1865, Dr. Billings, because of a bout of illness, was returned to Washington and assigned to the Office of the Surgeon General, U.S. Army. Dr. Billings remained in association with the surgeon general's office and especially with the development of its library and medical indexing tools until his retirement in 1895. At that time, Dr. Billings held the rank of colonel.

There is no need here to repeat the many accomplishments of Billings, since they have been included in many published accounts of his career. But we would be inclined to agree with Dr. William H. Welch, who said,

> I question whether America has made any larger contribution to medicine than that made by Billings in building up and developing the Surgeon-General's Library and in the publication of the Index Catalogue and the "Index Medicus." That in my judgment is America's greatest contribution to medicine[3].

Sir William Osler once said of his friend Billings, "There is no better float through posterity than to be the author of a good bibliography .... the great Index will remain an enduring monument to his fame[4]."

After retirement from the Army, Dr. Billings served as professor of hygiene at the University of Pennsylvania for a year before his appointment as director of the New York Public Library in 1896. He consolidated the three city libraries into one with the hope, which was realized, of a library worthy of the best in Europe. Billings persuaded the city to donate the land in the present central location, and the architects followed the plans that Billings originally sketched. Billings supervised the classification of the books and the arrangement. He also persuaded the Carnegie Foundation to provide $5 million for the building of the much-needed free circulating branch libraries. This great librarian continued to be active until his death on Mar. 11, 1913.

David Bishop was born on Sept. 23, 1928, in Newfoundland. He received a B.A. degree, majoring in economics, from Dalhousie University, Nova Scotia, Canada, in 1952. Deciding on a library career, Mr. Bishop studied at the Columbia University School of Library Service in New York City, where he received an M.S. in library science in 1958. From 1958 to 1961, Mr. Bishop was employed by the Los Angeles County Medical Association. First he was a junior librarian in cataloging and reference work and later, reference librarian. In October 1961, Mr. Bishop became associated with

the Biomedical Library at the University of California Medical School in Los Angeles. He spent the first 2 years as dental librarian, building up a library for the new dental school. During his last 2 years at UCLA, he served as serials librarian with special responsibility for the design of a computerized serials control system. He became a naturalized U.S. citizen in 1966.

From 1965 to 1971, Mr. Bishop was librarian of the Arizona Medical Center Library at the University of Arizona in Tucson. Here he developed the library for the new medical school and medical center. He also designed a medical library network for the state.

From 1971 to 1973, Mr. Bishop was medical librarian at the McGill University School of Medicine in Montreal, Canada. He developed a life science library encompassing seven libraries in seven fields relating to medicine.

From 1973 to 1977, Mr. Bishop served as director of the Library of Medicine of the Nebraska Medical Center in Omaha. He also succeeded to the position of his predecessor, director of the Midcontinental Regional Medical Library, and became associate director of the Clinical Neurology Information Center.

In the fall of 1977, Mr. Bishop became university librarian and coordinator of learning resources at the University of California in San Francisco. He also holds the rank of associate professor of history of th health sciences.

David Bishop has served on various committees of the Medical Librar Association. He was a member of the board of directors, 1971-197 chairman of the Medical Library Association/National Library Medicine Task Force on the Impact of MEDLARS on Cataloging a Classification; editorial consultant for the *Bulletin*, 1976 to present; a associate editor of the fourth edition of the *Handbook of Medical Libr Practice*, now in preparation.

Harold Bloomquist was born in Muskegan, MI, on Oct. 27, 1928. Bloomquist received an A.B. degree from Albion College in 1950 an M.S. degree from Columbia University School of Library Service in He studied under Professor Thomas Fleming, who inspired him to the medical library field. In 1958, Mr. Bloomquist joined the staff Harvard Medical Library as assistant librarian for resources and ac tion; in 1965, he advanced to associate librarian of the Countway L of Medicine. Merging the Boston Medical Library and the Lib Harvard College School of Medicine into the new Countway Libr planning the new library were partly his responsibility. In June 1 Countway Library became the nation's first Regional Medical

under the National Library of Medicine, encompassing the New England states. The library also serves as a MEDLARS search station for the medical institutions in the New England area.

Harold Bloomquist succeeded Ralph Esterquest, whose untimely death occurred in 1968, as librarian in 1969. Mr. Bloomquist has been active in the affairs of the Medical Library Association. For a number of years, he was associate editor of the *Bulletin,* and he served as chairman of the Committee on Continuing Education in 1964-1965.

As a result of illness, Hal Bloomquist, one of our favorite librarians, retired in 1976. He was made an honorary member and a fellow of the Medical Library Association in 1976.

Alfred N. Brandon was born on Sept. 10, 1922, in Ogden, UT. He attended Atlantic Union College (1947-1948), receiving a T.H.B. degree; University of Illinois (1950-1951), receiving an M.S. degree in library science; and the University of Michigan (1954-1956), receiving an M.A. degree in history. In 1954, Mr. Brandon was chosen librarian of the College of Medical Evangelists, Loma Linda, CA. In 1957, he was granted a leave of absence to continue his work on a Ph.D. in library science at the University of Michigan. That same year, he was named librarian of the University of Kentucky Medical Center in Louisville. He remained there until 1963, when he became director of the Welch Medical Library of the Johns Hopkins University in Baltimore, MD. Here he reorganized the library and made it a friendly and easy-to-use place to work. In 1969, he left the Welch Library to become director of the Mount Sinai School of Medicine Library in New York City. When the librarian position at the New York Academy of Medicine became vacant in 1973, Mr. Brandon was appointed.

Al Brandon is one of the bulwarks of our profession. He has served on many committees for the Medical Library Association and in 1961 became editor of the Association's *Bulletin.* He was president of the Association from 1965 to 1966. His most recent honor was being named recipient of the coveted Marcia Noyes award in 1977.

Estelle Brodman, born in New York City, received an A.B. degree from Cornell University and a Ph.D. from the Columbia School of Library Service. She began her library career at the Cornell University School of Nursing in New York City, 1936-1937, where she was assistant librarian. She then became assistant medical librarian at Columbia University, serving from 1939 until 1949.

Dr. Brodman continued her career as assistant librarian for reference services at the National Library of Medicine from 1949 to 1960. She then was placed in charge of extramural planning. In 1961, Dr. Brodman became librarian at Washington University Medical School in St. Louis,

MO. She was also appointed associate professor of medical history. In 1964, she was promoted to professor. Dr. Brodman has traveled widely. She was the first special librarian to teach at the Library School of Keio University in Tokyo (from February through July, 1962). She also has spent considerable time as a consultant on the continent and in India.

Dr. Brodman was the editor of the Medical Library Association's *Bulletin* for 10 years, 1947 to 1957. In 1954, she was the author of *Development of Medical Bibliography*, published under the sponsorship of the Medical Library Association.

Dr. Brodman has held many important offices in the Medical Library Association, including the presidency, 1964-1965. For her outstanding work as editor of the *Bulletin*, Dr. Brodman received a special award in 1957. In 1971, in recognition of her outstanding professional achievements, she received the Marcia Noyes award.

Glenn Brudvig was born in Kenosha, WI, on Oct. 14, 1931. He attended the University of North Dakota at Grand Forks, receiving a B.S. in education in 1954 and an M.A. in history in 1956. Previously (1951-1952), Mr. Brudvig served with the U.S. Army Medical Corps in the Korean war. He was a high school teacher in Mahnomen, MN, 1954-1955, and in Herman, MN, 1956-1958. From 1958 to 1963, Mr. Brudvig was a member of the library staff at the University of North Dakota. He was acquisitions librarian and archivist, 1958-1962; part-time library science instructor, 1962-1963; and assistant librarian, 1962-1963. During part of this time, Mr. Brudvig studied library science at the University of Minnesota, receiving an M.A. in 1962.

Since 1964, Mr. Brudvig has been associated with the University of Minnesota Libraries in Minneapolis. He was supervisor of departmental libraries from January to October, 1964, and director of the Biomedical Library from 1964 to the present. He has also been assistant director of the University Libraries for Research and Development since 1968. He holds the academic rank of professor.

Mr. Brudvig has memberships in the Medical Library Association, American Library Association, Minnesota Library Association, and Minnesota Health Sciences Library Association. He has served on many committees and held many offices. These include Biomedical Communications Network, Inc., board of directors, 1976 to present; Medical Library Association annual meeting co-chairman, Minneapolis, 1976; Midwest Health Science Library Network Assembly of Resource Libraries, 1973 to present; Medical Library Association Committee on Curriculum, 1972-1975; and National Library of Medicine, Biomedical Library Review Committee, 1971-1975. In the last-named appointment, Mr. Brudvig participated in visits to 23 health science institutions. He has held many offices, including the presidency of the North Dakota Library Association (1963-1964), and has served on several University of Minnesota committees, including the Biomedical Library Committee, Research Development Council, and Health Sciences Learning Resources Committee.

Arturo Castiglioni, famous medical historian and physician, was born in Trieste, Italy, on Apr. 10, 1874. He studied medicine at Rome, Paris, and Vienna. Dr. Castiglioni received his M.D. degree from the University of Vienna in 1896. He was a clinical assistant at the University of Vienna from 1896 to 1898. Dr. Castiglioni was head of the sanitary service of the *Lloyd Triestino* from 1899 to 1918. He was chief of the health department of the Italian Lines (ships) and served also as professor of the history of medicine at the University of Padua from 1918 to 1936. He was a member of the High Council for the Public Health of Rome (1922-1929) and professor of the University for Foreigners at the University of Perugia, 1934-1938.

Arturo Castiglioni came to the United States in 1939 and was naturalized in 1946. He was research associate and lecturer on the history of medicine at Yale University from 1939 to 1942 and professor from 1943 until 1947, when he retired at the age of 73. He was a brilliant lecturer, and his talks on medical history took him to the leading universities in the United States, Europe, and South America. He was an honorary professor at the University of Chile and held honorary memberships in the Royal Society of Medicine of London, the Academia Nacional of Buenos Aires, and the American Association of the History of Medicine. After his retirement from Yale, Dr. Castiglioni returned to Rome, where he died on Jan. 21, 1952.

Called by Dr. Henry Sigerist "Italy's most outstanding historian of medicine," Dr. Castiglioni was the author of many books and articles in his chosen field. Today his *History of Medicine* (translated into English and edited by the late Dr. E. B. Krumbhaar) is now recognized as perhaps the best book of its kind. It originally appeared in Italian in 1927.

When editor of the *Bulletin of the Medical Library Association*, one of us (T.E.K.), persuaded Dr. Castiglioni, long a friend of librarians, to prepare an article for the Vesalius issue (July 1943), and he graciously wrote a superb paper, "Three Pathfinders of Science in the Renaissance."

Mary Corning's professional experience has generally been in research and science administration, including policy and program development. She also has been involved in the planning of and negotiations for regional, national, and international activities, especially those related to biomedical communication. She is fluent in several languages, an accomplishment that has aided her understanding of international problems.

Miss Corning received a B.A. degree in 1947 from the Connecticut College for Women. She majored in chemistry and French. Miss Corning then attended Mount Holyoke College in South Hadley, MA, receiving an M.A. degree in chemistry in 1949. She spent the period from 1949 to 1958 with the National Bureau of Standards as a physical chemist and technical assistant to the associate director of chemistry. From 1958 to 1960, Mary Corning was special assistant to the science advisor to the Secretary of State. From 1960 to 1964, she was employed by the National Science Foundation in various capacities as project director, special assistant to the Office of International Science Activities, and later as associate program director.

Since 1964, Mary Corning has been with the National Library of Medicine. Here she has demonstrated her versatility by serving as chief of the Publications and Translation Division (1964-1966) and special assistant to the deputy director (1966-1967). She also was detailed to the Office of the Assistant Secretary for Health and Scientific Affairs of the Department of Health, Education, and Welfare. Miss Corning served as special assistant for international programs from 1967 to 1972, becoming assistant director in 1972. She also is a federal executive fellow of the Brookings Institution.

Miss Corning belongs to many professional societies, such as the Optical Society, American Chemical Society, Medical Library Association, and Gorgas Memorial Institute of Tropical and Preventive Medicine, and has served on numerous committees of the National Academy of Science. Many awards have come her way, including the silver medal for superior service, Department of Health, Education, and Welfare (1971), and the National Library of Medicine director's award (1974).

Helen Crawford was born in Sentinel Butte, ND. She attended the University of North Dakota, receiving an A.B. degree with a major in German in 1928. After a few years of secretarial work with the North Dakota Historical Society, Miss Crawford attended Simmons College in Boston (1930-1931), where she received a B.S. in library science. Returning to the Midwest, Miss Crawford was in charge of book classification at the Iowa State University Library, Iowa City, from 1931 to 1944. She then continued her graduate education at the University of Chicago.

In 1945, she was appointed librarian of the University of Wisconsin School of Medicine in Madison. Miss Crawford held this position, including an associate professorship, until 1971, when she retired to take a library consultantship involving the formation of the new Texas Tech University School of Medicine in Lubbock. She remained until a permanent medical librarian was appointed in 1972. Miss Crawford returned to Madison and served as president of the Medical Library Association, 1972-1973. During her tenure at the University of Wisconsin,

Miss Crawford developed a fine new medical library, the William S. Middleton Medical Library.

A member of Phi Beta Kappa, Miss Crawford served as secretary for the University of Wisconsin chapter at Madison for 7 years. She belongs to many library organizations. She has been a member of the American Library Association's Standards Committee of the Association of Hospital and Institutional Libraries and chairman of the State Networks Coordinating Committee for the Council of the Midwest Regional Health Sciences.

She has served the Medical Library Association well in many capacities. She taught a refresher course in 1959, served on the Bylaws Committee and the Certification Committee, was chairman of the Exchange Committee, was a member of the executive board, and, as already mentioned, achieved the presidency. An earlier honor was the receipt of the presidential citation of the State Medical Society of Wisconsin (1962).

Susan N. Young Crawford, a Canadian by birth, graduated with an A.B. degree from the University of British Columbia at Vancouver in 1948. Personal responsibilities brought her to Chicago. She attended the University of Chicago, receiving an M.A. degree in biological sciences in 1955. Also that year, she became a naturalized citizen of the United States. Attracted to librarianship, Mrs. Crawford became assistant librarian of the American Dental Association. In 1959, she was appointed director of the Archive-Library Department of the American Medical Association, Chicago, which subsequently became the Division of Library and Archives. Mrs. Crawford continued her graduate education at the University of Chicago and received a Ph.D.

Dr. Crawford has been involved with many activities in the Medical Library Association, such as Medical Society Libraries group chairman, 1965, and program chairman, 1978; consulting editor of the *Bulletin*, 1976-1979; Committee on Surveys and Statistics, appointed in 1966, chairman from 1975 to present; member of the Nominating Committee, 1975-1976; member of the Nominating Committee, 1975-1976; member of the Editorial Committee, *Handbook of Medical Library Practice*, 1971-1972; and annual meeting co-chairman, 1962.

Dr. Crawford also has been busy with other professional activities. These include member, the American Association for the Advancement of Science; member, Newcomb Prize Committee (1977); consultant, Office of Science Information, National Science Foundation (1977); and consultant, National Institute for Neurological and Communicable Diseases. Her professional honors include membership on the board of regents, National Library of Medicine, 1971-1974; certificate of recognition, United States Public Health Service; and recipient in 1975 of the Eliot prize, Medical Library Association.

Martin Marc Cummings, the amiable and efficient current director of the National Library of Medicine, has served in this important post since 1964. He attended Bucknell University, where he received an A.B. degree in 1941. His medical education was obtained from Duke University School of Medicine in Durham, NC. He interned at the Boston Marine Hospital from 1944 to 1945, was assistant resident there from 1945 to 1946, and spent the next year as a research fellow at the State Serum Institute, Copenhagen, Denmark. Dr. Cummings served as director of the Tuberculosis Evaluation Laboratory at the Communicable Disease Center in Atlanta, GA, from 1947 to 1949. From 1948 to 1953, he served on the faculty of medicine at Emory University School of Medicine in Atlanta, advancing to associate professor.

In 1953, Dr. Cummings was appointed director of research services at the Veterans Administration Central Office in Washington, DC, and he held this position until 1959. During these years, he also taught microbiology at George Washington University School of Medicine, Washington, DC. From 1959 to 1961, Dr. Cummings was chairman of and professor in the Department of Microbiology at the University of Oklahoma School of Medicine, Oklahoma City. In 1961, Dr. Cummings became chief of the Office of International Research at the National Institutes of Health, a position he held until 1963. At that time, he became associate director for research grants at the National Institutes of Health, and he continued in this capacity until he accepted his present position.

Dr. Cummings became a student and friend of the late Dr. Wilburt C. Davison, dean of the medical school at Duke University and a former Rhodes scholar. Dr. Davison was a former student of Sir William Osler at Oxford. Perhaps some of Dr. Cummings' interest in books, writing, and libraries stems from his friendship with Dr. Davison.

His memberships include the American Osler Society; Association of Research Libraries; Medical Library Association; Howard Florey Institute for Physiology and Medicine, Melbourne, Australia; honorary fellowship, Osler Club of London; and honorary member, World Health Organization.

Dr. Cummings' professional awards include many honorary doctorates, such as a D.Sc. degree from his alma mater, Bucknell University; a Doctor of Medicine from the Karolinska Institute in Stockholm, Sweden; and a Doctor Honoris Causa, Academy of Medicine, Lodz, Poland. He holds many other awards of distinction, including an alumnus membership in Phi Beta Kappa.

Dr. Cummings is the author of more than 100 scientific and historical publications and is a co-author of a textbook on tuberculosis.

No medical librarian was known better during her lifetime than **Eileen R. Cunningham**, who was for many years director of the library of the

Vanderbilt School of Medicine in Nashville, TN. Her impact upon our profession is still felt. Mrs. Cunningham had begun work on the fifth edition of the *Cunningham Classification for Medical Literature* before her death in 1965. Miss Eleanor Steinke, her successor, assisted by Miss Mary Louise Gladish, completed this revision, and it was published by the Vanderbilt University Press in 1967.

Born Eileen Roach in Baltimore, MD, she attended Roland Park School for Girls and later Johns Hopkins University. Much of her education, however, was received from private tutors, and she became proficient in foreign languages, especially French, Spanish, German, and Swedish. In 1921, Mrs. Cunningham put her scholarship and language knowledge to work in translating and abstracting foreign scientific literature for physicians. Attracted in this way to medical librarianship, she became associated with the newly developing Vanderbilt University School of Medicine. In 1929, she became chief librarian. Over the years under her guidance, Vanderbilt's medical library prospered and grew into one of the best medical libraries in the South. In addition, Mrs. Cunningham held the position of professor of library science, and when the new library was dedicated in 1964, she was recognized as the librarian "who had made the Vanderbilt Medical Library famous around the world."

Mrs. Cunningham was devoted to the affairs of the Medical Library Association. She chaired numerous committees and also served in other capacities, especially those concerning international cooperation both at home and abroad. She also prepared the excellent chapter on reference work in the first two editions of the Association's *Handbook*, together with its exhaustive list of references. Eileen Cunningham was elected president of the Medical Library Association in 1948 and the next year became the first recipient of the Marcia Noyes award. She was also responsible for aiding foreign medical librarians and got the Rockefeller Foundation to supply the funds for a 10-year period. Of interest, perhaps, to our readers, is the announcement in the *Bulletin* for July 1967, of her bequest to the Medical Library Association of $33,000, the money to be used to aid medical librarians from countries other than the United States to continue their medical library education in the United States.

Medical librarianship was greatly enhanced by the career of this remarkable woman.

Louise Darling was born in Los Angeles. She is related on her mother's side of the family to the famous surgeon and bibliophile Dr. Rudolf Matas of New Orleans. Her paternal grandfather, Dr. Andrew F. Darling, was a prominent early practitioner in the area around Los Angeles.

Miss Darling received an A.B. degree from the University of California,

Los Angeles, majoring in biology. She earned an M.A. in botany and then studied at the library school of the University of California in Berkeley. Miss Darling began her library career as assistant librarian of the Giannini Foundation of Agricultural Economics, University of California in Berkeley. After more library school courses, Miss Darling became librarian of the Acalanes Union High School nearby and then accepted the position of science reference assistant in the Library of Southern California, Los Angeles.

In 1944, Miss Darling joined the Army Library Service in Hawaii, where she worked in a variety of post and hospital libraries. After V-J Day, she was sent with a small group to organize Army libraries in the Philippines. She was then persuaded to return to her alma mater to organize the library of the life sciences departments of the newly organized medical center. Her zealous and thoughtful approach has brought into being one of America's most distinctive biomedical libraries, which is renowned for its fine collections and services. Miss Darling has been recognized for her achievements by her alma mater and by her colleagues in medical librarianship.

Louise Darling has contributed many publications to enrich medical librarians and physicians. She has held many offices in the Medical Library Association and served as its president from 1963 to 1964. The Association recognized her professional achievements by choosing her as the recipient of the Marcia Noyes award in 1974.

Janet Doe was born in South Newbury, VT, spent her childhood in Lexington, MA, and attended Wellesley College, where she majored in science. The profession of nursing interested Miss Doe, and she attended the Vassar Training School for Nurses. She continued nurses' training at Presbyterian Hospital in New York City. Because of a severe knee problem, Miss Doe reluctantly gave up nursing as a career. Finding librarianship exciting and to her liking, she studied this subject at the New York Public Library School. After receiving a certificate in librarianship, Miss Doe worked there briefly as a reviser of students' classwork and as a cataloger.

In 1923, Miss Doe became assistant librarian of the Rockefeller Institute for Medical Research. In 1926, she accepted the position as head of the Periodicals Department of the New York Academy of Medicine. It as at this institution that Miss Doe was to make her distinguished career. In 1929, she was appointed assistant librarian. In her new position as administrative associate to Dr. Malloch, the librarian, Miss Doe made the library run well, and her acumen and drive contributed much to the reputation of this great library. When Dr. Malloch resigned because of ill health, Miss Doe became the first female librarian of the Academy.

Miss Doe has made many contributions to medical librarianship. In 1936, she was elected secretary of the Medical Library Association, and she continued in this position for 4 years. She then became editor of the Association's first edition of the *Handbook of Medical Library Practice*. Published in 1943, the book was the result of much effort by her and the contributors. Probably more than any other publication of the Medical Library Association, this volume brought a professional status to medical librarianship. Previously, in 1937, after years of scholarly pursuit, Miss Doe's *A Bibliography of the Works of Ambroise Paré* had been issued. This volume established Miss Doe's reputation in medical history.

Miss Doe served as a member with other prominent librarians of a survey of the Army Medical Library. The report of the survey (1943) started the reutilization of the library to become the great National Library of Medicine. Miss Doe was appointed an honorary consultant to the Army Medical Library. When this organization was dissolved, she became a member of the smaller group of advisors to the library. Miss Doe was responsible, too, for preparing an index to the classification schedules (1945) for the Army Medical Library.

Miss Doe served as president of the Medical Library Association from 1948 to 1949, received the Marcia Noyes award in 1954, and was elected an honorary and fellow member upon her retirement in 1956. As mentioned in Chapter I, her professional colleagues thought so much of her as truly representative of the best in medical librarianship that they named a lecture in her honor. It is eagerly anticipated as the highlight of the annual meetings.

Merlin K. DuVal was born on Oct. 12, 1922, in Montclair, NJ. He received an A.B. from Dartmouth College in Hanover, NH, in 1943. He then attended Dartmouth Medical School, receiving their 2-year certificate in 1944. He continued his medical education at Cornell University Medical College in New York City, obtaining an M.D. degree in 1946. Dr. DuVal served his internships at New York Hospital (1946-1947) and at the Roosevelt Hospital, New York City (1949-1950). Dr. DuVal was on active duty with the U.S. Navy from 1947 to 1949 at two Navy hospitals. He then held a 4-year residency in surgery at the Veterans Administration Hospital, Bronx, NY.

Dr. DuVal spent 1954 to 1956 as an instructor and later assistant professor in surgery at New York State University College of Medicine. He also was attending surgeon at the Veterans Administration Hospital in Brooklyn as well as a consultant at St. Albans Naval Hospital.

From 1956 to 1961, Dr. DuVal was a Markle scholar in medical science. His research during this period involved many significant studies of diseases of the pancreas.

Dr. DuVal was called to the University of Oklahoma School of Medicine, Oklahoma City, as associate professor of surgery in 1957, advancing to professor in 1961. He also was assistant director of the University of Oklahoma Medical Center from 1962 to 1963.

In 1964, Dr. Du Val became the dean in charge of building a professional and paramedical staff at the new medical school at the University of Arizona in Tucson. One of the areas he concentrated on was building a medical library. During the next few years, Dr. DuVal was also appointed chairman of the Governor's Committee of Arizona's Regional Medical Programs and held many related appointments.

His work attracted the attention of the U.S. Department of Health, Education, and Welfare (HEW), and he served as a consultant to its Bureau of Health Manpower from 1966 to 1968. During these years, Dr. DuVal was project director of the National Library of Medicine study. He continued with HEW on the National Advisory Council on Education for the Health Professions from 1968 to 1971. His leadership qualities were recognized when he became, in 1971, assistant secretary for health for HEW. Dr. DuVal held this important post until 1973. It involved working with the American Medical Association and the Association of American Medical Colleges as liaison representative of the department. He also served as chief of the U.S. delegation to the World Health Organization meeting held in Geneva, Switzerland, in 1972 and as chief of the U.S. delegation to the Western Hemisphere meeting of the Ministers of Health held later that year.

In 1973, Dr. DuVal returned to the Medical School of the University of Arizona as acting dean and tht same year was appointed to his present position, vice-president of health sciences. He was also appointed consultant to the director of the Lister Hill National Center for Biomedical Communications of the National Library of Medicine (1975-1976).

Dr. DuVal holds memberships in many professional societies, including the American Medical Association, for which he served on the Advisory Committee on Undergraduate Medical Education from 1967 to 1971. He became a fellow in the American College of Surgeons in 1958 and later (1965-1968) a member of their board of governors and of the Committee on Undergraduate Education (1967-1970). He also received a membership in the American Surgical Association and has served on many of their committees. Dr. DuVal has held many positions with the Association of American Medical Colleges and for his work became a distinguished service member in 1974. His publications number more than 80, and many are on subjects relating to librarianship.

Jacqueline Williams Felter was born in Cleveland, OH, in 1909. She attended Western Reserve University in Cleveland, receiving a B.S. in library science in 1931. She then accepted the position of branch librarian of the Osterhout Free Library in Wilkes-Barre, PA. In 1936, she became librarian at Kingston (Pennsylvania) High School.

After marrying Irving Felter and moving to New York, Jacqueline began her career in medical librarianship as an assistant in the library of the New York Postgraduate Medical School and Hospital in 1943. When a change of administration took place in 1946, Mrs. Felter succeeded to the head librarian's position. In 1948, she became librarian at the Memorial Sloan-Kettering Cancer Center and transformed their meager library resources into a fine collection. In 1960, Mrs. Felter became librarian of the Medical Society of the County of Queens. Soon thereafter, in the fall of 1961, she accepted the position as director of the much-needed Union Catalog of Medical Periodicals.

Because of her spirit of cooperation with other libraries and librarians, she was chosen in 1967 to head the Medical Library Center of New York. She retired in 1974 but kept up her library interest by working on special projects for the Center until illness, which had plagued her for many years, forced her to stop early in 1976. She died on Sept. 19, 1976. In October, there was a memorial service at the New York Academy of Medicine. In tribute to Jacqueline, three addresses were given by her close friends Alfred Brandon, Estelle Brodman, and a fellow worker, Spencer C. Marsh.

Her quiet but incisive demeanor was noticed by the officers of the Medical Library Association, and she served from 1953 to 1956 on the Association's Committee on International Cooperation. From 1958 to 1961, Mrs. Felter was associate editor of the *Bulletin*. She declined the editorship on several occasions but consented to be editor pro tem from 1965 to 1966 during Mr. Brandon's presidency. Much was accomplished by her association with the *Bulletin*. Librarians can be grateful for the fine indexes she compiled covering volumes 1 through 50. With Gertrude Annan, Mrs. Felter was co-editor of the third edition of the *Handbook of Medical Library Practice*, published in 1969. She was elected to the presidency of the Medical Library Association for 1968-1969. She also was the Association's official representative at the Third International Congress on Medical Librarianship held in Amsterdam in 1969. Mrs. Felter served on many committees, and in recognition of her many accomplishments, she was made an honorary member of the Medical Library Association in 1974.

Max Harold Fisch was born in Elma, WI, on Dec. 21, 1900. He attended Butler University in Indiana and received an A.B. degree in 1924. From 1924 to 1928, he attended Cornell University in Ithaca, NY, where he received a Ph.D. Dr. Fisch began his academic career as instructor in philosophy at Cornell. He also became assistant to the editors of *The Philosophical Review* (1926-1928). During the summer of 1930, Dr. Fisch served at Cornell as assistant professor of Philosophy.

From 1928 to 1943, Dr. Fisch was assistant professor of philosophy at Western Reserve University, Cleveland, OH. During World War II, Dr. Fisch was appointed curator of rare books at the Cleveland Branch of the Army Medical Library. A great scholar with a fine knowledge of Latin and the Romance languages, he was an ideal choice for this position. Under his immediate supervision, about 10,000 rare medical books were carefully recataloged and restored, especially manuscripts and incunabula. During this time, too, he helped in the preparation of Blakiston's *New Gould Medical Dictionary* and was associate editor of the *Bulletin of the Medical Library Association.* Dr. Fisch served as chief of the History of Medicine Division of the U.S. Army in Cleveland from January to August 1946. Then he became professor of philosophy at the University of Illinois in Urbana, serving with distinction until 1969. He is now professor emeritus, but he has continued his career. At present, he is adjunct professor of philosophy at Indiana University-Purdue University at Indianapolis.

Sabbatical leaves took Dr. Fisch to Italy on two occasions—in 1939 and again from 1950 to 1951, when he was visiting professor on a Fulbright appointment at the University of Naples. Dr. Fisch had a second Fulbright appointment from 1958 to 1959 at Keio University in Tokyo, Japan. In 1960, he was appointed a George Santayana fellow at Harvard University. He also was an honorary research associate at Harvard, 1966-1967. He has served visiting professorships in philosophy in several American universities over the years. In 1955 and 1956, Dr. Fisch traveled in Egypt, Jordan, Lebanon, Turkey, and Syria—exploring the early philosophy of the great teachers of the past in his field.

His interest in medical history developed during his assignment with the Army Medical Library. One of us (T.E.K.) was editor of the *Bulletin of the Medical Library Association* at the time Dr. Fisch was associate editor. Our first issue, published in July 1943, was on Vesalius in celebration of the publication of the *Fabrica,* the first significant modern anatomy, superbly and handsomely produced. The issue was noticed with a favorable comment in *Time,* Aug. 9, 1943. To this number, Dr. Fisch contributed two scholarly articles, "Vesalius and His Book" and "The Printer of Vesalius's *Fabrica.*" Both are classics, and we have chosen to reproduce for our readers Fisch's first contribution. Dr. Fisch was also a member of the original board of editors of the *Journal of the History of Medicine and Allied Sciences,* published by the late Henry Schuman, as well as of Schuman's *Life of Science Library.*

Alderson Fry was born on Mar. 26, 1906, in Hawk's Nest, WV. Before settling into his two professions, law and librarianship, he roamed the country, taking odd jobs as he could find them, traveling by motorcycle. He lost a leg as a motorcycle stunt rider in a carnival. Very few people were aware of this loss, because he carried himself well. One of us (T.E.K.) didn't sense that Alderson had a wooden leg until, on a visit to Rochester, MN, he climbed a steep hill with some effort. That evening at my home, where he was an overnight guest, I played a Paul Whiteman record of "Rhapsody in Blue," since I knew of his love of jazz acquired in his 20's in New Orleans. Alderson said, "Tom, that isn't jazz!" His jazz was of a sophisticated caliber, and he pursued his avocation as well as a devotion to science fiction throughout his career.

Mr. Fry returned to West Virginia and attended Marshall College in Huntington, receiving a B.S. degree with a major in geology in 1928. He later attended George Peabody College in Nashville, TN, receiving a degree in librarianship in 1933. In 1939, he received a degree in law from Vanderbilt University in Nashville. While studying law at Vanderbilt, Mr. Fry worked part-time as a student assistant in the library. Sometime later, he became librarian of Meharry Medical College in Nashville. After graduating from Vanderbilt's law school, he left Meharry for a successful practice with a Nashville law firm. While at Meharry, he did much to improve the library structure as well as its services. Subsequently, these talents led to his appointment as librarian of the University of Washington's new medical center in Seattle.

At the University of Washington he had the opportunity of planning a new library from start to finish. He often disagreed with the architects and generally won them over. The library is a good facility, but no account was taken of the enormous expansion of the literature. The library outgrew its facilities and has had to be remodeled. But it had many innovative features, and the word got around.

Mr. Fry returned to West Virginia in 1955 to plan and to build (one imagines that here, too, the architects needed persuasion) the library for the new University of West Virginia Medical Center in Morgantown. From 1955 until 1971, Alderson Fry was their librarian and stayed on the staff until his retirement in 1972. He died in 1976.

Scott Adams[5] pointed out that Fry was the first to use the term "health sciences library." Alderson was colorful, unconventional, outspoken, and argumentative, but he possessed good common sense and a salty humor. For many years he served the Medical Library Association as its parliamentarian (beginning in 1958 with the meeting in Rochester, MN).

Mr. Fry's publications were well written and interesting. Many were on library planning, including his fine chapter in the third edition of the Medical Library Association's *Handbook.* These abilities were noticed by some organizations, especially the Pan American Health Association and the Rockefeller Foundation. Consequently, he served as visiting consultant to help plan the National Library of Medicine of Chile. He assisted in the planning of the National Library of Medicine of India at New Delhi. And as a consultant, he also gave his advice to medical libraries in Japan, Hong Kong, Malaya, and Greece. As mentioned by Scott Adams, Alderson was called on again by the Pan American Health Organization for advice on medical library development in Jamaica, Trinidad, and Venezuela.

Eugene Garfield is the founder and president of the Institute for Scientific Information housed in Philadelphia, PA. This institute is of invaluable help to librarians in medicine and allied fields. Dr. Garfield has more than 400 people in the employment and distribution of the publications of this computerized approach to the literature of scientific and technical information. Helping Garfield from the start was the late Dr. Chauncey Leake, whose advice and encouragement were of great significance. Dr. Garfield met Dr. Leake in 1951 while working in the Welch Medical Library on an indexing project under the late Dr. Sanford Larkey. Garfield often discussed his problems with Dr. Leake. A feeling of friendship and understanding grew up between the scientist and the librarian interested in the retrieval of the literature. Dr. Leake became chairman of the editorial advisory board for *Current Contents,* now issued in six fields. Dr. Leake also was a member of the editorial board for Garfield's *Index to Scientific Reviews.* Recently, Garfield published a two-volume work, *Essays of an Information Scientist,* in which he reviews progress in many fields. Garfield also operates many computerized services.

Dr. Garfield attended Columbia University in New York City, where he received a B.S. degree in chemistry (1949) and an M.S. in library science (1954). He later received a Ph.D. degree (1961) in structural linguistics from the University of Pennsylvania in Philadelphia. He was the first fellow of the Grolier Society, 1953-1954.

Dr. Garfield belongs to many organizations, including the American Society for Information Science, Medical Library Association, Special Libraries Association, Institute of Electric and Electronic Engineers, Association for Computer Machinery, American Chemical Society, Authors' League and Guild, and American Association for the Advancement of Science, in which he currently (1978) serves as chairman-elect of Section T (Information, Computing, and Communication). He is also a fellow of the Institute of Information Scientists of London and has served on several committees of the National Academy of Sciences.

Murray Gottlieb, a scholarly bookdealer and owner with his wife, Johanna, of the Old Hickory Bookshop, originally located in New York City, died suddenly of a cerebral hemorrhage on July 16, 1954. Mr. Gottlieb was known and admired by medical librarians, and many sought his advice in building up their rare book collections, be they large or small. To honor Mr. Gottlieb's memory, his widow, Mrs. Ralph Grimes of Brinklow, MD, where Old Hickory Bookshop is now located, gives an award annually for the best article written by medical librarians on some aspect of the history of medicine or allied sciences. This award is sponsored by the Medical Library Association, and its presentation is one of the highlights of the Association's annual meeting.

Gertrude Annan and Estelle Brodman in tribute wrote:

> It has been traditional since the time of Henry Stevens of Vermont that the dealer be a mentor, a guide, a friend. No one exemplified this tradition more than Murray Gottlieb of the Old Hickory Bookshop. To him selling books was not a business but a way of life. It was his pleasure to be able to give advice and encouragement. It was his aim not to get the highest price for a book but to see it go into the collection it would most fittingly grace[6].

Oliver Wendell Holmes was born in Cambridge, MA, on Aug. 29, 1809. His father, the Reverend Abiel Holmes, was the minister of the First Church before it became Unitarian. It is thought that Holmes' exposure to good reading and the companionship of thoughtful elders greatly benefited his subsequent career. He has had considerable influence as a distinguished poet and essayist. When he was 21, his poem "Old Ironsides" brought him into prominence and resulted in the saving of the famous ship the U.S. Constitution. Later, his "Chambered Nautilus" brought him acclaim as a serious poet. His masterpiece of light verse is "The Wonderful One Hoss Shay." He made many more contributions as an essayist and novelist. But here we are concerned with his library interests and medical accomplishments.

Holmes attended Phillips Academy in Andover, MA, and then studied at Harvard College, graduating in 1829. After studying law for a year, Holmes decided on a medical career. He first went to a private medical school in Boston and then took some courses at the Harvard Medical School. In 1833, Mr. Holmes sailed to Europe and studied medicine in the hospitals in Paris under the famous physicians and surgeons Larrey and Louis. In 1835, Holmes returned to Boston, and in 1836, he received his M.D. degree from Harvard.

As a writer, lecturer, and anatomist, Holmes brought distinction to medicine. His paper "The Contagiousness of Puerperal Fever," now a great medical classic, was originally published in 1843. It attracted little attention, but Holmes persisted in his efforts, and the article was reprinted with additions in 1855. At this time, he had his supporters but also detractors, but at a later date, 1891, in again reprinting his article, he convinced the American obstetricians of the value of antisepsis in postpartum care. Meanwhile, Dr. Ignaz Semmelweis (1818-1965) of Hungary, unaware of Holmes' paper, came to the same conclusion. Semmelweis was bitterly attacked by his European colleagues and died, presumably from an infection due to streptococcus cellulitis, after confinement in a mental asylum. Another interesting accomplishment was Holmes's suggesting the word "anaesthesia" in a letter to Dr. William T. G. Morton, Nov. 21, 1846. The term is still in use to signify insensibility to pain in surgical procedures when an anesthetic agent is used.

For 3 months a year from 1839 to 1849, Dr. Holmes served at Dartmouth College as professor of anatomy. In 1847, he was appointed Parkman Professor of Anatomy in Harvard Medical School. At Harvard, he was also dean of the medical school from 1847 to 1853. He was gifted as a lecturer, especially to medical students, who always applauded him before his talks. Holmes continued at Harvard, becoming an emeritus professor in 1882.

Long a collector of medical classics, Holmes presented his personal library of 2,000 volumes to the Boston Medical Library in 1889 and described it in an "Address Before the Boston Medical Library Association" (Boston Med Surg J 120:129-130, 1889). We have decided to reprint, however, his "Dedicatory Address" delivered at the opening of the Boston Medical Library, Dec. 3, 1878, during Holmes' presidency. The article, eloquent and of great significance, describes Holmes' collection as well as the importance of medical libraries. Sir William Osler called Oliver Wendell Holmes "the most successful combination the world has ever seen of physician and man of letters." Dr. Holmes died on Oct. 7, 1894, just after his 85th birthday.

Mildred McMillan Jordan was born on Aug. 11, 1908, in Hartsville, SC. She attended Winthrop College in Rock Hill, SC, receiving a B.A. degree in 1929. Miss Jordan continued her education at Emory University in Atlanta, GA, receiving a B.A. in library science in 1930 and an M.A. degree from the department of history in 1942. Miss Jordan became librarian and professor of medical bibliography at Emory University School of Medicine in Atlanta in 1933. Here she continued until her death from cancer on Oct. 7, 1965.

She had charm, spunk, and indomitable courage—especially in the face of her illness, which she fought hard to overcome. She was an excellent presiding officer, especially during her presidency of the Medical Library Association (1959-1960). She was a distinguished member of the Association, serving on many committees and the board of directors. Miss Jordan served her country during World War II as southern regional director of medical library service for the Armed Forces.

She was very much concerned about the need to recruit desirable young people to medical librarianship. To aid this worthy objective, she developed and taught a Medical Library Association-approved course in medical librarianship at Emory University from 1951 through 1965. In 1961, Miss Jordan was awarded a 5-year U.S. Public Health Service grant to establish and conduct an internship program for medical librarians. Her interest in medical librarianship became international when she was invited to participate in a symposium on education and training for medical librarianship at the First International Congress on Medical Librarianship held in London in 1953. She was also appointed lecturer at the first Seminar on Medical Librarianship held in Medellin, Colombia, South America, in 1960.

Mildred Jordan received the Medical Library Association's highest honor, the Marcia Noyes award, in September 1964. Her interest in her profession was furthered by her many contributions to the literature of medical librarianship, including Chapter 4 in the second edition of the Association's *Handbook of Medical Library Practice*, published in 1956.

Always interested in the history of Georgia and the Confederacy, she published many articles on these subjects.

Jack D. Key was appointed librarian at the Mayo Clinic in March 1970. He is also an instructor in the history of medicine and an assistant professor of biomedical communications at the Mayo Medical School. Mr. Key received a B.A. degree from Phillips University in 1958, an M.A. from the University of New Mexico in 1960, and an M.S. from the University of Illinois in 1962. He was certified by the Medical Library Association in 1962, and, before joining the Mayo Clinic, served as staff supervisor at the University of Illinois Graduate Library, pharmacy librarian at the University of Iowa, and medical librarian for the Lovelace Foundation, Albuquerque, NM.

Mr. Key has published approximately 80 articles on medical history, librarianship, and library automation in various professional journals; edited a book entitled *Library Automation—The Orient and South Pacific LARC Press*, 1975; edited a monographic series entitled *Automated Activities in Health Sciences Libraries*, 1975-1978; and traveled as a consultant or speaker to Japan, Hong Kong, Singapore, New Zealand, Australia, Iceland, and Egypt.

Mr. Key is a member of the Medical Library Association, American Association for the History of Medicine, American Institute for the History of Pharmacy, American Medical Writers Association, American Osler Society, and various other organizations on local, state, and national levels.

Thomas E. Keys graduated from Beloit College, Beloit, WI, in 1931 with a B.A. degree and received an M.A. degree from the Graduate Library School of the University of Chicago in 1934. He was library assistant at the Newberry Library in Chicago in 1931 and 1932. Keys attended the University of Chicago as a Carnegie fellow in the Graduate Library School in the fall of 1932. In 1933, he held an assistantship at the Graduate Library School.

Tom Keys joined the library staff at the Mayo Clinic in Rochester, MN, in 1934 as assistant librarian and served from 1935 to 1942 as reference librarian. In June 1942, he entered the Army as a first lieutenant in the Medical Administration Corps and was assigned as assistant to the librarian of the Army Medical Library. Later that year, he was appointed officer-in-charge of the Cleveland Branch of the Army Medical Library. During his Army career, he was responsible for the restoration of more than 8,000 rare books in medicine and the allied sciences. He returned to civilian life in 1946 after having attained the rank of lieutenant colonel. He was awarded the Army Commendation Ribbon by the Secretary of War. His alma mater, Beloit College, presented him their Distinguished Service citation in 1956 and in 1972 conferred upon him an honorary Sc.D. In 1966, he was the recipient of the Marcia Noyes award.

In 1946, he returned to the Mayo Clinic as librarian, and in 1957, he was appointed assistant professor of medical history in the Mayo Graduate School of Medicine. He advanced to associate professor in 1963 and to professor in 1969. He was an organizer of and, from 1964 to 1967, president of the Mayo Foundation History of Medicine Society.

Dr. Keys held the post of librarian at the Mayo Clinic until 1969 and was senior library consultant from 1969 to 1972. He retired in December 1972 after 38 years of distinguished service.

He is a member of the American Association for the History of Medicine, International Society for the History of Medicine, Medical Library Association (president, 1957-1958), Special Libraries Association, Sigma Xi, Pi Kappa Alpha, Beta Phi Mu (national honorary library fraternity), and Phi Beta Kappa. He is a charter member of the American Osler Society, an honorary member of the American Society of Anesthesiologists, and a former member of the board of regents of the National Library of Medicine, having been appointed to the board by President Eisenhower and having served under both Eisenhower and Kennedy. He is also a corresponding member of the Swedish Medical Association Section on Medical History.

Dr. Keys was editor of the *Bulletin of the Medical Library Association* (1942-1945), has served as a member of the editorial board of Blakiston's *New Gould Medical Dictionary*, and has been an advisory member of the Committee to Survey Biological Abstracts. He was compiler of *Cardiac Classics* (1941, in association with Dr. F. A. Willius) and of the two-volume *Foundations in Anesthesiology* (1965, with Dr. Albert Faulconer, Jr.). He is author of *The Development of Anesthesia* (1943), *The History of Surgical Anesthesia* (1945) and revised edition (1963), and *Applied Medical Library Practice* (1958). Dr. Keys has lectured extensively in the United States, the Far East, and Europe. He has contributed numerous papers on medical library work and on the history of medicine. *The History of Surgical Anesthesia* was translated into Japanese (1966) and into German (1968).

As a colleague said about him in 1957, equally true today,

> to the present, his footsteps have not deviated from the primrose path of librarianship. With like restraint, and good fortune, he has needed but two libraries, in this near quarter of a century, as theatres of operation. If they happened to be good ones, he has made them better[7].

David Kronick was born in Connelsville, PA, on Oct. 5, 1917. He attended Western Reserve University, Cleveland, OH, from 1936 to 1939, where he received a B.A. degree with a major in American literature. From the same university, he received a B.L.S. degree in 1940. After holding various positions, Mr. Kronick became librarian of the Western Reserve University School of Medicine (1946-1950). He then continued his higher education at the University of Chicago, receiving a Ph.D. from the Graduate Library School in 1953.

Dr. Kronick served as library assistant at the National Library of Medicine in Bethesda, MD, from 1953 to 1955. Then he became librarian of the University of Michigan School of Medicine, serving until 1959. In that year, he accepted the directorship of the Cleveland Medical Library. From 1964 to 1965 he was chief of the reference division of the National Library of Medicine. Dr. Kronick was then named professor of medical bibliography and director of medical communications at the University of Texas Medical School in San Antonio, his present position.

Dr. Kronick has on many occasions been appointed as medical library consultant. Chief among these appointments were those for the University of Oklahoma, the University of Florida, and the National Library of Medicine. Dr. Kronick surveyed medical libraries in South America in 1965 and in Texas in 1967.

For the Medical Library Association, he has served as business manager and held a 3-year appointment to its board of directors. He has been president of the Texas Council of Health Science Librarians and has held other offices. He has written articles on medical library practice and on the historical aspects of the profession. In 1962, he published a book entitled *A History of Scientific and Technical Periodicals.*

Mildred Crowe Langner was born in Chattanooga, TN, and attended the University of Chattanooga, receiving an A.B. degree in 1933 after majoring in English literature. In 1935, she became head of cataloging and acquisition librarian for the branches of the Chattanooga Public Library, and from 1940 to 1944 she served as librarian of the Chattanooga Medical Society. She then became assistant under Mrs. Eileen Cunningham at the Vanderbilt Medical Library in Nashville, TN. At the same time, she was the Medical Library Association's first intern (1944-1945). Simultaneously, Miss Crowe studied at Peabody College for Teachers in Nashville, receiving a B.S. degree in library science in 1945.

Miss Crowe was appointed chief librarian and assistant professor at the University of Alabama Medical Center in Birmingham in 1945. In her tenure of 10 years, Miss Crowe built up a fine collection of books and journals, and even after leaving this position, she maintained her interest in the library at Alabama Medical Center. She played an important role in helping Dr. Lawrence Reynolds, a Detroit roentgenologist, decide to give an exceptionally fine library of rare medical books to the University of Alabama Medical Center, including a small building to house the rare books.

Miss Crowe left Birmingham in 1955 to become librarian and assistant professor of medical bibliography at the newly opened University of Miami School of Medicine in Miami, FL. Here she had the dual responsibility of administering the basic science library housed in Coral Gables and the new clinical collection housed in Miami. She continued to build up both libraries, and finally they were combined. Soon after coming to Miami, Miss Crowe married Julian Langner, who had become one of the leading economic research consultants in southern Florida. The marriage was cut short 4 years later by Mr. Langner's death.

In 1961, Mrs. Langner became chief of the reference services division of the National Library of Medicine in Bethesda, MD. Everywhere she worked saw an improvement in library service, and her disarming but decisive manner and her friendly and attractive ways have endeared her to the profession. Mrs. Langner returned to the University of Miami School of Medicine to head the library again in 1963. In 1967, she achieved the rank of professor of medical bibliography. Under her leadership, a beautiful new library, the Louis Calder Memorial Library, named in honor of a prominent benefactor, was built, aided by a large grant from the Health Manpower Bureau; it was dedicated in 1972.

Mrs. Langner has been active in the affairs of the Medical Library Association. She was editor of the Association's *Bulletin* from 1957 to 1961, later serving on the publication committee. She was secretary to the Medical Library Association from 1948 to 1949. She also served as the Association's chairman of its standards Committee and as the first chairman of the Refresher Course Committee for the courses in continuing education for medical librarians from 1958 to 1959. For many years, too, she was chairman of the Honors and Awards Committee. She was elected president of the Association for the years 1966 and 1967. For her leadership in many fields of medical librarianship, Mrs. Langner received the Marcia Noyes award in 1976. Upon her retirement in 1978, Mrs. Langner was named an honorary member and fellow of the Medical Library Association.

Sanford V. Larkey was born in Oakland, CA, on May 11, 1898. He attended the University of California in Berkeley, receiving a B.A. in 1921. Then he studied medicine in San Francisco at the University of California, graduating in 1925 at the head of his class. He greatly enjoyed English literature and spent 2 years at Oxford University in England, earning both B.A. and M.A. degrees, the latter in 1931.

In 1930, Dr. Larkey was appointed assistant professor of medical history and librarian of the University of California School of Medicine (San Francisco). Except for a period at the Huntington Library, in Pasadena, CA, where he held an international fellowship in Tudor science, Dr. Larkey remained at his position until 1935. He then was chosen to succeed Fielding H. Garrison, M.D., as director of the William H. Welch Library of the Johns Hopkins University in Baltimore, M.D. Dr. Larkey was also appointed as lecturer at the Johns Hopkins Institute of the History of Medicine. Following his retirement from the directorship of the Welch Medical Library in 1963, Dr. Larkey continued as lecturer in the history of medicine. He also served on the advisory council of the Folger Library in Washington, DC, and continued his research on public health and medicine during the times of Tudor England.

During World War I, Dr. Larkey served as a second lieutenant in the U.S. Army, and in World War II, he was in the Army Medical Corps, achieving the rank of colonel. Dr. Larkey traveled widely in Europe between 1942 and 1946, laying the groundwork for the history of the medical department. For his endeavors he was the recipient of the Bronze Star medal.

Dr. Larkey belonged to several societies, including the Medical Library

Association, American Association for the History of Medicine, and History of Science Society. He also was a member of the Bohemian Club (San Francisco) and the Charaka Club (New York City). Dr. Larkey became a member of the Medical Library Association in 1933, wrote many articles for the *Bulletin*, and served the Association in several capacities, including the presidency (1949-1950). He was elected to honorary membership in 1964. His death occurred on Apr. 16, 1969.

With the death of Dr. **Chauncey D. Leake** in San Francisco on Jan. 11, 1978, medicine, pharmacology, and medical librarianship lost a distinguished colleague.

Chauncey Leake was born in Elizabeth, NJ, on Sept. 5, 1896. He attended Princeton, receiving a B.A. degree in 1917. He served with the chemical warfare service of the U.S. Army during World War I. He then continued his education at the University of Wisconsin, where he obtained an M.S. degree in 1917 and a Ph.D. in philosophy, chemistry, and biology in 1923. Dr. Leake remained at the University of Wisconsin, teaching pharmacology and engaging in research, until 1928. Dr. Leake then accepted the opportunity at the reorganized University of California Medical School in San Francisco to develop the department of pharmacology and to become its professor. Because of his interest in libraries, Dr. Leake also served as honorary librarian of the medical school.

In 1942, Dr. Leake accepted the post of executive vice-president of the University of Texas to head the Medical Branch in Galveston. Here, too, he improved its library facilities. In 1955, Dr. Leake left Galveston to become professor of pharmacology, lecturer on the history of medicine, and assistant dean of the Ohio State University College of Medicine in Columbus. Dr. Leake returned to San Francisco in 1962, where he was appointed senior lecturer in pharmacology and in the history and philosophy of medicine at the University of California. He also taught medical jurisprudence at the Hastings College of Law in San Francisco. Dr. Leake held these positions until his death.

He was a member of the honorary consultants of the Army Medical Library from 1946 to 1950, serving as president in 1948. He subsequently advised the staff during the transition period when the Armed Forces Medical Library became the National Library of Medicine. Dr. Leake was an honorary member of the Medical Library Association and the Association's honorary vice-president when the meeting took place in Galveston in 1949.

Besides writing many scientific and historical articles and books, Dr. Leake translated William Harvey's *De Motu Cordis* in 1928, published by Charles C Thomas, and the *Hearst Medical Papyrus*, published in 1952 by the University of Kansas.

Miriam Hawkins Libbey was born in Loganville, GA. She attended Shorter College in Rome, GA, receiving a B.A. degree in 1942. Deciding on librarianship as a career, Miriam attended Emory University's division of librarianship in Atlanta, receiving an M.A. in 1950. While at Emory, Miriam Libbey came under the influence of the late Mildred Jordan, who was one of her teachers in library school. Miss Jordan recognized Mrs. Libbey's potential in medical librarianship and, at the completion of her education in librarianship, hired her as reference librarian and chief of services to the public at the A. W. Calhoun Medical Library of Emory University School of Medicine. From 1955 to 1963, Mrs. Libbey became successively reference librarian, assistant head of the reference section, and head of the indexing section of the National Library of Medicine in Bethesda, MD. She was then appointed librarian of the Health Sciences Library of the State University of New York at Buffalo. In 1966, Mrs. Libbey succeeded the late Mildred Jordan as librarian at the A. W. Calhoun Medical Library at Emory University, her present post. Since 1969, in addition, she has directed the Southeastern Regional Medical Library Program, with headquarters in her own library.

Mrs. Libbey has been active in the affairs of the Medical Library Association, serving on many of its committees, including the Legislative Committee (1972-1977) and the Committee on Future Developments. She has been chairman of the Medical Library Education Group (1975-1976) and of the Medical Library Group and has been an instructor in the Association's continuing education programs.

Although Mrs. Hutton, known professionally as **Mary Louise Marshall**, was a Northerner by birth (Salem, IL), she is a Southerner by choice, spending most of her academic career in New Orleans, LA. Miss Marshall received her early academic education at Illinois Woman's College. She then attended Southern Illinois Normal University, now Southern Illinois University, and then the library school of the University of Wisconsin.

Her career in librarianship covered 45 years. She was employed first in public and school libraries. In 1920, Miss Marshall was placed in charge of the library of the Orleans Parish Medical Society, and in 1928, she was appointed also as librarian of Tulane University Medical School. Upon her appointment, the medical school entered into an agreement with the Orleans Parish Medical Society whereby the libraries of the two organizations, both housed in the same building, should be combined under Miss Marshall's administration. From this time on, she worked closely with Dr. Rudolf Matas, the famous surgeon. Dr. Matas built up a large personal library, which he later gave to the Tulane University Medical Library.

Because of the gift and Dr. Matas' continued financial support and untiring interest, the library was named for Dr. Matas in 1937. When Dr. Matas died in 1957, he left, in addition to thousands of his medical volumes, a bequest of $1 million to the library. During the years of Miss Marshall's administration, the library collected not only a large number of medical books and journals but also portraits of physicians, medical bookplates, pictures illustrative of medicine and art, postage stamps of medical interest, and medals. Upon her retirement in 1959, she was named emeritus professor of medical bibliography and emeritus librarian of Tulane University School of Medicine.

Miss Marshall is the author of more than 100 articles on medical librarianship and medical history. Her book, *The Physician's Own Library: Its Development, Care and Use* (1957), is still very useful. She has received many professional appointments and awards. One appointment she cherished was to be named, with a few other leading librarians, to a committee to survey the Army Medical Library. This survey, conducted in 1943 and 1944 under the leadership of Keyes D. Metcalf, was momentous in implementing the development of the National Library of Medicine. Miss Marshall served as honorary consultant to this library from 1947 to 1952. She served in other capacities, including the chairmanship of the Army Medical Library Committee on Classification. In 1957, she was appointed by President Eisenhower to the board of regents of the National Library of Medicine, and she served until 1959.

The Medical Library Association is greatly indebted to Miss Marshall, who held many important assignments from 1927 to 1959. After becoming treasurer and later chairman of the Executive Committee, Miss Marshall was elected president of the Association (1941). As a result of the war, she kept the presidency until 1946. Miss Marshall contributed the chapter on classification to the first edition of the Medical Library Association's *Handbook* and served as joint editor with Janet Doe of the second edition (1956). For these accomplishments and many others, Miss Marshall was chosen the recipient of the Marcia Noyes award in 1953.

Since her retirement, she has been involved in genealogy and has been active in many patriotic and heritage societies, such as the Daughters of the American Revolution and the Society of Mayflower Descendants. She recently compiled an ancestor index containing names of more than 6,000 17th-century settlers in our first 12 colonies.

When T. E. Keys gave a paper on the medical books of William Worrall Mayo, the father of Dr. **William James Mayo**, at the Mayo Clinic general staff meeting on July 6, 1938, Dr. W. J. Mayo discussed this presentation, saying:

I believe that the atmosphere of books is one of the most important formative factors in the development of young minds. The family library in our home was the living-room; there were books from the floor to the ceiling, and our mother and father gave us books to read which were appropriate to our age[8].

William James Mayo was born on June 29, 1861, at Le Sueur, MN. He received an M.D. degree from the University of Michigan, Ann Arbor, and then engaged in the private practice of medicine and surgery with his father and later with his younger brother, Charles Horace Mayo. From this surgical practice evolved the cooperative group clinic later to be known as the Mayo Clinic. From 1907 until his death on July 28, 1939, Dr. Mayo served on the Board of Regents of the University of Minnesota.

Dr. Mayo's medical reading habits and ideas are interesting. He urged systematic study for surgeons and said:

I began by charging myself with one hour's study a day, and I did not give myself credit for advance work; that is, if I put in three hours, I took credit for one. I was scrupulous, however, in making up the deficit when it happened that I was unable to study. It is surprising how much one can accomplish by adherence to this type of program. The reading should be catholic. To the young surgeon I would say, do not read all surgery and technique, for technique is constantly changing.... Along with surgical literature, read medical articles in high class medical journals. Do not skim, but here and there select certain articles and read them with care[9].

Erich Meyerhoff was born in Braunschweig, Germany, on Nov. 24, 1919. He emigrated to New York City and attended the College of the City of New York, receiving a B.S. degree in sociology in 1943. From 1943 to 1945, Mr. Meyerhoff served as a staff sergeant in the United States Army, where he was associated with military intelligence. From 1946 to 1949, he attended the New York School of Social Work. He then studied at Columbia University in New York City, receiving an M.S. in library science in 1951. In 1974, Mr. Meyerhoff received the certificate of advanced librarianship from Columbia University. From 1951 to 1957, he worked in the medical library at Columbia University, advancing to the position of reference librarian. In 1957, Mr. Meyerhoff was appointed librarian and assistant professor at the Downstate Medical Center of the State University of New York in Brooklyn. He held this position until 1961, when he became director of the Medical Library Center of New York. In 1967, he became librarian of the Health Sciences Library, State University of New York at Buffalo. Mr. Meyerhoff held this position until 1970, when he was appointed librarian of the Cornell University Medical College in New York City.

Greatly esteemed by his medical colleagues, Mr. Meyerhoff, in addition to his library duties, was appointed assistant dean for information resources at Cornell Medical College in 1977. In making this appointment, the dean of the medical school, Dr. Thomas H. Miekle, said, "The new appointment represents a richly deserved recognition of (Mr. Meyerhoff's) many contributions."

Erich Meyerhoff has also worked long and hard for the Medical Library Association. He was chairman of the Committee on Continuing Education from 1963 to 1964 and chairman of the Ad Hoc Committee to Review the Goals and Structure of the Medical Library Association (1968-1971). Mr. Meyerhoff became a member of the board of directors of the Medical Library Association in 1972, serving in this capacity until 1975. He is also a member of the American Association for the Advancement of Science and the American Association of University Professors and is a former chairman of the Executive Committee of the New York Regional Group of the Medical Library Association.

His bibliography includes many outstanding publications. In addition, Mr. Meyerhoff has held many medical library consultantships and given many lectures.

Wilhelm Moll was born in Austria in 1920. After graduation from the realgymnasium, he emigrated to the United States and obtained a B.A. degree from Denison University, Granville, OH. Mr. Moll then attended the University of Chicago Law School, receiving a Doctor of Law degree in 1945. For the next 10 years he was employed by various agencies of the U.S. government, including the departments of War and State. In 1956, Wilhelm Moll received an M.A. in library science from Catholic University in Washington, DC. His first library position was that of assistant documents librarian at Indiana University in Indianapolis in 1956. He remained there until 1960, when he was appointed assistant medical librarian at the University of Kentucky in Louisville. He left this position in 1962 to become medical librarian at the University of Virginia Medical Center in Charlottesville. Dr. Moll was director and professor of the Claude Moore Health Sciences Library until his death in 1979.

Dr. Moll served on various committees of the Medical Library Association and made many contributions to medical librarianship. He was also active in the American Association for the History of Medicine and was a member of the International Association for the History of Medicine. In 1977 Wilhelm Moll was awarded a sabbatical leave and spent it at the University of Vienna, studying their medical giants of the 19th century.

Peter Olch was born on Apr. 10, 1930, in St. Louis, MO. He attended Pomona College in Claremont, CA, receiving an A.B. degree in 1951. Deciding on a medical career, Mr. Olch attended Johns Hopkins School of Medicine in Baltimore, MD, where he was awarded an M.D. degree in 1955. After a surgical internship at Johns Hopkins Hospital (1955-1956), Dr. Olch was senior assistant surgeon at the National Cancer Institute in Bethesda, MD (1956-1958). From 1958 to 1959, Dr. Olch was a surgical resident at the University of Washington Medical School, performing his duties in the King County Hospital as well as working 6 months in pathology at the Swedish Hospital. He was a research assistant in the Department of Surgery at the University of Washington from 1959 to 1960. Dr. Olch served as a resident in clinical anatomy at the National Institutes of Health from 1960 to 1962 and as a resident in clinical pathology from 1962 to 1964. Since Dr. Olch's interest was in the history of medicine, he spent a year as a fellow at the Institute of the History of Medicine at Johns Hopkins School of Medicine. Since that time, having been special assistant to the director of the National Library of Medicine from 1964 to 1965, Dr. Olch has been deputy chief of their History of Medicine Division.

Dr. Olch holds memberships in many scientific societies, including the American Osler Society (Board of Governors, 1975-1978), American Society of Clinical Pathologists, Oral History Association (president, 1970-1971), and Washington Academy of Medicine (Board of Directors, 1974 to present). He has been active, also, in the Medical Library Association. He was chairman of the Association's Hafner Award Committee (1968-1969) and the Murray Gottlieb Prize Essay Committee (1971-1972) and was a member of the Editorial Committee (1975-1977).

Dr. Olch has lectured extensively and has received the U.S. Public Health Service's commendation medal (1971), and the National Library of Medicine's director's award (1977).

Gerald J. Oppenheimer was born in Frankfurt, Germany, on May 8, 1922. He received B.A. and M.A. degrees from the University of Washington, Seattle. Mr. Oppenheimer later attended the School of Library Service, Columbia University, in New York City, receiving an M.S. in 1953. He was appointed junior librarian in the technology department of the Seattle Public Library in 1953, serving in this position until 1955. He became fisheries-oceanography librarian later that same year and continued in this position until 1960. During the next 3 years, Mr. Oppenheimer was manager of information services of the Boeing Research Laboratories and also chairman of their library committee. In 1963, he became the director of the Health Sciences Library and assistant director of libraries at the University of Washington, Seattle. In addition, he has been director of the Pacific Northwest Regional Health Sciences Library since 1968. Mr. Oppenheimer's honors include Phi Beta Kappa and Delta Phi Alpha, cum laude.

Mr. Oppenheimer holds memberships in the Association for Symbolic Logic, American Society for Information Science, Special Libraries Association, Medical Library Association, Association of Academic Health Sciences Library Directors (president, 1978-1979), and the American Association of University Professors.

His offices with the Medical Library Association include: director, 1974-1977; chairman, Finance Committee, 1974-1977; chairman, Medical Library Association/National Library of Medicine Liaison Committee, 1976-1977; and member, Executive Committee, 1974-1977.

Miss Marcia C. Noyes put it well: "No one man has so left his imprint on the libraries of two continents as has **Sir William Osler**[10]." While alive, he generously aided libraries and librarians. To librarians, his magnum opus, *The Bibliotheca Osleriana,* which his librarian Dr. W. W. Francis and others perfected, is one of the most important reference tools for describing significant historical medical books.

William Osler was born at Bond Head, Ontario, in the wilderness of Canada, on July 12, 1849. He prepared for college at Trinity College School and then became a student at Trinity University in 1867. Attracted to medicine, he left liberal arts and enrolled in Toronto Medical School in 1868. He decided to change schools and to study medicine at McGill Medical School, which he attended from 1870 until his graduation in 1872. Osler then spent 2 years of postgraduate study in Great Britain. Later he traveled on the continent, studying at the medical centers in Berlin and Vienna. After going back to London for a short time, Osler returned to Canada, receiving an appointment at McGill as lecturer in medicine in 1874. Because of his interest in pathology, Osler accepted the newly created post as pathologist at the Montreal General Hospital. In 1878, he became the hospital's full-time physician. That same year, Osler made a short visit to London, where he qualified for and received membership in the Royal College of Physicians. In 1881, Osler, with Dr. R. Palmer Howard, represented McGill at the meeting of the International Congress of Medicine held in London. Here he heard many excellent addresses by many of medicine's top leaders, especially Paget, Virchow, Huxley, Pasteur, and John Shaw Billings. Probably Osler's contact with Billings kindled his awakening interest in medical libraries and their importance not only for undergraduate study but also as a means of continuing a physician's lifelong postgraduate training.

In 1884, Osler was chosen to assume the chair of clinical medicine at the University of Pennsylvania. He remained in Philadelphia until 1889, when he accepted an offer to be physician-in-chief at the newly opened Johns Hopkins Hospital. Wherever he went, libraries were of great importance to him.

He served for 5 years as a member of the library committee at the College of Physicians in Philadelphia. During his tenure, many precious books were added to their famous library. In Baltimore, he continued his library interest not only at Johns Hopkins but also at the Medical and Chirurgical Faculty of the State of Maryland. Here he aided in the library's rebirth and saw the small collection of a few hundred volumes grow to 15,000 volumes before his departure.

The Johns Hopkins School of Medicine, which had been in the planning stages for several years, was opened in 1893 with Osler as physician-in-chief. Meanwhile, he had prepared his masterwork, *The Principles and Practice of Medicine,* first published in 1892. The first edition is now a rare book and is much sought after by librarians and medical collectors. For years, the book continued to be published in many editions. Under the editorship of many outstanding physicians since Osler's death, it still is the standard text in many schools.

Osler kept a keen interest in books and libraries throughout his life. Although he did not attend the first meeting of the Medical Library Association in 1898, he is considered a founder along with Dr. George Milbry Gould and Miss Margaret Charlton. He has been memorialized in many ways and is included on the medal prepared for the annual meeting of the Medical Library Association in 1976.

In August 1904, Osler accepted the position of Regius Professor of Medicine at the University of Oxford. He began his new position in May 1905. This new assignment allowed him some freedom, and during his remaining days, he found time to build up his great library, which he willed to McGill, and, with the help of others, to prepare a catalog of the collection. He also prepared several papers and gave many talks on the history of medicine and wrote articles on books and librarianship. Because of his many contributions, Dr. Osler was created a baronet in 1911 at the coronation of King George V. He died in 1919.

Osler served as president of the Medical Library Association from 1901 to 1904 and received honorary membership in 1915.

Among the many individuals influenced by Sir William Osler was Dr. **Francis Randolph Packard**[11] (1870-1950) of Philadelphia, PA. Packard was asked by Osler in 1893 to work with him at the Johns Hopkins Hospital in Baltimore. Here Dr. Packard observed Osler's skill as a pathologist as well as his ward work. The impact of Osler on Packard resulted in many articles and book reviews about Osler, especially concerning his contributions to medical literature and to medical history. Several were published in the *Annals of Medical History*, which Packard edited.

Francis Packard was born in Philadelphia, PA, on Mar. 23, 1870. He graduated with a major in biology from the University of Pennsylvania in Philadelphia in 1889 and received an M.D. degree from the same institution in 1892, which honored him in 1939 with an LL.D. degree. For several months in 1893, as mentioned above, Packard worked with Osler until accepting the position as a resident physician in the Pennsylvania Hospital (1893-1895). Dr. Packard served in the Department of Otology at the Postgraduate School of the University of Pennsylvania, later becoming a full professor as well as chief of otolaryngology at the Pennsylvania Hospital. In the Spanish-American War, Dr. Packard became a first lieutenant and served as an assistant surgeon. He also served his country in World War I from 1917 to 1919, achieving the rank of major. He saw duty overseas as chief consultant in otolaryngology of the District of Paris (1918-1919).

Dr. Packard was president of many societies and organizations: American Laryngological Association (1930), American Otological Society (1936), College of Physicians of Philadelphia (1931-1934), Library Company of Philadelphia (1936-1941). He is well known for his work *History of Medicine in the United States*. In addition, he was the author of many medical and historical papers and other books, including *Diseases of the Ear, Nose, and Throat, The School of Salerno, The Life and Times of Ambroise Paré, and The Gold Headed Cane.*

Vern M. Pings was born on Apr. 10, 1923, in Sauk City, WI. He attended the University of Chicago, receiving a Ph.B. degree in 1946. He continued his education at the University of Wisconsin, where he received a B.A. in 1947. From 1948 to 1952, Mr. Pings attended Columbia University, receiving an M.A. in 1952. He then returned to the University of Wisconsin and obtained an M.A. in library science (1955) and a Ph.D. (1958).

Dr. Pings has had a varied and stimulating career in the United States and in foreign countries. He has worked for the Chicago Health Department and the Englewood Hospital School of Nursing (Chicago). He was sanitation officer for the American Friends Service Committee, United Nations Relief for Palestine Refugees, Gaza and Palestine (1949-1950). He was works officer for the United Nations Relief and Works Agency in Beirut, Lebanon, from 1950 to 1951 and director of the University Farms at the American University of Beirut (1952-1954). From 1955 to 1958, Dr. Pings was assistant engineering librarian for the University of Wisconsin.

He then, after receiving his doctorate, became librarian of Ohio Northern University in Ada, OH.

In 1960, Dr. Pings accepted the position of associate professor at the University of Denver School of Librarianship. From 1961 to 1971, Dr. Pings was medical librarian at the Wayne State University School of Medicine in Detroit. He had additional duties as professor in the medical school as well as director (from 1969 to 1975) of the Regional Medical Library encompassing Michigan, Kentucky, and Ohio. In 1972, Dr. Pings became the director of University Libraries at Wayne State University, his present position.

Over the years, Dr. Pings has served as project director and visiting lecturer in many institutions both in the United States and in other countries. He has also been involved with many associations and been active in committee assignments. For the Medical Library Association, Dr. Pings was a member of the Committee on Surveys and Statistics (1965-1968) and the Committee on Goals and Structure (1969-1972) and from 1974 to 1975 was consulting editor. He also served as a member of the Executive Council of the Medical Library Association's Midwest Regional Group (1964-1965). At present (1978), Dr. Pings is in Romania consulting on library matters in connection with Wayne State University's involvement with new programs in that area.

Dr. Pings has contributed more than 200 articles and many studies to the enrichment of librarianship.

William Dosite Postell was born in Plaquemine, LA. He received a B.S., an M.S., and a B.S. in library science from Louisiana State University. He is certified in three fields: medical librarianship, public librarianship, and public school teaching. After working in various capacities at Louisiana State University, Mr. Postell served from 1933 to 1934 as assistant librarian of Sabine Parish Library. He then became librarian of the Mansfield Public Schools. He held this position until 1938, when he was appointed medical librarian of the Louisiana State University School of Medicine. He was also appointed professor of medical bibliography and served as secretary to the Faculty Council.

In 1959, Mr. Postell became librarian and professor of medical bibliography at the Tulane University Medical School. He taught library science at Loyola University during the summers of 1934, 1936, and 1937. He directed a refresher course for U.S. Veterans Administration librarians in Kansas City, KS, in 1959 and in Minneapolis, MN, in 1962. Mr. Postell presented the first and second refresher courses on architecture preceding the 1958 and 1959 conventions of the Medical Library Association. He has acted as medical library consultant for many universities, clinics, hospitals, and academies. In 1955, Mr. Postell spent a year at the Medical School of the University of Taiwan in Taipei, where he was asked to initiate and to build a medical library in the existing facilities. He also helped to plan their new library. He retired from the librarian's position in 1974.

Besides his professional writings, especially his book, *Applied Medical Bibliography for Students* (1955), Mr. Postell has written on the history of medical problems of the South, in particular on the health of the slaves of the southern plantations.

After serving in many official capacities for the Medical Library Association, Mr. Postell was named president for the years 1953 and 1954. In recognition of his professional achievements, he received the Marcia Noyes award in 1958. He has subsequently been awarded Medical Library Association honorary and fellow memberships.

L. Margueriete Prime was born in Nebraska, but her family soon moved to Oak Park, IL, which was her home for many years. While working during the summers in the Oak Park Public Library, Margueriete became interested in librarianship. She attended the University of Chicago, where she received a Ph.B. degree. For several years after graduation, Miss Prime taught in high schools in Minnesota and Indiana. She became assistant principal of a school in Indiana but also taught most of the subjects in the curriculum. During this time, too, she attended a business school and later did secretarial work for the Society for Visual Education. From here, Miss Prime became a library assistant and soon thereafter was put in charge of the library and Department of Literary Research of the American College of Surgeons in Chicago (1931). Miss Prime continued her career with the American College until her retirement in 1960. After retirement, she kept up her ties with the College and in 1965 prepared the index for *Surgery, Gynecology and Obstetrics,* their official publication. An interest in history of the United States has kept Miss Prime active in study classes and lately in the history of political science.

When active with her library work at the American College of Surgeons, Miss Prime helped to raise the standards for hospital medical libraries and was especially interested in adequate medical libraries properly administered for the medical staffs. She served as chairman of the Library Section of the Tri-State Hospital Assembly of the American College of Surgeons from 1941 to 1948. From 1943 to 1950, she lectured on the history and development of the hospital library to students in the program in hospital administration at the Northwestern University School of Commerce. She has written many fine articles relating to her work.

Miss Prime attended the annual meetings of the Medical Library

Association regularly and served a 3-year term on its board of directors. She was a member of the Publications Committee for many years, 1 year as its chairman. Miss Prime was a member and a chairman of the Subcommittee on Certification. She was an advisor to regional groups of the Medical Library Association and was especially interested in promoting the cause of the small medical library. She wrote the chapter on cataloging in the first edition of *The Handbook of Medical Library Practice* (1943) and served on many joint committees, such as Hospital Libraries (1943-1944) and Medical Library Service for the Armed Forces Service of the Army of the United States (1942-1944). For her fine and loyal service to her library, Miss Prime was honored in 1957 by the College at the annual president's dinner. Miss Prime was president of the Medical Library Association from 1951 to 1952. In 1960, she was made an honorary member of the Association in recognition of her outstanding achievements in medical librarianship.

Among the top innovators and contributors to medical librarianship is Dr. **Frank Bradway Rogers**, now in early retirement in Denver, CO, but still involved in many activities, including the binding of rare books. After receiving a B.A. degree from Yale in 1936, he pursued a course in medicine, obtaining his M.D. degree from Ohio State University in 1942. Dr. Rogers served his internship at the Letterman General Hospital in San Francisco from 1942 to 1943. He joined the U.S. Army Medical Corps in 1943, advancing from first lieutenant through the grades to colonel in 1959.

Dr. Rogers read an announcement in 1948 that the directorship of the Army Medical Library was vacant. Because of his interest in scholarship, this possible assignment appealed to him. He applied and was accepted. Dr. Rogers then attended Columbia University School of Library Service and received an M.S. degree in 1949. After graduation he was appointed director of the National Library of Medicine at the early age of 34. Background, training, and drive provided Dr. Rogers with the talents necessary to carry out a national library program of utmost significance to medical librarianship. The present-day elegant but modern National Library of Medicine in Bethesda, MD, was created through the efforts of Dr. Rogers.

Dr. Rogers was president of the Medical Library Association from 1962 to 1963, having received the coveted Marcia Noyes award in 1961. In 1963, Dr. Rogers left the exhausting work entailed in organizing and implementing innovative programs from the National Library of Medicine. He then accepted the position of librarian at the University of Colorado Medical Center in Denver, where he remained until retirement in 1973.

Charles W. Sargent was born on Dec. 18, 1925, in Shelburn, IN. He received B.A. and M.A. degrees in history from Michigan State University, Lansing, in 1951, graduating with honors. Deciding on librarianship as a career, Mr. Sargent attended library school at the University of Michigan, Ann Arbor, receiving an M.A. in library science in 1953. He continued his studies and in 1964 received a Ph.D. in economic history at the University of New Mexico. Dr. Sargent's honors include Phi Kappa Phi, Phi Alpha Theta, and Beta Phi Mu and also honorary membership in the National Library of Science.

Dr. Sargent's library career began at Michigan State University, where he was assistant circulation librarian from 1949 to 1951. From 1952 to 1953, he served as assistant manuscript cataloger at the William L. Clements Library at the University of Michigan, and from 1952 to 1953, he was curator of the Kansas Historical Collections and university archivist of the University of Kansas at Lawrence. Dr. Sargent was chief of the Cataloging Department of Sandia Corporation's Technical Library in Albuquerque, NM, from 1954 to 1962. From 1962 to 1966, he was information scientist of the Department of Aerospace Medicine and Bioastronautics of the Lovelace Foundation for Medical Education and Research in Albuquerque. Dr. Sargent then joined the faculty of the University of New Mexico, Library of the Medical Sciences, School of Medicine, as deputy librarian and assistant professor of medical bibliography. From 1968 to 1969, he was associate professor in the Department of Community Health and Medical Practice and assistant director of the Medical Computer Center at the University of Missouri at Columbia. In 1969, Dr. Sargent was promoted to associate professor in the Department of Information Science and deputy director of the Union Book Catalog Project at the university as well as director of the Audio Message Center at the University of Missouri School of Medicine. From 1971 to 1972, Dr. Sargent served as chairman of the Department of Information Sciences at the University of Missouri.

From 1972 to 1974, Dr. Sargent was director of the Library of Health Sciences at Texas Tech University School of Medicine. Since 1974 he has been director of the Educational Resources Division at the same medical school in Lubbock, TX, as well as professor of health communications. Since 1977, in addition to his other duties, he has been chairman of the Health Communications Department.

Dr. Sargent has had many academic assignments besides those mentioned as well as many consultantships. He holds membership in several organizations related to his work. Some of his activities with the Medical Library Association should be mentioned: Board of Directors (1972-1975), Parliamentarian (1971-1974), Bylaws Committee (1971-1974),

Finance Committee (1972-1975), and Central Office Committee (1972-1974). He has been especially active in continuing education programs.

Henry Schuman was born in Russia in 1899. His family moved to the United States and lived successively in Brockton, MA, New York City, and Detroit, MI. Henry Schuman engaged in various enterprises and ultimately founded a ballbearing business. Like many other businesses, especially during the depression years, his were unsuccessful. Meanwhile, he collected books, gathering together many first editions of modern writers. Using his own collection, Mr. Schuman went into the book trade. He was joined by his wife, Ida, in these book activities.

One of Schuman's early visitors to his store was the late Dr. Lawrence Reynolds, a roentgenologist from Detroit. After locating a copy of the first edition of Laennec's *De l'auscultation mediate* (2 vol, 1819) for Dr. Reynolds, Schuman decided to become an antiquarian book dealer. He subsequently helped Dr. Reynolds put together a magnificant rare book collection, now the proud possession of the University of Alabama Medical Center.

In the bookstore, the Schumans met Dr. and Mrs. Josiah Trent. Dr. Trent in 1938 was an intern at the Henry Ford Hospital and much interested in rare items in the history of his profession. Mrs. Trent also developed an interest in rare medical books and helped her husband acquire a collection that, after Dr. Trent's premature death in 1948, she presented to the Duke University Medical Library. The Schumans assisted the Trents in this endeavor.

Gradually, Mr. Schuman became interested in the publication of fine limited-edition books—historical medicine and science. He initiated the *Life of Science Library*, a series of nontechnical monographs written to inform the intelligent lay reader about the past accomplishments of medicine. Altogether, Schuman published more than 350 books. In 1946, he issued the periodical *Journal of the History of Medicine and Allied Sciences*. It was taken over in 1951 by Dr. John Fulton and continues to maintain a vigorous and lively approach to the history of medicine and its allied sciences.

In the fall of 1953, the Abelard Press absorbed the Schuman publishing business. The Schumans continued their rare book business. Mr. Schuman died in 1962, and Mrs. Schuman carried on the business until her death in 1977.

Katherine J. Sholtz has a B.S. degree (1952) from the University of Illinois and an M.S. degree in biochemistry (1953) from the same institution. In 1967, she was granted an M.L.S. degree from the State University of New York at Albany.

From 1953 to 1955, Mrs. Sholtz was a research associate in the Department of Nutrition at the Harvard University School of Public Health. In 1955, she became a researcher for the department of nutrition at Iowa State University; she held that position until 1957.

Mrs. Sholtz was librarian for the International Business Machines facility in Rochester, MN, during 1967. That year, she joined the Mayo Clinic in Rochester as computer applications librarian. Since 1972, she has been associate librarian at the Mayo Clinic Medical Library.

Owsei Temkin was born in Minsk, Russia, on Oct. 6, 1902. The family moved to Leipzig, Germany, in 1905. Mr. Temkin attended the gymnasium in Leipzig and then studied medicine at the University of Leipzig from 1922 to 1927, when he received his M.D. degree. He was an intern at the St. Jacob Hospital, Leipzig, from 1928 to 1932. He served, from 1931 to 1933, as "Privat Dozent" for the Institute of the History of Medicine in Leipzig.

In 1932, Dr. Temkin came to the United States; he was naturalized in 1938. He was an associate in the history of medicine (1932-1935) and associate professor (1935-1937) at the Johns Hopkins University in Baltimore, MD. He then became William H. Welch Professor of the History of Medicine and director of the Institute of Medicine, Johns Hopkins University. Dr. Temkin also was lecturer in the history of science on the Hopkins faculty of philosophy and later their professor of the history of medicine in the Department of the History of Science. From 1948 to 1968, Dr. Temkin in addition was the editor of the *Bulletin of the History of Medicine.*

Since 1968, Dr. Temkin has been William H. Welch Professor Emeritus of the History of Medicine. From 1943 to 1944, he was civilian advisor with the Division of Medical Sciences of the National Research Council. Dr. Temkin has given many lectures. He was the Hideyo Noguchi lecturer in 1969 at the Johns Hopkins University and the Messenger lecturer in 1970 at Cornell University. Owsei Temkin holds membership in several learned societies, including the National Academy of Sciences, American Philosophical Society, American Academy of Arts and Sciences, International Academy of the History of Medicine, and History of Science Society. He is a fellow of the American Association for the Advancement of Science and has long been associated with the American Association for the History of Medicine (president, 1958-1960).

For his outstanding contributions, Dr. Temkin was recipient of the William H. Welch medal (1952), the Sarton medal (1960), and the 1962 Prize for Distinguished Scholarship in the Humanities, American Council of Learned Societies. He has been awarded honorary doctorates by Johns Hopkins University (1973) and by the Medical College of Ohio at Toledo (1975). Phi Beta Kappa, the Dutch Society for the History of Medicine,

Mathematics, and Science, the Israeli Society for the History of Medicine, the Swiss Society for the History of Medicine and Science, the Worshipful Society of Apothecaries of London, and the Faculty of History of Medicine and Pharmacy have bestowed honorary or corresponding memberships on Dr. Temkin.

Dr. Temkin is the author of many essays and books. His main publications are *The Falling Sickness* (1945, revised in 1971), *Soranus' Gynecology* (1956), *Galenism: Rise and Decline of Medical Philosophy* (1973), and *The Double Face of Janus and Other Essays on the History of Medicine* (1977).

Stanley Durham Truelson, Jr., was born in Cambridge, MA, on Mar. 19, 1929. He attended Harvard College, receiving an A.B. cum laude in 1951. From 1951 to 1954, he served in the U.S. Army. He received an M.A. in teaching from the Harvard Graduate School of Education in 1955. Mr. Truelson then studied librarianship at Simmons College in Boston, receiving an M.S. in library science in 1956. He served as an assistant at Harvard College Library (1955-1956) and librarian at John Hay High School in Cross River, NY (1956-1957). Mr. Truelson was circulation librarian and instructor in library science at Tufts University Library, Medford, MA (1957-1958), and then became librarian and assistant professor of the library of Tufts University Schools of Medicine and Dentistry in Boston. In 1960, he became librarian and assistant professor of medical bibliography at the State University of New York Upstate Medical Center, Syracuse. From 1963 to 1966, Mr. Truelson was medical librarian and associate professor of medical bibliography at the University of Rochester, Rochester, NY.

In 1966, Mr. Truelson became librarian of Yale Medical Library, and he remained there until 1976. He was then appointed director of the Alaska Health Science Library, Anchorage, his present position.

Mr. Truelson has served on many committees and in other ways aided the cause of medical librarianship: Ad Hoc Panel on the Selection of Journals for the *Index Medicus* (1965-1966); vice-chairman, Library Task Force, Connecticut Regional Medical Progress (1967-1968); Advisory Committee, New England Regional Medical Library Service (1967-1976); consultant, Division of Regional Medical Progress of the U.S. Public Health Service (1969); chairman, Upstate New York Regional Group, Medical Library Association (1965); chairman, Medical Library Association Publication Committee (1966-1970); Eliot Prize Essay Committee (1967-1968); Special Joint Committee on Libraries in International Education (1967 to present); and associate editor of the *Bulletin of the Medical Library Association* (1962-1964).

Martha Jane Koontz Zachert was born in York, PA. She attended Lebanon Valley College in Annville, PA, receiving an A.B. degree in 1941. From 1941 to 1946, Mrs. Zachert worked in the Enoch Pratt Free Library in Baltimore, MD, as an assistant. In 1947, she became librarian at the Wood Research Institute in Atlanta, GA. From 1950 to 1952, she was school librarian of the De Kalb County Schools in De Kalb County, Georgia. From 1952 to 1963, Mrs. Zachert was head librarian and professor of the history of pharmacy at the Southern College of Pharmacy, Mercer University, Atlanta. During this time, she continued her library education, and in 1953, she received an M.A. in librarianship from Emory University. In the summers from 1955 to 1959 and for the academic years 1956-1957 and 1959-1960, she was also visiting instructor in librarianship at Emory. From 1962 to 1963, Mrs. Zachert was instructor in librarianship at Georgia State College in Atlanta. During the summer of 1961, Mrs. Zachert was visiting instructor in the library school at Florida State University in Tallahassee. From 1963 to 1969, she served as assistant professor at the same school.

Meanwhile, she had completed her requirements for the D.L.S. degree, which she received from Columbia University in 1968.

Dr. Zachert was associate professor at Florida State University from 1969 to 1973 and then was appointed professor. After a leave of absence for a year, Dr. Zachert was named professor of library science at the University of South Carolina in Columbia, which is her present position.

Dr. Zachert holds memberships in many library organizations, including the Medical Library Association, Association of American Library Schools, American Library Association, and Special Libraries Association (president, Florida chapter, 1973-1974). She is also a member of the American Institute of the History of Pharmacy, the Oral History Association, and the honorary library association, Beta Phi Mu (president, 1973-1974).

Dr. Zachert was associate editor of the *Journal of Library History* (1966-1971), managing editor (1971-1973), and associate editor again (1973-1976). She has served as consultant to many institutions, including the Southern Regional Medical Library, Emory University (1976-1977), and the Mid-Atlantic Regional Medical Library (1977 to present).

Author of more than 50 articles relating to her professional career, Dr. Zachert was honored by the Medical Library Association in 1978 when she was named the Janet Doe lecturer.

REFERENCES

1. McDaniel WB 2d: James Francis Ballard, 1878-1955 (obituary). Bull Med Libr Assoc 44: 92-97, 1956.

2. Fund in Memory of JAMES F. BALLARD. Bull Med Libr Assoc 43: 563, 1955.
3. WELCH WH: Papers and Addresses. Vol 3. Baltimore, Johns Hopkins Press, 1920, p. 400.
4. OSLER W: Bibliotheca Osleriana: A Catalogue of Books Illustrating the History of Medicine and Science. Oxford, Clarendon Press, 1929, p. 568.
5. ADAMS S: ALDERSON FRY, 1906-1976 (obituary). Bull Med Libr Assoc 65: 317-318, 1977.
6. ANNAN G, BRODMAN E: Murray Gottlieb stricken suddenly (obituary). Bull Med Libr Assoc 42: 538-539, 1954.
7. McDANIEL WB 2d: THOMAS E. KEYS: President, Medical Library Association, 1957-58. Bull Med Libr Assoc 45: 575-580, 1957.
8. MAYO WJ: Discussion of Mr. T. E. Keys' paper. Bull Med Libr Assoc 31: 128-132, 1943.
9. BALFOUR DC: WILLIAM JAMES MAYO (1861-1939) and CHARLES HORACE MAYO (1865-1939). Surgery 8: 170-175, 1940.
10. NOYES MC: Osler's Influence on the Library of the Medical and Chirurgical Faculty of the State of Maryland. Johns Hopkins Hosp Bull 30: 212-213, 1919.
11. PACKARD FR: William Osler in Philadelphia, 1884-1889. Arch Intern Med 84: 18-25, 1949.

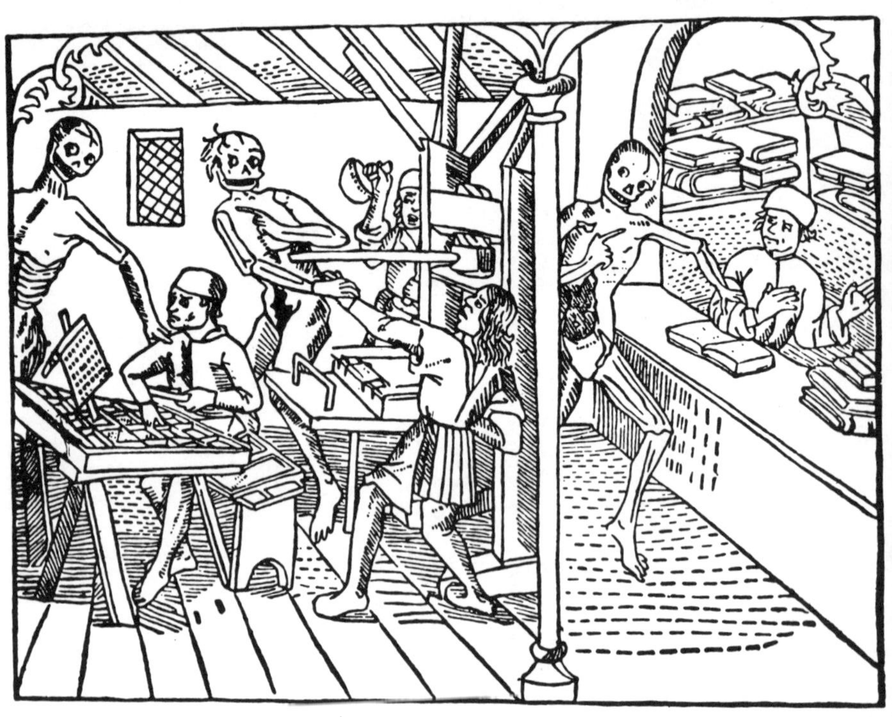

The earliest representation of a printing press. From a Dance of Death, Lyons, 1499. (After Dieterichs.)